Textbook of Pediatric Asthma
An International Perspective

Textbook of Pediatric Asthma
An International Perspective

Edited by

CHARLES K NASPITZ, MD
Professor of Pediatrics
Division of Allergy, Clinical Immunology and Rheumatology
Department of Pediatrics
Federal University of São Paulo/Escola Paulista de Medicina
São Paulo, Brazil

STANLEY J SZEFLER, MD
Professor of Pediatrics and Pharmacology
University of Colorado Health Sciences Center
Helen Wohlberg and Herman Lambert Chair in Pharmacokinetics
Director of Clinical Pharmacology
National Jewish Medical and Research Center
Denver, Colorado, USA

DAVID G TINKELMAN, MD
Professor of Pediatrics
University of Colorado Health Sciences Center
Staff Physician
National Jewish Medical and Research Center
Denver, Colorado, USA

JOHN O WARNER, MD, FRCPCH
Professor of Child Health & Director
Allergy & Inflammation Sciences Division
School of Medicine
University of Southampton
Southampton, UK

*With a foreword by Dr Gro Harlem Brundtland,
Director-General, World Health Organization*

MARTIN DUNITZ

© 2001, Martin Dunitz Ltd, a member of the Taylor & Francis group

First published in the United Kingdom in 2001 by
Martin Dunitz Ltd
The Livery House
7–9 Pratt Street
London NW1 0AE

Tel: +44-(0)20-7482-2202
Fax: +44-(0)20-7267-0159
E-mail: info.dunitz@tandf.co.uk
Website: http://www.dunitz.co.uk

All rights reserved. No part of this publication may be reproduced, stored in a retrieval system, or transmitted, in any form or by any means, electronic, mechanical, photocopying, recording or otherwise, without the prior permission of the publisher or in accordance with the provisions of the Copyright, Designs and Patents Act 1988, or under the terms of any licence permitting limited copying issued by the Copyright Licensing Agency, 90 Tottenham Court Road, London W1P 0LP.

Although every effort has been made to ensure that all owners of copyright material have been acknowledged in this publication, we would be glad to acknowledge in subsequent reprints or editions any omissions brought to our attention.

Although every effort has been made to ensure that drug doses and other information are presented accurately in this publication, the ultimate responsibility rests with the prescribing physician. Neither the publishers nor the authors can be held responsible for errors or for any consequences arising from the use of information contained herein. For detailed prescribing information or instructions on the use of any product or procedure discussed herein, please consult the prescribing information or instructional material issued by the manufacturer.

A CIP catalogue record for this book is available from the British Library

ISBN 1-85317-789-X

Distributed in the United States by:
Blackwell Science Inc.
Commerce Place, 350 Main Street
Malden MA 02148, USA
Tel: 1-800-215-1000

Distributed in Brazil by:
Ernesto Reichmann Distribuidora de Livros, Ltda
Rua Coronel Marques 335, Tatuape 03440-000
Sao Paulo
Brazil

Cover photograph: Giovanna Ceroni
Cover design: Minuche Mazumdar Farrar

Composition by Wearset, Boldon, Tyne and Wear
Printed and bound in Spain by Grafos, S.A.

Contents

Foreword vii
Preface ix
Contributors x
List of abbreviations xiv

1. Lung function and development   *Peter N Le Souëf* 1
2. Asthma—basic mechanisms   *John O Warner* 19
3. Pediatric asthma: epidemiology and natural history   *Jonathan M Samet,*
   Denise G Wiesch, Iqbal H Ahmed 35
4. Risk factors for the development of asthma   *Fernando D Martinez* 67
5. Relationship of viral and bacterial infections to the development and course of asthma
   Amjad Tuffaha, William W Busse 83
6. Chronic cough and/or wheezing in infants and children less than 5 years old: diagnostic
   approaches   *Andrew Bush* 99
7. Pharmacologic management of asthma in infants and small children
   Joseph D Spahn, Ronina A Covar, Melanie C Gleason, David G Tinkelman, Stanley J Szefler 121
8. Management of chronic asthma in children between 5 and 18 years of age
   John O Warner, Charles K Naspitz, Maria C Rizzo 149
9. Assessment and treatment of acute asthma in children and adolescents   *Gary L Larsen,*
   Giuseppe N Colasurdo 189
10. Exercise-induced asthma in children and adolescents and its relationship to sports
    Kai-Håkon Carlsen 211
11. Upper airways disease and asthma   *Jonathan Corren, Gary Rachelefsky* 223
12. Nonpharmacologic approaches to the management of asthma
    Robert A Wood, Peyton A Eggleston 237
13. Indoor and outdoor allergens   *L Karla Arruda, Martin D Chapman* 257
14. Food allergy and asthma in children   *S Allan Bock, Hugh A Sampson* 279
15. Psychosocial factors mediating asthma treatment outcomes   *Bruce G Bender* 293
16. Education programs   *Virginia S Taggart* 309
17. Delivery of aerosol to children: devices and inhalation techniques
    Myrna B Dolovich, Mark L Everard 327
18. Economics in pediatric asthma   *Sean D Sullivan, Paula Lozano, Kevin B Weiss* 347

19. Prediction and prevention of asthma   *John O Warner* 359
20. Childhood asthma in developing countries   *Pakit Vichyanond, Eugene G Weinberg, Dirceu Solé* 377

Index 391

Foreword

Asthma is a chronic inflammatory disease of the airways that affects all human societies and erodes the health and well-being of its victims. There is growing evidence that the prevalence of asthma is rising in all age groups—particularly in children—and among populations in countries of widely differing lifestyles and ethnic groups. The causes of these international trends are unclear and are currently a major focus for asthma researchers worldwide. The toll of asthma in the developing countries is incalculable: in some countries the disease has reached almost the same proportions as in the developed countries. As infectious diseases come under control, asthma is emerging as a major chronic disease in children.

The World Health Organization (WHO) recognizes the importance of asthma as a widespread public health problem and is making major efforts to promote programmes that will enhance the health and well-being of people with this condition. In close association with major national and international institutions and organizations in the area of respiratory and allergic diseases, the WHO has developed joint activities and action programmes that emphasize the two key issues of management and prevention.

The importance of empowering children with asthma and their carers to play an effective role in self-management cannot be overemphasized. When one considers the network of parents, friends and community health care workers around the asthmatic child, one recognizes that an enormous potential for the promotion of good health can be mobilized. Physicians will often have the challenge and privilege of organizing, motivating and supervising this network.

Prevention of asthma is a principal focus. While efforts to prevent asthma are still in the research phase, there are proven areas where the application of simple, direct methods at the primary health care level can postpone or prevent the long-term ravages of the disease. One example is reducing exposure to tobacco smoke, as maternal smoking during gestation and parental smoking during early childhood are associated with reduced respiratory function and recurrent wheezing. Another major issue is the need to organize available health care resources optimally, to create an informed and educated team of which the asthmatic child is an integral and essential member.

Textbook of Pediatric Asthma: An International Perspective aims to provide a comprehensive repository of knowledge to which the health professional can turn as a major resource. I hope it will serve as a key source of information and of inspiration to those who are fighting the battle against childhood asthma and its complications.

Gro Harlem Brundtland, MD, MPH
Director-General
World Health Organization
Geneva, Switzerland

Preface

Asthma is the most common chronic disease of childhood and its prevalence continues to increase throughout the world. This disease accounts for a large and increasing proportion of total health care costs. Children with asthma have frequent school absences and often drop out of sporting activities, and their parents miss excessive days of work to take care of them.

The present burden of asthma on patients and on the whole society is so high that the World Health Organization (WHO) considers asthma as a major public health problem. As a consequence of this concern, the WHO in collaboration with a number of other international organizations, is producing reports and guidelines addressing the primary issue of asthma prevention.

As the vast majority of patients develop their symptoms of asthma in the first five years of life, asthma is predominantly a pediatric problem. The impact of asthma in the developing child is not yet fully understood; however, there are indications that early interventions in the management of pediatric asthma may minimize its manifestations in adult life.

As in other chronic disorders, the prevention of asthma is the ideal approach. Although recent advances in the early origins of asthma are available and we remain committed to developing prevention strategies, we do not yet have the necessary information to develop a method for primary prevention. In the meantime, we pediatricians must understand and use the best methods to diagnose and manage asthma in children. To provide the information for pediatricians to be able to do these things is the purpose of this textbook. We assembled and integrated into one volume the latest basic and clinical knowledge related to pediatric asthma. The chapters were written by recognized experts from all continents, offering an international perspective on the preferred and alternative approaches for the management of children with both acute and chronic asthma. We believe that we are offering our readers a wealth of knowledge and a broad perspective from years of research and clinical experience.

We have enjoyed the challenge of not only assembling the work of so many authorities into one text, but also negotiating the varying opinions and strategies of these experts into unified concepts that can be used on a daily basis by pediatricians treating infants, children and adolescents with asthma. We sincerely thank our contributing authors from around the world, for their time and effort in writing their chapters.

Charles K Naspitz
Stanley J Szefler
David G Tinkelman
John O Warner

Contributors

Iqbal H Ahmed MB ChB MSc MPH
Director of Respiratory Services
The Richmond Hospital
560–6091 Gilbert Road
Richmond
British Columbia V7C 5L9
Canada

L Karla Arruda MD
Assistant Professor
Departments of Pediatrics and Cell and
Molecular Biology
University of São Paulo School of Medicine of
Ribeirão Preto
Av. Bandeirantes 3900
Riberão Preto
São Paulo 14049-900
Brazil

Bruce G Bender PhD
Professor of Psychiatry
University Colorado School of Medicine, and
Head, Pediatric Behavioral Health
National Jewish Medical and Research Center
1400 Jackson Street, Room J-212
Denver, CO 80206
USA

S Allan Bock MD
Staff Physician
Department of Pediatrics
National Jewish Medical and Research Center,
and
Clinical Professor
Department of Pediatrics
University of Colorado Health Sciences Center
Boulder Valley Asthma and Allergy Clinic
3950 Broadway
Boulder, CO 80304
USA

Andrew Bush MB BS (Hons) MA MD FRCP FRCPCH
Reader in Paediatric Respirology
Imperial School of Medicine at National Heart
and Lung Institute, and
Honorary Consultant Paediatric Chest
Physician
Royal Brompton Hospital
Sydney Street
London SW3 6NP
UK

William W Busse MD
Professor of Medicine and Head
Section of Allergy/Clinical Immunology
University of Wisconsin-Madison
600 Highland Avenue
Madison, WI 53792-2454
USA

Kai-Håkon Carlsen MD PhD
Director General and Professor
Voksentoppen National Hospital of Asthma,
Allergy and Chronic Lung Diseases in Children
Ullveien 14
N-0791 Oslo
Norway

Martin D Chapman PhD
Professor
Departments of Medicine and Microbiology
Asthma and Allergic Diseases Center
University of Virginia
300 Lane Road
MR4 Building, room 5060
Charlottesville, VA 22908
USA

Giuseppe N Colasurdo MD
Associate Professor and Head
Division of Pulmonary Medicine
Department of Pediatrics
University of Texas Health Science Center
6431 Fannin
Houston, TX 77030
USA

Jonathan Corren MD
Medical Co-Director
Allergy Research Foundation Inc.
11620 Wilshire Blvd, #200
Los Angeles, CA 90025
USA

Ronina A Covar MD
Staff Physician
National Jewish Medical and Research Center
1400 Jackson Street
Denver, CO 80206
USA

Myrna B Dolovich PEng
McMaster University
1200 Main St West, HSC 1V18
Hamilton
Ontario L8N 3Z5
Canada

Peyton A Eggleston MD
Professor of Pediatrics
Division of Allergy and Immunology
The Johns Hopkins University School of Medicine
CMSC 1102
Johns Hopkins Hospital
600 North Wolfe Street
Baltimore, MD 21287
USA

Mark L Everard MB ChB MRCP DM
Consultant Paediatrician
Paediatric Respiratory Unit
Sheffield Children's Hospital
Western Bank
Sheffield S10 2TH
UK

Melanie C Gleason PA
National Jewish Medical and Research Center
1400 Jackson Street
Denver, CO 80206
USA

Gary L Larsen MD
Senior Faculty Member
Professor and Head
Division of Pediatric Pulmonary Medicine
National Jewish Medical & Research Center
1400 Jackson Street
Denver, CO 80206
USA

Peter N Le Souëf MD MRCP(UK) FRACP
Professor of Paediatrics
University of Western Australia, and
Respiratory Physician
Department of Respiratory Medicine
Princess Margaret Hospital for Children
GPO Box D184
Perth
Australia 6001

Paula Lozano MD MPH
Assistant Professor
Department of Pediatrics
University of Washington
1730 Minor Avenue
Seattle, WA 98101
USA

Fernando D Martinez MD
Swift-McNear Professor of Pediatrics, and Director
Respiratory Sciences Center
University of Arizona
PO Box 24-5030
Tucson, AZ 85724-5030
USA

Charles K Naspitz MD
Professor of Pediatrics
Division of Allergy, Clinical Immunology and Rheumatology
Department of Pediatrics
Federal University of São Paulo/Escola Paulista de Medicina
Rua dos Otonis, 725
São Paulo 04025-002
Brazil

Gary Rachelefsky MD
Medical Co-Director
Allergy Research Foundation Inc.
11620 Wilshire Blvd, #200
Los Angeles, CA 90025
USA

Maria C Rizzo MD
Associate Researcher
Division of Allergy, Clinical Immunology and Rheumatology
Department of Pediatrics
Federal University of São Paulo/Escola Paulista de Medicina
Rua dos Otonis, 725
São Paulo 04025-002
Brazil

Jonathan M Samet MD MS
Professor and Chairman
The Johns Hopkins School of Public Health
Department of Epidemiology
615 N Wolfe Street, Suite 6041
Baltimore, MD 21205
USA

Hugh A Sampson MD
Kurt Hirschhorn Professor of Pediatrics & Biomedical Sciences,
Chief, Pediatric Allergy and Immunology, and Professor of Pediatrics
The Elliot and Roslyn Jaffe Food Allergy Institute
Division of Allergy and Immunology
Department of Pediatrics
Mount Sinai School of Medicine
PO Box 1198, One Gustave Levy Place
New York, NY 10029
USA

Dirceu Solé MD
Professor of Pediatrics
Department of Pediatrics
Federal University of São Paulo/Escola Paulista de Medicina
Rua Mirassol 236, apto 72
São Paulo 04044-010
Brazil

Joseph D Spahn MD
Associate Professor
University of Colorado Health Sciences Center, and
Staff Physician
National Jewish Medical and Research Center
1400 Jackson Street
Denver, CO 80206
USA

Sean D Sullivan PhD
Associate Professor
Departments of Pharmacy and Health Services
Adjunct Associate Professor
Division of Allergy
Director, Pharmaceutical Outcomes Research and Policy Program
Department of Pharmacy
Box 357630
University of Washington
Seattle, WA 98195
USA

Stanley J Szefler MD
Professor of Pediatrics and Pharmacology
University of Colorado Health Sciences Center
Helen Wohlberg and Herman Lambert Chair in Pharmacokinetics, and
Director of Clinical Pharmacology
National Jewish Medical and Research Center
1400 Jackson Street
Denver, CO 80206
USA

Virginia S Taggart MPH
Health Scientist Administrator
Division of Lung Diseases
National Heart, Lung and Blood Institute
Rockledge Center II – suite 10018
6701 Rockledge Drive MSC 7952
Bethesda, MD 20892
USA

David G Tinkelman MD
Professor of Pediatrics
University of Colorado Health Sciences Center,
and
Staff Physician
National Jewish Medical and Research Center
1400 Jackson Street
Denver, CO 80206
USA

Amjad Tuffaha MD
Clinical Fellow
Section of Allergy/Clinical Immunology
University of Wisconsin-Madison
600 Highland Avenue
Madison, WI 53792-2454
USA

Pakit Vichyanond MD
Professor of Pediatrics
Department of Pediatrics
Faculty of Medicine Siriraj Hospital
Mahidol University
2 Prannok Street
Bangkok 10700
Thailand

John O Warner MD FRCPCH
Professor of Child Health and
Director of Allergy & Inflammation Sciences
Division
School of Medicine
Level G (803), Centre Block
Southampton General Hospital
Tremona Road
Southampton SO16 6YD
UK

Eugene G Weinberg MB ChB FCPaeds(SA)
Red Cross Children's Hospital and Institute of
Child Health
University of Cape Town
Rondebosch 7700
South Africa

Kevin B Weiss MD
Director, Center for Healthcare Studies
Northwestern Medical School
Northwestern University
680 N. Lake Shore Drive
Chicago, IL 60611
USA

Denise G Wiesch PhD
Program Officer
Division of Allergy, Immunology and
Transplantation
National Institute of Allergy and Infectious
Diseases
National Institutes of Health
4700-B Rockledge Drive, Room 5253
Bethesda, MD 20892-7640
USA

Robert A Wood MD
Associate Professor of Pediatrics
Division of Allergy and Immunology
The Johns Hopkins University School of
Medicine
CMSC 1102
Johns Hopkins Hospital
600 North Wolfe Street
Baltimore, MD 21287
USA

List of abbreviations

2-D	two-dimensional	CysLT	cysteinyl leukotriene
3-D	three-dimensional	DB	double blind
ABPA	allergic bronchopulmonary aspergillosis	DBPCFC	double-blind, placebo-controlled food challenge
ACTH	adrenocorticotrophic hormone	DNA	deoxyribonucleic acid
AHR	airway hyperresponsiveness	DPI	dry powder inhaler
ALLSA	Allergy Society of South Africa	DSCG	disodium cromoglycate
APC	antigen-presenting cell	DZ	dizygotic
ATS	American Thoracic Society		
BAL	bronchoalveolar lavage	ECP	eosinophilic cationic protein
BCG	bacille Calmette-Guérin	ED	emergency department
BDP	beclomethasone dipropionate	EGA	estimated gestational age
BHR	bronchial hyperresponsiveness	EIA	exercise-induced asthma
bid	twice daily	EIB	exercise-induced bronchospasm, bronchoconstriction
BLT-receptor	leukotriene B_4 receptor		
BN	Brown Norway	ELISA	enzyme-linked immunosorbent assay
BPD	bronchopulmonary dysplasia		
BUD	budesonide	EPA	Environmental Protection Agency
CAM	complementary and alternative medicine	EPR-2	Expert Panel Report 2
		ERV	expiratory reserve volume
CAMP	Childhood Asthma Management Program	ETAC	Early Treatment of the Atopic Child
cAMP	cyclic 3',5' adenosine monophosphate	ETS	environmental tobacco smoke
		F	female
cDNA	complementary DNA	FAPESP	Fundação de Amparo a Pesquisa Estado de São Paulo
CF	cystic fibrosis		
CFC	chlorofluorocarbon	FDA	Food and Drug Administration
CI	confidence interval	FEF_{25-75}	forced expiratory flow from 25% to 75% of FVC
Cl⁻	chloride ion		
CNS	central nervous system	$FEV_{0.5}$	forced expiratory volume in 0.5 second
COPD	chronic obstructive pulmonary disease		
		$FEV_{0.75}$	forced expiratory volume in 0.75 second
CPK-MB	creatine phosphokinase, MB isozyme		
		FEV_1	forced expiratory volume in 1 second
CS	corticosteroid		
CsA	cyclosporin A	FLAP	5-lipoxygenase activating protein
CT	computed tomography		
CWD	chest wall distortion		
CXR	chest X-ray	FOB	fibreoptic bronchoscopy

FRC	functional residual capacity	IL-8	interleukin-8
FVC	forced vital capacity	IL-9	interleukin-9
		IL-10	interleukin-10
GA	gestational age	IL-11	interleukin-11
GC	glucocorticoid	IL-12	interleukin-12
GCR	glucorticoid receptor	IL-13	interleukin-13
GER	gastro-oesophageal reflux	IRV	inspiratory reserve volume
GI	gastrointestinal	ISAAC	International Study of Asthma and Allergy in Children
GINA	Global Initiative for Asthma		
GM-CSF	granulocyte macrophage colony-stimulating factor	ISS	immunostimulatory sequences
		ISS-ODN	oligonucleotide immunostimulatory sequences
GST	glutathione-S-transferase		
		IUIS	International Union of Immunological Societies
H and E	haematoxylin and eosin		
H_2O	water	IV	intravenous
HEPA	High-efficiency particle air filter system	IVIG	intravenous immunoglobulin
HFA	hydro-fluoro-alkane	LFA-1	lymphocyte function associated antigen 1
HFC	hydro-fluoro-carbon		
HIV	human immunodeficiency virus	5-LO	5-lipoxygenase
		LPS	lipopolysaccharide
HLA	human leukocyte antigen	LRI	lower respiratory illness or infection
HPA axis	hypothalamic-pituitary-adrenal axis		
		LTA_4	leukotriene A_4
5-HPETE	5-hydroperoxy-eicosatetraenoic acid	LTB_4	leukotriene B_4
		LTC_4	leukotriene C_4
HVSD	height velocity standard deviation	LTD_4	leukotriene D_4
		LTE_4, LTE4	leukotriene E_4
		LTRA	leukotriene receptor antagonist
ibd	identity by descent		
IC	inspiratory capacity	M	male
ICAM-1	intercellular adhesion molecule 1	M_2 receptors	type 2 muscarinic receptors
ICD	International Classification of Diseases	ma	mean age
		MDI	metered dose inhaler
ICR	International Consensus Report	MEFR	maximal expiratory flow rate
ICS	inhaled corticosteroids	MEFV	maximal expiratory flow–volume
ICU	intensive care unit		
IFN	interferon	MHC	major histocompatibility complex
IFR	inspiratory flow rate		
IgA	immunoglobulin A	MIP-1α	macrophage inflammatory protein-1α
IgE	immunoglobulin E		
IgG	immunoglobulin G	MMAD	mass median aerosol diameter
IgM	immunoglobulin M	MMP	matrix metalloproteinase
IL-1	interleukin-1	MPn	methylprednisolone
IL-2	interleukin-2	mRNA	messenger RNA
IL-3	interleukin-3	MTX	methotrexate
IL-4	interleukin-4	MZ	monozygotic
IL-5	interleukin-5		
IL-6	interleukin-6	Na^+	sodium ion

NAEPP	National Asthma Education and Prevention Program	PES	oesophageal pressure
NAMCS	National Ambulatory Medical Care Survey	PET	positron emission tomography
		PFT	pulmonary function test
NANC	non-adrenergic, non-cholinergic	PGE2	prostaglandin E2
		PIF	peak inspiratory flow
NF-κB	nuclear factor kappa B	PIV	parainfluenza virus
NHAMCS	National Hospital Ambulatory Medical Care Survey	pMDI	pressurized metered dose inhaler
NHANES	National Health and Nutrition Examination Survey	po	oral
		PPRU	Pediatric Pharmacology Research Unit
NHDS	National Hospital Discharge Survey	PPV	parts per volume
		PUFA	polyunsaturated fatty acid
NHIS	National Health Interview Survey	QD, qd	once daily
NHLBI	National Heart, Lung and Blood Institute	qid	four times daily
NICHHD	National Institute of Child Health and Human Development	r	range
		RAE	renal adverse effects
		RAST	radioallergosorbent test
NIH	National Institutes of Health	RDS	respiratory distress syndrome
NK	natural killer	REM	rapid eye movement
NMES	National Medical Expenditure Survey	rhIL-12	recombinant human interleukin-12
NO	nitric oxide	rhuMAb-E25	recombinant human anti-IgE monoclonal antibody
NO_2	nitrogen dioxide		
		RNA	ribonucleic acid
O_2^-	superoxide	RR	relative risk
OSA	obstructive sleep apnoea	RSV	respiratory syncytial virus
		RT-PCR	reverse transcription polymerase chain reaction
$PaCO_2$	arterial carbon dioxide tension		
PaO_2	arterial oxygen tension	RV	residual volume
PAT	Preventive Allergy Treatment	RV	rhinovirus
PC	placebo-controlled		
PC20	provocative concentration of methacholine causing a 20% fall in forced expiratory volume in 1 second	s-ECP	soluble eosinophilic cationic protein
		s-MPO	soluble myeloperoxidase
		SACAWG	South African Childhood Asthma Working Group
PD_{20}	provocative dose of methacholine causing a 20% fall in forced expiratory volume in 1 second	SAY	Support for Asthmatic Youth
		SBFC	single-blind food challenge
		sd	standard deviation
PCD	primary ciliary dyskinesia	SDS	standard deviation score
PCR	polymerase chain reaction	SE	standard error
PDE	phosphodiesterase	sICAM-1	soluble intercellular adhesion molecule 1
PEEP	positive end-expiratory pressure		
		SPECT	single photon emission computed tomography
PEF	peak expiratory flow		
PEFR	peak expiratory flow rate		

$t_{1/2}$	elimination half-life	UK	United Kingdom
TAO	troleandomycin	URI	upper respiratory tract infection
TB	tuberculosis		
TBB	transbronchial biopsy	US, USA	United States of America
Tc$_2$ cell	type 2 CD8+ T cell		
TGF	transforming growth factor	VC	vital capacity
Th-1 cell	type 1 T-helper cell	VCAM-1	vascular cell adhesion molecule 1
Th-2 cell	type 2 T-helper cell		
TH$_1$ cell	type 1 T-helper cell	VCD	vocal cord dysfunction
TH$_2$ cell	type 2 T-helper cell	VEGh	von Ebner's gland protein
tid	three times daily	V'_{maxFRC}	maximal flow at functional residual capacity
TIMP	tissue inhibitor of matrix metalloproteinase		
		VOC	volatile organic compounds
TLC	total lung capacity		
TNF-α	tumour necrosis factor-α	WHO	World Health Organization
T_{ptef}/T_E	time to peak tidal expiratory flow divided by total time of expiration	yr	year
TV	tidal volume		

1

Lung function and development

Peter N Le Souëf

Introduction • Respiratory system development • Measurement of lung function in infants • Data on airway function in infants • Measurement of lung function in children between 2 and 5 years of age • Measurement of lung function in children aged over 5 years • Lung function in asthmatic children

INTRODUCTION

To understand asthma in children, a thorough knowledge of the development and physiology of the lung from fetal life through childhood to adulthood is essential. Knowledge of the stages of the development of the airway and the relationships between airway size and lung gas volume is needed to interpret clinical signs in normal and asthmatic children. It is also needed to interpret lung function data from children, along with familiarity with the methodologies for measuring lung function. To look after sick asthmatic children, a sound basis in respiratory physiology is especially important. Recognizing early signs of respiratory failure and implementing appropriate strategies require an appreciation of the basic mechanisms of moving gas in and out of the lung and gas exchange within the lung. For physicians training during the last decade, it has not been easy to gain an appropriately in-depth knowledge of these processes owing to the current research emphasis on cellular and molecular aspects of asthma. For non-physician asthma researchers, knowledge of the physiology contributing to changes in lung function data is helpful, since such data are frequently used in outcome assessments of research studies. This chapter will summarize important elements in the development of the lung, and techniques for objectively assessing lung and airway function in infants and children.

RESPIRATORY SYSTEM DEVELOPMENT

In utero lung development

During fetal life, the airways develop earlier than the air spaces in the lung. Around the end of the first month of the first trimester, the lung bud appears as an outpouching from the endoderm of the foregut. Soon after, the first airway branch appears and by the middle of the first trimester, all segmental bronchi have been formed. Branching of the bronchi is complete early in the 16th week of gestation.[1] At that time, the future gas-containing elements of the lung begin to appear, but they are not present in sufficient number to allow life-sustaining gas exchange until around 22 weeks of gestation. The number of alveoli continues to increase from near the end of the second trimester and

Table 1.1 Developmental problems in chest wall physiology in early life

Physiological difference	Physiological consequence
Ribs set horizontally	Bucket-handle action lost
Diaphragm more horizontal	Poor elevation of rib cage on inspiration
Increased rapid-eye-movement sleep	Loss of stabilizing effect on rib cage
Low % type 1 muscle fibres in diaphragm	Diaphragm prone to fatigue
High chest wall compliance	Wasted inspiratory effort distorting chest wall

through the third trimester. At birth, approximately 8% of the adult number of alveoli are present and the number continues to increase until around 8–10 years of age.[2] The diameter of the airway increases in a linear fashion from the middle of the second trimester of fetal life until the end of the first year of life. The relative rate of increase of all the components of the airway is constant during this period.[2]

Chest wall development

The chest wall does more than encase the lungs. More importantly, it is a pump that moves gas in and out of the lungs. In fetal life, it is ill-prepared for this role for several reasons (Table 1.1). Firstly, the configuration of the rib cage is suboptimal. The ribs are more horizontally placed, reducing the bucket-handle capability that comes with having them placed obliquely to the spine.[3] Secondly, the diaphragm is also more horizontally placed and this causes it to pull the lower margin of the rib cage inwards during inspiration rather than elevating the ribs as would happen if it were more obliquely placed. Thirdly, the stabilizing effect of the intercostal muscles on the chest wall is reduced in the fetus, as they spend more of their time in rapid-eye-movement (REM) sleep. During REM sleep, intercostal muscle activity is markedly reduced and the rib cage moves inwards rather than outwards on inspiration. Thus, effort is expended in sucking in the rib cage rather than fresh air (Figure 1.1). Newborn infants spend about half of their sleep time in REM sleep, and this probably drops to adult levels at around 3 years of age.[6] Fourthly, the diaphragm has a reduced percentage of fatigue-resistant type 1 muscle fibres (Figure 1.2),[7] so it is less able to operate for sustained periods at a higher work load. In preterm infants, the diaphragm is more prone to fatigue and can develop electromyographic evidence of fatigue during spontaneous breathing in the absence of lung disease.[4,5] Finally, the rib cage structure itself is less stiff because it is more cartilaginous. The compliance of the chest wall is three times that of the lung at birth, but chest wall compliance decreases and is the same as lung compliance during the second year of life, a situation that is the same as in adults.[8]

These problems with function are particularly relevant in preterm infants, but they also compromise breathing in the first few years of life. Paradoxical motion of the rib cage on inspiration during REM sleep reflects the mechanical problems of the chest wall. This motion does not disappear until about 3 years of age, when it becomes minimal or absent,[6] as occurs in adults. The problems with the pumping action of the chest wall are likely to contribute to an increased tendency to develop respiratory failure in infants with asthma.

Airway smooth muscle development

Early studies suggested that young infants' airways have very little smooth muscle.[9] Later studies have shown that this is not true, since airway smooth muscle is present almost as soon as the airway is formed *in utero* (Figure 1.3)[10] and its bronchoconstriction in response to

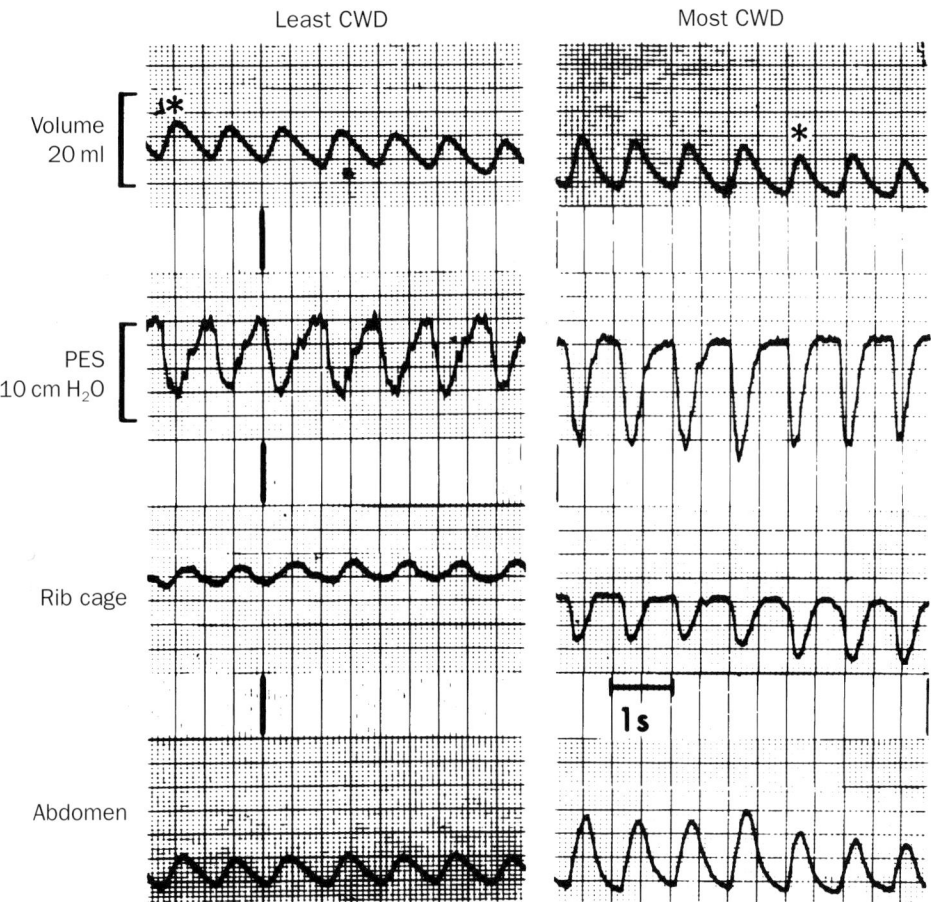

Figure 1.1 Sections of trace are shown for one preterm infant with magnetometer pairs to detect motion of the rib cage and abdomen. Breaths were matched for tidal volume. The left panel shows minimal chest wall (CWD) distortion and is consistent with quiet sleep. The right panel shows marked chest wall distortion consistent with rapid-eye-movement (REM) sleep. In REM sleep, unproductive effort is expended in sucking in the rib cage rather than fresh air. PES = oesophageal pressure. (From ref 33 with permission.)

pharmacological agonists is similar to that in older individuals.[11–14] Despite this, response to bronchodilators is poor or absent in the first year or two of life[15,16] and gradually becomes established during the first 5 years of life.[17] The reason for the lack of response in early life is unclear. It is not due to a lack of β_2-adrenoreceptors, since salbutamol has been shown to block the bronchial response to histamine[14,18] in infants and to speed the return to normal lung function after a bronchial response to histamine has been recorded.[19] In infants, the bronchial response of agents such as histamine could be taken as evidence that the airway smooth muscle in infants can constrict the airway, but not as proof, since a change in airway wall oedema could produce airway narrowing.

Development of the lung in childhood

From birth to adulthood, the increase in lung volume occurs with an exponent of approximately 2.75 with respect to height.[20] This is a

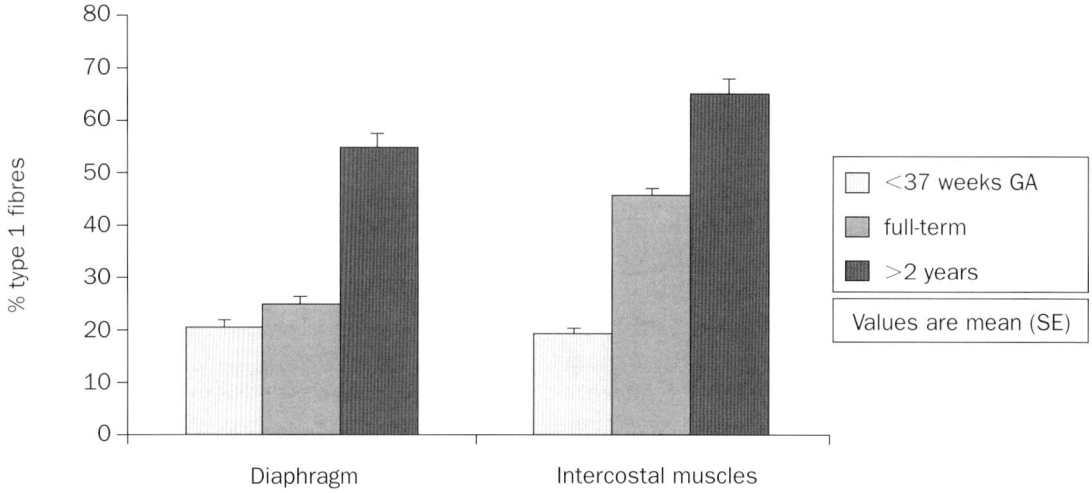

Figure 1.2 Relationship between age in early life and mean (SE) % type 1 slow-twitch, high-oxidative muscle fibres in the diaphragm and intercostal muscles. GA = gestational age; SE = standard error. (Derived from data from ref 7 with permission.)

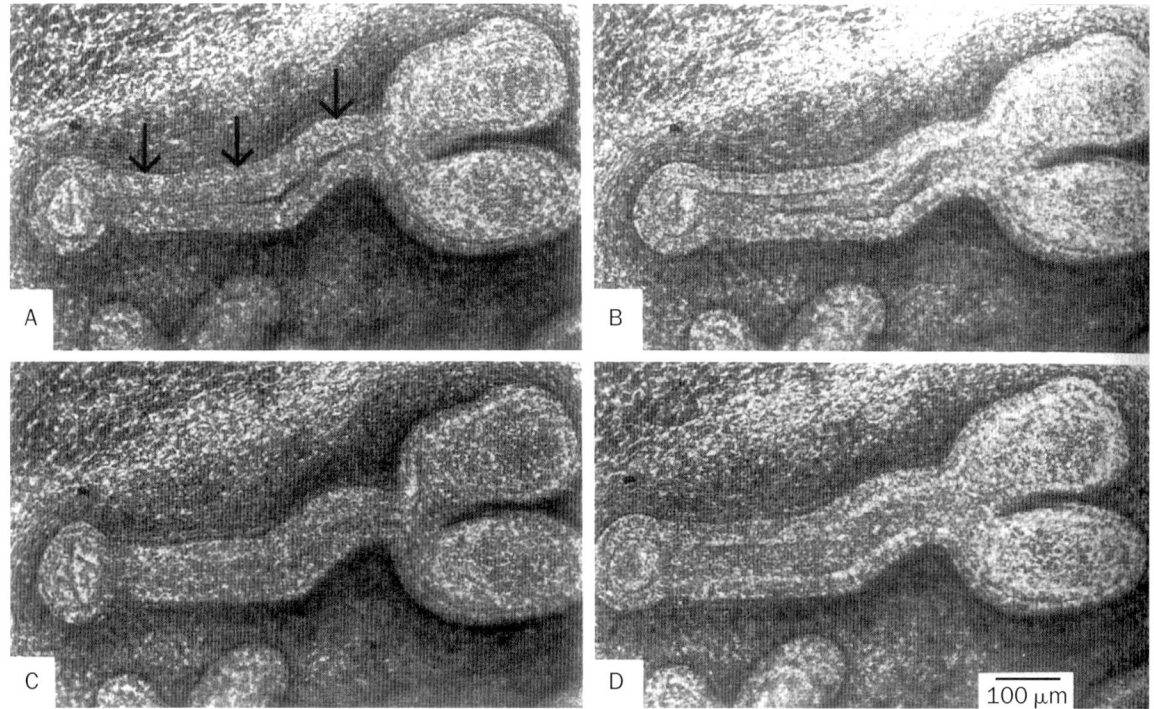

Figure 1.3 Responses of a human airway from a first trimester fetus. (A) Control, contracted; (B) control, relaxed; (C) after the addition of carbachol; (D) after the atropine had reversed the effects of carbachol. (From ref 10 with permission.)

similar figure to that found in all mammals and reflects the fact that the lungs do not increase in volume in all dimensions as would be the case with a cube, with an exponent of 3. The increase in height of the lung is likely to be greater than the increase in width or depth. Compliance increases with an exponent closer to 2 with respect to height.[21]

In infant girls the airways may be both relatively and absolutely larger than in infant boys. Maximal flow at functional residual capacity (V'_{maxFRC}) is higher in female than in male infants.[22] However, whether these differences reflect larger airways in girls or more compliant airways in boys is not known. A higher level of airway compliance could reduce V'_{maxFRC} by allowing the airway wall to collapse during expiration. The physiological differences between infant boys and girls may explain why wheeze is more likely to develop in boys in response to a viral respiratory tract infection.

Increases in airway size and lung volume occur at different rates during childhood, leading to the concept of dysanapsis.[23] From infancy onwards, boys of a given height have larger lungs than girls, and the rate of increase in lung volume is higher for boys.[24] However, there are limited data on the rate of increase of airway size. In older children, the difference between girls and boys with respect to height-corrected maximal flows is no longer evident, since the forced expiratory volume in 1 second (FEV_1) is not different between the two genders.[25] So in older children, airway size may not be different between boys and girls of the same height. There are two ways to interpret the data. One is that among younger children, girls have bigger or less compliant airways than boys, but this difference disappears with increasing age. The other is that the rate of increase of lung volume in boys is greater than the rate of increase in airway size, leading to relatively small airways for the size of their lungs. In the absence of good direct assessments of airway size, the relative importance of these two interpretations is unclear.

MEASUREMENT OF LUNG FUNCTION IN INFANTS

Assessing function in infants

Over the last 20 years, more accurate and reliable techniques for assessing lung and particularly airway function in infants have become available. These techniques have allowed a much better understanding of airway physiology in healthy infants and in those with airway disease.

Earlier methodologies produced data that are a reflection more of large rather than small airway function.[26] The techniques include: lung volume and airway resistance techniques that employ a body plethysmograph,[27-30] dynamic compliance and resistance measurements using oesophageal manometry,[27-33] and respiratory conductance measurements using forced oscillation.[34,35]

Tidal volume forced expiration

More recent approaches have employed forced expiration to produce data that are more likely to reflect small airway function,[36] although direct assessment to support this view is lacking. Assessments of forced expiration became available in infants in the early 1980s, after the publication of the first technique to describe forced expiration using a plethysmograph[37] and its subsequent modification using an inflatable jacket.[36] The tidal volume forced expiratory method has provided much of the current knowledge regarding airway function in infants.[38-50]

As in most assessments of respiratory function in infants, the tidal volume forced expiration technique requires the infant to be *asleep*. The hypnotic agent that has been used for most of these studies is chloral hydrate and most parents find that this approach is acceptable.[51] Once the infant is asleep, the jacket is inflated at end-inspiration and the forced expiratory flow at functional residual capacity (FRC) is measured from a facemask using a suitable flow meter. To obtain V'_{maxFRC} (Figure 1.4), the

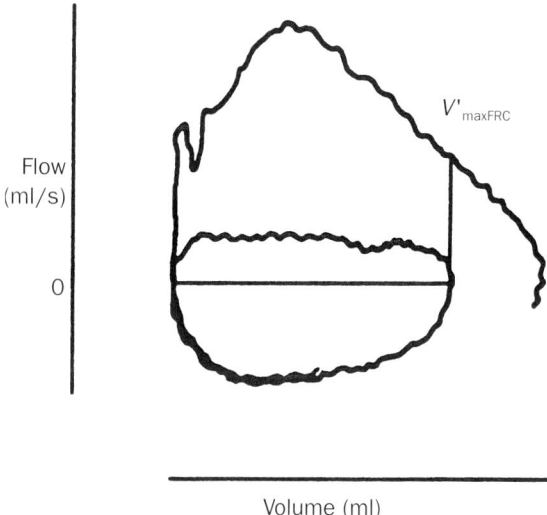

Figure 1.4 Tidal flow–volume loops showing a spontaneous expiration, a spontaneous inspiration followed by a forced expiration. The derivation of maximal flow at functional residual capacity (V'_{maxFRC}) is shown.

pressure in the jacket is gradually increased for repeated forced expirations until no further increases in flow are observed. Whether normal infants can reach maximal flow using this approach has been controversial.[26] Most laboratories choose an arbitrary maximal compression pressure.

Assessing the efficacy of the inflatable jacket in *transmitting pressure* across the chest wall to the pleural space is important, since it allows the relative efficiency of jackets in different studies to be compared. This can be done non-invasively by occluding the infant's airway at end-inspiration and, when the mouth pressure has plateaued, inflating the jacket.[47] The increase in mouth pressure from jacket inflation is equivalent to the increase in pleural pressure from jacket inflation. The efficiency of the jacket in transmitting pressure is equivalent to the ratio between the increase in airway pressure attributed to the jacket and the increase in jacket pressure.[47]

The major drawback in the use of tidal volume forced expirations is the lack of a reliable *volume landmark*. The main parameter, V'_{maxFRC}, relies on the stability of FRC from breath to breath. Functional residual capacity in infants is not at the same volume as the relaxed expiratory volume, which is the volume that would be reached at the end of a passive expiration, since infants usually breathe in before a full passive expiration is completed.[52] The problem with this 'dynamic elevation of FRC' is that inspiration does not occur at the same volume for every breath. Factors known to affect the timing of inspiration and, therefore, FRC include sleep state, changes in the degree of airway obstruction and changes in the volume of dead space.[47,52-55] The result is that FRC is highly variable. This may be the main reason why V'_{maxFRC} is a highly variable parameter with intra-subject coefficients of variation (CV) of over 10%.[38-43,47,49,56,57]

In addition, changes in airway calibre are accompanied by *changes in FRC* that are likely to affect measurements of V'_{maxFRC} in a way that masks the underlying airway changes. For example, if a bronchodilator response occurs in an individual with significant airways obstruction, FRC could be expected to end up at a lower lung volume. Since V'_{maxFRC} is highly volume dependent, the shift to a lower lung volume would mean that a lower value would be recorded than would have been noted if FRC had not shifted. In this way, bronchodilation could be missed in infants assessed with this technique.[38]

The reverse may be the case in agonist-induced airway narrowing in tests of airway responsiveness.[12] In this situation, FRC is likely to increase during the course of the test, since expiration will be slowed by the narrowed airways and inspiration will occur before lung volume has had a chance to drop to its pretest levels. An increase in FRC has been noted in infants during testing of airway responsiveness.[58] Since increases in FRC mean that the recorded V'_{maxFRC} will be increased, the true drop that would have been noted if FRC had not changed will be missed and the change in V'_{maxFRC} underestimated. This means that a higher dose of agonist will be needed to produce a given change in V'_{maxFRC}.

Tidal breathing assessments

Non-invasive assessments of flow–volume data obtained during spontaneous tidal breathing can provide data on airway function in infants. The most useful parameter has proven to be the time to peak tidal expiratory flow divided by the total time of expiration (T_{ptef}/T_E). This can be measured using a conventional flow meter attached to a facemask[50] or derived from uncalibrated respiratory inductance plethysmograph bands around the chest and abdomen.[59] In infants with airway disease, the peak expiratory flow is reached more quickly with respect to the total expiratory time compared with normal infants. Airway disease is associated with values of T_{ptef}/T_E of approximately 0.15 versus 0.45 in normal infants. The reason for the lower ratio with airway disease is unclear, but may relate to a combination of quicker release of postinspiratory respiratory muscle tone and prolongation of expiration. The usefulness of the technique has been demonstrated by low values of T_{ptef}/T_E predicting adverse outcome in a longitudinal study of infants[50] and associated with maternal smoking in a study of breathing patterns in newborn infants.[60]

Raised volume forced expiration

To counter the problem of a lack of reliable lung volume landmark, the raised volume forced expiration technique has been developed[61] (Figure 1.5) and is now being used increasingly in clinical studies in infants.[26] The use of raised volume forced expiration to quantify function is in line with practice in older children and adults, in whom this approach has for many years been the most useful parameter for assessing respiratory function.[62,63] Advantages and disadvantages of the raised volume technique in infants are summarized in Table 1.2, in which the tidal and raised volume techniques are compared.

The raised volume approach has several advantages:

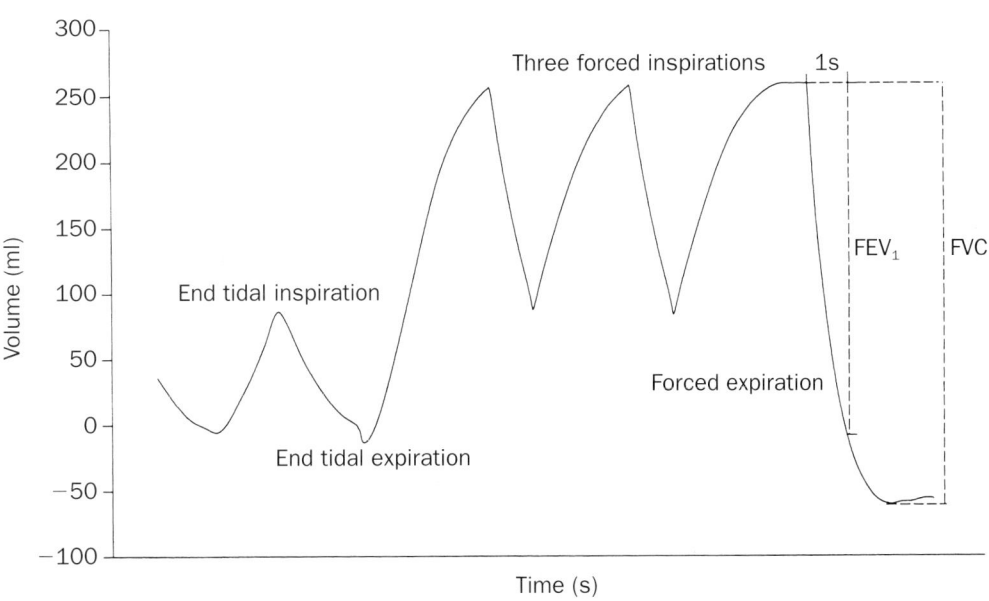

Figure 1.5 A volume–time plot of a raised-volume forced expiration. This begins with a tidal spontaneous inspiration and expiration, followed by three raised-volume cycles and finally a forced expiration. The derivation of FEV_1 and FVC is shown. (From Hayden MJ, MD thesis, Leicester University, 2000.)

Table 1.2 Comparison of tidal and raised volume forced expiratory flow–volume

	Tidal volume forced expiration	Raised volume forced expiration
Volume landmarks	End-inspiratory volume, FRC	End-inflation lung volume
Inspiratory/inflation pressure	Determined by infant	Preset (20 or 30 cm H_2O)
Intrapleural compression pressure	Minimum needed for V'_{maxFRC}	Preset (20 cm H_2O change in intrapleural pressure at end-inflation)
Main parameters	V'_{maxFRC}	Volume–time (e.g., $FEV_{0.5}$) Flow at given expiratory volume (e.g., FEF_{25-75})
Coefficient of variation	10–15% (V'_{maxFRC})	4–5% ($FEV_{0.5}$)
Advantages	Simpler equipment	Controlled volume landmarks Controlled compression force Reduced variability of measurements Better reflection of physiology
Disadvantages	Variable volume landmarks Less reliable data	More complex equipment More care needed to hold mask on

1. *Lung volume* can be standardized by a given inflation pressure. In the tidal volume technique, the inflation pressure reflects the inspiratory effort of the infant. The level of effort can vary greatly in an infant, so the volume of the forced expiration will also vary.
2. Reliable *lung volume landmarks* are available, particularly end-inflation lung volume. Within-test variability could be expected to be very small. Between-test variability might be greater, since factors such as atelectasis or airway closure can produce changes in lung volume.
3. *Compression pressure* can be standardized. This can be done using the non-invasive, airway occlusion method.[47]

Inflation pressure

Standardizing inflation pressure provides a reliable, reproducible, within-test lung volume landmark. Some authorities recommend using 20 cm H_2O and others recommend using 30 cm H_2O for inflating the lung.[26] These two suggestions have advantages and disadvantages. Using 20 cm H_2O has several advantages. First, this pressure is well tolerated by infants, and is less likely to wake them or to push gas down the oesophagus into the stomach.[26] It is also sufficient to produce a lung volume close to 'total lung capacity' (TLC). With 30 cm H_2O inflation pressure, lung volume could be considered closer to TLC, but in normal infants there is little difference in lung volume between inflation pressures of 20 and 30 cm H_2O. The concept of TLC comes from adult physiology, in which there is no control over inflation pressure and TLC is defined as the lung volume achieved with the greatest inspiratory effort. However, since pressures greater than 30 cm H_2O will produce further increases in lung volume in infants and adults, the claim that 30 cm H_2O will produce TLC cannot really be justified. An inflation pressure of 30 cm H_2O is less well tolerated by infants, so a higher level of sedation might be needed to complete the study. In addition, a few infants will have air pushed into their stomachs with the higher pressure in the facemask. Thus, there are theoretical advantages in using 30 cm H_2O to standardize inflation, but the use of 20 cm H_2O is more practical and more likely to produce data in a greater number of infants.

Compression pressure
Using the same compression pressure for all infants is sensible since it should produce better separation between normal and abnormal infants. As long as the compression pressure is high enough, infants with normal airways will be at or very close to maximal flow. Infants with abnormal airways would need little or no increase in compression pressure above passive expiration to produce maximal expiratory flow[48] and the level of maximal flow would be reduced due to the airway disease. Using the standardized compression pressure in these infants could be expected to produce submaximal flows, owing to negative-effort dependence.[47] In this way, the difference between normal and abnormal would be maximized.

The efficiency of the transmission of pressure from the jacket to the pleural space at end-inflation lung volume is measured in the same way as mentioned above in relation to the tidal volume forced expiration technique.[47,64–66] This information is essential to allow the adequacy of the jacket to be assessed and to allow comparisons to be made between infants at given levels of compression force.[67] Although the information on the efficiency of transmission of pressure provided at end-inflation does not provide direct information on the change in pleural pressure throughout the forced expiration, it does allow the efficiency of the jacket to be determined and the initial compression force to be accurately preset. However, the compression force during expiration is not likely to vary greatly between jackets and between infants. A problem would occur only if the jacket had been so poorly designed that it was unable to maintain a compressive force during expiration. Given the relatively small change in volume of the infant compared with the volume in the jacket, this would occur only if the jacket had a markedly limited ability to change volume itself.

Some investigators recommend attempting to obtain 'maximal expiratory flow–volume curves' in every infant in the belief that this will produce better data owing to flow limitation. There is a potential problem with this concept, since a maximal flow–volume curve may not be attainable. The reason is that maximal flow is achieved at a different compression force in different parts of the flow–volume curve. At a high lung volume, flow is effort dependent, so that the higher the compression force, the higher the flow, and maximal flows cannot be obtained.[47,48] At mid lung volume, flow is no longer effort dependent, provided a comparatively high compression force is needed to achieve maximal flow (i.e., flow limitation). In contrast, at low lung volumes, a lower compression force is needed to achieve maximal flow, and lower flows will be produced with higher compression forces owing to negative-effort dependence.[48] The concept of flow limitation is more acceptable in adults, since there is no practical way to control compression force in conscious adults.

Recommended standardized pressures
A benefit of standardizing both inflation and compression pressure has been that more reliable comparisons can be made both between infants and between results from different laboratories. The use of an inflation pressure of 20 cm H_2O and a compression pressure of 20 cm H_2O (increase in pleural pressure of 20 cm H_2O at end-inflation) has recently been advocated.[67] The sum of these two driving pressures at the commencement of forced expiration is 40 cm H_2O, which is the initial full driving pressure.

Parameters used to quantify airway function
Either volume–time or flow at a particular lung volume can be used. For *volume–time* measurements, the forced expiratory volume (FEV) in 1 second ($FEV_{1.0}$) is not as useful as FEV in 0.75 second ($FEV_{0.75}$) or 0.5 second ($FEV_{0.5}$) owing to

the shorter expiratory time in infants. Expiratory time will exceed 1 second in only a few young infants. In other words, $FEV_{1.0}$ and forced vital capacity (FVC) would be the same in most infants. The total expiratory time will exceed 0.75 second in the majority of infants, so $FEV_{0.75}$ could be used. To avoid missing meaningful data in any infants, $FEV_{0.5}$ should be used, since few if any infants are not still expiring at 0.5 second. Both $FEV_{0.75}$ and $FEV_{0.5}$ have low coefficients of variation (CV), of approximately 4–5%. Alternatively, *flow* can be measured at a fraction of the forced expiratory lung volume. This approach has the advantage of providing measurements of flow at a low lung volume, where flow is likely to be most affected by airway disease.

Practical considerations

Inflation pressure can be generated by either a pump[61,66,68] or an external gas source.[69] The use of a pump and an appropriate circuit allows the flow sensor to remain at atmospheric pressure.[61] When the flow sensor is a pneumotachograph employing a differential pressure transducer, artifactual transient changes in flow can be avoided if a pump is used and the pneumotachograph is kept at atmospheric pressure. If an external gas supply is used, the airway is occluded during inflation and the differential transducer will be pressurized on both sides of its diaphragm. When the airway occlusion is released, there is a sudden drop in pressure to atmospheric levels, and, at the time that this is happening, the transducer is expected to provide accurate flow signals. Fortunately, the differential transducer can be properly balanced, so that the transient flow signal produces results with an insignificant change in volume.[26]

Several rapid full inflations before the measured forced expiration provide better respiratory muscle relaxation[26,69] presumably owing to improving the Hering–Breuer reflex by washing out carbon dioxide. An improved Hering–Breuer reflex means that the period of apnoea produced by the inflation will be longer and that the residual volume can be obtained.[69]

Measuring airway responsiveness in infants

Airway responsiveness to an inhaled agonist such as histamine or methacholine is a useful research measurement and has led to new understanding of airway disease in infants. Cold air was used in a few early studies[13] but there are problems in quantitating the dose of cold air which have precluded the test being used in more recent studies. For histamine or methacholine, a response is usually recorded as a significant change in a respiratory parameter after inhalation of a known concentration of the agonist. A significant change for an individual is usually taken as a multiple of the parameter's coefficient of variation. For example, for V'_{maxFRC}, the change would need to be 30%, since this would be equivalent to at least two coefficients of variation,[14] so that there would be a 95% chance that the change had not occurred by chance. However, some researchers choose to use more stringent criteria, and wish to approximate a three coefficients of variation change. Hence for V'_{maxFRC}, a 40% change is used to signify a response. Agonists are usually administered in increasing concentration of the agonist, the dose doubling with each increase until a response is recorded.

The level of airway response in an infant or young child cannot be compared with that of an older child or an adult. The reason for this is that there are no data on how to provide an infant with a dose of agonist that is equivalent to the dose for an adult.[70–72] Meaningful data can be obtained only in infants or children of a similar age or body size.

DATA ON AIRWAY FUNCTION IN INFANTS

Relation between lung function data and respiratory symptoms

Some apparently normal infants demonstrate flow limitation on tidal expiration within weeks of birth and these infants have a much higher incidence of respiratory symptoms during the first 2 years of life.[73] Whether this predisposition to increased symptoms occurs after this age is unknown. The level of V'_{maxFRC} measured soon after birth is an important predictive factor for respiratory outcome in the first few years of life. V'_{maxFRC} is reduced in infants who are destined to wheeze in the first few years of life in response to a viral respiratory infection, but this predictive effect is much less obvious by the time the children reach 6 years of age.[74] In wheezy infants, V'_{maxFRC} is lower than in controls.[75] The raised volume technique should be able to provide more accurate data on infants with airway disease, since $FEV_{0.75}$ is better than V'_{maxFRC} at differentiating between infants with recurrent wheeze[66] or cystic fibrosis[61] and controls.

Bronchodilator responsiveness

As noted in the discussion of airway smooth muscle development, bronchodilator response is poor or absent[15,51] during infancy and gradually develops during the first 5 years of life.[68] Many studies in wheezy infants with an acute or recent diagnosis of asthma or bronchiolitis have noted no bronchodilator response.[27,28,31,34,35,76] One study has suggested that a bronchodilator response can be expected in the second year of life.[76] After 2 years of age, the response appears to gain in strength and is fully established by around 5 years of age.[17] A few studies have reported a positive bronchodilator response in infancy. In one such study, the results are not convincing owing to confounding effects of age and gender,[77] and in the other, the post-bronchodilator results are statistically insignificantly different from baseline values.[78] The reason for the poor or absent bronchodilator response at this age is not clear.

Airway responsiveness

Studies on airway responsiveness in infants have established that the level of airway responsiveness in infants at 1 month of age is increased if there is a family history of asthma.[49] This suggests that there is a genetic factor that affects airway function in those destined to become asthmatic and that this factor is present from birth. The fact that it is detectable so soon after birth suggests that the difference is genetic rather than environmental. Airway responsiveness is unlikely to be acting as a surrogate for atopy, since atopic responses to inhalant allergens are not usually present in the first year or two of life. Wheezy infants do not have an increased level of airway responsiveness compared with control infants.[60] These data clearly suggest that wheeze in infants is caused by factors other than an inherent increase in airway responsiveness. The findings at this age are unique in that wheeze at all other ages is invariably associated with increased airway responsiveness.

The level of airway responsiveness measured soon after birth is predictive of respiratory outcome in early childhood.[79,80] In preliminary work, the level of airway responsiveness at 1 month of age correlated with the level of $FEV_{1.0}$ and the presence of a doctor diagnosis of asthma at 6 years of age.[80] This association was noted to be independent of IgE responses at 6 years of age, suggesting again that the mechanism by which increased airway responsiveness produces airway disease is separate from IgE responses.

MEASUREMENT OF LUNG FUNCTION IN CHILDREN BETWEEN 2 AND 5 YEARS OF AGE

For some years, a number of researchers have attempted to develop a practical assessment of airway function in this age group. Partial forced expiratory flow–volume procedures have been able to provide some useful data,[81] but the problems of lack of cooperation and difficulty with sedation have precluded the establishment of an acceptable method.

MEASUREMENT OF LUNG FUNCTION IN CHILDREN AGED OVER 5 YEARS

There are several accurate and technically valid techniques for assessing airway function in children. The same techniques used in adults can be employed in children once they reach around 5 or 6 years of age, since they can then cooperate with the testing procedures. Tests that are available include the measurement of absolute lung volume, the resistance of the airway, maximal inspiratory flow and maximal expiratory flow.

Lung volume

An understanding of the subdivisions of lung volume is essential for a clinician looking after asthmatic children (Figure 1.6). *Total lung capacity* (TLC) is the volume of the gas in the lung at the end of a maximal inspiratory effort. *Residual volume* (RV) is the volume of gas in the lung at the end of a maximal expiratory effort. *Forced vital capacity* (FVC) is the maximal volume that can be expired after a maximal inspiratory effort. *Functional residual capacity* (FRC) is the volume of gas in the lung at the end of a spontaneous expiration. $FEV_{1.0}$ is the maximal volume that can be expired from TLC in 1 second.

Absolute lung volume can be measured by either plethysmography or gas dilution. With plethysmography, a body box is employed and Boyle's law is used to determine the volume based on measurements of box pressure. The problem with this technique is that trapped gas cannot be distinguished from gas in communication with the atmosphere. This means that gas trapped behind occluded airways will be recorded as part of the lung volume. With gas dilution, a known volume of gas is inhaled and the lung volume can be calculated by the drop in concentration of the inhaled gas. The problem with this approach is that it underestimates lung volume in children with significant airway obstruction.

In asthmatic children, hyperinflation is reflected by an increase in TLC or FRC. This can occur acutely within minutes with a stimulus such as exercise or with an acute exacerbation of asthma. In some children, hyperinflation can remain between exacerbations and, in this situation, chronic asthma is very likely to be pre-

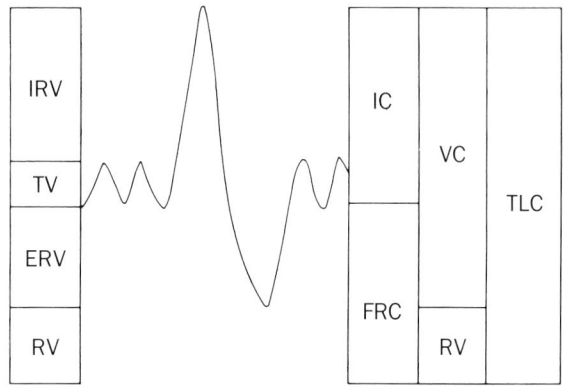

Figure 1.6 Schematic representation of subdivisions of lung volume. IRV = inspiratory reserve volume; TV = tidal volume; ERV = expiratory reserve volume; RV = residual volume; IC = inspiratory capacity; FRC = functional residual capacity; VC = vital capacity; TLC = total lung capacity. (With permission from Phelan PD, Landau LI, Olinsky AO. *Respiratory Illness in Children*. Oxford: Blackwell, 1982.)

sent. Since hyperinflation is expected with acute asthma, the measurement of lung volume is probably of most use in apparently well children to detect the presence of chronic airflow limitation.

Airway resistance

This can be measured using plethysmography and is calculated from absolute lung volume and the change in pressure in the box (which reflects changes in alveolar pressure and alveolar volume) and flow at the mouth during rapid breathing. Children may need to be aged 8 years or more to perform this technique reliably.

Forced expiration

To evaluate asthma, the maximal expiratory flow–volume technique has been by far the most useful and informative test in this age group and $FEV_{1.0}$ has been the best parameter for quantitating airway function. The key to the reliability of spirometry is the physiological phenomenon of flow limitation. Flow limitation means that maximum flow on expiration is reached using a submaximal expiratory effort and further increases in effort (i.e., pleural pressure) produce no further increase in flow. The resulting forced expiratory flow–time (or its derived flow–volume) relationship is highly reproducible. $FEV_{1.0}$ is the best parameter for reflecting airway disease because it has the most favorable combination of sensitivity and specificity. Other spirometric parameters such as flow at a fraction of forced vital capacity (FVC) can be more sensitive, but are also more variable and therefore less specific.

In recent years, peak expiratory flow (PEF) has been examined in the context of its accuracy and utility in providing information about airways in children. In general, studies have found that it is a relatively poor predictor of $FEV_{1.0}$ and of exacerbations of asthma.[82,83] Peak expiratory flow is effort dependent and this may be the reason for its lack of accuracy. These findings may have resulted in a decline in the use of PEF for monitoring.

$FEV_{1.0}$ can be measured reliably in most children from 5 or 6 years of age, although some younger children can perform the technique adequately.

Airway responsiveness

Several agents have been used to measure airway responsiveness and a number of techniques have been developed to measure the response.[84,85] A response is usually taken as the concentration of agonist producing a fall of 20% in $FEV_{1.0}$ (PC20). The inhalational agonists histamine and methacholine have been used the most and studies using them have generated a great deal of interesting information. However, other inhalational agents, including cold air, dry air, mannitol and hypertonic saline, have been used to assess airway responses. Exercise has also been used as a general test of airway response, but it is also useful to investigate the clinical problem of exercise-induced asthma.

With all tests of airway responsiveness in children, there is a problem with quantitating the level of response. For agents such as histamine, using the same dose in children as used in adults to determine the level of responsiveness is not acceptable. This is because the dose would need to be matched precisely to the size of the child, and there is no known way that this can be done. Clearly, giving an adult dose to a small child and seeing a greater response is not an indication of increased responsiveness. The effect of this has been demonstrated in a study of New Zealand children in which the same dose of agonist was given to children of various ages.[72] The difference in level of responsiveness between children of different age and size was best explained by the effect of dose. That is, smaller children responded more as a result of receiving a greater dose for their size. These problems mean that comparisons are possible between similar-sized or similar-aged children but not between children of different age, particularly where the younger children are substantially smaller than the older children.[71] For other provocations, quantitation is also a problem. For example, with exercise, in comparing a 5-year-old child with a 15-year-old, one would need to know that raising the heart rate of the 5-year-old to a particular level would have exactly the same stimulating influence on the airway as raising the heart rate to the same amount in the older child.

LUNG FUNCTION IN ASTHMATIC CHILDREN

Variability

Lung function in asthmatic children is highly variable for several reasons. Firstly, asthma is characterized by the variability of airway narrowing, so that in almost all children with asthma there will be a higher variability of baseline lung function than in normal children.[86] Secondly, the degree of airway narrowing during an attack of asthma is highly variable, at times from minute to minute, spontaneously and in response to acute treatment.

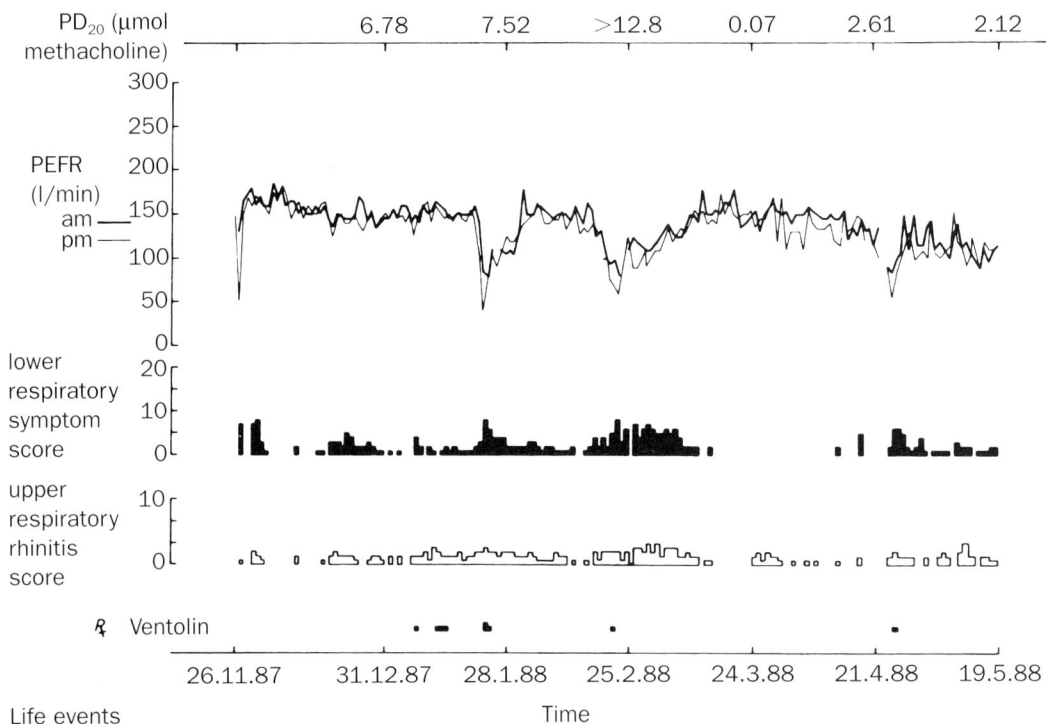

Figure 1.7 Typical variability of asthma-related variables demonstrated by data obtained over a 6-month period from a 7-year-old boy with wheeze who was symptomatic on most days. He was treated with occasional inhaled salbutamol only and his PD_{20} was >6.4 µmol on three of six occasions. (From ref 87 with permission.)

Thirdly, the severity of asthma is highly variable within subjects from month to month[87] (Figure 1.7) and from year to year. Finally, asthma varies greatly in severity between individuals, with the majority having very mild disease with little or no abnormality of lung function most of the time. Airway responsiveness is also highly variable in asthmatic children both within subject and between subjects.

Changes during childhood

Lung function tends to track through childhood. In a longitudinal study of 406 asthmatic children, the level of lung function in early childhood was the best predictor for lung function in adulthood.[88] In this study, lung function ($FEV_{1.0}$ percent predicted) also tended to improve with time (mean interval for follow-up was 14.8 years) in subjects with and without current respiratory symptoms.[88] This suggests that there is a general improvement in respiratory status in asthmatics across childhood. At the same time, the number of children responding to a given concentration of histamine declined, but whether this is a true decline in airway responsiveness or simply a reflection of a difference in dose for size, as mentioned above, is unclear. Over an even longer term, lung function in asthmatics depends more on severity of current asthma. In the Melbourne study, 268 subjects were followed up over 28 years and those with continuing asthma had lower lung function than those whose symptoms had decreased or disappeared (Figure 1.8).[89] Similar results were reported in a Californian study of 1041 children in whom

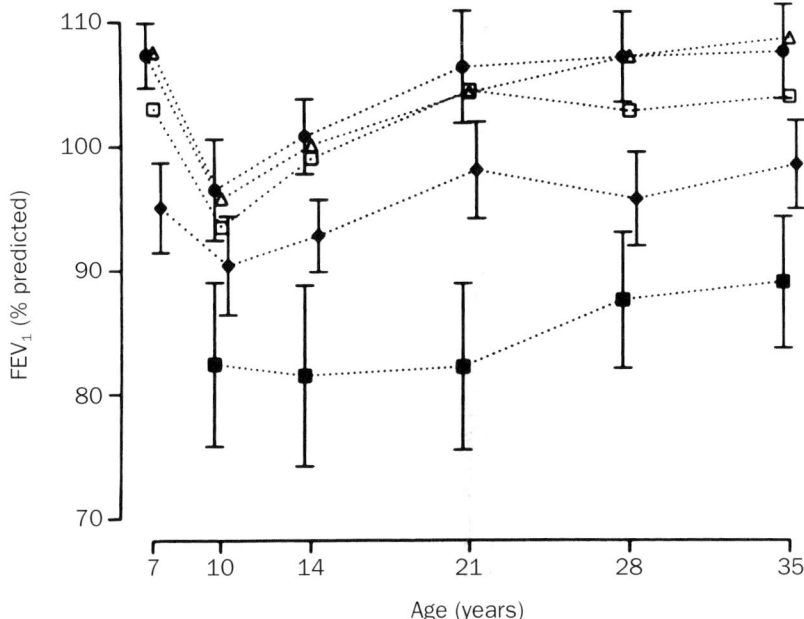

Figure 1.8 Lung function in adulthood predicted from asthma severity in childhood. Data from 268 subjects from the long-term, longitudinal asthma study from Melbourne. Those with the worst asthma at entry to the study continue to have the worst lung function throughout the 28 year follow-up period. At entry to the study: ● controls; △ mild wheezy bronchitis; □ wheezy bronchitis; ◆ asthma. (From ref 89 with permission.)

longer asthma duration was associated with lower lung function and greater airway responsiveness.[90] The implications of childhood asthma on lung function in later adulthood are still unknown, since no longitudinal study has covered this age span.

REFERENCES

1. Hislop AA, Haworth SG. Airway size and structure in the normal fetal and infant lung and the effect of premature delivery and artificial ventilation. *Am Rev Respir Dis* 1989; **140**: 1717–26.
2. Hislop A, Wigglesworth JS, Desai R, Aber V. The effects of preterm delivery and mechanical ventilation on human lung growth. *Early Hum Dev* 1987; **15**: 147–64.
3. Openshaw P, Edwards S, Helms P. Changes in rib cage geometry during childhood. *Thorax* 1984; **39**: 624–7.
4. Lopes JM, Muller NL, Bryan MH, Bryan AC. Synergistic behavior of inspiratory muscles after diaphragmatic fatigue in the newborn. *J Appl Physiol* 1981; **51**: 547–51.
5. Bryan H, Le Souëf PN, England SJ, Fisher J, Bryan C. Respiratory mechanics in newborn infants. In: Stern L, Oh W, Friis-Hansen B, eds. *Physiological Foundations of Perinatal Care* Vol II. New York: Elsevier, 1987, 82–90.
6. Gaultier C, Praud JP, Canet E, Delaperche MF, D'Allest AM. Paradoxical inward rib cage motion during rapid eye movement sleep in infants and young children. *J Dev Physiol* 1987; **9**: 391–7.
7. Keens TG, Bryan AC, Levison H, Ianuzzo CD. Developmental pattern of muscle fiber types in human ventilatory muscles. *J Appl Physiol* 1978; **44**: 909–13.
8. Papastamelos C, Panitch HB, England SE, Allen JL. Developmental changes in chest wall compliance in infancy and early childhood. *J Appl Physiol* 1995; **78**: 179–84.
9. Matsuba K, Thurlbeck WM. A morphometric study of bronchial and bronchiolar walls in children. *Am Rev Respir Dis* 1972; **105**: 908–13.
10. McCray PB. Spontaneous contractility of human fetal airway smooth muscle. *Am J Respir Cell Mol Biol* 1993; **8**: 573–80.
11. Tepper RS. Airway reactivity in infants; a positive response to methacholine and metaproterenol. *J Appl Physiol* 1987; **62**: 1155–9.
12. Le Souëf PN, Geelhoed GC, Turner DJ, Morgan SEG, Landau LI. Response of normal infants to inhaled histamine. *Am Rev Respir Dis* 1989; **139**: 62–6.

13. Geller DE, Morgan WJ, Cota KA, Wright AL, Taussig LM. Airway responsiveness to cold, dry air in normal infants. *Pediatr Pulmonol* 1988; **4**: 90–7.
14. Prendiville A, Green S, Silverman M. Bronchial responsiveness to histamine in wheezy infants. *Thorax* 1987; **42**: 92–9.
15. Hughes DM, Le Souëf PN, Landau LI. Effect of salbutamol on respiratory mechanics in bronchiolitis. *Pediatr Res* 1987; **22**: 83–6.
16. Hayden MJ, Wildhaber JH, Sly PD, Le Souëf PN. Bronchodilator responsiveness testing using raised volume forced expiration in recurrently wheezing infants. *Pediatr Pulmonol* 1998; **26**: 35–41.
17. Turner DJ, Landau LI, Le Souëf PN. The effect of age on bronchodilator responsiveness. *Pediatr Pulmonol* 1993; **15**: 98–104.
18. Clarke JR, Aston H, Silverman M. Delivery of salbutamol by metered dose inhaler and valved spacer to wheezy infants: effect on bronchial responsiveness. *Arch Dis Child* 1993; **69**: 125–9.
19. Henderson AJW, Young S, Stick SM, Landau LI, Le Souëf PN. The effect of salbutamol on histamine-induced broncho-constriction in healthy infants. *Thorax* 1993; **48**: 317–23.
20. Hibbert ME, Lannigan A, Landau LI, Phelan PD. Lung function values from a longitudinal study of healthy children and adolescents. *Pediatr Pulmonol* 1989; **7**: 101–9.
21. Cook CD, Helliesen PJ, Agathon S. Relationship between mechanics of respiration, lung size, and body size from birth to young adulthood. *J Appl Physiol* 1958; **13**: 348–52.
22. Tepper R, Morgan W, eds. *Infant Pulmonary Function—A Practical Guide*. New York: Wiley-Liss, 1996, 379–410.
23. Mead J. Dysanapsis in normal lungs assessed by the relationship between maximal flow, static recoil pressure and vital capacity. *Am Rev Respir Dis* 1980; **121**: 339–42.
24. Thurlbeck WM. Postnatal human lung growth. *Thorax* 1982; **37**: 564–71.
25. Schwartz J, Katz SA, Fegley RW, Tockman MS. Sex and race differences in the development of lung function. *Am Rev Respir Dis* 1988; **138**: 1415–21.
26. Le Souëf PN, Castile R, Turner DJ, Motoyama E, Morgan WJ. Forced expiratory maneuvers. In: Stocks J, Sly P, Tepper R, Morgan W, eds. *Infant Pulmonary Function—A Practical Guide*. New York: Wiley-Liss, 1996, 379–410.
27. Phelan PD, Williams HE. Sympathomimetic drugs in acute viral bronchiolitis. Their effect on pulmonary resistance. *Paediatrics* 1969; **44**: 493–7.
28. Radford M. Effect of salbutamol in infants with wheezy bronchitis. *Arch Dis Child* 1975; **50**: 535–8.
29. Hodges RL, Groggins RC, Milner AD, Stokes GM. Bronchodilator effect of inhaled ipratropium bromide in wheezy toddlers. *Arch Dis Child* 1981; **56**: 729–32.
30. Kreiger I. Mechanics of respiration in bronchiolitis. *Pediatrics* 1964; **33**: 45–54.
31. Stokes GM, Milner AD, Hodges IGC et al. Nebulized therapy in acute severe bronchiolitis in infancy. *Arch Dis Child* 1980; **58**: 279–83.
32. Asher MI, Coates AL, Collinge J-M, Milic-Emili J. Measurement of pleural pressure in neonates. *J Appl Physiol* 1982; **52**: 491–4.
33. Le Souëf PN, Lopes JM, England SJ, Bryan MH, Bryan AC. Influence of chest wall distortion on esophageal pressure. *J Appl Physiol* 1983; **55**: 353–8.
34. Soto ME, Sly PD, Uren E, Taussig LM, Landau LI. Bronchodilator response during acute viral bronchiolitis in infancy. *Pediatr Pulmonol* 1985; **2**: 85–90.
35. Rutter N, Milner AD, Hiller E. Effect of bronchodilators on respiratory resistance in infants and young children with bronchiolitis and wheezy bronchitis. *Arch Dis Child* 1975; **50**: 719–22.
36. Taussig LM, Landau LI, Godfrey S, Arad I. Determinants of forced expiratory flows in newborn infants. *J Appl Physiol* 1982; **53**: 1220–7.
37. Adler S, Wohl ME. Flow–volume relationship at low lung volumes in healthy term newborn infants. *Pediatrics* 1978; **61**: 636–40.
38. England SJ. Current techniques for assessing pulmonary function in the newborn and infant: advantages and limitations. *Pediatr Pulmonol* 1988; **4**: 48–53.
39. Morgan WJ, Geller DE, Tepper RS, Taussig LM. Partial expiratory flow–volume curves in infants and young children. State of the art review. *Pediatr Pulmonol* 1988; **5**: 232–43.
40. Phelan PD, Sly PD. International pediatric respiratory meeting. Terrigal, Australia, March 10–13. *Pediatr Pulmonol* 1989; **6**: 603.
41. Allen J, Castile RG. Conference report: Infant Pulmonary Function Testing Workshop 1. *Pediatr Pulmonol* 1991; **10**: 214–18.
42. Allen J, Bashir N, Brown R, Castile R. Infant pulmonary function testing workshop, Anaheim, California, May 1991. *Pediatr Pulmonol* 1992; **12**: 236–69.

43. American Thoracic Society, European Respiratory Society. Respiratory mechanics in infants: physiologic evaluation in health and disease. *Am Rev Respir Dis* 1993; **147:** 474–96.
44. Kraemer R. Practical interest in the detection of functional abnormalities in infants and children with lung disease. *Eur J of Pediatr* 1993; **152:** 382–6.
45. Kraemer R. Assessment of functional abnormalities in infants and children with lung disease. *Agents and Actions* 1993; **40**(suppl): 41–55.
46. Pfaff JK, Morgan WJ. Pulmonary function in infants and children. *Pediatr Clinics N Am* 1994; **41:** 401–23.
47. Le Souëf PN, Hughes DM, Landau LI. Effect of compression pressure on forced expiratory flow in infants. *J Appl Physiol* 1986; **61:** 1639–47.
48. Le Souëf PN, Hughes DM, Landau LI. Shape of forced expiratory flow volume curves in infants. *Am Rev Respir Dis* 1988; **138:** 590–7.
49. Young S, Le Souëf PN, Geelhoed GC, Stick SM, Turner KJ, Landau LI. The influence of a family history of asthma and parental smoking on airway responsiveness in early infancy. *New Engl J Med* 1991; **324:** 1168–73.
50. Martinez FD, Morgan WJ, Holberg CJ, Taussig LM. Diminished lung function as a predisposing factor for wheezing respiratory illness in infants. *New Engl J Med* 1988; **319:** 1112–17.
51. Hayden MJ, Wildhaber J, Le Souëf PN. Parental attitudes to infant pulmonary function testing. *Pediatr Pulmonol* 1998; **25:** 309–13.
52. Stark AR, Cohlan BA, Waggener TB, Frantz ID, Kosch PC. Regulation of end-expiratory lung volume during sleep in premature infants. *J Appl Physiol* 1987; **62:** 1117–23.
53. Le Souëf PN, England SJ, Bryan AC. Passive respiratory mechanics in infants and children. *Am Rev Respir Dis* 1984; **129:** 552–6.
54. Turner DL, Morgan SEC, Landau LI, Le Souëf PN. Methodological aspects of flow–volume studies in infants. *Pediatr Pulmonol* 1990; **8:** 289–93.
55. Steinbrugger B, Lanigan A, Raven JM, Olinsky A. Influence of the 'squeeze jacket' on lung function in young infants. *Am Rev Respir Dis* 1988; **138:** 1258–60.
56. Tepper RS, Morgan WJ, Cota K, Wright A, Taussig LM. Physiologic growth and development of the lung during the first year of life. *Am Rev Respir Dis* 1986; **134:** 513–19.
57. Mallol J, Hibbert ME, Robertson CF, Olinsky A, Phelan PD, Sly PD. Inherent variability of pulmonary function tests in infants with bronchiolitis. *Pediatr Pulmonol* 1988; **5:** 152–7.
58. Maxwell DL, Prendiville A, Rose A, Silverman M. Lung volume changes during histamine-induced bronchoconstriction in recurrently wheezy infants. *Pediatr Pulmonol* 1988; **5:** 145–51.
59. Stick SM, Ellis E, Le Souëf PN, Sly PD. Validation of respiratory inductance plethysmography ('Respitrace') for the measurement of tidal breathing parameters in newborns. *Pediatr Pulmonol* 1992; **14:** 187–91.
60. Stick SM, Burton PR, Gurrin L, Sly PD, Le Souëf PN. Respiratory function in newborn infants: effects of maternal smoking during pregnancy and a family history of asthma. *Lancet* 1996; **348:** 1060–4.
61. Turner DJ, Stick SM, Le Souëf KL, Sly PD, Le Souëf PN. A new technique to generate and assess forced expiration from raised lung volume in infants. *Am J Resp Crit Care Med* 1995; **151:** 1441–50.
62. Pride NB. The assessment of airflow obstruction: role of measurements of airways resistance and tests of forced expiration. *Br J Chest* 1971; **65:** 155–69.
63. Takishima T, Grimby G, Graham W, Knudson R, Macklem P, Mead J. Flow–volume curves during quiet breathing, maximum voluntary ventilation and forced vital capacities in patients with obstructive lung disease. *Scan J Respir Dis* 1967; **48:** 384–93.
64. Stick SM, Turner DJ, Le Souëf PN. Transmission of pressure across the chest wall during the rapid thoracic compression technique in infants. *J Appl Physiol* 1994; **76:** 1411–16.
65. Turner DJ, Lanteri CJ, Le Souëf PN, Sly PD. Improved detection of abnormal respiratory function using forced expiration from raised lung volume in infants with cystic fibrosis. *Eur Respir J* 1994; **7:** 1995–9.
66. Turner DJ, Lanteri CJ, Le Souëf PN, Sly PD. Pressure transmission across the respiratory system at raised lung volumes in infants. *J Appl Physiol* 1994; **77:** 1015–20.
67. Hayden MJ, Sly PD, Devadason SG, Gurrin LC, Wildhaber J, Le Souëf PN. Influence of driving pressure on raised-volume forced expiration in infants. *Am J Resp Crit Care Med* 1997; **156:** 1876–83.
68. Turner DJ, Sly PD, Le Souëf PN. Assessment of forced expiratory volume–time parameters in detecting histamine-induced bronchoconstriction in wheezy infants. *Pediatr Pulmonol* 1993; **15:** 220–4.

69. Feher A, Castile R, Kisling J, Angelicchio C, Filbrun D, Flucke R et al. Flow limitation in normal infants: a new method for forced expiratory maneuvers from raised lung volumes. *J Appl Physiol* 1996; **80**: 2019–25.
70. Le Souëf PN. Validity of airway responsiveness testing in children. *Lancet* 1992; **339**: 1282–4.
71. Le Souëf PN. Can measurements of airway responsiveness be standardised in children? *Eur Respir J* 1993; **6**: 1085–7.
72. Le Souëf PN, Sears MR, Sherrill D. The effect of size and age of subject on airway responsiveness in children. *Am J Resp Crit Care Med* 1995; **152**: 576–9.
73. Young S, Arnott J, Le Souëf PN, Landau LI. Flow limitation during tidal expiration in asymptomatic infants and the subsequent development of asthma. *J Pediatr* 1994; **124**: 681–8.
74. Martinez FD, Wright AL, Taussig LI et al. Asthma and wheezing in the first six years of life. *New Eng J Med* 1995; **332**: 133–8.
75. Stick SM, Arnott J, Turner DJ, Young S, Landau LI, Le Souëf PN. Bronchial responsiveness and lung function in recurrently wheezing infants. *Am Rev Respir Dis* 1991; **144**: 1012–15.
76. Lenny W, Milner AD. Alpha and beta adrenergic stimulants in bronchiolitis and wheezy bronchitis in children under 18 months of age. *Arch Dis Child* 1978; **53**: 707–9.
77. Tepper RS, Rosenberg D, Eigen H, Reister T. Bronchodilator responsiveness in infants with bronchiolitis. *Pediatr Pulmonol* 1994; **17**: 81–5.
78. Seidenberg J, Mir Y, von der Hardt H. Hypoxaemia after nebulised salbutamol in wheezy infants: the importance of aerosol acidity. *Arch Dis Child* 1991; **66**: 672–5.
79. Rye PJ, Palmer LJ, Young S, Gibson NA, Landau LI, Goldblatt J et al. The association between infant lung function and respiratory symptoms during the first 6 years of life [abstract]. *Am J Resp Crit Care Med* 1997; **155**: A77.
80. Palmer LJ, Rye PJ, Gibson NA, Judge V, Young S, Burton PR et al. Airway responsiveness (AR) and lung function at 1 month of age predict airway responsiveness, lung function, asthma and atopy at 6 years of age. *Am J Resp Crit Care Med* 1999; **157**: A44.
81. Taussig L. Maximal expiratory flows at functional residual capacity: a test of lung function for young children. *Am Rev Respir Dis* 1977; **116**: 1031–8.
82. Sly PD. Peak expiratory flow monitoring in pediatric asthma: is there a role? *J Asthma* 1996; **33**: 277–87.
83. Sly PD. Relationship between change in PEF and symptoms: questions to ask in paediatric clinics. *Eur Respir J* 1997; **24**(suppl): 80S–83S.
84. Yan Yan K, Salome C, Woolcock AJ. Rapid method for measurement of bronchial responsiveness. *Thorax* 1983; **38**: 760–5.
85. Cockroft DW, Killan DN, Mellon JJA, Hargreave FE. Bronchial reactivity to inhaled histamine: a method and clinical survey. *Clin All* 1977; **7**: 235–43.
86. Timonen KL, Nielsen J, Schwartz J, Gotti A, Vondra V, Gratziou C et al. Chronic respiratory symptoms, skin test results, and lung function as predictors of peak flow variability. *Am J Respir Crit Care Med* 1997; **156**: 776–82.
87. Clough JB, Williams JD, Holgate ST. Effect of atopy on the natural history of symptoms, peak expiratory flow, and bronchial responsiveness in 7-year-old and 8-year-old children with cough and wheeze. A 12-month longitudinal study. *Am Rev Respir Dis* 1991; **143**: 755–60.
88. Roorda RJ, Gerritsen J, van Aalderen WM, Schouten JP, Veltman JC, Weiss ST et al. Follow-up of asthma from childhood to adulthood: influence of potential childhood risk factors on the outcome of pulmonary function and bronchial responsiveness in adulthood. *J Allergy Clin Immunol* 1994; **93**: 575–84.
89. Oswald H, Phelan PD, Lanigan A, Hibbert M, Carlin JB, Bowes G et al. Childhood asthma and lung function in mid-adult life. *Pediatr Pulmonol* 1997; **23**: 14–20.
90. Zeiger RS, Dawson C, Weiss S. Relationships between duration of asthma and asthma severity among children in the Childhood Asthma Management Program. *J Allergy Clin Immunol* 1999; **103**: 376–87.

2

Asthma—basic mechanisms

John O Warner

Introduction • Gene by environment interaction • BHR, atopy, airway inflammation and asthma • Ontogeny of airway inflammation in asthma • Proinflammatory cells • Airway remodelling • Non-invasive markers of airway inflammation

INTRODUCTION

Asthma is now considered to be a disorder associated with chronic inflammation in the airways. This has been a result of extensive research utilizing fibreoptic bronchoscopy in adults with relatively mild asthma. Indeed, the insight gained by studying airway histopathology has created a remarkable paradigm shift which has fundamentally altered the therapeutic approach to the disease. A mere 30 years ago, the fundamental component of the disease was considered to be bronchial hyperresponsiveness (BHR) and most treatment was directed at controlling bronchospasm. However, since chronic inflammation is believed to underlie BHR, it has followed that therapy directed at the inflammation has been considered paramount.[1]

It is interesting to note, however, that as early as 1769 John Miller described a child who had died of asthma 'with an abundance of gelatinous secretions obstructing the bronchi'.[2] The first information on the pathology of asthma was gained from post-mortem examinations and is detailed in Osler's *Textbook of Medicine* published in 1892.[3] He described the widespread mucosal plugging of airways resulting in air trapping and hyperinflated lungs. Subsequent studies confirmed that the plugs contain not only plasma protein and sloughed epithelial cells but also inflammatory cells.[4] It was also appreciated that the airway wall was affected with thickening of the smooth muscle and sub-basement membrane fibrosis as well as accumulation of inflammatory cells.[5–8] These changes were subsequently also identified in the airways of even mild asthmatics with particular accumulation of eosinophils and mast cells in the lamina propria.[1,9] However, this had already been highlighted from post-mortem studies in which death had not been caused by asthma.[10] The very first suggestion that airway inflammation even underlay mild asthma came from paediatricians. In 1978, Cutz and colleagues published information on ultrastructural examination of the airways of two asthmatic children undergoing open lung biopsies who by chance had asthma that was in remission and compared them with the lung tissue from two children who had died of *status asthmaticus*. All four had submucosal cellular infiltrates, especially with eosinophils and had sloughing of airway epithelium.[11] This chapter will, therefore, elaborate on the concepts that explain the inflammatory response and the implications of this for management of the disease.

GENE BY ENVIRONMENT INTERACTION

There is a strong hereditary component to asthma, many gene polymorphisms having been identified as associated with either the disease or some of its associated features, namely, atopy and BHR (these are discussed in Chapter 4). However, the large geographical differences in incidence and the rising trends in prevalence primarily associated with an affluent Western lifestyle suggest a strong environmental influence.[12] Many would view the genetic predisposition as being a tendency to respond to allergens, with a more aggressive allergy promoting lymphocyte response. Thus sensitized T-helper lymphocytes generate peptide regulatory factors (cytokines) which promote gene deletional switching in B-lymphocytes from IgM to IgE production (mediated by IL-4 and -13) as well as cytokines which promote eosinophil production, activation and survival, IL-5 and GMCSF.[13] The above cytokines are all genetically encoded in a cluster on the long arm of chromosome 5q[31–33], where polymorphisms associated with atopy and asthma have been described.[12]

Many environmental factors have been identified to interact with genetic predisposition in the genesis of both atopy and asthma. These include allergen exposure particularly in early life; both protective and inducing effects of different infections; nutritional aberration; and some forms of air pollution, of which environmental tobacco smoke figures most prominently.[14] However, although the gene by environment interaction in relation to the generation of allergy is fairly coherent, it remains to be understood how this ultimately leads to airway disease. Furthermore not all asthmatics have associated atopy, though all do have very similar pathology in the airways and, conversely, many atopic individuals do not develop asthma.[15]

BHR, ATOPY, AIRWAY INFLAMMATION AND ASTHMA

The *sine qua non* of asthma in the 1950s, 1960s and 1970s was BHR and this concept was encompassed in the definition which indicated that asthma was a condition of variable airflow limitation which altered over short periods of time, either spontaneously or under the influence of treatment.[16] Although BHR can be demonstrated in the majority of asthmatics, it also occurs transiently in normal individuals in association with intercurrent viral infection.[17] Furthermore, the effect of drugs on BHR did not necessarily predict their efficacy in the management of asthma, despite the fact that the degree of hyperresponsiveness was to a certain extent associated with the severity of the disease and varied over time in relation to the disease activity (see Figure 2.1).[18]

Much of the confusion about BHR has occurred because a wide range of different non-specific provoking factors have been employed to detect it. There are very different receptor and cell targets for the various provocants such as histamine, methacoline, cold air, exercise, hypertonic saline, ultrasonic nebulized water and adenosine. Most challenge protocols identify a provocation dose that will produce a 15% or 20% fall in lung function, this threshold being estimated by extrapolation between points either

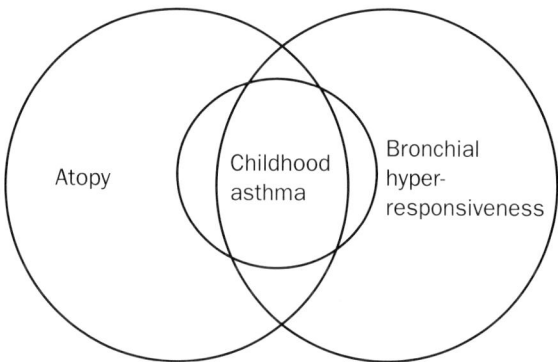

Figure 2.1 Venn diagram indicating the associations between atopy, asthma and BHR. It can be seen that the majority of childhood asthmatics are atopic and have BHR, but either can occur in isolation with or without asthma.

Table 2.1 Allergen-induced airway responses

	Immediate reaction	Late reaction
Timing after challenge	10–60 minutes	3–48 hours
Airway generations involved	Large only	Large and small
Response to β-agonists	Complete resolution	Variable effect
Response to corticosteroid prophylaxis	No effect	Effectively prevented
Effect on BHR	None	Increased
Correlation with degree of BHR	Good	None
Pathology	Bronchospasm	Neutrophil and eosinophil influx

side of the critical lung functional fall. Some have suggested, however, that the slope of the dose–response curve, known as 'bronchial reactivity', may be more important, since higher degrees have been associated with an increased risk of death from asthma in children.[19,20]

In allergic asthmatics, inhalation of allergen induces an immediate bronchial response that in many respects is similar to pharmacologically induced bronchospasm. Indeed, the magnitude of the immediate response to allergen can to a certain extent be predicted by the degree of non-specific BHR.[21] Furthermore, the immediate allergen-induced response like BHR is completely prevented by predosing with a β-agonist and in the short term is uninfluenced by predosing with steroids. However, many patients when challenged with allergen have not only an immediate response but also a late reaction which develops 3–6 hours after challenge. This late reaction is more prolonged, often more severe and has many more characteristics of severe asthma.[22] There is more evidence of small airway involvement in the response which is associated with less bronchodilator responsiveness but appreciable prevention from predosing with steroids and also, to a lesser extent, with sodium cromoglycate and leukotriene receptor antagonists.[23] Furthermore, the late allergen-induced reaction increases non-specific BHR for days or even weeks after challenge.[24] Effective allergen avoidance can be shown to reduce symptoms of asthma, drug requirements and BHR, this intervention even influencing the effect of the allergen-induced late reaction on non-specific BHR.[25] Conversely, high allergen exposure of allergic asthmatics increases symptoms, BHR and risk of hospital admission with acute exacerbation (see Table 2.1).[26,27]

These data explain why atopy and BHR are commonly associated. Indeed, an atopic reaction in the airway can induce an increase in BHR. However, a component additional to atopy must dictate whether an allergic reaction will influence the course of asthma and induce BHR. Perhaps a predisposition to both is necessary for asthma to be manifest.

The immunopathological link between allergic airway reaction and BHR is airway inflammation. The late reaction has very similar immunopathological characteristics to asthma, with influx of neutrophils and eosinophils during the evolution of the late reaction.[28] The way in which this inflammation affects BHR could be by damage to the airway epithelium thereby increasing access of stimuli directly to autonomic reflex arcs and airway smooth muscle; or by a reduction in the production of epithelial-derived relaxant factor (nitric oxide); but is also likely to be influenced by the many mediators released during the inflammatory process which have direct effects on smooth muscle.[29]

ONTOGENY OF AIRWAY INFLAMMATION IN ASTHMA

The development of airway inflammation in allergic asthma has been well characterized. How this occurs in individuals who do not appear to have any allergy remains unclear, though all forms of the disease are characterized by a similar process. There are several steps in the evolution of airway inflammation, starting with primary sensitization followed by the establishment of an allergic phenotype of immune response, which eventually localizes in the airways. Subsequent exposures then result in activation of sensitized cells with the production of a range of mediators inducing both bronchospasm and chronic inflammation.

The chapter on prediction and prevention will elaborate on the primary sensitization process and factors that influence it. In brief, allergen that is presented at mucosal surfaces is picked up by antigen-presenting cells (APCs), of which the dendritic cell and alveolar macrophage in the airway are particularly important.[30] The APCs then migrate to regional lymph nodes, where they present antigens in association with class II major histocompatability complex (MHC) molecules to T-lymphocytes. Two main classes of T-lymphocytes are identified by surface molecule characteristics, CD4+ (T-helper cells) and CD8+ (cytotoxic or suppressor cells). CD8 cells have antigen presented to them via Class I MHC molecules and CD4 by Class II. The interaction is between the MHC molecule and the T-cell receptor with a variety of co-stimulatory signals involving adhesion molecules and interactions with a variety of other surface receptors and ligands. In addition, cytokines produced by the APCs also influence the response, of which IL-10 and IL-12 are particularly important in relation to allergy. IL-12 promotes the production of IFN-γ, which is associated with inhibition of allergic-type responses. IL-10 inhibits the production of IL-12 and thereby indirectly promotes an allergic pattern of response. The characteristic of the allergen exposure—both in terms of dose and whether it is particulate or soluble, as well as the root of exposure, which, in turn, relates to the predominant APC type in different tissues—has profound influences on the characteristic of the APC stimulus to T-cells and thereby whether the response is immunizing or allergic in nature.[31] Naïve CD4+ T-helper lymphocytes polarize towards one of two phenotypic responses. Th-1 is associated with the generation of IL-2 and IFN-γ, which mediates cellular immune responses and T-cell cytotoxicity. This is the normal response associated with infection. Th-2, on the other hand, is associated with the generation of IL-4, IL-5, IL-10 and IL-13, which promote humoral immunity, IgM isotype switching to IgE production and eosinophil activation. These, as indicated, are the hallmarks of allergic inflammation.

The primary sensitization process described could occur at any epithelial surface, whether this be the skin, gastrointestinal tract or respiratory tract. Strong evidence points to there being a primary route of sensitization in the fetus through the gut (see chapter Prediction & Prevention). How the sensitized cells subsequently traffic to the target organ, namely the respiratory tract, is not clear. However, APCs having picked up antigens will migrate to regional lymphoid accumulations and regional lymph nodes. There, sensitized T-cells can be released via the lymphatics into the circulation. Subsequent aeroallergen exposure may be important in localizing specifically sensitized T-cells, which then following further allergen exposure will activate a local inflammatory process, including upregulation of endothelial adhesion molecules to facilitate trafficking of both neutrophils and eosinophils into the mucosa. There, activation will lead to the release of a wide array of mediators that enhance inflammation (see Figure 2.2).

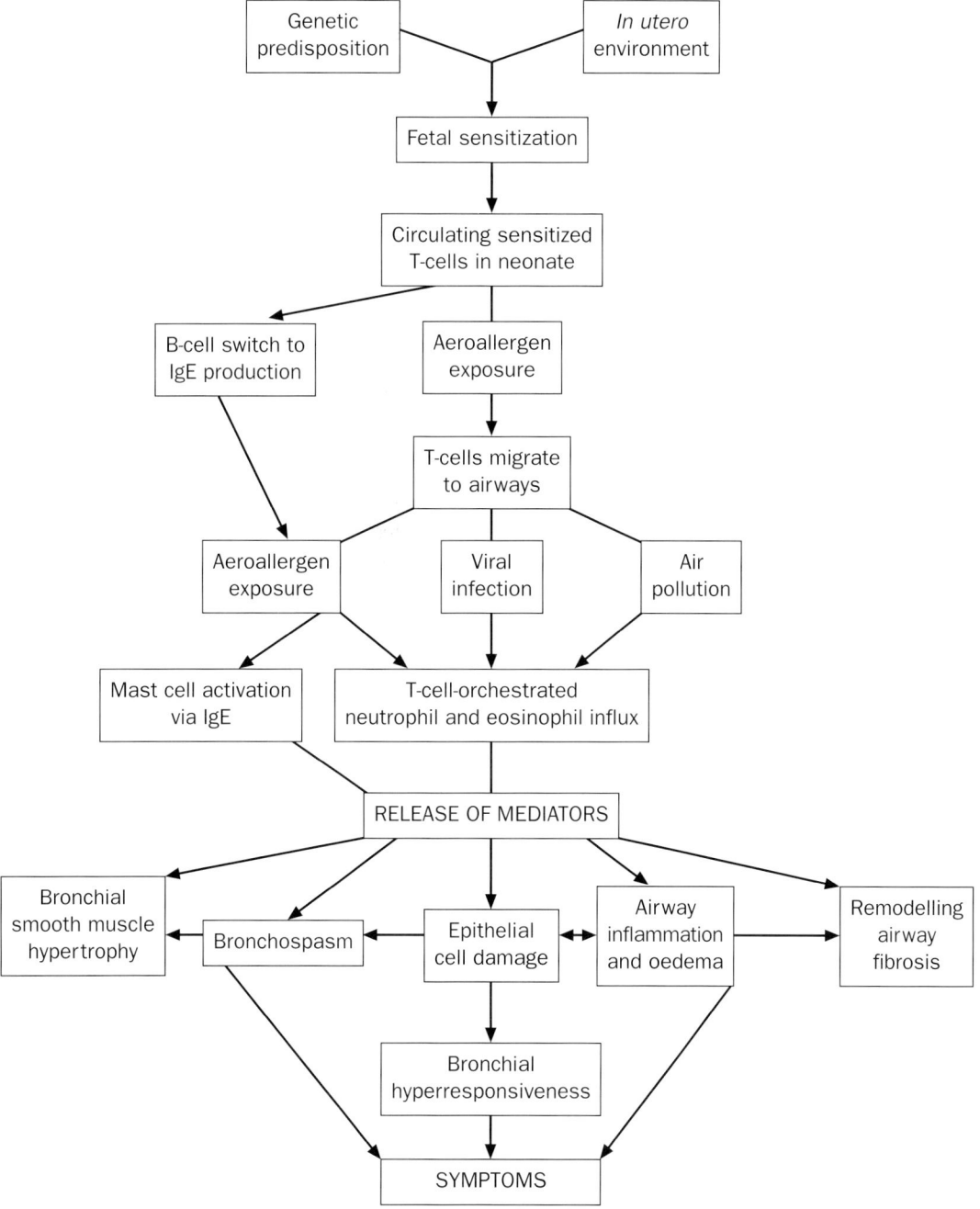

Figure 2.2 Algorithm indicating the way in which early life immunological sensitization to allergen evolves into airway inflammation, following activation of a variety of proinflammatory cells which contribute to the various components of the immunopathology of asthma.

PROINFLAMMATORY CELLS

Eosinophils

The eosinophil proteins (eosinophil cationic protein, major basic protein, eosinophil peroxidase, eosinophil-derived neurotoxin otherwise known as eosinophil protein X) that are present in the cytoplasmic granules are damaging to airway epithelium and probably are the major contributors to epithelial shedding. Additionally, these proteins may contribute to promoting mast cell degranulation. Furthermore, the eosinophil also generates a range of other mediators, including leukotrienes which, among other effects, are eosinophil chemoattractant themselves. This provides feedback loops that enhance inflammation.[13]

Neutrophils

The neutrophils generate, among other mediators, oxygen radicals which also will be toxic to tissues, particularly if not adequately counteracted by the antioxidant systems. One mechanism whereby nutritional aberration might affect the degree of inflammation in asthma is through reduction in intake of fresh vegetables and fruits, which are a significant source of antioxidant.[32]

Mast cells

Mast cells are also clearly involved in allergic airway inflammation, being increased in numbers in the asthmatic airway.[33] Mast cells discharge their contents of granules once cross-linked cell surface IgE on high affinity IgE receptors combines with specific allergen. The preformed mediators released include histamine, tryptase, chemotactic factors for eosinophils and neutrophils, and also heparin. Furthermore, newly synthesized mediators from activation of the arachidonic acid pathway include bradykinin, prostaglandins and leukotrienes. These mediators induce bronchospasm and also promote inflammation. Furthermore, it has now been shown that mast cells are also capable of generating cytokines which in asthma particularly focus on Th-2 patterns of IL-4 and IL-5 production.[34] Prostaglandin D_2 is seen as a pivotal mediator from mast cells in that deletion of its receptor in mice appreciably reduces the accumulation of Th-2 lymphocytes and their cytokines, eosinophils and BHR induced by allergen despite the presence of increased levels of IgE.[35]

However, although in the past mast cells have been seen as the pivotal cells in allergic asthmatic inflammation, it is likely that eosinophils and possibly neutrophils play a more important role in the chronicity of the disease. Indeed, there may even be a downregulatory influence of mast-cell-derived heparin, which has been shown to inhibit late, but not early, antigen-induced reactions.[36] Furthermore, heparin can be shown to inhibit antigen-induced airway hyperresponsiveness.[37] The mode of action of the heparin is likely to be through binding, and thereby inactivation, of proinflammatory mediators, which indeed is probably its role when the mediators are stored within the mast cell granules. As β-agonists are potent mast cell stabilizers, it has even been tentatively proposed that one of the mechanisms by which β-agonists might sometimes promote allergic inflammation is through inhibition of the release of heparin.[38] Interestingly, there is now evidence accumulating that heparin might also have an impact on the so-called airway remodelling process in that it inhibits the proliferation of airway smooth muscle *in vitro*.[39] Heparin can also inhibit fibroblast proliferation and the secretion of collagen by fibroblasts.[40] This raises the prospect of a new therapeutic intervention.

Alveolar macrophage

Although asthma histopathology focuses primarily on eosinophils and mast cells, with lymphocytes as the orchestrators of the response, other cells are also involved including alveolar macrophages and the respiratory epithelium. The alveolar macrophage and also, indeed, circulating monocytes have low affinity IgE receptors, and increased surface IgE on such cells has been particularly identified in asthmatics.[41] Macrophages are a source of leukotrienes, prostanoids and other mediators. Thus they are not only involved with antigen presentation but also can contribute to the promotion of inflammatory responses. Although steroids, as part of their anti-inflammatory reaction, can inhibit the release of prostanoids, they do not have any effect on a stimulated release of cysteinyl leukotrienes. These observations have been made in alveolar macrophages harvested from very young children with wheezing illnesses.[42] Alveolar macrophages from wheezy infants also release larger quantities of tumour necrosis factor (TNF-α) and thromboxane (B_2), compared with controls, both of which are inhibited by prior dexamethasone treatment.[43] The absence of an effect of steroids on cysteinyl leukotriene generation provides one credible argument for combining leukotriene receptor antagonists with inhaled steroids to improve asthma control. Furthermore, the lack of effect of steroids on the lipoxygenase pathway might explain why neutrophilic inflammation characterizes steroid-resistant asthma.[44,45] Leukotriene B_4, one of the products of this pathway, is a powerful neutrophil chemoattractant. This effect may also be relevant to asthma in early life, with neutrophil counts in bronchoalveolar lavage from infant wheezers and childhood asthmatics correlating with disease activity.[46]

Bronchial epithelium

In asthma, the bronchial epithelium shows evidence of significant damage with the separation of the columnar epithelial cells from their basal attachments.[47] The bronchial epithelium, when damaged in asthma, becomes an important source of many proinflammatory mediators including various cytokines[48] as well as arachidonic acid metabolites and growth factors.[49] Epithelial cells are potent sources of eotaxin, rantes and IL-8, which have chemotactic and activation effects on eosinophils, lymphocytes and neutrophils, respectively.[48] The key issue yet to be elaborated in asthma is whether the epithelial cells are more susceptible to damage and thereby to the generation of proinflammatory mediators.

AIRWAY REMODELLING

A pathognemonic feature of asthma is the deposition of interstitial collagens, types 1, 2, 5 and 6, fibronectin, β-laminin and tenascin-c in the lamina reticularis beneath the true epithelial basement membrane.[50,51] This is but one component of the remodelling process (see Figure 2.3). In the past, it has been proposed that the epithelial damage consequent upon the release of mediators from inflammatory cells such as eosinophils induced a compensatory remodelling process which was an attempt to repair the damage. The primary abnormality could conceivably rest either in the airway epithelium or in the remodelling process and this has been proposed as the additional factor linking atopy and other proinflammatory processes in the airway to asthma.[52] However, other components of the remodelling process include smooth muscle hyperplasia.[8] Furthermore, airway smooth muscle cells are themselves a source of proinflammatory signals including cytokines and chemokines, such as eotaxin, rantes, GM-CSF and IL-5 as well as growth factors and lipid mediators,[53] and in addition there is increased collagen deposition throughout the lamina propria.

The prevailing paradigm in relation to remodelling is that this is a slowly evolving process consequent upon the inflammation and respiratory epithelial damage. Thus the inevitable putative therapeutic consequence is that the longer that prophylactic therapy is delayed, the greater the degree of remodelling and thereby irreversibility of airflow limitation. This is certainly apparent from adult inhaled corticosteroid intervention studies.[54] However, data on bronchial biopsies from a small number of children who were bronchoscoped at a time when their respiratory diagnosis was uncertain would suggest otherwise. Subsequent follow-up characterized two groups of children—those with definite asthma and those definitely with-

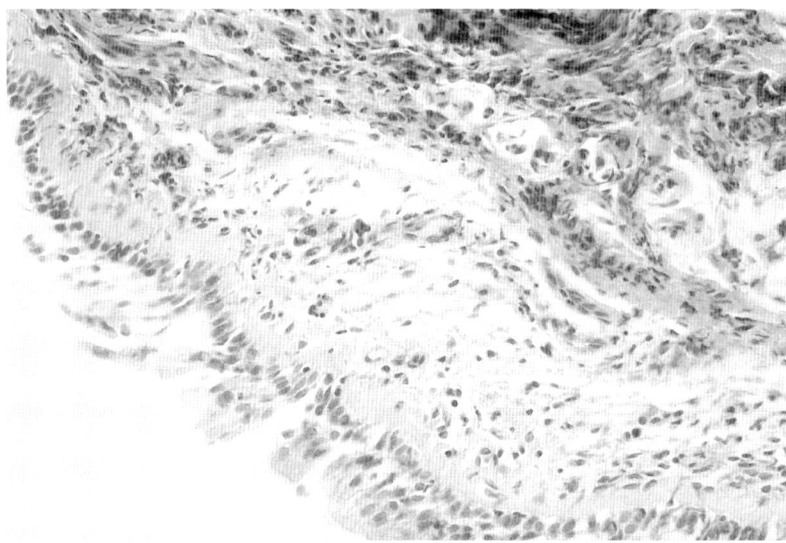

Figure 2.3 An H and E stained bronchial biopsy from an 8-year-old child with a short history of recurrent cough and wheeze who was subsequently identified as having clear-cut asthma. The biopsy shows some damage to the bronchial epithelium, marked thickening of the lamina reticularis, prominent collagen deposition in the lamina propria and smooth muscle hypertrophy.

out asthma. Irrespective of atopic status, the subsequent asthmatics had significantly thicker lamina reticularis and also, indeed, activated eosinophil numbers in the lamina propria. There was no correlation between either the degree of eosinophil infiltration or the thickness of the lamina reticularis and the duration of the symptoms up to the time of biopsy.[18] This suggests that at least some of the remodelling process is not a consequence of chronic long-standing inflammation but occurs early if not simultaneously with the inflammation. In view of the lack of correlation with disease severity, which has indeed been shown in adults[55] as well as children, or the duration of symptoms,[18] this suggests that airway inflammation and remodelling may well have evolved very early if not before the onset of first symptoms. This being the case, early intervention after the onset of symptoms may already be too late to modify the natural history of the disease.

The process by which airway remodelling is initiated has yet to be elaborated. Following epithelial damage, release of growth factors may well be important.[52] Many growth factors have been implicated in contributing to the remodelling process. The best studied is transforming growth factor beta, whose main source is the bronchial epithelium. It has certainly been noted to be increased in some studies on asthma. Furthermore, its levels have been correlated with both thickness of the reticular basement membrane and the number of fibroblasts in asthma. Epidermal growth factor immunoreactivity has also been increased in bronchial biopsies from asthmatics and this may increase the synthesis of protein such as fibronectin. Endothelins are also increased in asthma and will activate fibroblasts as well as contributing to the inflammatory process. GM-CSF, which has effects in activating eosinophils and promoting survival, probably also has a profibrotic effect and is increased in asthma. (This is well summarized by Vachier and colleagues[56].) Furthermore, there may well be a role for matrix metalloproteinases (MMPs) and their associated regulators, the tissue inhibitors of matrix metalloproteinases (TIMPs). In severe chronic asthma in adults, MMP9 is specifically increased.[57] Our preliminary studies from bronchoalveolar lavage of asthmatic children compared with non-asthmatics has shown an excess of MMP9 compared with its inhibitor, TIMP-1. Indeed MMP9/TIMP-1 ratios were higher in child than adult asthmatics.[58] The matrix proteolysis induced by MMPs with incomplete

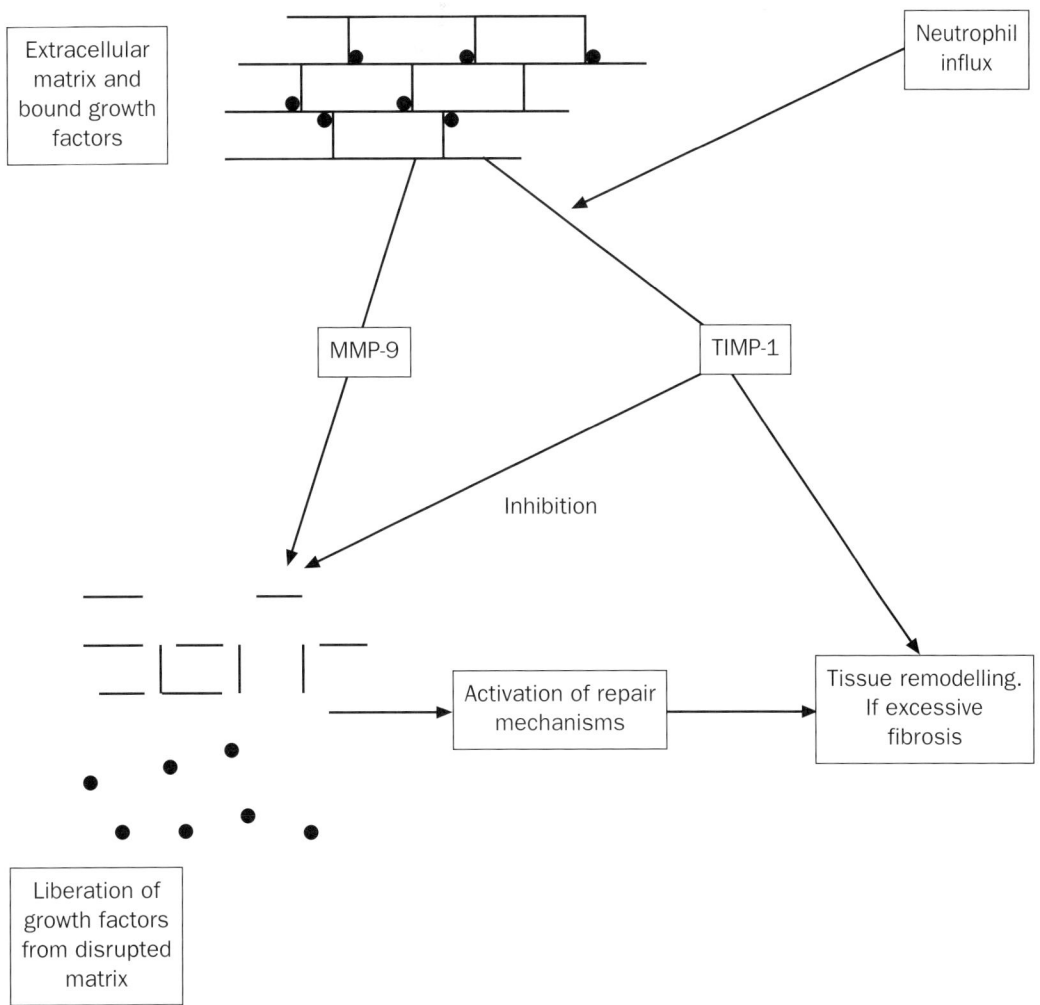

Figure 2.4 The effect of matrix metalloproteinase 9 (MMP-9) and its tissue inhibitor of matrix metalloproteinase 1 (TIMP-1) on the extracellular matrix and growth factors that contribute to fibrosis and tissue remodelling.

TIMP-1 inhibition will release growth factors which are bound to the extracellular matrix, thereby promoting fibroblast proliferation.[59] TIMP-1 may also directly contribute to stimulation of repair and remodelling (see Figure 2.4). The source of MMP9 is probably inflammatory cells, such as neutrophils and macrophages. Therefore, one possible hypothesis is that infiltrating neutrophils break down the extracellular matrix, which, in turn, activates inappropriate repair mechanisms leading to remodelling. Given the early appearance of neutrophils in the airway at the onset of allergen-induced late phase reactions[28] and the appearance of neutrophils in more severe asthma,[44–46] this suggests that neutrophils may be a primary stimulus for airway remodelling and that eosinophils appearing later during the course of a late phase reaction damage the respiratory epithelium. This generates a new paradigm for airway immunopathology in asthma in which remodelling and inflammation are simultaneous processes (see Figure 2.5).[60]

28 TEXTBOOK OF PEDIATRIC ASTHMA: AN INTERNATIONAL PERSPECTIVE

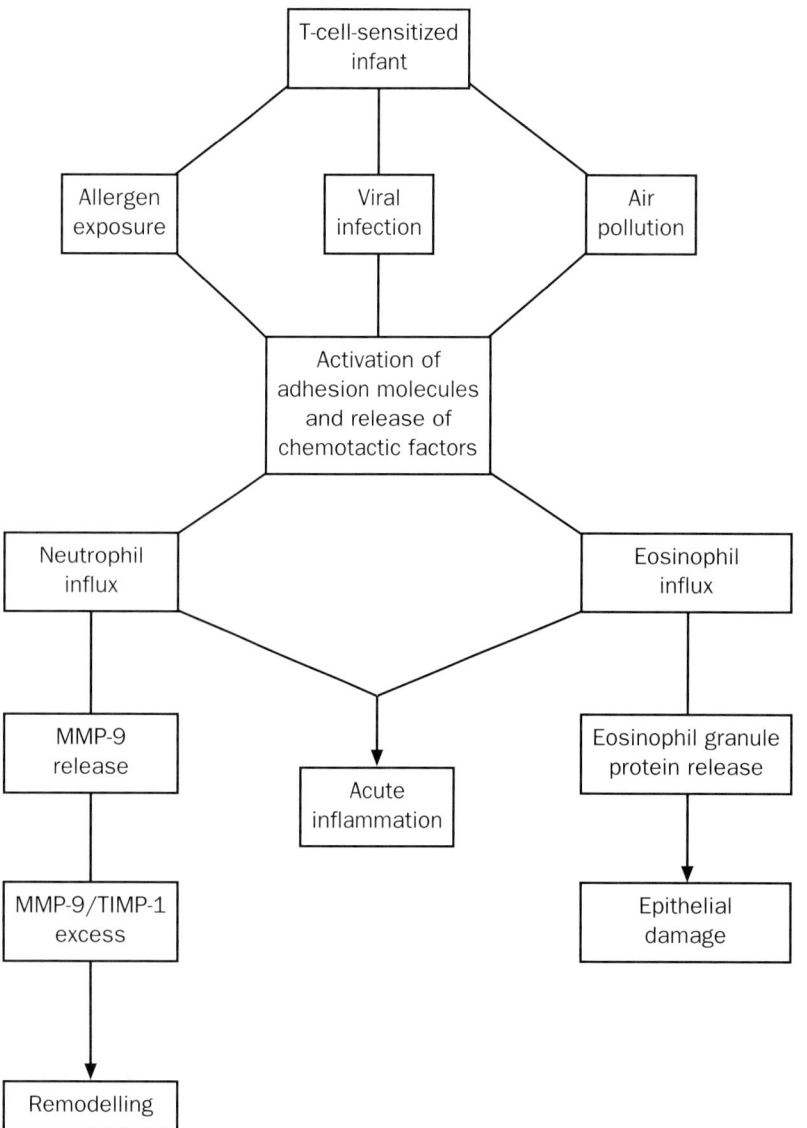

Figure 2.5 A new paradigm for the evolution of airway immunopathology in asthma, indicating the parallel development of tissue remodelling, acute inflammation and epithelial damage. This is distinct from the old paradigm suggesting inflammation and particularly eosinophilic damage to the epithelium was the primary stimulus for remodelling.

Adhesion molecules

Since cell migration from the vasculature into the airway is a key component of the evolving pathology in asthma, upregulation of glycoprotein adhesion molecules is an important feature. Upregulation of intercellular adhesion molecule 1 (ICAM-1), a member of the immunoglobulin super-gene family, has been seen as a particularly prominent feature in the airways of asthmatics and is overexpressed on airway mucosal cells as well as endothelium.[61] Interestingly, the Th-1 cytokine, IFN-γ, is strongly involved in the upregulation of ICAM-1.[62] IFN-γ also potentiates the release of TNF-α[62] and we have found raised levels of soluble ICAM-1 and IFN-γ in alveolar lavage from asthmatics compared with non-asthmatic children, and in infant wheezers there was a linear correlation between IFN-γ and sICAM-1 levels.[63] Indeed in this study, sICAM-1 levels correlated to some extent with disease activity, suggesting they may play an important role in the evolution of airway inflammation. The role of IFN-γ as a Th-1 cytokine is somewhat confusing in that it both contributes to the inflammatory process and inhibits it by antagonizing the effect of IL-4 and IL-13 on IgE production. The adhesion molecules are also important in cell to cell signalling such as between the antigen-presenting cell and T-lymphocytes; indeed, the latter study showed a correlation between sICAM-1 and lymphocyte numbers in bronchoalveolar lavage.[63]

ICAM-1 is but one of the cell adhesion molecules that may be important in asthma. Its expression on the endothelium facilitates leukocyte adhesion via ligands on the leukocytes including lymphocyte function associated antigen 1 (LFA-1), complement receptor 3 (Mac-1). However, vascular cell adhesion molecule 1 (VCAM-1) is also important for cell adhesion and ligates very late antigen 4 on leukocytes. VCAM-1 expression is also increased not only in pulmonary endothelium but also in epithelium in asthmatics after allergen provocation.

Before cell adhesion to the endothelium, there is a process known as 'rolling' in which leukocytes roll along the endothelium. Molecules involved in this process are primarily the selectins, with L-selectin on both neutrophils and eosinophils interacting with E-selectin on the endothelium. Increased expression of E-selectin has also been shown in bronchial epithelium as well as endothelium in asthmatics.[64]

These adhesion molecules provide yet another target for therapeutic intervention. Thus corticosteroids can inhibit upregulation of many of the molecules, which clearly is another route by which this group of drugs has an impact in asthma.[65] It is interesting to note that the antihistamine cetirizine has an inhibitory effect on allergen-induced upregulation of ICAM-1.[66] This might explain the beneficial effects of cetirizine given long term to babies with atopic dermatitis in preventing the onset of asthma in those sensitized to grass pollen or house dust mite.[67]

Relevance of airway inflammation to childhood asthma

As is apparent, although the majority of studies of airway inflammation in asthma have been conducted on adults, there is now accumulating evidence that at least in older children with asthma, identical processes occur.[13] Both from lavage studies and now biopsies, it is clear that eosinophilic infiltration is characteristic of the disease[46,68] and remodelling occurs early in the ontogeny of the disease (see Figure 2.6). This may well account for the observation that the prognosis of asthma from childhood to adulthood is influenced by the degree of lung function abnormality and BHR at presentation and that the outcome is uninfluenced by the use of inhaled corticosteroid.[69]

There is very little information on the airway immunopathology of infant wheeze. Many infant wheezers do not progress to atopic asthma and may well have a very different underlying pathology.[68] It is suggested that many infant wheezers have geometric differences in their airways caused by maternal smoking in pregnancy, prematurity and low birth weight.[70,71] Such infants do not need treatment with inhaled steroids,[72] because there is potential for this to interfere with alveolar development and there is some association between low birth weight, abnormal lung function in infancy and chronic obstructive lung disease in late adult life.[73] However, the infants destined to develop asthma cannot be discriminated from those with transient problems, other than by pre-existing atopy or an atopic family history. It is possible that bronchial lavage and biopsy appearance would distinguish the future asthmatic but the procedure is relatively invasive. One study has assessed the clinical utility of bronchoscopy and lavage in wheezing infants. It was deemed that in 28 of the 30 children studied, useful information was derived in just over half with airway structural abnormalities and in 40% with abnormal differential cell counts in the bronchoalveolar lavage.[74]

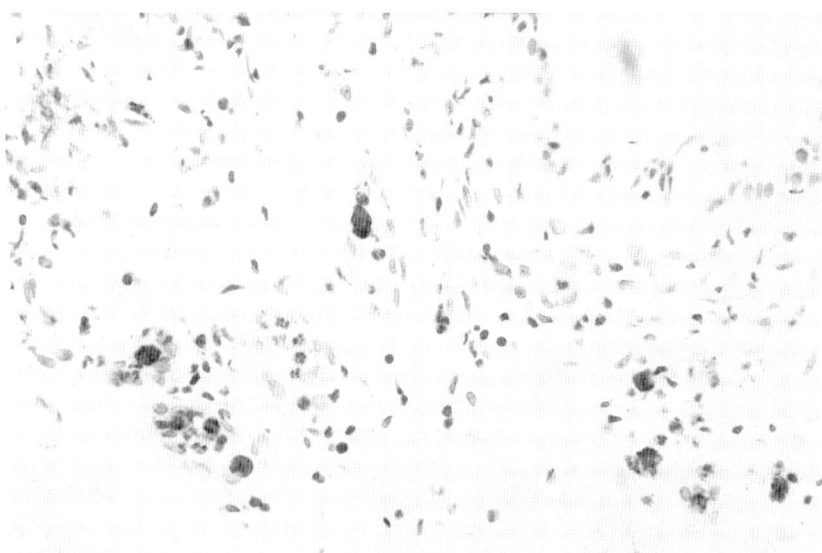

Figure 2.6 Bronchial biopsy from a 5-year-old child with asthma, stained with a monoclonal antibody against eosinophil cationic protein. The brown stain cells are positive and indicate activated eosinophils which are increased in number in the lamina propria.

NON-INVASIVE MARKERS OF AIRWAY INFLAMMATION

There has been a drive to identify circulating markers of airway inflammation which might indicate those in need of early introduction of prophylaxis. An Oslo birth cohort study has shown that in infant wheezers compared with matched controls there was a higher probability of salbutamol responsiveness which correlated with the level of serum, eosinophil cationic protein, as a marker of eosinophil activation.[75] One might predict that the bronchodilator-responsive individuals with eosinophilic activation would be asthmatics. Follow-up studies are awaited. We have also shown that a circulating marker of lymphocyte activation, soluble IL-2 receptor, may be a useful indicator of future asthma in infant wheezers.[76] Indeed, we have also shown that this marker is dramatically upregulated in the fatality-prone childhood asthmatic.[20] Many more longer-term follow-up studies will be required to identify whether any circulating markers or other non-invasive markers, such as those that can be obtained from induced sputum, will prove to have any utility in clinical practice.[77]

With regard to the monitoring of disease activity using circulating markers, hitherto the most detailed studies have been of the eosinophil activation proteins. Although there is some correlation between levels, lung function and disease severity, these are not good enough to have any clinical utility.[78] Thus far, exhaled nitric oxide has proved to have more value in characterizing the severity of disease in asthmatic children and may prove to be a more robust marker to employ in clinical practice.[79]

REFERENCES

1. Laitinen LA, Heino M, Laitinen A, Kava T, Hachtera T. Damage to the airway epithelium and bronchial reactivity in patients with asthma. *Am Rev Respir Dis* 1985; **131**: 599–606.
2. Miller J. Observations on the asthma and the hooping cough. London: T Cadell, 1769.
3. Osler W. Bronchial asthma. In: *Principles and Practice of Medicine* 1st edn. New York: Appleton, 1892, 497–501.
4. James AL, Pare PD, Hogg JC. The mechanics of airway narrowing in asthma. *Am Rev Respir Dis* 1989; **139**: 242–6.
5. Dunnell MS. The pathology of asthma with special reference to changes in the bronchial mucosa. *J Clin Pathol* 1960; **13**: 27–33.

6. Dunnell MS, Massarella GR, Anderson JA. A comparison of the quantitative anatomy of the bronchi in normal subjects and status asthmaticus in chronic bronchitis and emphysema. *Thorax* 1969; **24:** 176–9.
7. Bentley AM, Menz G, Storz C et al. Identification of T-lymphocytes, macrophages and activated eosinophils in the bronchial mucosa. *Am Rev Respir Dis* 1992; **146:** 500–6.
8. Hossain S, Third BE. Hypoplasia of bronchial muscle in asthma. *J Pathol* 1970; **101:** 171–84.
9. Beasley R, Roche WR, Roberts JA, Holgate ST. Cellular events in the bronchi in mild asthma and after bronchial provocation. *Am Rev Respir Dis* 1989; **139:** 806–17.
10. Sobonya RE. Concise clinical study: quantitative changes in long standing allergic asthma. *Am Rev Respir Dis* 1984; **130:** 289–92.
11. Cutz F, Levison H, Cooper DM. Ultra-structure of airways in children with asthma. *Histopathology* 1978; **2:** 407–21.
12. Holgate ST. Genetic and environmental interaction in allergy and asthma. *J Allergy Clin Immunol* 1999; **104:** 1139–46.
13. Rao RK, Warner JO. Airway inflammation: is it relevant to childhood asthma? In: Phelan PD, ed. *Clinical Paediatrics—Asthma.* London: Bailliere Tindall 1995, 277–96.
14. Warner JO. Worldwide variations in the prevalence of atopic symptoms. What does it all mean? *Thorax* 1999; **5**(suppl 2): S46–S51.
15. Pearce N, Pekkanen J, Beasley R. How much asthma is really attributable to atopy? *Thorax* 1999; **54:** 268–72.
16. CIBA Foundation Study Group. *Identification of Asthma.* Edinburgh: Churchill Livingstone, 1971, 58.
17. NPDW, Laitinen LA, Jacobs L et al. Mechanisms of bronchial hyper-reactivity in normal subjects after upper respiratory tract infection. *Am Rev Respir Dis* 1976; **113:** 131–9.
18. Warner JO. Bronchial hyperresponsiveness, atopy, airway inflammation and asthma. *Pediatr Allergy Immunol* 1998; **9:** 56–60.
19. Zach MA, Karner U. Sudden death in asthma. *Arch Dis Child* 1989; **64:** 1446–51.
20. Warner JO, Nikolaizik WH, Besley CR, Warner JA. A childhood asthma death in a clinical trial; potential indicators of risk. *Eur Respir J* 1998; **11:** 229–33.
21. Cockcroft DW, Ruffin RE, Frith PA. Determinants of allergen induced asthma: dose of allergen, circulating IgE antibody concentration and bronchial responsiveness to inhaled histamine. *Am Rev Respir Dis* 1979; **120:** 1053–9.
22. Warner JO. The significance of late reactions following bronchial challenge with house mite. *Arch Dis Child* 1976; **51:** 905–11.
23. Friedmann BS, Bell EH, Buntinx A. Oral leukotriene inhibitor (MK-866) blocks allergen induced airway responses. *Am Rev Respir Dis* 1993; **143:** 839–44.
24. Cockcroft DW, Ruffin RE, Dolovich J, Hargreave FE. Allergen induced increase in non-allergic bronchial reactivity. *Clin Allergy* 1977; **7:** 503–13.
25. Peroni DG, Boner AL, Vallone G et al. Effective allergen avoidance at high altitude reduces allergen induced bronchial hyperresponsiveness. *Am J Respir Crit Care Med* 1994; **149:** 1442–6.
26. Sporik R, Platts-Mills TAE, Cogswell JJ. Exposure to house dust mite allergen of children admitted to hospital with asthma. *Clin Exp Allergy* 1993; **23:** 740–6.
27. Peat JK, Tovey E, Toelle BG et al. House dust allergens: a major risk factor for childhood asthma in Australia. *Am J Respir Crit Care Med* 1996; **153:** 141–6.
28. Montefort S, Gratzious C, Goulding D et al. Bronchial biopsy evidence for leukocyte infiltration and upregulation of leukocyte endothelial cell adhesion molecules 6 hours after local allergen challenge of sensitized asthmatic airways. *J Clin Invest* 1994; **93:** 1411–21.
29. Folkerts G, Broeke RT, Fischer A et al. Nitric oxide control of airway smooth muscle. *Eur Respir Rev* 2000; **1073:** 249–52.
30. Holt PG. Regulation of antigen presenting cell functions in lung and airway tissue. *Eur Respir J* 1993; **6:** 120–9.
31. Semper AE, Hartley JA. Dendritic cells in the lung: what is their relevance to asthma? *Clin Exp Allergy* 1996; **26:** 485–90.
32. Butland BK, Strachan DP, Anderson HR. Fresh fruit intake and asthma symptoms in young British adults: confounding or effect of modification by smoking. *Eur Respir J* 1999; **13:** 744–50.
33. Tomiaka M, Ida S, Yuriko S et al. Mast cells in bronchoalveolar lumen of patients with bronchial asthma. *Am Rev Respir Dis* 1984; **129:** 1–27.
34. Roberts JA, Holgate ST. Asthma basic mechanisms. In: Tinkelman DG, Naspitz CK, eds. *Childhood Asthma: Pathophysiology and Treatment* 2nd edn. New York: Marcel Dekker, 1993, 1–28.
35. Matsuoka T, Harata M, Tanaka H et al. Prostaglandin D_2 as a mediator of allergic asthma. *Science* 2000; **287:** 2013–17.

36. Diamant Z, Timmers MC, Van der Venn H et al. Effect of inhaled heparin on allergen induced early and late asthmatic responses in patients with atopic asthma. *Am J Respir Crit Care Med* 1996; **153**: 1790–5.
37. Molinari JF, Campo C, Shakir S, Ahmed T. Inhibition of antigen induced airway hyperresponsiveness by ultra low molecular weight heparin. *Am J Respir Crit Care Med* 1998; **157**: 887–93.
38. Green WF, Konnaris K, Woolcock AJ. Effect of salbutamol, fenoterol and sodium cromoglycate on the release of heparin from sensitized human lung fragments challenged with *Dermatophagoides pteronyssinus* allergen. *Am J Respir Crit Care Med* 1993; **8**: 518–21.
39. Johnson PR, Armour CL, Carey D, Black JL. Heparin and PGE_2 inhibit DNA synthesis in human airway smooth muscle cells and culture. *Am J Physiol* 1995; **269**: L514–L519.
40. Karnovsky MJ, Edelman ER. Heparin-heparan sulphate regulation of vascular smooth muscle behaviour. In: Page CP, Black J, eds. *Airways and Vascular Remodelling in Asthma and Cardiovascular Diseases—Implications for Therapeutic Intervention.* London: Academic Press, 1994, 41–77.
41. Capron M, Jouault T, Prin C et al. Functional study of a monoclonal antibody to IgE F_c receptor of eosinophils, platelets and macrophages. *J Exp Med* 1986; **164**: 72–89.
42. Azevedo I, de Blic J, Scheinmann P, Vargaftig BB, Bachelet M. Enhanced arachidonic acid metabolism in alveolar macrophages from wheezy infants: modulation by dexamethasone. *Amer J Respir Crit Care Med* 1995; **152**: 1208–14.
43. Azevedo I, de Blic J, Dumarey CH. Increased spontaneous release of tumen necrosis factor by alveolar macrophages from wheezy infants. *Eur Respir J* 1997; **10**: 1767–73.
44. Wenzel SE, Szefler SJ, Leung DWM et al. Bronchoscopic evaluation of severe asthma: persistent inflammation despite high dose glucocorticoids. *Am J Respir Crit Care Med* 1997; **156**: 737–43.
45. Jataknon A, Uasuf C, Maziak W et al. Neutrophilic inflammation in severe persistent asthma. *Am J Respir Crit Care Med* 1999; **160**: 1532–9.
46. Marguet C, Jouen-Boedes F, Dean TP, Warner JO. Bronchoalveolar cell profiles in children with asthma, infantile wheeze, chronic cough or cystic fibrosis. *Am J Respir Crit Care Med* 1999; **159**: 1533–40.
47. Montefort S, Roberts JA, Beasley R et al. The site of disruption of the bronchial epithelium in asthmatic and non-asthmatic subjects. *Thorax* 1992; **47**: 499–503.
48. Chung KF, Barnes PJ. Cytokines in asthma. *Thorax* 1999; **54**: 825–57.
49. Knobil K, Jacoby DB. Mediator functions of epithelial cells. In: Holgate ST, Busse WW, eds. *Inflammatory Mechanisms in Asthma.* New York: Marcel Dekker, 1998, 469–95.
50. Altraja A, Laitinen A, Virtanen I et al. Expression of laminens in the airways in various types of asthmatic patients: a morphometric study. *Am J Respir Cell Mol Biol* 1996; **15**: 482–8.
51. Laitinen A, Altraja A, Kampe M et al. Tenascin is increased in airway basement membrane of asthmatics and decreased by an inhaled steroid. *Am J Respir Crit Care Med* 1997; **156**: 951–8.
52. Holgate ST. The inflammation–repair cycle in asthma: the pivotal role of the airway epithelium. *Clin Exp Allergy* 1998; **28**(suppl 5): 103–9.
53. Chung KF. Airway smooth muscle cells: contributing to and regulating airway mucosal inflammation? *Eur Respir J* 2000; **15**: 961–8.
54. Laitinen LA, Laitinen A, Haahtella TA. A comparative study of the effects of an inhaled corticosteroid, budesonide, and a β_2-agonist, terbutaline, on airway inflammation in newly diagnosed asthma: a randomised double blind placebo group controlled trial. *J Allergy Clin Immunol* 1992; **90**: 32–42.
55. Sont JK, Han J, van Krieken JM et al. Relationship between the inflammatory infiltrate in bronchial biopsy specimens and clinical severity of asthma in patients treated with inhaled steroids. *Thorax* 1996; **51**: 496–502.
56. Vachier I, Vignola AM, Bousquet J. Growth factors in the remodelling of asthma. *Eur Respir Rev* 2000; **1073**: 319–23.
57. Dahlen B, Shute J, Howarth P. Immunohistochemical localization of the matrix metalloproteinases MMP3 and MMP9 within the airways in asthma. *Thorax* 1999; **54**: 590–6.
58. Parker HM, Mander A, Perks B et al. Potential mechanisms of airway remodelling in childhood asthma. *Eur Respir J* 1999; **14**(suppl 30): 36S.
59. Redington AE, Roche WR, Holgate ST, Howarth PH. Co-localization of immunoreactive transforming growth factor beta-1 and decorin in bronchial biopsies from asthmatic and normal subjects. *J Pathol* 1998; **186**: 410–15.
60. Warner JO, Marguet C, Rao R et al. Inflammatory mechanisms in childhood asthma.

Clin Exp Allergy 1998; **28**(suppl 5): 179–83.
61. Vignola AM, Campbell AM, Chanez P et al. HLA-DR and ICAM-1 expression on bronchial epithelial cells in asthma and chronic bronchitis. *Am Rev Respir Dis* 1993; **148**: 689–94.
62. Dery RE, Bissonnette EY. IFN-γ potentiates the release of TNF-α and MIP-1α by alveolar macrophages during allergic reactions. *Am J Respir Cell Mol Biol* 1999; **20**: 407–12.
63. Marguet C, Dean TP, Warner JO. Soluble intercellular adhesion molecule 1 (sICAM-1) and IFN-γ in bronchoalveolar lavage fluid from children with airway diseases. *Am J Respir Crit Care Med* 2000; **162**: 1016–22.
64. Bloemen PGM, Henricks PAJ, Nijkamp FP. Cell adhesion molecules in asthma. *Clin Exp Allergy* 1997; **27**: 128–41.
65. Henriks PAJ, Nijkamp FP. Modulation of cell adhesion molecules. *Eur Respir Rev* 2000; **10**: 329–32.
66. Ciprandi G, Passalacqua G, Canonica GW. Effects of H1 antihistamines on adhesion molecules: a possible rationale for long term treatment. *Clin Exp Allergy* 1999; **29**(suppl 3): 49–53.
67. ETAC Study Group. Allergic factors associated with the development of asthma and the influence of cetirizine in a double blind randomised placebo controlled trial: first results of ETAC. *Pediatr Allergy Immunol* 1998; **9**: 116–24.
68. Stevenson EC, Turner G, Heaney LG et al. Bronchoalveolar lavage findings suggest two different forms of childhood asthma. *Clin Exp Allergy* 1997; **9**: 1027–35.
69. Gerritsen J, Koeter GH, Postma DS et al. Prognosis of asthma from childhood to adulthood. *Am Rev Respir Dis* 1989; **140**: 1325–30.
70. Martinez FD, Wright AL, Taussig LM et al. Asthma and wheezing in the first 6 years of life. *New Engl J Med* 1995; **332**: 133–8.
71. Dezateux C, Stocks J, Dundas I, Fletcher ME. Impaired airway function and wheezing in infancy: the influence of maternal smoking and a genetic predisposition to asthma. *Am J Respir Crit Care Med* 1999; **159**: 403–10.
72. Pedersen S, Warner JO, Price JF. Early use of inhaled steroids in children with asthma. *Clin Exp Allergy* 1997; **27**: 995–1006.
73. Barker DJP, Godfrey KM, Fall C et al. Relation of birthweight and childhood respiratory infection to adult lung function and death from chronic obstructive airways disease. *Brit Med J* 1991; **303**: 671–5.
74. Schellhase DE, Fawcett DD, Schutze GE et al. Clinical utility of flexible bronchoscopy and bronchoalveolar lavage in young children with recurrent wheezing. *J Pediatr* 1998; **132**: 312–18.
75. Lödrup-Carlsen KC, Ragnhild H, Ahlstedt S, Carlsen K-H. Eosinophilic cationic protein and tidal flow volume loops in children 0–2 years of age. *Eur Respir J* 1995; **8**: 1148–54.
76. Clough JB, Keeping KA, Edwards LC et al. Can we predict which wheezy infants will continue to wheeze? *Am J Respir Crit Care Med* 1999; **160**: 1473–80.
77. Jayaram L, Parameswaran K, Sears MR, Hargreave FE. Induced sputum cell counts: their usefulness in clinical practice. *Eur Respir J* 2000; **16**: 150–8.
78. Rao KR, Frederick JM, Enander I et al. Airway function correlates with circulating eosinophil but not mast cell markers of inflammation in childhood asthma. *Clin Exp Allergy* 1996; **26**: 789–93.
79. Lanz MJ, Leung DYM, McCormick DR et al. Comparison of exhaled nitric oxide, serum eosinophilic cationic protein and soluble interleukin-2 receptor in exacerbations of pediatric asthma. *Pediatr Pulmonol* 1997; **24**: 305–11.

3

Pediatric asthma: epidemiology and natural history

Jonathan M Samet, Denise G Wiesch, Iqbal H Ahmed

Introduction • Problems in the epidemiological investigation of childhood asthma • Descriptive epidemiology • Prevalence • Summary

INTRODUCTION

For prevention and management of asthma, information is needed on patterns of disease occurrence, risk factors, and natural history, including the impact of therapy on disease outcome. Much of this information is obtained through epidemiologic investigation. Epidemiology is defined as the scientific methods used to study disease occurrence in human populations. Although formal definition of this discipline has been difficult, the emphasis on human populations differentiates epidemiology from conventional clinical research that addresses patient groups. Epidemiology may be considered to have two distinct components: description of disease occurrence, most often by person, place, or time; and the identification of risk factors for disease.[1] Experimental study designs, such as the controlled clinical trial, are also used to evaluate therapeutic modalities and to conduct health services research.

Incidence, mortality, and prevalence rates describe the occurrence of disease in a population.[1] The incidence rate during a specified time period is the ratio of the number of new cases to the population at risk. Incidence data for asthma are not readily available because of the difficulty of identifying new cases. Mortality is a similar ratio, with the number of deaths as the numerator. In most countries, cause-specific mortality, including asthma-specific mortality, is closely tracked. Prevalence is the most widely used index of asthma occurrence because it can be ascertained in surveys using questionnaires. Because prevalence is determined by both the incidence rate and the disease duration, it reflects the natural history of a disease. Diseases with a longer duration but a low case-fatality rate, like asthma, have a higher prevalence.

Cross-sectional surveys—for example, the International Study of Asthma and Allergy in Children (ISAAC)—are used to measure disease prevalence. To identify risk factors for disease, epidemiologists conduct case–control and cohort studies. The case–control design involves the identification of a case series, such as persons with asthma, and an appropriate control group, followed by comparison of the proportions of cases and controls exposed to the risk factor(s) of interest. In the cohort design, study subjects are followed over time and observations are made concerning risk factors for disease or concerning natural history. For example, a cohort study of atopy and asthma might involve follow-up of persons with and without atopy and ascertainment of new cases of asthma in the two groups. The Tucson study of respiratory health in children is a well-known example of a prospective cohort study.[2] In this study, a group of children were enrolled at birth and respiratory illness experience was prospectively documented, as were putative risk factors for asthma.

These epidemiological approaches have provided important information about the occurrence, causes, and natural history of childhood asthma. The epidemiological data complement data from clinical series, which are generally based on children who are ill or receiving medical care. This chapter reviews the epidemiology of childhood asthma and emphasizes the accumulating evidence on the natural history and the risk factors of this disorder.

PROBLEMS IN THE EPIDEMIOLOGICAL INVESTIGATION OF CHILDHOOD ASTHMA

Definitions

Clinical, physiological, and questionnaire approaches can be used to identify asthma in study participants in the context of an epidemiological investigation. The difficulty of defining asthma in operational terms has frustrated the study of childhood asthma, regardless of the approach for identifying the disease. Both expert groups (Table 3.1)[3-10] and individuals have prepared definitions, but none of these has led to specific, operational criteria for differentiating asthmatic from non-asthmatic children. In fact, participants in the 1971 Ciba Study Group on the Identification of Asthma concluded that the then-available information was inadequate for developing a satisfactory definition of asthma;[9] more recent information does not alter this conclusion. Although the definition of asthma has evolved to incorporate contemporary concepts of pathogenesis, we are no closer to having definition-based criteria for clinical or research purposes. Furthermore, the syndrome of asthma spans a range of severity from intermittent and mild to continuous and severe, and any boundary along this spectrum is arbitrary.

The present terminology for major diseases associated with airflow obstruction, including asthma, follows that formulated in 1959 by participants in a Ciba symposium.[3] That group addressed diseases in the adult, including chronic bronchitis, emphysema, chronic airflow obstruction, and asthma, and wrote a definition of asthma that emphasized varying physiological dysfunction (Table 3.1). Subsequent definitions have added hyperresponsiveness of the airways as a fundamental abnormality and the more recent definitions have added inflammation as the hallmark of pathogenesis. Although not prepared specifically for childhood asthma, these definitions are conceptually appropriate for children and are used for research purposes. Their application is difficult, however, because ventilatory function and airway responsiveness cannot be readily assessed in younger children and we do not yet have useful, non-invasive markers of inflammation.

Questionnaires

Because children may be unable to cooperate adequately with physiological testing, for reasons of feasibility, questionnaires are the most widely used method for classifying subjects as affected in epidemiological studies of childhood asthma. A number of instruments have been developed, including several specific to children. One of the first standardized respiratory symptoms questionnaires for children was developed by the American Thoracic Society.[10] The questionnaire includes questions on major respiratory symptoms and diseases; some of the questions relate to asthma, but the questionnaire is not comprehensive in covering the symptoms of this disease. New instruments have been developed that are more specific for childhood asthma. A brief, standardized instrument was developed for the ISAAC study.[11] This questionnaire covers key symptoms of

Table 3.1 Asthma definitions

ATS[4]	1962	Asthma is a disease characterized by an increased responsiveness of the trachea and bronchi to various stimuli and manifested by a wide-spread narrowing of the airways that changes in severity either spontaneously or as a result of therapy.
CIBA[3]	1959	The condition of subjects with widespread narrowing of the bronchial airways, which changes its severity over short periods of time either spontaneously or under treatment.
World Health Organization[6]	1975	A chronic condition characterized by recurrent bronchospasm resulting from a tendency to develop reversible narrowing of the airway lumina in response to stimuli of a level or intensity not inducing such narrowing in most individuals.
ATS[28]	1987	A clinical syndrome characterized by increased responsiveness of the tracheobronchial tree to a variety of stimuli. Major symptoms are paroxysms of dyspnea, wheezing and cough, which may vary from mild and almost undetectable to severe and unremitting (status asthmaticus). The primary physiologic manifestation of this hyperresponsiveness is variable airways obstruction. This can take form of fluctuations in the severity of obstruction, following bronchodilators or corticosteroids, or increased obstruction caused by drugs or other stimuli. . . . evidence of mucosal edema of the bronchi, infiltration of the bronchial mucosa or submucosa with inflammatory cells, especially eosinophils; shedding of epithelium, obstruction of peripheral airways with mucus.
NHLBI/NIH[152]	1991	A lung disease with the following characteristics: 1) airway obstruction that is reversible (but not completely so in some patients) either spontaneously or with treatment; 2) airway inflammation; and, 3) increased airway responsiveness to a variety of stimuli.
NHLBI/NIH[140,153,154]	1993/1995/1997	A chronic inflammatory disorder of the airways in which many cells play a role, in particular mast cells, eosinophils, and T lymphocytes. In susceptible individuals this inflammation causes recurrent episodes of wheezing, breathlessness, chest tightness, and cough in early morning. These symptoms are usually associated with widespread but variable airflow limitation that is at least partly reversible either spontaneously or with treatment. The inflammation also causes an associated increase in airway responsiveness to a variety of stimuli.

asthma and other allergic diseases. The core questions on asthma cover wheezing, nocturnal cough, and report of asthma. A video version was also developed and validated against the conventional instrument.[12]

In many studies using questionnaires, epidemiologists have considered a parent's report of asthma, with or without a physician's diagnosis, as affirmative evidence. This type of estimate of the disease occurrence is affected by patterns of use of medical care and the choice of diagnostic labels by individual physicians. For children, the terminology used by clinicians may not match that of epidemiologists; this may have been particularly true in the past when there was a general tendency not to use the label 'asthma'. In the late 1970s, Taussig et al.[13] questioned physicians in Tucson, Arizona, about their diagnostic criteria for chronic bronchitis in children. For most of the physicians, wheezing and allergy were important considerations, and bronchodilator therapy was frequently given to children with chronic bronchitis. The authors concluded that the diagnoses of chronic bronchitis and asthma overlap considerably in children. About the same time in England, Speight et al.[14] identified children with a history of wheezing episodes and then confirmed the clinical significance of the wheezing by bronchial challenge testing with histamine, examination of school absenteeism, and treatment responses. Although most of the children with wheezing had been evaluated by a physician, only a small proportion had been diagnosed as having asthma. These past labeling trends, however, probably no longer prevail in many developed countries.

Prevalence estimates based on questionnaires may be affected by the wording of questions on asthma. For example, Table 3.2 provides US prevalence rates for different indicators of asthma: physician report, current disease, and the symptom of wheezing.[15] For all ages, physician-diagnosed asthma is less frequent than wheezing and about half of those with a physician-diagnosis have active asthma. There is also variation of prevalence estimates by age, with the youngest age group having less reported doctor-diagnosed disease relative to nonspecific wheeze in comparison with the pattern at older ages.

In infants and younger children, the terms 'wheezy bronchitis' and 'asthmatic bronchitis' have been used for patients who wheeze when provoked by a respiratory infection, but the labels do not differentiate these patients distinctly from those diagnosed with asthma. For example, Williams and McNicol[16] showed that the natural histories of disease in children diagnosed with asthma and wheezy bronchitis were the same. Thus, to assess completely the frequency of asthma, a questionnaire must include all labels that may be used locally by physicians. However, even a comprehensive questionnaire may not detect all cases of asthma, and some false-positive cases must be anticipated because of the imperfect sensitivity of questionnaires.

DESCRIPTIVE EPIDEMIOLOGY

Methods

Most of the information concerning the occurrence of asthma is prevalence data collected in cross-sectional surveys; many surveys have been carried out throughout the world. In the United States, periodic surveys conducted by the National Center for Health Statistics provide prevalence estimates from nationwide probability samples. In contrast to the abundant data on prevalence, only a few cohort studies provide incidence rates. Further insights into the occurrence of asthma may be gained from mortality and hospitalization rates. However, these measures integrate the frequency of the disease with variations in severity, diagnosis and treatment patterns, and classification.

Prevalence

The prevalence of asthma has been described in many populations and tracked over time in a number of developed countries, including the United States. The prevalence of asthma has been estimated from surveys using question-

Table 3.2 Estimates of prevalence of asthma by selected criteria, by age, from the second National Health and Nutrition Examination Survey of the United States, 1976–1980[15]

Question	Total	6 months–2 years	3–5 years	6–11 years	12–17 years
Did a doctor ever tell you that you had asthma?	6.2	4.0	6.5	7.6	6.6
Do you still have asthma?	3.0	2.3	3.9	3.9	3.2
During the past 12 months, not counting colds or the flu, have you frequently had trouble with wheezing?	6.5	7.2	6.2	5.9	4.5
Have you ever been told you have asthma and/or wheezing?	10.5	8.8	9.8	10.4	8.7
Do you still have asthma and/or wheezing?	7.7	7.8	7.6	7.4	5.7

naires, spirometry, and assessment of airways hyperresponsiveness. The National Health Interview Survey (NHIS) and the National Health and Nutrition Surveys (NHANES), conducted by the National Center for Health Statistics on random samples of the entire US population, provide periodic prevalence estimates, and data are now available for a span of 40 years.

The NHIS, a population-based interview survey of households across the United States, is a key source of longitudinal information on the prevalence of asthma. The latest data available, 1995 information from 116 179 people in 45 705 households, indicate that 5.6% of US residents, or 14.6 million people, have asthma.[17] Prevalence estimates were based on a positive response to the question 'During the past 12 months did you have asthma?' The survey results showed that asthma was most prevalent in the youngest age groups and that 4.8 million (6.9%) children under age 18 years have the disease, making asthma the most common chronic illness of childhood in the US. Geographically, asthma prevalence rates were highest in the West and Northeast (5.9%) and slightly lower in the South (5.5%) and Midwest (5.2%).

Review of data from the NHIS back to 1982 shows that the prevalence of asthma has been increasing in all age and racial groups. Prevalence rates vary among racial and ethnic groups; this variation likely reflects differences in genetic, environmental, social, and cultural influences among population groups.[18] Figure 3.1 shows the rising prevalence of asthma for blacks and whites in persons aged 5–34 years old. Overall, for both groups together, the prevalence rate increased 52% during this time period from 34.6 to 52.6 per thousand.[19]

Asthma is a worldwide problem that has been considered to be more common in the more affluent and the developed countries than in the less affluent and the developing countries.[20] Prevalence estimates in children range from 0%

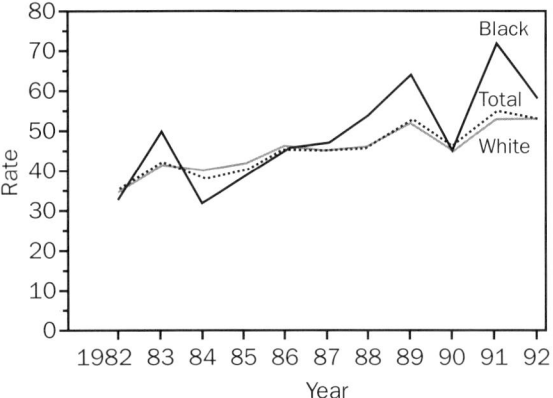

Figure 3.1 Age-adjusted prevalence rates of self-reported asthma for persons aged 5–34 years, by race and year—United States, 1982–1992.[19]

to 30% and data for this age range are less subject to misclassification, since chronic obstructive pulmonary disease, which may be mislabeled as asthma in older persons, does not affect children.

Prevalence rates for children and young adults in countries around the world differ substantially. The ISAAC study provides the most extensive information on variation in asthma prevalence throughout the world.[11] In 1998, the ISAAC Steering Committee reported findings for 463 801 children, aged 13–14 years, from 155 collaborating centers in 56 countries.[11] Figure 3.2 provides the prevalence figures for a positive response to the question 'Have you had wheezing or whistling in the chest in the last 12 months?' Across the countries, there was an approximate 20-fold range of prevalence with the highest rates generally in more developed countries. Patterns for other allergic diseases were generally similar.

In addition to the substantial variation across countries, worldwide data also show rising prevalence. Table 3.3 shows data for a number of countries for which prevalence rates have been measured at least twice, as well as representative survey data from a single point in time for other countries. There is no clear pattern of variation by economic status, and methods of assessment vary considerably.

Within-country comparisons, however, indicate rising prevalence in recent decades, as in the United States. In Sweden, asthma in 18-year-old military conscripts increased by 47% between 1971 and 1981.[21] Asthma diagnosis was based on an interview by the examining doctor and on the patient's history. Another study of military conscripts in Finland showed a five-fold increase of asthma prevalence from 1966 to 1989.[22] Data from England, Australia, New Zealand, France, and Tahiti also indicate an increase in asthma in the past two decades (Table 3.3).[23–26] The study in Melbourne schoolchildren[24] yielded notably elevated prevalence rates; the outcome measure, any history of asthma or wheeze, is likely to provide an upwardly biased measure of asthma occurrence. Nonetheless, with this possibly biased method, there was a substantial increase in prevalence over 26 years.

In the Far East, as well, asthma prevalence has been on the rise (Table 3.3). Other parts of the world and the less affluent regions of Asia report less asthma. Japan is the exception to the pattern, being the wealthiest country in the Pacific area but having a relatively low prevalence rate of asthma.[27]

Measurement of airways responsiveness has the potential to provide an objective measure of the frequency of asthma. Airways responsiveness has been measured in communities and standardized protocols are available for its determination.[28–30] Table 3.4 shows prevalence data on increased airways responsiveness for children in different countries. Methacholine, histamine, exercise, or cold air were used in the different studies to induce bronchial hyperresponsiveness (BHR). The table reveals that the prevalence rates of BHR were different from those for doctor-diagnosed asthma but were neither consistently higher nor lower. BHR, however, is only a component of the asthma phenotype; many people with BHR never experience asthma attacks or symptoms. Nevertheless, it is an important component and valuable in unbiased prevalence estimations of asthma. In the study of Chinese adolescents,[31] for example, 93% with severe to moderate BHR also had a current doctor's diagnosis of asthma

Table 3.3 International prevalence estimates of asthma

Region/population studied	Age (years)	Number studied	Definition of asthma	Year	Prevalence (%)
England /schoolchildren[23]	4–12	5806 6056	Self-reported diagnosis of asthma	1973 1986	2.0 4.1
Scotland /schoolchildren[155]	8–13	3403 4034	Self-reported diagnosis of asthma	1989 1994	10.2 19.6
Australia /Melbourne schoolchildren[24]	7 12 15	— 3325 2899 2968	Self-reported 'ever has asthma' or 'ever had wheeze'	1964 1990	19.1 46.0 39.7 40.3
New Zealand[25]	12–18 12–18	715 435	Previous diagnosis of asthma	1975 1989	2.9 5.3
Sweden /military conscripts[21]	17–20 17–20	55 393 57 150	Doctor diagnosis based on personal interview	1971 1981	1.9 2.8
Finland /military conscripts[22]	19 19	900 000	Doctor diagnosis of asthma	1966 1989	0.3 1.8
France /young adults[26]	21 21	8140 10 559	Self-reported 'ever has asthma'	1968 1982	3.3 5.4
Tahiti /adolescents[156]	16 13	3870 6731	Self-reported 'ever had asthma'	1979 1984	11.5 14.3
Hong Kong[27]	16–28 17–33	1610 1573	Self-reported 'ever had asthma'	1989 1994	4.8 7.2
Japan[27]	Children Children	55 388 45 675	Self-reported 'ever had asthma'	1982 1992	3.3 4.6
Taiwan[27]	7–15 7–15	23 678 92 471	Self-reported 'current asthma'	1974 1991	1.3 5.8

Continued

Region /population studied	Age (years)	Number studied	Definition of asthma	Year	Prevalence (%)
Table 3.3 continued					
Singapore[27]	4–17	22 268	Self-reported 'ever had asthma'	1967	3–5.5
	6–14	2457		1994	19.5
Morocco /schoolchildren[157]	6–14	1804	Self-reported asthma	1986?	3.1
Algeria /schoolchildren[157]	6–14	5200	Self-reported asthma	1986?	3.5
Chile[158]	6–14	2759	Self-reported asthma	1979	2.7
Uruguay[158]	11–16	4296	Self-reported asthma	1981	7.5

and 73% had a previous diagnosis. Of those with normal levels of airways responsiveness, none had a current doctor's diagnosis and only 0.5% had a previous diagnosis. For people with mild BHR, 56% had a current doctor's diagnosis and 38% had a previous diagnosis, reflecting, perhaps, uncertainty in diagnosis and disease status at this level of pulmonary reactivity.

Incidence

Asthma incidence data are available from several cohort studies in the United States (Table 3.5) and from a few studies in other countries.[32] Some of the most comprehensive data are available for 1964–1983 for Rochester, Minnesota, the site of the Mayo Clinic (Figure 3.3).[33] Using the comprehensive records of the Mayo Clinic, it has been possible to capture virtually all incident cases of asthma in the Rochester population. As expected from prevalence figures, asthma incidence rates are highest in the youngest age groups and among boys.[33] There is little new asthma during the teenage and young adult years. Although the highest asthma incidence rates are in early childhood, these rates may be biased upwards by the labeling of wheezing during infections as asthma. Martinez et al.[2] followed children from birth through 6 years and found that a substantial proportion of children with wheezing during the first 3 years of life did not have wheezing at 6 years.

Morbidity/hospitalization data

Indicators of morbidity include measures of medical service utilization, such as hospitalizations, medication usage, and quality of life. Information on asthma hospitalizations from the National Hospital Discharge Survey (NHDS) provides a picture of asthma preva-

Table 3.4 Prevalence of bronchial hyperresponsiveness (BHR) in children and doctor-diagnosed asthma

Country	Study year	Number	Age (years)	Doctor-diagnosed asthma Prevalence (%)	BHR Prevalence (%)	Method of BHR testing
Germany[159]	1992	5697	9–11	7.9	13.3	Cold air
Australia[160]	1986	1217	8–12	17.3	15.3	Histamine
Australia[161]	1982	1487	8–10	11.1	10.1	Histamine
Denmark[162]	1987	495	7–16	5.6	16.0	Histamine
New Zealand[163]	1981	813	9–13	27.0	22.0	Methacholine
New Zealand[164]	1989	873	12	16.8	12.0	Exercise
Kenya[165]	1991	402	9–12	11.4	10.7	Exercise
Spain[166]	1990	2216	9–14	—	6.9	Exercise
China[31]	1988	3067	11–17	2.4	4.1	Histamine
Papua New Guinea[167]	1985	257	6–20	—	0.8	Histamine

lence and severity based on hospital records of inpatients discharged from short-stay (less than 30 days) non-federal hospitals. In 1993 asthma accounted for 198 000 hospitalizations among people less than 25 years old in the US. In addition, an increase in hospitalizations by 28% from 1980 to 1993 was seen in this age group. Most of this increase was accounted for by admissions for persons less than 5 years old (Figure 3.4). Moreover, the report indicated that rates were consistently higher among blacks, who were 3.5 times more likely than whites to be hospitalized for asthma.[34]

Counts of ambulatory care visits due to asthma offer an additional index of asthma morbidity. For the US in 1993–1994, there were approximately 13.7 million visits annually with asthma as the principal diagnosis.[35] The characteristics of persons with asthma vary by the type of medical care setting. Patients relying

Table 3.5 Estimates of incidence of asthma in the United States from various studies

Region	Follow-up period	Age (years)	Incidence in males	Incidence in females	Definition of asthma	Total population
US National Cohort[168]	1971–1975 to 1982–1984	25–74	2.1/1000 per year		Self-reported doctor diagnosis or hospitalization due to asthma (determined by hospital records)	14 404
Tecumseh, MI[169]	1959–1960 to 1962–1965	0–4	3.2%	1.7%	Doctor-diagnosed asthma	6563
		5–9	1.1%	2.1%		
		10–15	1.1%	1.5%		
		16–25	0.5%	0		
		25–34	1.4%	0		
		35–44	0.9%	0		
		45–54	0	0.4%		
		55–64	0	0.9%		
		65–74	0	0.9%		
		75+	1.0%	1.5%		
		All ages		1.1%		
Tucson, AZ[170]	1970 to 1974	0–4	1.4%	0.9%	Self-reported doctor diagnosis of asthma	3432
		5–9	1.0%	0.7%		
		10–14	0.2%	0.3%		
		15–19	0	0		
		20–29	0.2%	0.4%		
		30–39	0	0.4%		
		40–49	0	0.5%		
		50–59	0.3%	0.8%		
		60–69	0.2%	0.6%		
		70+				

Table 3.5 continued

Region	Follow-up period	Age (years)	Incidence in males	Incidence in females	Definition of asthma	Total population
Lebanon, CT[72]	1972 to 1978	7–17 18+	3% 1%	1% 0%	Self-reported asthma	1303
Rochester, MN[47]	1964 to 1983	<1 1–4 5–9 10–14 15–29 30–49 >50 All ages	3.9% 1.1% 0.4% 0.2% 0.08% 0.08% 0.1% 0.3%	2.3% 0.6% 0.2% 0.2% 0.1% 0.1% 0.09% 1.9%	Doctor diagnosis of asthma or the presence of asthma symptoms	58 000
Rochester MN[171]	1964 to 1983	65–74 75–84 ≥85	0.14% 0.12% 0.07%	0.08% 0.07% 0.06%	Doctor diagnosis of asthma or the presence of asthma symptoms	3622
Tucson, AZ[2]	1980–1984 to 1986–1990	0–6	48.5%		Parents' report of wheeze on questionnaire or physician history taking and auscultation	826

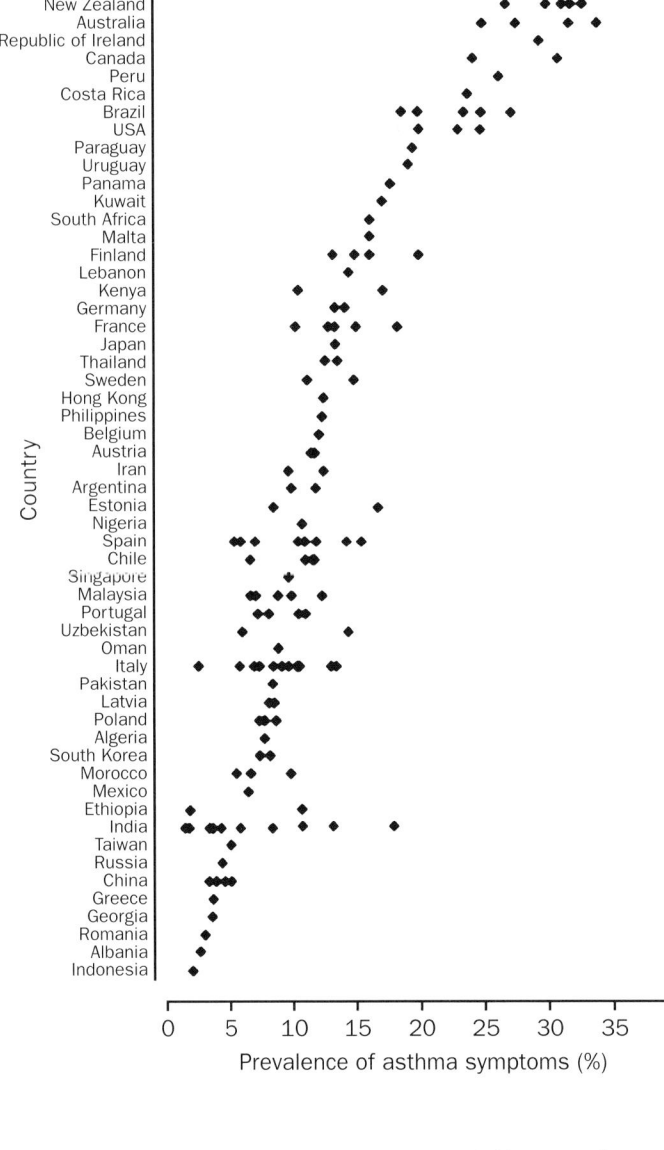

Figure 3.2 12 month prevalences of self-reported asthma symptoms from written questionnaires.[11]

on emergency room treatment may have different severity, receive different treatment, and have different outcomes compared with patients using office-based physicians. In order to characterize visits for asthma in the US, data were analyzed for 1993–1994 from the National Ambulatory Medical Care Survey (NAMCS), a national survey of visits to office-based physicians in the US, and from the National Hospital Ambulatory Medical Care Survey (NHAMCS), a national survey of visits to hospital emergency and outpatient departments in the US.[35] Physician office visits accounted for 80.5% of all visits for asthma, followed by emergency room visits at 12%, and outpatient departments with 7.5%. Age was shown to be significantly related to type of provider, with persons 15–24 years old having the lowest rate of office visits and the highest rate of emergency room visits.

Race was also significantly associated with type of visit, with blacks being more likely to use emergency rooms and hospital outpatient departments than whites, and less likely to use physicians' offices. The acute care nature of

EPIDEMIOLOGY AND NATURAL HISTORY **47**

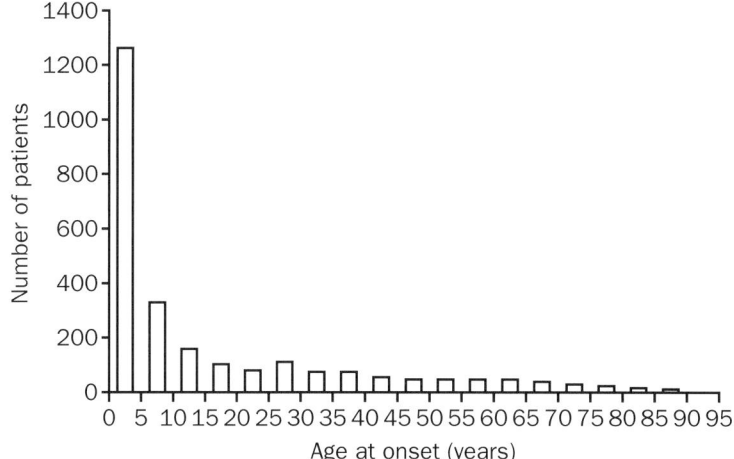

Figure 3.3 Distribution of ages at the onset of asthma among 2499 residents of Rochester, MN. The bars represent age ranges (0–4 years, 5–9 years, 10–14 years, and so forth).[33]

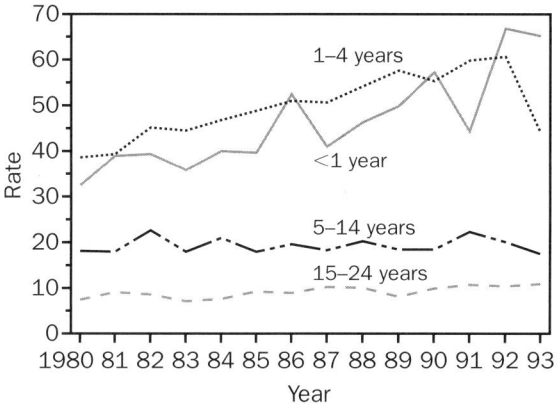

Figure 3.4 Hospital discharge rates per 10 000 population for asthma as the first-listed diagnosis among persons aged 0–24 years, by age group and year—United States, 1980–1993.[34]

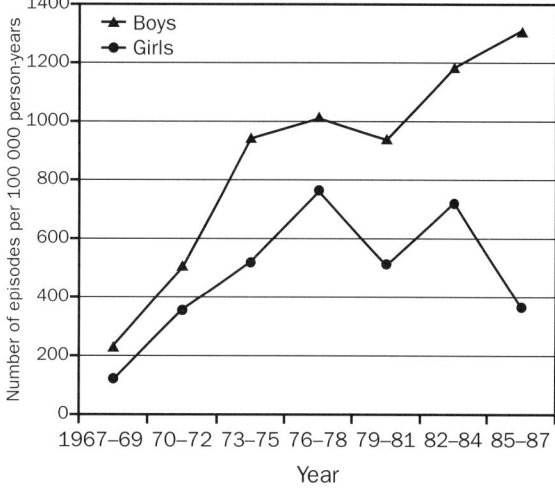

Figure 3.5 Estimated rate of asthma episodes among boys and girls 0–4 and 5–14 years of age.[36]

these former settings imply a lack of good preventive asthma management for black persons with possible barriers to effective medical treatment.

Other studies have demonstrated an increase in asthma using health care databases for the US. Vollmer et al.[36] examined 20 year trends in 'episodes of asthma' for the members of the Portland, Oregon population served by Kaiser Permanente. The total population was 86 200 in 1966, and grew to 310 800 by 1987. Vollmer and colleagues presented a methodology for defining episodes of asthma in order to counter potential biases in asthma morbidity estimates that may result from temporal changes in health care utilization and administration. For example, as health maintenance organizations grow and change, erroneous conclusions about asthma morbidity based on hospital admission rates could result from economic incentives to reduce hospital stays. Furthermore, asthma hospital admissions represent only a small fraction of total acute asthma health care utilization. Episodes of asthma were therefore defined to capture severe occurrences of asthma and included hospital admissions, emergency room visits, and hospital-based 'urgency care clinic' utilizations. Figure 3.5[36] displays the results for males and females 0–14 years of age, the age group with the most consistent patterns of change for the time period studied. The increase in asthma episodes was most pronounced in boys but the time trend was also statistically significant in girls. When this age group was further separated, boys 0–4 years old had the steepest rate of increase from 285 per 100 000 during 1965–1967 to 2025 per 100 000 during 1985–1987. Among age groups older than 14 years, no consistent pattern of change in episodes of asthma was observed.

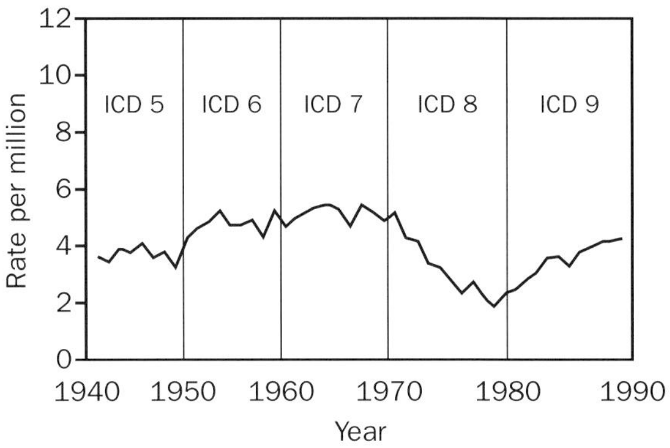

Figure 3.6 US age-adjusted, sex-adjusted, and race-adjusted asthma mortality rates by ICD (International Classification of Disease) revision, 1941–1989.[41]

Mortality

Although death from asthma is relatively rare, mortality rates are closely watched as an indicator of the impact of the disease on the population, and of the consequences of management, whether favorable or unfavorable. There have been substantial increases in asthma mortality periodically in recent decades and the causes of so-called asthma epidemics have been intensely investigated.[37]

Asthma deaths are coded according to the International Classification of Disease (ICD), which is revised approximately every 10 years. Mortality rates can be affected by coding changes from one revision to another and may account entirely or in part for the observed increases or decreases. In the United States, for example, the change from the eighth to the ninth revision in 1979 has been estimated to have increased the overall deaths of asthma by 35%.[38] For persons under age 45 years, however, the estimated effect is less than 5%.[39] The increase due to coding likely occurred because under the eighth revision 'bronchitis with mention of asthma' was coded as 'bronchitis,' whereas in the ninth revision the same was recorded as 'asthma'.[40] The tenth revision, soon to be implemented, also records coexistent bronchitis and asthma as 'asthma.' The validity of death certificate listings of asthma has been examined, but primarily in adults because of the potential for misclassification of chronic obstructive pulmonary disease (COPD).

An examination of long-term trends in the US from 1941 to 1989 described three distinct periods of asthma mortality in people 5–34 years of age; the patterns were the same in those 5–14 years old and 15–34 years of age. A gradual increase was seen from 1941 to 1964. From 1965 to 1977 a marked decline in mortality rates was observed, but from 1978 to 1989 asthma mortality nearly doubled (Figure 3.6).[41] These temporal changes need to be interpreted with recognition of the changing ICD codes, but there is general agreement for childhood asthma that the recent rise does not reflect changes in coding alone.[40]

Another time trend analysis looked at the recent period of increase in asthma mortality from 1980 to 1993 for US residents less than 25 years old (Figure 3.7).[34] During this period, blacks had consistently higher rates than whites in all age groups, and within each race the 15–24 age group also had the highest rates for every year observed. In 1993, blacks aged 15–24 were six times more likely to die of asthma than were whites, and blacks aged 5–14

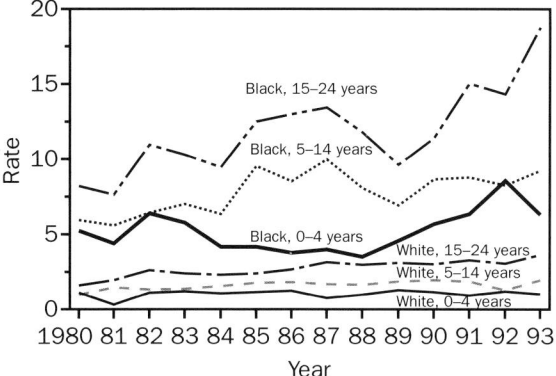

Figure 3.7 Death rates for asthma, by race, age group, and year—United States, 1980–1993.[34]

were four times more likely than whites to die of asthma.

As shown by these national data, patterns of asthma mortality have been shown to differ markedly between ethnic groups.[18] A study to identify target populations of children and young adults within the US at high risk of dying from asthma found that New York City and Cook County, Illinois had disproportionately high mortality rates.[42] Within New York City, Carr et al.[43] demonstrated large variations of asthma mortality with the highest rates concentrated in the poorest neighborhoods. Moreover, death rates among blacks and Hispanics were shown to be 3–5.5 times those of whites. In Chicago (Cook County), Targonski et al.[44] examined trends in asthma mortality between 1968 and 1991 for persons aged 5–34 years. They also found an inverse relationship between asthma mortality and income and found blacks to have consistently higher death rates and a steeper rate of increase than whites during this time period. Similar findings were observed in Philadelphia for persons aged 5–34 years,[45] where asthma mortality rates were higher than expected based on the whole of Pennsylvania.[46]

Results from the Rochester, Minnesota, cohort study of asthma,[47] suggest that the increasing mortality rates observed may be due to increasing incidence of asthma. A marked rise in the annual incidence rate from 1964 to 1983 was observed in all age groups less than 15 years except for children younger than 1 year old, for whom annual incidence rates remained constant. Annual incidence rates also rose to a lesser degree in the 15–29, 30–49 and ≥50 age groups. This study supports the idea that it is the increase in the prevalence of asthma, rather than mismanagement of the disease, that is leading to the observed rise in asthma deaths.

Direct comparisons of asthma mortality between countries can be difficult to interpret, since practices in diagnosis and certification may differ.[48] Also, asthma mortality rates are not widely available for many countries, particularly the less developed nations.[20] However, worldwide estimates show the US, Canada, Hong Kong, and The Netherlands to have relatively low rates across all ages in comparison with other developed countries (Figure 3.8).[49]

Analyses of recent trends indicate an increase in asthma mortality rates (Figure 3.9).[50] Of note is the dramatic rise of asthma deaths observed in New Zealand between 1976 and 1980, including younger persons, and the consistently high rates reported thereafter until 1989. After formal investigation, it was concluded that this epidemic appeared to be real and not a result of changes in classification or inaccuracies of death certificates. Several factors were found to be associated with fatal asthma including lack of appreciation by the patient, family, and doctor of severity and risk of death. Implementation of self-management strategies led to the decrease in asthma mortality rate subsequently observed after 1980.[37] These management factors alone, however, could not account for the entire increase in asthma deaths that occurred, nor was there evidence that any of these factors had increased or worsened during this time period. The beta agonist fenoterol, which was introduced in 1976 and gained a 30% share of the New Zealand market during the same five-year period that mortality increased three-fold, was considered by some New Zealand researchers to be the main cause

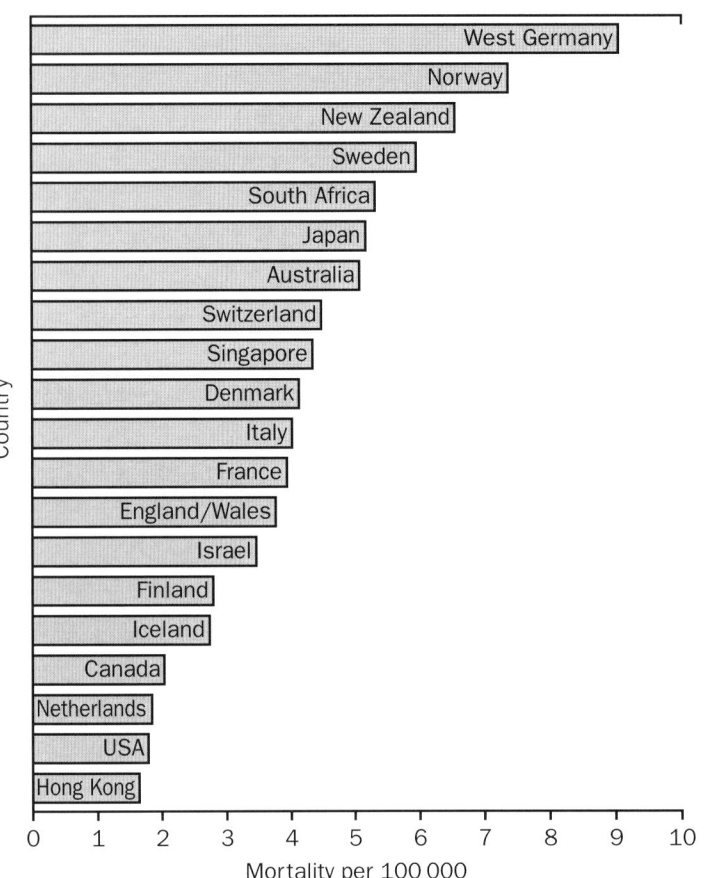

Figure 3.8 Asthma mortality in 20 countries, rate per 100 000 population, mean for 1985–1987.[49]

of the epidemic.[37] Subsequent withdrawal of the drug in 1989 was followed by a two-thirds drop in asthma mortality in a 12 month period and a return to mortality rates consistent with other countries.[37] However, this conclusion about asthma deaths and fenoterol remains controversial.

Summary

Data through the mid-1990s show a changing picture of asthma occurrence. Prevalence is rising and mortality figures show a slight upward trend. There is substantial variation by region and across countries in the frequency of the disease. The rising prevalence has been of great public health concern; hypotheses have been advanced but have not yet been fully tested.[40] The rising prevalence does not appear to reflect methodologic changes alone. Indoor air pollution has been considered as a potential factor, with emphasis placed on bioallergens. The role of pharmacologic agents in determining mortality patterns remains very controversial.

Risk factors for asthma

Risk factors are personal characteristics, acquired or genetic, that may increase the probability of disease. Information on risk factors can be used by clinicians to counsel patients and identify individuals likely to develop disease. An understanding of risk factors is also the basis for preventive strategies. A number of risk factors have been identified in the many epidemiologic studies conducted to date on the etiology of asthma: male sex, family history, respiratory infections in early life, indoor and

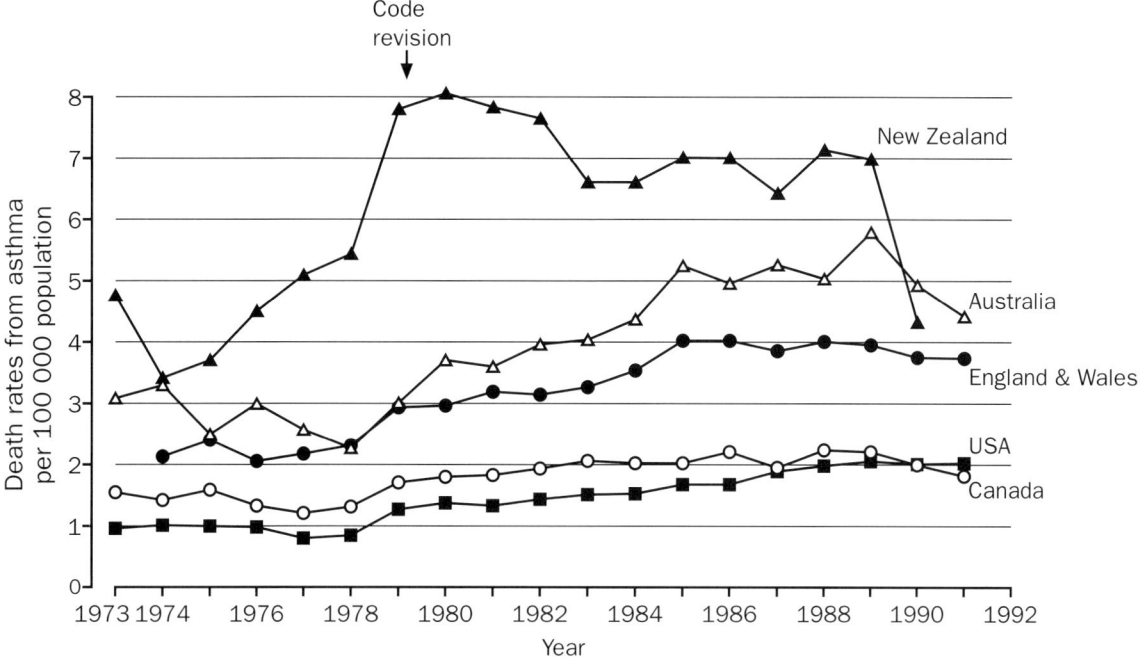

Figure 3.9 Rates of death from asthma per 100 000 general population by year in New Zealand, Australia, England and Wales, Canada, and the United States.[50]

outdoor allergens, and exposure to tobacco smoke. The evidence is primarily cross-sectional in time and the currently rising rates of asthma have not been readily explained by the available evidence, which does not provide the needed longitudinal perspective. Hypotheses for the rising asthma incidence abound, including changing patterns of respiratory infection, indoor air pollution, diet, and sedentary lifestyle, as examples. This section will review the major risk factors for asthma.

Role of gene–environment interactions

Asthma has long been held as a disease in which both genetic susceptibility and environmental factors determine the onset and the clinical picture of the disease. With the recent explosion of information on the human genome, genetic elements are now widely incorporated into research on asthma and are soon likely to be relevant to care of patients with asthma. Current concepts of asthma pathogenesis postulate that onset of the disease and its clinical course are determined by gene–environment interactions; that is, those persons who develop asthma both are genetically susceptible and receive an appropriate environmental stimulus. Across the range of asthmatics in the population, the relative influence of genes and environmental factors probably varies.

Gene–environment interactions can be assessed in case–control and cohort studies as well as in family-based genetic studies. The conceptual model assumed for gene–environment interaction is that individuals with different asthma-related genotypes will have different sensitivities to environmental exposures. Khoury et al.[51] suggested several possible patterns for gene–environment interaction. First, both the presence of a given asthma susceptibility gene and an environmental exposure are necessary to produce excess risk of disease. The second pattern is that an environmental factor could produce an increased risk of disease in all individuals, but a much greater risk in individuals with the susceptible genotype. The third possible pattern of gene–environment interaction is that the environmental exposure alone does not produce increased risk, but in individuals with the susceptible genotype the presence of the environmental factor increases the risk of asthma more than does the genotype alone. A fourth pattern is that both the genotype and the environmental exposure produce increased risk. Finally, the effect of a particular genotype may depend on whether the environmental factor is present.

Genetic/familial factors
A potential genetic component of asthma has long been hypothesized based initially on the observation that asthma tends to cluster in families, as is well known to clinicians. Subsequently, familial aggregation, twin, linkage, and association studies have provided evidence to support this hypothesis.

Family aggregation studies compare disease occurrence between different family members. The presence of disease aggregation between siblings and between parents and children supports a hereditary component, whereas increased aggregation between spouses suggests that environment is more important. However, the presence of aggregation among related individuals may represent either shared genes or a common household environment. Evidence of a hereditary component of asthma has been demonstrated in numerous family-based studies.[52–56] In addition, population-based studies have shown increased prevalence of asthma in first-degree relatives of index cases.[57–61]

Twin studies compare disease frequency in monozygotic (MZ) twins, who share 100% of their genes, versus dizygotic (DZ) twins, who share, on average, 50% of their genes. This is another method to determine the relative contribution of genetic and environmental factors. A greater occurrence of disease in MZ than in DZ twins is evidence for a genetic component to the disease, since both types of twins are assumed to share environmental factors similarly. Significantly higher concordance rates in MZ twins have been observed in some small studies.[62,63] Larger studies of twin registries also suggest a significant genetic contribution to asthma. In 6996 twin pairs from the Swedish twin registry, Edfors-Lubs[64] found the prevalence of asthma to be 3.8%. The higher concordance of asthma in MZ pairs (19.8%) over DZ (4.8%) implies that genetic factors contribute to asthma. Similarly, Duffy and coworkers[65] observed 30% concordance in MZ versus 12% in DZ twins in a total of 2902 Australian pairs.

Genetic linkage analysis is another method to elucidate underlying genetic mechanisms and find chromosomal locations of disease susceptibility genes. Several chromosomal regions have been implicated in the genetic regulation of asthma, including 5q, 6p, 11q, 12q, 13q, and 14q. In a multi-center US study, a recent screen of the entire human genome for asthma confirmed the importance of these chromosomal regions and suggested other regions (2q, 5p, 11p, 17p, 19q, and 21q) that may also be important.[66] Subsequent fine mapping of these regions promises to reveal underlying major and minor asthma susceptibility genes. Different types of association studies (including linkage disequilibrium studies) can be used to assess the importance of specific candidate genes as risk factors for asthma. Preliminary evidence from association and linkage analyses suggests the possible connection of several different genes in asthma and asthma-related phenotypes including the IgE receptor, T-cell antigen receptor, HLA class II antigens, and the β_2-adrenergic receptor.[67–71] However, causative involvement of these candidate genes has not been demonstrated and further research is needed to resolve their role in the pathogenesis of asthma.

Male sex
Data from epidemiologic studies consistently reveal male gender to be a risk factor for asthma in children. Before the age of 14 years, the prevalence of asthma in boys has been shown to be as much as twice that of girls.[60,72] As age increases, however, the difference between the sexes narrows.

One hypothesized explanation for the excess of asthma seen in boys is differing airways geometry. Boys have been shown to have smaller airways for a given lung size than girls; lower flow rates in boys age 4–6 years were found[73] in addition to higher airways resistance in comparison with girls of the same age.[74] This difference in airways anatomy could predispose boys to more wheezing and lower respiratory tract illnesses. In fact, boys have been shown to have a higher incidence of lower respiratory tract infections.[75,76]

Martinez et al.[77] also suggested that reduced lung function was a key determinant of wheezing in both boys and girls. In the Tucson study, lung function was measured within weeks of birth in 124 healthy infants. The subsequent incidence of wheezing illness over the first 6 years of life was increased in boys with high respiratory resistance and in girls with a low functional residual capacity.

Atopy
Most children with asthma have respiratory allergies, particularly to indoor allergens, and asthma and atopy are closely linked.[78] Atopy is a state of allergic response to environmental allergens, mediated by IgE.[79] Allergy plays a strong role in childhood asthma and some have hypothesized that sensitization *in utero* may occur and shape future immune responses.[78] There is no standardized definition of atopy and it is assessed in epidemiological studies in a number of ways, including total serum IgE, allergen-specific IgE, and positive skin-test reaction to allergens, or by questionnaire evaluation of diseases associated with atopy, such as infantile eczema, and allergic rhinitis. We briefly address the relationship of atopy to asthma.

Epidemiologic studies consistently show an association between atopy and asthma, although the strength of the association varies with the index used and the study population. Burrows et al.[80] assessed this association in a random sample selected from Tucson, Arizona, using skin tests with local antigens as an index of atopic status. In children age 3–14 years, atopy was strongly associated with attacks of wheezing and dyspnea, regardless of whether asthma had been diagnosed. Later analyses of the Tucson population indicated that total serum IgE was more strongly associated with the prevalence of asthma.[81] Another study using self-reported diagnosis of hay fever in a population sample from western Pennsylvania showed atopy to be more common in asthmatic than non-asthmatic children.[82] Several other studies demonstrated parental atopy and asthma as risk factors for asthma in the children.[83,84] Their results also demonstrated a complex interaction between these factors and the sex of the child.

Clearly asthma and atopy are closely linked, and their causal relationships are seemingly complex. Furthermore, causal mechanistic pathways remain elusive and require more investigation. Nonetheless, atopy in parents and children does increase the risk of asthma and can be used as an empiric predictor of likelihood of asthma.

Environmental factors
Although genetic factors may characterize the child most susceptible to developing asthma, this susceptibility may only manifest as asthma after exposure to environmental triggers. The major environmental factors that have been investigated as risk factors for asthma include aeroallergens, respiratory tract infections, outdoor or ambient air pollution, and environmental tobacco smoke.

Aeroallergens
Allergens are well-known causes of asthma exacerbations, but their role in the development of asthma has been only recently examined. A recent report from the Institute of Medicine in the United States provides a comprehensive review of the role of indoor allergens as a cause of asthma. A number of epidemiologic studies have addressed the potential role of aeroallergens, particularly indoor allergens, but most of these studies have been cross-sectional and not informative on the role of allergens in causing new cases.

Using parents' reports of dampness and mold in the home as surrogates for allergen exposure, Brunekreef et al.[85] found among a cohort of 4625 children 8–12 years of age, living in six US cities, relative risks of 1.42 (95% confidence interval 1.04–1.94) and 1.27 (95% confidence interval 0.93–1.74), respectively, for doctor-diagnosed asthma. A more direct examination of the role of allergens was conducted by Sporik et al.,[86] who enrolled 93 infants who had one parent with asthma or hay fever, and obtained baseline measurements of house-dust mite antigen in their homes. After 11 years, 67 children were re-evaluated, and 17 had asthma. The relative risk for development of asthma was 19.7 for children with skin-test sensitivity to house-dust mite, and 4.8 among children with high levels of exposure to the mite antigen during infancy. These results suggest that allergen exposure may be an important risk factor for development of childhood asthma, a conclusion supported by the Institute of Medicine review.

Respiratory tract infections

Viral infections of the lower respiratory tract occur frequently in childhood and are known to provoke wheezing in children with and without asthma.[87] Less certain, however, is the role of viral or other respiratory infections in the etiology of asthma. The inflammatory response of the airways is mediated by T-helper lymphocytes, which may be classified in Th1 or Th2 subgroups on the basis of the cytokines they generate when activated. Viral antigens have been shown to stimulate the production of cytokines associated with Th1 lymphocytes. However, studies of airways of persons with asthma show the presence of cytokines associated with the Th2 rather than the Th1 profile. Respiratory infections are hypothesized to play a role in setting the immune response phenotype and the balance between Th1 and Th2 responses.[78,88] The Th2 response leads to IgE production, eosinophilia, and airways responsiveness, whereas the Th1 response is self-limiting and results in low-level IgE only.

The 'hygiene hypothesis' proposes that slow maturation of the Th2 to the Th1 phenotype, because of lesser exposure to infectious pathogens in early life, leads to a shift towards the T2 phenotype and greater risk for asthma.[79,88–90] One consequence of a trend of declining infections may have been a shift towards a lung immunophenotype associated with greater risk for asthma. This hypothesis, although attracting substantial attention, remains untested.

Lower respiratory tract infections in children, caused by respiratory syncytial virus, parainfluenza viruses, or other pathogens, are universal in childhood. A community-based study in Tecumseh, Michigan, estimated that children experience on average 2.1 lower respiratory infections in the first year of life, and 1.5 infections between age 1 and 2 years.[76] Another cohort study of respiratory illnesses from birth through 18 months in Albuquerque, New Mexico,[91] adapted a surveillance system similar to the one used in Tecumseh and found quite comparable incidence rates from 1988 through 1992. Incidence of severe episodes of viral respiratory infections was captured in another study using surveillance through a pediatric group practice. This study showed that 25% of children were affected in the first year of life, that 12% had annual occurrences by age 5 years, and that 8% of children aged 6–8 years old experienced annual episodes of infection.[75]

Follow-up studies of children with a history of hospitalization for respiratory infections suggest these illnesses may predispose to the development of asthma. Children with past hospitalizations tended to have abnormal lung function in several studies that were indicative of airflow obstruction, including hyperinflation, increased respiratory resistance, and reduced spirometric flow rates.[92–99] In children with past hospitalizations, increased airway reactivity has also been shown after assessment by exercise, cold air inhalation, or methacholine or histamine inhalation challenge.[94–96] Since most children are not hospitalized for lower respiratory tract disease, however, these results apply only to the more severe infections. Still, a population-based study of children in East Boston, Massachusetts, also found that a history of bronchiolitis or croup was a predictor of increased airway responsiveness.[100]

The Tucson Children's Respiratory Study

offers the most relevant data in a follow-up interval that has spanned from birth to the teenage years.[101] Respiratory illnesses requiring medical treatment were tracked during the participants' first 3 years of life and respiratory symptoms and lung function were then tracked over time. Stein et al.[101] examined infection with respiratory syncytial virus infection as a predictor of subsequent wheezing and lung function level. Infection with the virus was found to be a predictor of wheezing up to age 10 years, but not at age 13 years. Infection did not predict atopic status, but another cohort study suggests that children with atopy may have higher rates of more severe respiratory illnesses.[102] Lung function was significantly lower in those with a past history of respiratory syncytial virus as well.

Mechanisms have been proposed to describe the potential relationship between viral respiratory infections and the subsequent development of asthma. A current hypothesis involves the ability of viral infections to enhance airway inflammation, a component of the asthma phenotype.[87] In the past the hypothesis has also been proposed that respiratory syncytial virus infection may promote allergic sensitization, but the supporting data are limited, and the recent report from the Tucson study does not link respiratory syncytial virus infection and atopy.[103] Several decades ago, Welliver and colleagues[104] in a study of 79 children with documented respiratory syncytial virus infection showed that some respiratory viruses can stimulate an IgE-specific response. In addition, the level of this response and the level of histamine and leukotriene C4 in nasal secretions was associated with the degree of airway obstruction in lower airway disease. Moreover, when 38 infants with respiratory syncytial virus (RSV) infection were prospectively followed for 48 months, only 20% with undetectable RSV-specific IgE titers developed episodes of wheeze, compared with 70% with high RSV IgE antibodies. This finding suggested that the ability to generate a virus-specific IgE response may be a marker for individuals with a genetic susceptibility to develop bronchial hyperresponsiveness.[105] However, whether virus-specific generation of IgE is a marker or a cause of subsequent asthma has not been established.[87]

Another similar mechanistic hypothesis suggests that viral respiratory infections increase subsequent airway hyperresponsiveness and the pattern of airway response to inhaled allergen. Results from a small group,[106] examined before and following rhinovirus infection, indicated that eight of 10 subjects experienced airway obstruction 4–8 hours after antigen inhalation (late-phase reaction) during rhinovirus infection when only one of the 10 subjects had a late-phase reaction before infection. Furthermore, five of the seven available for testing still had evidence of airway obstruction four weeks after rhinovirus inoculation. These observations suggest that viral respiratory infections may have an extended effect on factors involved in the pathogenesis of asthma.[87] However, the role of viral respiratory antigens in the etiology of asthma remains unclear and may be indirect as proposed in the 'hygiene hypothesis.'

Outdoor air pollution

Outdoor air pollutants can be classified by origin as natural or human-made. Naturally occurring air pollutants comprise particulate matter, including bioaerosols, volatile organic compounds, and ozone. The key human-made pollutants result from combustion of fossil fuels in cars, power plants, heating devices, and industrial point sources, and also emissions of chemicals from manufacturing facilities, storage tanks, and accidental releases. In the United States, air pollutants have been categorized on the basis of their regulation under the Clean Air Act as 'criteria pollutants' (lead, nitrogen dioxide, sulfur dioxide, particulate matter, ozone, and carbon monoxide) and air toxins. The latter were specified under the Clean Air Act Amendments of 1990 as a specific list of 189 chemicals, some of concern as potential causes of asthma. These same types of pollutants are generally of concern throughout the world's polluted cities and regions. Comprehensive reviews of the health effects of these pollutants have been recently published and these should be examined for in-depth review of the data on exposures and health effects.[107–109]

Outdoor air pollution is principally considered as a factor that exacerbates but does not cause asthma. There are examples of several air pollutants, however, that have been linked to the initiation of asthma. These agents have been identified through the occurrence of clusters of asthma. Responsible agents have included castor beans and soybeans.

The widespread combustion-related pollutants have not been associated with onset of asthma at current concentrations. A large body of evidence links outdoor air pollution to exacerbation of asthma.[110,111] Experimental studies have shown that the oxidant pollutants nitrogen dioxide and ozone may enhance the effects of allergens, possibly by increasing airways permeability.[112,113]

Indoor air pollution

In the home and other indoor environments, children and adults inhale diverse pollutants that may be associated with asthma risk. These pollutants include combustion-source emissions from cooking stoves and ovens, space heaters fueled by gas or kerosene, wood-burning stoves and fireplaces, and tobacco smoking; volatile and semi-volatile organic compounds released from household products, furnishings, and other sources; and allergens coming from insects and mites, rodents, pets, and other sources.[114] Whether these exposures by themselves, without underlying genetic susceptibility, can cause asthma is uncertain. However, there is mounting evidence that maternal smoking is associated with increased risk for onset of asthma as well as for exacerbation of asthma, and that levels of allergen exposure affect the incidence of asthma and wheezing.[115–117] In fact, the Environmental Protection Agency of the State of California[116] and the Scientific Committee on Tobacco in the United Kingdom[118] have concluded that tobacco smoke exposure is associated with asthma prevalence.

To date, however, there have been only limited investigations of indoor air pollution and incidence of asthma for factors other than passive exposure to tobacco smoke. With regard to combustion sources other than cigarette smoking, a number of investigations have addressed the prevalence of asthma and exposure to nitrogen oxides from cooking stoves. Homes with natural gas or propane fueled cooking stoves tend to have levels of nitrogen dioxide substantially above those of homes with electric stoves.[119] Some investigations indicate increased risk of respiratory symptoms, including wheezing, in households with gas stoves; however, the data are inconsistent and not indicative of an effect of nitrogen oxides in increasing asthma incidence. The myriad exposures to volatile and semi-volatile organic compounds that can occur in homes and other locales have not been investigated as risk factors for childhood asthma.

Studies of indoor allergens have largely focused on the status of children with asthma in relation to levels of allergen, rather than on levels of allergens as predictors of asthma.[120] A prospective cohort study in the United Kingdom reported by Sporik and colleagues[86] indicated that risk of asthma may depend on level of exposure to house dust mites across childhood. In this prospective study, 93 children were enrolled who were at high risk for asthma on the basis of having a parent with asthma or hay fever. Levels of house dust mites in the home were predictive of the later development of asthma and children with higher levels of house dust mite antigen in their homes tended to wheeze at a younger age. One prevention trial showed that reduction of allergen exposure during early childhood could postpone the appearance of allergic diseases, including asthma.[121] Further prevention trials are in progress.

A case–control study of asthma conducted by Infante-Rivard[122] examined multiple risk factors for onset of asthma, including environmental exposures and family history. In this study, characteristics of children presenting to emergency rooms with new onset of asthma were compared with those of appropriate controls. Increased risk was found for family history, as expected from the data on exacerbation, and also for certain types of indoor heating and for exposure to cigarette smoke.

Environmental tobacco smoke

The non-smoking child is exposed to environmental tobacco smoke (ETS), a name given to the mixture of the sidestream smoke released by the burning cigarette and the mainstream smoke exhaled back into the air by the smoker. Smoking adds respirable particles and gases to indoor air and it represents one the major sources of fine particles in the air of US homes.[123] Exposure of children to particles and gases in tobacco smoke has been documented by measuring personal exposures and also using biomarkers that provide an indication of the levels of tobacco smoke components that have actually been absorbed into the body. Cotinine, a major metabolite of nicotine, has been extensively investigated in children in relationship to parental smoking. Compared with children living in households where there is no smoking, children living with smokers tend to have substantially higher cotinine levels.[124,125]

Exposure to environmental tobacco smoke could both contribute to the causation of asthma and exacerbate the status of children who do have asthma. Passive smoking might exert its effect on increasing the risk for asthma by increasing risks for more severe lower respiratory tract infections during the first years of life.[126] Second, ETS might have direct toxicity and thereby induce and maintain the heightened nonspecific airways responsiveness found in asthmatic children. Third, a substantial proportion of children have ETS exposure both during gestation and after birth. Exposure to ETS might cause asthma as a long-term consequence of the increased occurrence of lower respiratory infection in early childhood or through other pathophysiological mechanisms including inflammation of the respiratory epithelium.[127,128] Assessment of airways responsiveness shortly after birth has shown that infants whose mothers smoke during pregnancy have increased airways responsiveness compared with those whose mothers do not smoke.[129] Maternal smoking during pregnancy also reduced ventilatory function measured shortly after birth.[130] These observations suggest that *in utero* exposures from maternal smoking may affect lung development, perhaps reducing relative airways size. There is evidence suggesting that *in utero* exposure to tobacco smoke components may affect airways responsiveness after birth. Young et al.[129] assessed nonspecifc airways responsiveness using histamine challenge and 63 normal infants at a mean age of 4.5 weeks. Even at this young age, parental smoking and a family history of asthma were associated with an increased level of airways responsiveness. In a similar prospective investigation, Hanrahan and colleagues found that children whose mothers smoked during pregnancy had a lower level of airways function shortly after birth.[130]

There is an extensive literature on passive smoking and childhood asthma. An early case report described an infant whose asthma was difficult to manage until the child was removed from exposure to any tobacco smoke.[131] Some studies have shown that children exposed to smoke from smoking at home have an increased frequency of wheezing, although the evidence on this association is not uniform.[126] In its 1992 risk assessment of ETS,[132] the Environmental Protection Agency reviewed the evidence on ETS as a cause and exacerbating factor for asthma. It found the evidence to be sufficient to identify parental smoking as a factor that could worsen the status of children with asthma. For example, children with parents who smoked were found to have greater bronchial responsiveness and to use medical care for their asthma more frequently. There was suggestive evidence that passive smoking could also cause asthma, although the evidence was not regarded as sufficient to warrant a labeling of this association as causal.

More recently, the California Environmental Protection Agency reviewed the evidence available through 1996, identifying 37 relevant investigations.[116] The investigations were pooled using meta-analysis with a finding of an approximately 50% increased risk for clinically diagnosed asthma and a similar increase in risk for other wheezing syndromes associated with parental smoking. A similar synthesis by Cook and Strachan[133] shows a significant excess of childhood asthma if both parents or the mother smoke. Thus, the weight of evidence increasingly indicates a causal association of childhood asthma with ETS exposure.

Evidence also indicates that involuntary smoking worsens the status of those with asthma. The possibility that ETS adversely affects children with asthma was described as early as 1950 in a case report entitled 'Bronchial asthma due to allergy to tobacco smoke in an infant'.[131] More recently Murray and Morrison[134,135] evaluated asthmatic children followed in a clinic. Level of lung function, symptom frequency, and responsiveness to inhaled histamines were adversely affected by maternal smoking. Population studies have also shown increased airways responsiveness for ETS-exposed children with asthma.[136,137] The increased level of airway responsiveness associated with ETS exposure would be expected to increase the clinical severity of asthma. In this regard exposure to smoking in the home has been shown to increase the number of emergency room visits made by asthmatic children.[138] Asthmatic children with smoking mothers are more likely to use asthma medications,[139] a finding that confirms the clinically significant effects of ETS on children with asthma. Guidelines for the management of asthma all urge reduction of ETS exposure at home.[140]

Determinants of the natural history of asthma

Gender
Asthma is more frequent in boys than in girls but gender does not appear to affect the course of the disease. In the early studies of Rackenmann and Edwards[141] and Blair,[142] clinical course was comparable over 20 year follow-up intervals in males and females. Findings of the Australian cohort study, initiated by McNicol and Williams,[143] suggested that the course in early adulthood might be more favorable in women.[144] Between age 21 and 28 years, significantly more men than women had moved to a more severely symptomatic group.

Age and severity of onset
The early clinic-based studies provided conflicting information regarding age of onset and the course of childhood asthma.[145] More recent prospective cohort studies have shown that wheezing in infancy and early childhood has a different natural history from wheezing of later onset and does not necessarily constitute asthma.[2,146] In the follow-up study of the 1958 birth cohort in the United Kingdom, at age 33 years, those with the most recent onset of wheezing tended to be more symptomatic than those whose wheezing was first reported before age 7 years. Although age of onset may not be a strong predictor of the course of childhood asthma, initial severity may be a useful clinical marker.[142,143]

Atopic status
Indicators of atopy have been associated with poorer prognosis in several studies. In the early study of Buffum and Settipane,[147] children with eczema and positive skin tests had more severe asthma. Persistence of eczema has also been associated with persistence of asthma.[142] The findings were similar in the follow-up of the 1958 United Kingdom birth cohort.[148] Of those with asthma or wheezy bronchitis by age 16, a report of wheezing during the past year was approximately twice as common in those with a report of hay fever, allergic rhinitis, or eczema compared with those with this history. Atopy was also associated with persistent wheezing in the cohort study of babies at high risk for allergic diseases conducted by Sporik and colleagues.[149]

Family history
A family history of asthma has been shown to increase a child's risk for persistent disease in several studies.[142,150] These limited data will undoubtedly be followed by more informative studies of genotype and prognosis in the future.

Smoking
Smoking during adolescence and young adulthood has been associated with increased risk for the persistence of symptoms. In the 1958 birth cohort study in the United Kingdom,

relapse at age 33 years was more common among current smokers.[148] In a 25 year follow-up study of children originally enrolled in a school survey in Aberdeen, smoking was associated with an increased risk for wheezing and other symptoms.[151]

Treatment

Although treatment has been shown to substantially benefit the status of children with asthma, there are no data available to indicate that the natural history of the disease is altered by early intervention or intensive therapy. In the study in Australia, severity of asthma at age 21 years was not related to intensity of therapy reported at earlier evaluations.[144] The Childhood Asthma Management Program (CAMP), a randomized trial funded by the National Heart, Lung and Blood Institute, is presently testing the hypothesis that intensive and regular treatment may favorably affect the natural history of childhood asthma.

SUMMARY

Epidemiologic data have provided substantial insights into the patterns of occurrence of pediatric asthma and the factors that determine risks for the disease. Incidence has been described and its natural history has been evaluated. Striking variation in the frequency of childhood asthma has been demonstrated, comparing urban, inner-city areas and suburban and rural areas in the United States, and across countries. The prevalence of pediatric asthma has been convincingly shown to be rising in a number of developed countries. Methodologic differences in the techniques used to identify persons as having asthma do not appear to be the sole explanation. Mortality from asthma has again risen in a number of countries.

The rising prevalence of asthma has sparked speculation about changes in risk factors for asthma, particularly related to indoor air pollution and respiratory infections. However, definitive research has not yet been conducted to test these hypotheses; neither have the periodic fluctuations of asthma mortality been fully explained. The epidemic asthma mortality of the 1960s was attributed to the use of specific, potent bronchodilators, and similar concerns about therapeutic agents have been raised in relation to the more recent rise in asthma mortality. Epidemiologic studies have provided an indication that drug therapy could be playing a role, although observational data have inherent limitations for isolating the effects of therapy, since the more severe asthmatics tend to be treated more aggressively.

A number of risk factors have been identified for the development of asthma. For some—indoor allergens and tobacco smoke exposure—the evidence is sufficient to warrant programs of intervention. Current concepts of the pathogenesis of asthma emphasize gene–environment interaction; we do not yet know, however, how genes and environmental factors act together to determine asthma risks. Future research, incorporating genetic marks of susceptibility, will ultimately be informative for clinicians and for those concerned with preventing asthma.

REFERENCES

1. Gordis L. *Epidemiology* 2nd ed. Philadelphia: WB Saunders, 2000.
2. Martinez FD, Wright AL, Taussig LM, Holberg CJ, Halonen M, Morgan WJ. Asthma and wheezing in the first six years of life. The Group Health Medical Associates. *N Engl J Med* 1995; **332**(3): 133–8.
3. Fletcher CM, Gilson JG, Hugh-Jones P, Scadding JG. Terminology, definitions, and classification of chronic pulmonary emphysema and related conditions. A report of the conclusions of a CIBA guest symposium. *Thorax* 1959; **14**: 286–99.
4. American Thoracic Society. Chronic bronchitis, asthma, and pulmonary emphysema. *Am Rev Respir Dis* 1962; **85**: 762–8.
5. American College of Chest Physicians, American Thoracic Society. Pulmonary terms and symbols. *Chest* 1975; **67**: 583–93.
6. World Health Organization. Epidemiology of chronic nonspecific respiratory diseases. *Bull World Health Organ* 1975; **52**: 251–9.
7. American Thoracic Society, American Lung

Association, Medical Section. Standards for the diagnosis and care of patients with chronic obstructive pulmonary disease (COPD) and asthma. *Am Rev Respir Dis* 1987; **136:** 225–44.
8. National Institutes of Health. *Expert Panel Report on Guidelines for Diagnosis and Management of Asthma.* Bethesda, MD: National Heart, Lung, and Blood Institute Information Center, 1991.
9. Ciba Foundation Study Group. *Identification of Asthma.* Edinburgh: Churchill Livingstone, 1971.
10. Ferris BG. Epidemiology standardization project. *Am Rev Respir Dis* 1978; **188:** 1–53.
11. Beasley R, Keil U, Von Mutius E, Pearce N, ISAAC Steering Committee. Worldwide variation in prevalence of symptoms of asthma, allergic rhinoconjunctivitis, and atopic eczema: ISAAC. *Lancet* 1998; **351:** 1225–32.
12. Asher MI, Keil U, Anderson HR, Beasley R, Crane J, Martinez F et al. International study of asthma and allergies in childhood (ISAAC): rationale and methods. *Eur Respir J* 1995; **8:** 483–91.
13. Taussig LM, Smith SM, Blumenfeld R. Chronic bronchitis in childhood: what is it? *Pediatrics* 1981; **67**(1): 1–5.
14. Speight ANP, Lee DA, Hey EN, McDonald JC. Underdiagnosis and undertreatment of asthma in childhood. *Br Med J* 1983; **286:** 1253–6.
15. Evans R 3rd, Mullally DI, Wilson RW, Gergen PJ, Rosenberg HM, Grauman JS et al. National trends in the morbidity and mortality of asthma in the US. Prevalence, hospitalization and death from asthma over two decades: 1965–1984. *Chest* 1987; **91**(6 suppl): 65S–74S.
16. Williams H, McNicol KN. Prevalence, natural history, and relationship of wheezy bronchitis and asthma in children. An epidemiological study. *Br Med J* 1969; **4:** 321–5.
17. Benson V, Marano MA. Current estimates from the National Health Interview Survey, 1995. *Vital Health Stat* 1998; **199:** 1–428.
18. Coultas DB, Gong H Jr, Grad R et al. Respiratory diseases in minorities of the United States. *Am J Resp Crit Care Med* 1993; **149:** S93–S131.
19. Current trends asthma—United States, 1982–1992. *MMWR* 1995; **43**(51): 952–5.
20. National Heart, Lung and Blood Institute. Global Initiative for Asthma. Washington, DC: US Government Printing Office, 1995.
21. Aberg N. Asthma and allergic rhinitis in Swedish conscripts. *Clin Exp Allergy* 1989; **19:** 59–63.
22. Haahtela T, Lindholm H, Bjorksten F, Koskenvuo K, Laitinen LA. Prevalence of asthma in Finnish young men. *Br Med J* 1990; **301:** 266–8.
23. Burney PGJ, Chinn S, Rona RJ. Has the prevalence of asthma increased in children? Evidence from the national study of health and growth 1973–1986. *Br Med J* 1990; **300:** 1306–10.
24. Robertson CF, Heycock E, Bishop J, Nolan T, Olinsky A, Phelan PD. Prevalence of asthma in Melbourne schoolchildren: changes over 26 years. *Br Med J* 1991; **302:** 1116–18.
25. Shaw RA, Crane J, O'Donnell TV. Prevalence of asthma in children. *Br Med J* 1990; **300:** 1652–3.
26. Perdrizet S, Neukirch F, Cooreman J, Liard R. Prevalence of asthma in adolescents in various parts of France and its relationship to respiratory allergic manifestations. *Chest* 1987; **91**(6 suppl): 104S–106S.
27. Lai CKW, Douglass SS, Chan J, Lau J, Wong G, Leung R. Asthma epidemiology in the Far East. *Clin Exp Allergy* 1996; **26:** 5–12.
28. American Thoracic Society. Standardization of spirometry—1987 update. *Am Rev Respir Dis* 1987; **136:** 1285–98.
29. American Thoracic Society, American Lung Association, Medical Section. ATS statement—Snowbird workshop on standardization of spirometry. *Am Rev Respir Dis* 1979; **119:** 831–8.
30. Chatham M, Bleecker ER, Smith PL, Rosenthal RR, Mason P, Norman PS. A comparison of histamine, methacholine, and exercise airway reactivity in normal and asthmatic subjects. *Am Rev Respir Dis* 1982; **126:** 235–40.
31. Zhong NS, Chen RC, O-yang M, Wu JY, Fu WX, Shi LJ. Bronchial hyperresponsiveness in young students of southern China: relation to respiratory symptoms, diagnosed asthma, and risk factors. *Thorax* 1990; **45:** 860–5.
32. Larsson L. Incidence of asthma in Swedish teenagers: relation to sex and smoking habits. *Thorax* 1994; **50:** 260–4.
33. Silverstein MD, Reed CE, O'Connell EJ, Melton LJ III, O'Fallon WM, Yunginger JW. Long-term survival of a cohort of community residents with asthma. *N Engl J Med* 1994; **331:** 1537–41.
34. Centers for Disease Control and Prevention (CDC). Asthma mortality and hospitalization among children and young adults—United States, 1980–1993. *MMWR* 1996; **45:** 350–3.
35. Burt CW, Knapp DE. Ambulatory care visits for

asthma: United States, 1993–94. *Adv Data* 1996; Sept 27(277): 1.
36. Vollmer WM, Osborne ML, Buist AS. Temporal trends in hospital-based episodes of asthma care in a health maintenance organization. *Am Rev Respir Dis* 1993; **147:** 347–53.
37. Beasley R, Burgess C, Crane J, Pearce N. A review of the studies of the asthma mortality epidemic in New Zealand. *Allergy Proc* 1995; **16:** 27–32.
38. Klebba AJ, Scott JH. *Estimates of Selected Comparability Ratios Based on Dual Coding of 1976 Death Certificates by the Eighth and Ninth Revisions of the International Classification of Diseases.* DHEW Publication No. 80-1120. Washington, DC: Superintendent of Documents, G.P.O., 1980.
39. Stewart CJ, Nunn AJ. Are asthma mortality rates changing? *Br J Dis Chest* 1985; **79:** 229–34.
40. Weiss KB, Gergen PJ, Wagener DK. Breathing better or breathing worse? The changing epidemiology of asthma morbidity and mortality. In: Omenn GS, Lave LB, eds. *Annual Review of Public Health.* Palo Alto: Annual Reviews, 1993, 491–513.
41. Arrighi MH. US asthma mortality: 1941 to 1989. *Ann Allergy Asthma Immunol* 1995; **74:** 321–6.
42. Weiss KB, Wagener DK. Changing patterns of asthma mortality. Identifying target populations at high risk. *JAMA* 1990; **264**(13): 1683–7.
43. Carr W, Zeitel L, Weiss K. Variations in asthma hospitalizations and deaths in New York City. *Am J Public Health* 1992; **82:** 59–65.
44. Targonski P, Persky V, Orris P, Addington W. Trends in asthma mortality among African-Americans and whites in Chicago, 1968 through 1991. *Am J Public Health* 1994; **84:** 1830–3.
45. Lang DM, Polansky M. Patterns of asthma mortality in Philadelphia from 1969 to 1991. *N Engl J Med* 1994; **331**(23): 1542–6.
46. Kaplan KM. Epidemiology of deaths from asthma in Pennsylvania, 1978–87. *Public Health Rep* 1993; **108:** 66–9.
47. Yunginger JW, Reed CE, O'Connell CJ III et al. A community-based study of the epidemiology of asthma, incidence rates, 1964–1983. *Am Rev Respir Dis* 1992; **146**(4): 888–94.
48. Burney PGJ, Clark TJH, Godfrey S, Lee HH, eds. *Asthma.* London: Chapman & Hall, 1992, 254–307.
49. Sears MR. Worldwide trends in asthma mortality. *Bull Int Union Tuberc Lung Dis* 1991; **66:** 79–83.
50. Sly M. Changing asthma mortality. *Ann Allergy* 1994; **73:** 259–68.
51. Khoury MJ, Beaty TH, Cohen BH. *Fundamentals of Genetic Epidemiology.* New York: Oxford University Press, 1993.
52. Longo G, Strinati R, Poli F, Fumi F. Genetic factors in nonspecific bronchial hyperreactivity. An epidemiologic study. *Am J Dis Child* 1987; **141**(3): 331–4.
53. Holberg CJ, Elston RC, Halonen M, Wright AL, Taussig LM, Morgan WJ et al. Segregation analysis of physician-diagnosed asthma in Hispanic and non-Hispanic white females. A recessive component? *Am J Resp Crit Care Med* 1996; **154:** 144–50.
54. Martinez FD, Holberg CJ. Segregation analysis of physician diagnosed asthma in Hispanic and non-Hispanic white families. *Respiratory Sciences* 1995; **14:** 2–8.
55. Townley RG, Bewtra A, Wilson AF et al. Segregation analysis of bronchial response to methacholine inhalation challenge in families with and without asthma. *J Allergy Clin Immunol* 1986; **77:** 101–7.
56. Panhuysen CIM, Xu J, Postma DS et al. Evidence for a major locus for bronchial hyper-responsiveness independent of the locus regulating total serum IgE levels. *Am J Hum Genet* 1996; **59:** A231.
57. Higgins M, Keller J. Familial occurrence of chronic respiratory disease and familial resemblance in ventilatory capacity. *J Chronic Dis* 1975; **28:** 239–51.
58. Lebowitz MD, Knudson RJ, Burrows B. Family aggregation of pulmonary function measurements. *Am Rev Respir Dis* 1984; **129:** 8–11.
59. Leeder SR, Corkhill R, Irwig LM, Holland WW, Colley JRT. Influence of family factors on the incidence of lower respiratory illness during the first year of life. *Br J Prev Soc Med* 1976; **30:** 203–12.
60. Horwood LJ, Fergusson DM, Shannon FT. Social and familial factors in the development of early childhood asthma. *Pediatrics* 1985; **75:** 859–68.
61. Sibbald B, Turner-Warwick M. Factors influencing the prevalence of asthma among first degree relatives of extrinsic and intrinsic asthmatics. *Thorax* 1979; **34:** 332–7.
62. Redline S, Tishler PV, Lewitter FI, Tager IB, Muñoz A, Speizer FE. Assessment of genetic and nongenetic influences on pulmonary function. A twin study. *Am Rev Respir Dis* 1987; **135**(1): 217–22.

63. Hopp RJ, Bewtra AK, Watt GD, Nair NM, Townley RG. Genetic analysis of allergic disease in twins. *J Allergy Clin Immunol* 1984; **73**: 265–70.
64. Edfors-Lubs ML. Allergy in 7000 twin pairs. *Acta Allergol* 1971; **26**: 249–85.
65. Duffy DL, Nicholas MG, Battistutta D, Hopper JL, Mathews JD. Genetics of asthma and hay fever in Australian twins. *Am Rev Respir Dis* 1990; **142**: 1351–8.
66. Collaborative Study on the Genetics of Asthma. A genome-wide search for asthma susceptibility loci in ethnically diverse populations. *Nature Genetics* 1997; **15**(4): 389–92.
67. Reihsaus E, Innis M, MacIntyre N, Liggett SB. Mutations in the gene encoding for the beta2-adrenergic receptor in normal and asthmatic subjects. *Am J Respir Cell Mol Biol* 1993; **8**: 334–9.
68. Sandford AJ, Shirakawa T, Moffatt MF et al. Localisation of atopy and beta subunit of high-affinity IgE receptor on chromosome 11q. *Lancet* 1993; **341**: 332–4.
69. Postma DS, Bleecker ER, Amelung PJ et al. Genetic susceptibility to asthma: bronchial hyperresponsiveness coinherited with a major gene for atopy. *N Engl J Med* 1995; **333**(14): 894–900.
70. Cookson WOCM, Young RP, Sandford AJ, Moffatt MF, Shirakawa T, Sharp PA et al. Maternal inheritance of atopic IgE responsiveness on chromosome 11q. *Lancet* 1992; **340**: 381–4.
71. Moffatt MF, Hill MR, Cornelis F et al. Genetic linkage of T-cell receptor complex to specific IgE responses. *Lancet* 1994; **343**: 1597–600.
72. Schachter EN, Doyle CA, Beck GJ. A prospective study of asthma in a rural community. *Chest* 1984; **85**(5): 623–30.
73. Taussig LM. Maximal expiratory flows at functional residual capacity: a test of lung function for young children. *Am Rev Respir Dis* 1977; **116**: 1031–8.
74. Doershuk CF, Fisher BJ, Matthews LW. Specific airway resistance from the perinatal period into adulthood. Alterations in childhood pulmonary disease. *Am Rev Respir Dis* 1974; **109**: 452–7.
75. Glezen WP, Denny FW. Epidemiology of acute lower respiratory disease in children. *N Engl J Med* 1973; **288**:(10): 498–505.
76. Monto AS, Ullman BM. Acute respiratory illness in an American community. The Tecumseh study. *JAMA* 1974; **227**(2): 164–9.
77. Martinez FD, Morgan WJ, Wright AL, Holberg CJ, Taussig LM, Group Health Medical Associates. Diminished lung function as a predisposing factor for wheezing. Respiratory illness in infants. *N Engl J Med* 1988; **319**: 1112–17.
78. Gern JE, Lemanske RF, Jr, Busse WW. Early life origins of asthma. *J Clin Invest* 1999; **104**(7): 837–43.
79. Shirakawa T, Enomoto T, Shin-inchiro S, Hopkin JM. The inverse association between tuberculin responses and atopic disorder. *Science* 1997; **275**: 77–9.
80. Burrows B, Lebowitz MD, Barbee RA. Respiratory disorders and allergy skin-test reactions. *Ann Intern Med* 1976; **84**(2): 134–9.
81. Burrows B, Martinez FD, Halonen M, Barbee RA, Cline MG. Association of asthma with serum IgE levels and skin-test reactivity to allergens. *N Engl J Med* 1989; **320**(5): 271–7.
82. Schenker MB, Samet JM, Speizer FE. Risk factors for childhood respiratory disease: the effect of host factors and home environmental exposures. *Am Rev Respir Dis* 1983; **128**: 1038–43.
83. Davis JB, Bulpitt CJ. Atopy and wheeze in children according to parental atopy and family size. *Thorax* 1981; **36**: 185–9.
84. Fergusson DM, Horwood LJ, Shannon FT. Parental asthma, parental eczema, and asthma and eczema in early childhood. *J Chronic Dis* 1983; **36**(7): 517–24.
85. Brunekreef B, Dockery DW, Speizer FE. Home dampness and respiratory morbidity in children. *Am Rev Respir Dis* 1989; **140**: 1363–7.
86. Sporik R, Holgate ST, Platts-Mills TA, Cogswell JJ. Exposure to house-dust mite allergen (Der p 1) and the development of asthma in childhood. A prospective study. *N Engl J Med* 1990; **323**(8): 502–7.
87. Busse WW, Lemanske RF Jr, Dick EC. The relationship of viral respiratory infections and asthma. *Chest* 1992; **101**: 385S–388S.
88. Martinez FD, Holt PG. Role of microbial burden in aetiology of allergy and asthma. *Lancet* 1999; **354**(suppl 2): 12–15.
89. Holgate ST. Asthma genetics: waiting to exhale. *Nature Genetics* 1997; **15**: 227–9.
90. Cookson WOC, Moffatt MF. Asthma: an epidemic in the absence of infection? *Science* 1997; **275**: 41–3.
91. Samet JM, Cushing AH, Lambert WE, Hunt WC, McLaren LC, Young SA et al. Comparability of parent-reported respiratory illnesses to clinical diagnoses. *Am Rev Respir Dis*

1993; **148:** 441–6.
92. Stokes GM, Milner AD, Hodges IGC, Groggins RC. Lung function abnormalities after acute bronchiolitis. *Pediatrics* 1981; **98:** 871–4.
93. Kattan M, Keens TG, Lapierre JG, Levison H, Bryan C, Reilly BJ. Pulmonary function abnormalities in symptom-free children after bronchiolitis. *Pediatrics* 1977; **59**(5): 683–8.
94. Sims DG, Downham MAPS, Gardner PS, Webb JKG, Weightman D. Study of 8-year-old children with a history of respiratory syncytial virus bronchiolitis in infancy. *Br Med J* 1978; **1:** 11–14.
95. Gurwitz D, Mindorff C, Levison H. Increased incidence of bronchial reactivity in children with a history of bronchiolitis. *J Pediatr* 1981; **98:** 551–5.
96. Pullan CR, Hey EN. Wheezing, asthma, and pulmonary dysfunction 10 years after infection with respiratory syncytial virus in infancy. *Br Med J* 1982; **284:** 1665–9.
97. Henry RL, Hodges IGC, Milner AD, Stokes GM. Respiratory problems 2 years after acute bronchiolitis in infancy. *Arch Dis Child* 1983; **58:** 713–16.
98. Hall CB, Hall WJ, Gala CL, MaGill FB, Leddy JP. Long-term prospective study in children after respiratory syncytial virus infection. *J Pediatr* 1984; **105:** 358–64.
99. McConnochie KM, Hall CB, Barker WH. Lower respiratory tract illness in the first two years of life: epidemiologic patterns and costs in a suburban pediatric practice. *Am J Public Health* 1988; **78**(1): 34–9.
100. Weiss ST, Tager IB, Muñoz A, Speizer FE. The relationship of respiratory infections in early childhood to the occurrence of increased levels of bronchial responsiveness and atopy. *Am Rev Respir Dis* 1985; **131:** 573–8.
101. Stein RT, Sherrill D, Morgan WJ, Holberg CJ, Halonen M, Taussig LM et al. Respiratory syncytial virus in early life and risk of wheeze and allergy by age 13 years. *Lancet* 1999; **354:** 541–5.
102. Bosken CH, Hunt WC, Lambert WE, Samet JM. A parental history of asthma is a risk factor for wheezing and non-wheezing respiratory illnesses in infants younger than 18 months of age. *Am J Resp Crit Care Med* 2000; **161:** 1810–15.
103. Everard ML. What link between early respiratory viral infections and atopic asthma? *Lancet* 1999; **354**(9178): 527–8.
104. Welliver RC, Wong DT, Sun M. The development of respiratory syncytial virus specific IgE and the release of histamine in nasopharyngeal secretions. *N Engl J Med* 1981; **305:** 841–6.
105. Welliver RC, Sun M, Rinaldo D. Predictive value of respiratory syncytial virus-specific IgE response for recurrent wheezing following bronchiolitis. *J Pediatr* 1986; **109:** 776–80.
106. Lemanske RF Jr, Dick EC, Swenson CA. Rhinovirus upper respiratory infection increases airway reactivity in late asthmatic reactions. *J Clin Invest* 1989; **83:** 1–10.
107. American Thoracic Society, Committee of the Environmental and Occupational Health Assembly, Bascom R, Bromberg PA, Costa DA, Devlin R, Dockery DW, Frampton MW et al. Health effects of outdoor air pollution. Part 2. *Am J Resp Crit Care Med* 1996; **153:** 477–98.
108. Denison D, Mallick B, Smith A. Automatic Bayesian curve fitting. *J Royal Stat Soc Series B* 1998; **60:** 333–50.
109. Holgate ST, Samet JM, Koren HS, Maynard RL, eds. *Air Pollution and Health.* San Diego: Academic Press, 1999.
110. Thurston GD, Ito K. Epidemiological studies of ozone exposure effects. In: Holgate ST, Samet JM, Koren HS, Maynard RL, eds. *Air Pollution and Health.* San Diego: Academic Press, 1999, 485–510.
111. Pope CA III, Dockery DW. Epidemiology of particle effects. In: Holgate ST, Samet JM, Koren HS, Maynard RL, eds. *Air Pollution and Health.* San Diego: Academic Press, 1999, 673–705.
112. Molfino NA, Wright FC, Katz I et al. Effect of low concentrations of ozone on inhaled allergen responses in asthmatic subjects. *Lancet* 1991; **338:** 199–203.
113. Devalia JL, Rusznak C, Herdman MJ, Trigg CJ, Tarraf H, Davies RJ. Effect of nitrogen dioxide and sulfur dioxide on airway responses of mild asthmatic patients to allergen inhalation. *Lancet* 1994; **344:** 1668–71.
114. Spengler JD. Sources and concentrations of indoor air pollution. In: Samet JM, Spengler JD, eds. *Indoor Air Pollution. A Health Perspective.* Baltimore: Johns Hopkins University Press, 1991, 33–67.
115. Strachan DP, Cook DG. Health effects of passive smoking. 1. Parental smoking and lower respiratory illness in infancy and early childhood. *Thorax* 1997; **52**(10): 905–14.
116. California Environmental Protection Agency, Office of Environmental Health Hazard Assessment. *Health Effects of Exposure to Environmental Tobacco Smoke.* Sacramento, CA:

California Environmental Protection Agency, 1997.
117. WHO. *International Consultation on Environmental Tobacco Smoke (ETS) and Child Health. Consultation Report.* Geneva: World Health Organization, 1999.
118. Scientific Committee on Tobacco and Health. *Report of the Scientific Committee on Tobacco and Health.* London: HMSO, 1998.
119. Samet JM, Spengler JD, eds. *Indoor Air Pollution. A Health Perspective.* Baltimore: Johns Hopkins University Press, 1991, 170–86.
120. Institute of Medicine, Committee on the Health Effects of Indoor Allergens, Division of Health Promotion and Disease Prevention, Pope AM, Patterson R, Burge H, eds. *Indoor Allergens: Assessing the Controlling Adverse Health Effects.* Washington: National Academy Press, 1993.
121. Hide DW. Matthews S, Tariq S, Arshad SH. Allergen avoidance in infancy and allergy at 4 years of age. *Allergy* 1996; **51:** 89–93.
122. Infante-Rivard C. Childhood asthma and indoor environmental risk factors. *Am J Epidemiol* 1993; **137**(8) 834–44.
123. Guerin MR, Jenkins RA, Tomkins BA, Center for Indoor Air Research, eds. *The Chemistry of Environmental Tobacco Smoke: Composition and Measurement.* Chelsea, MI: Lewis Publishers, 1992.
124. Pirkle JL, Flegal KM, Bernert JT, Brody DJ, Etzel RA, Maurer KR. Exposure of the US population to environmental tobacco smoke. The Third National Health and Nutrition Examination Survey, 1988 to 1991. *JAMA* 1996; **275**(16): 1233–40.
125. Samet JM, Wang SS. Environmental tobacco smoke. In: Lippmann M, ed. *Environmental Toxicants: Human Exposures and Their Health Effects,* 2nd edn. New York: Van Nostrand Reinhold, 2000, 319–75.
126. US Department of Health and Human Services. *U.S. Public Health Services: The Health Consequences of Involuntary Smoking. Report of the Surgeon General.* Public Health Service, Office of the Assistant Secretary of Health, Office of Smoking and Health. Washington, DC: Government Printing Office, 1986.
127. Samet JM, Tager IB, Speizer FE. The relationship between respiratory illness in childhood and chronic airflow obstruction in adulthood. *Am Rev Respir Dis* 1983; **127:** 508–23.
128. Tager IB. Passive smoking-bronchial responsiveness and atopy. *Am Rev Respir Dis* 1988; **138:** 507–9.
129. Young S, Le Souef PN, Geelhoed GC, Stick SM, Turner KJ, Landau LI. The influence of a family history of asthma and parental smoking on airway responsiveness in early infancy. *N Engl J Med* 1991; **324**(17): 1168–73.
130. Hanrahan JP, Tager IB, Segal MR, Tosteson TD, Castile RG, Van Vunakis H et al. The effect of maternal smoking during pregnancy on early infant lung function. *Am Rev Respir Dis* 1992; **145:** 1129–35.
131. Rosen FL, Levy A. Bronchial asthma due to allergy to tobacco smoke in an infant: a case report. *JAMA* 1950; **144**(8): 620–1.
132. US Environmental Protection Agency. *Respiratory Health Effects of Passive Smoking: Lung Cancer and Other Disorders.* Washington: US Government Printing Office, 1992.
133. Cook DG, Strachan DP. Parental smoking and prevalence of respiratory symptoms and asthma in school age children. *Thorax* 1997; **52**(12): 1081–94.
134. Murray AB, Morrison BJ. The effect of cigarette smoke from the mother on bronchial responsiveness and severity of symptoms in children with asthma. *J Allergy Clin Immunol* 1986; **77**(4): 575–81.
135. Murray AB, Morrison BJ. Passive smoking by asthmatics: its greater effect on boys than on girls and on older than on younger children. *Pediatrics* 1989; **84**(3): 451–9.
136. O'Connor GT, Weiss ST, Tager IB, Speizer FE. The effect of passive smoking on pulmonary function and nonspecific bronchial responsiveness in a population-based sample of children and young adults. *Am Rev Respir Dis* 1987; **135:** 800–4.
137. Martinez FD, Antognoni G, Macri F, Bonci E, Midulla F, DeCastro G et al. Parental smoking enhances bronchial responsiveness in nine-year-old children. *Am Rev Respir Dis* 1988; **138:** 518–23.
138. Evans D, Levison MJ, Feldman CH, Clark NM, Wasilewski Y, Levin B et al. The impact of passive smoking on emergency room visits of urban children with asthma. *Am Rev Respir Dis* 1987; **135:** 567–72.
139. Weitzman M, Gortmaker S, Walker DK, Sobol A. Maternal smoking and childhood asthma. *Pediatrics* 1990; **85**(4): 505–11.
140. US Department of Health and Human Services, Public Health Service, National Institute of

Health et al. *Practical Guide for the Diagnosis and Management of Asthma.* Bethesda, MD: NIH, 1997.
141. Rackemann FM, Edwards MC. Asthma in children. A follow-up study of 688 patients after an interval of twenty years. *N Engl J Med* 1952; **246:** 815–23.
142. Blair H. Natural history of childhood asthma. 20-year follow-up. *Arch Dis Child* 1977; **52:** 613–19.
143. McNicol KN, Williams HB, Spectrum of asthma in children. I. Clinical and physiological components. *Br Med J* 1973; **4:** 7–11.
144. Kelly WJ, Hudson I, Phelan PD, Pain MC, Olinsky A. Childhood asthma in adult life: a further study at 28 years of age. *Brit Med J [Clin Res Ed]* 1987; **294:** 1059–62.
145. Coultas DB, Samet JM. Epidemiology and natural history of childhood asthma. In: Tinkelman DG, Naspitz CG, eds. *Childhood Asthma.* New York: Marcel Dekker, 1993, 71–114.
146. Silverman M. Out of the mouths of babes and sucklings. Lessons from early childhood asthma. *Thorax* 1993; **48:** 1200–4.
147. Buffum WP, Settipane GA. Prognosis of asthma in childhood. *Am J Dis Child* 1966; **112:** 214–17.
148. Strachan DP, Butland BK, Anderson HR. Incidence and prognosis of asthma and wheezing illness from early childhood to age 33 in a national British cohort. *BMJ* 1996; **312:** 1195–9.
149. Sporik R, Holgate ST, Cogswell JJ. Natural history of asthma in childhood—a birth cohort study. *Arch Dis Child* 1991; **66**(9): 1050–3.
150. Foucard T, Sjoberg O. A prospective 12-year follow-up study of children with wheezy bronchitis. *Acta Paediatr Scand* 1984; **73:** 577–83.
151. Godden D, Ross S, Abdalla M et al. Outcome of wheeze in childhood. Symptoms and pulmonary function 25 years later. *Am J Resp Crit Care Med* 1994; **149:** 106–12.
152. US Department of Health and Human Services. *Guidelines for the Diagnosis and Management of Asthma. National Asthma Education Program Expert Panel Report.* Bethesda, MD: US Government Printing Office, 1991.
153. National Heart, Lung and Blood Institute and World Health Organization. *Global Initiative for Asthma.* Washington: US Government Printing Office, 1993.
154. National Heart, Lung and Blood Institute and National Institute of Health. *Guidelines for the Diagnosis and Management of Asthma.* Bethesda, MD: Department of Health and Human Services, 1995.
155. Omran M, Russell G. Continuing increase in respiratory symptoms and atopy in Aberdeen schoolchildren. *Br Med J* 1996; **312:** 34.
156. Liard R, Chansin R, Neukirch F, Levallois M, Leproux P. Prevalence of asthma among teenagers attending school in Tahiti. *J Epidemiol Community Health* 1988; **42**(2): 149–51.
157. Chaulet P. Asthma and chronic bronchitis in Africa. Evidence from epidemiologic studies. *Chest* 1989; **96:** 334S–339S.
158. Carrasco E. Epidemiologic aspects of asthma in Latin America. *Chest* 1987; **91**(6 suppl): 93S–97S.
159. Nicolai T, Mutius EV, Reitmeir P, Wjst M. Reactivity to cold-air hyperventilation in normal and in asthmatic children in a survey of 5,697 schoolchildren in southern Bavaria. *Am Rev Respir Dis* 1993; **147:** 565–72.
160. Hurry VM, Peat JK, Woolcock AJ. Prevalence of respiratory symptoms, bronchial hyperresponsiveness and atopy in school children living in the villawood area of Sydney. *Aust N Z J Med* 1988; **18:** 745–51.
161. Peat JK, Britton WJ, Salome CM, Woolcock AJ. Bronchial hyperresponsiveness in two populations of Australian schoolchildren. The relationship between asthma and skin reactivity to allergens in two communities. *Int J Epidemiol* 1986; **15:** 202–9.
162. Backer V, Bach-Mortensen N, Dirksen A. Prevalence for the predictors of bronchial hyperresponsiveness in children aged 7–16 years. *Allergy* 1989; **44:** 214–19.
163. Sears MR, Herbison GP, Holdaway MD, Hewitt CJ, Flannery EM, Silva PA. The relative risks of sensitivity to grass pollen, house dust mite and cat dander in the development of childhood asthma. *Clin Exp Allergy* 1989; **19:** 419–24.
164. Barry DMJ, Burr ML, Limb ES. Prevalence of asthma among 12 year old children in New Zealand and South Wales: a comparative study. *Thorax* 1991; **46:** 405–9.
165. Ng'ang'a LW, Odhiambo JA, Gicheha NM et al. The prevalence of bronchial asthma in primary school children in Nairobi, Kenya. *Am Rev Respir Dis* 1992; **145**(suppl 2): A537.
166. Bardagi S, Agudo A, Gonzalez CA et al. Prevalence of exercise induced bronchial hyperreactivity in schoolchildren and indoor pollutants. *Am Rev Respir Dis* 1992; **145**(suppl 2): A533.
167. Turner KJ, Dowse GK, Stewart GA, Alpers MP. Studies on bronchial hyperreactivity, allergic responsiveness, and asthma in rural and

urban children of the highlands of Papua New Guinea. *J Allergy Clin Immunol* 1986; **77:** 558–65.
168. McWhorter WM. Occurrence, predictors, and consequences of adult asthma in NHANES I and follow-up survey. *Am Rev Respir Dis* 1989; **139:** 721–4.
169. Broder I, Higgins MW, Mathews KP, Keller JB. Epidemiology of asthma and allergic rhinitis in a total community, Tecumseh, Michigan IV. Natural history. *J Allergy Clin Immunol* 1974; **54**(2): 100–10.
170. Dodge RR, Burrows B. The prevalence and incidence of asthma and asthma-like symptoms in a general population sample. *Am Rev Respir Dis* 1980; **122**(4): 567–75.
171. Bauer BA, Reed CE, Yunginger JW, Wollan PC, Silverstein MD. Incidence and outcomes of asthma in the elderly. *Chest* 1997; **111:** 303–10.

4

Risk factors for the development of asthma

Fernando D Martinez

Methodological issues • Genetic factors • Gender • Maternal effects • Atopy • Respiratory infections as risk factors for asthma • Microbial burden in early life as a protective factor against atopic asthma

During the last ten years, significant progress has been made in our understanding of the factors that are associated with the development of childhood asthma. In spite of these advances, essential aspects of the etiology of asthma remain unresolved. For example, there is ample evidence that the prevalence of asthma is increasing and that only a small proportion of these changes in prevalence can be explained by reporting biases.[1] Although many hypotheses have been proposed to explain these increases, what is causing this 'asthma epidemic' is largely unknown.

In this chapter we will review the most important advances that have recently occurred in our understanding of the factors that predispose an individual who does not have asthma to develop the disease. We will not address here the environmental exposures that may trigger asthma attacks in individuals who already have the disease.

METHODOLOGICAL ISSUES

Although the objective of establishing the factors that determine the inception of asthma seems to be clearcut, there are several methodological obstacles that make this task quite cumbersome. Since there is no clear accepted definition of asthma, it is often difficult to determine when exactly the disease really begins. For example, it may be useful from an epidemiologic point of view to define the beginning of asthma as the time at which an individual who will go on to have chronic disease has their first episode of airway obstruction. Studies that have defined the beginning of asthma in this manner almost invariably reach the same conclusion: most cases of asthma begin in early life.[2,3] However, an important potential bias is introduced by this rather simple definition. Airway obstruction associated with viral infection is a frequent phenomenon in early life, and both subjects who will and those who will not go on to develop asthma develop their first wheezing episodes in early childhood and, more specifically, during the first year of life.[4] It could thus be argued that this first episode of 'asthma-like symptoms' is not the true beginning of asthma, but simply the expression of a condition with symptoms that are similar to those of asthma but the pathogenesis of which is completely different from that of asthma. In fact, when a different definition of the beginning of asthma is used, namely the time at which the diagnosis of asthma is first made by a physician, the age of onset is usually markedly greater: mean age at the onset of childhood asthma is usually between 3 and 5 years.[5] The explanation for this discrepancy is quite straightforward: most pediatricians are aware of the fact that many children who wheeze in early life will not go on to develop asthma and are thus reluctant to assign this label to all wheezy infants and young children. However, once the disease becomes more chronic and particularly when symptoms become more frequent, the need to justify more intense therapy with daily anti-inflammatory medicines supports the assignment of the new diagnostic label. In agreement with this explanation, we have found in our longitudinal studies in Tucson, Arizona, that if the beginning of childhood asthma is considered to be the time at which parents report for the first time more than 3 episodes of wheezing during the previous year, peak incidence shifts to the age of 3–6 years and overlaps with the time at which the diagnosis is first made by a physician (Martinez, unpublished observation).

Which of these two criteria should be used to define the beginning of asthma is far from being an academic issue. Considerable interest has developed in the development of strategies for the primary and secondary prevention of asthma. If the first episodes of asthma are truly those first wheezing lower respiratory illnesses (LRI) with viral infections, then primary/secondary prevention would need to begin either before or shortly after those episodes, that is, very early during childhood. If, on the contrary, asthma really starts at the time in which more chronic symptoms develop, primary prevention could also be considered treatment that is targeted toward children at high risk for the development of asthma who have already had their first wheezing illnesses but who, presumably, have not yet developed the chronic changes in the airways that are characteristic of established asthma.

Although these issues have not been solved, several new lines of evidence strongly suggest that asthma is indeed a progressive disease. Therefore, there are risk factors that influence the initiation of the disease process but there are additional factors that may influence the passage from this initial phase into a more chronic phase (Figure 4.1).

Therefore, when analyzing risk factors for the inception of asthma it is important to take into account both the pre-asthma phase and a potential initial phase of the disease during which it has not yet acquired its chronic connotations. For the purpose of this analysis, we will consider that, in most cases of asthma, the initial phase of the disease—i.e. that phase in which the individual presents with the first symptoms of current airway obstruction—occurs during the first years of life.[2]

GENETIC FACTORS

Assessing the relative importance of genetic and environmental factors as determinants of disease risk is complex. The most reliable approach seems to be the comparison of concordance of disease between monozygotic and dizygotic twins.[6] Since monozygotic twins have identical genetic material whereas dizygotic twins share only 50% of their backgrounds, the excess concordance potentially observed among the former compared with the latter should be attributable exclusively to their common genetic background. These studies assume that the degree of concordance in environmental exposures between monozygotic and dizygotic twins is comparable. Unfortunately, this assumption is not always justified. Several lines

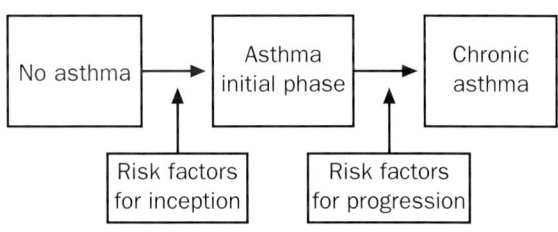

Figure 4.1 Risk factors acting at different times during the natural history of asthma.

of evidence suggest that monozygotic twins do share more environmental exposures than dizygotic twins do, essentially because they are culturally 'expected' to do so. Nevertheless, these studies are useful to assess the potential significance of genetic background as a determinant of disease risk. Most published studies in this area have shown that anywhere between 40% and 70% of the determination of asthma is attributable to genetic factors.[7]

Studies of the familial aggregation and segregation of asthma have confirmed that asthma indeed has a strong genetic component.[8,9] However, no particular pattern of familial segregation has been found. In other words, the disease does not seem to behave in a classical Mendelian fashion.[10] This means that no genetic variant in the human genome seems to have an influence that is strong enough to emerge as a 'major gene' for the disease. Simply stated, there is no 'asthma gene'. Most of the available evidence indicates that, on the contrary, asthma behaves like a polygenic disease. Given the strong genetic influence on the susceptibility to asthma, this observation strongly suggests one of two conclusions: either there is no single pathogenetic mechanism that is crucial for the expression of asthma, or if such a mechanism exists its expression is not controlled by a single gene or a small number of genes. Given the large proportion of the population that is apparently susceptible to asthma, the former conclusion seems more realistic than the latter. Asthma is therefore a genetically heterogeneous disease, and it is thus very unlikely that one or a few genetic markers will be discovered in the future which could identify most asthmatic subjects in the population.

What is to be expected is a distribution of risk ratios like that shown in Figure 4.2, a suggestion of Sing and co-workers.[11] There will be genetic variants in the population which will show a strong association with certain forms of asthma that are caused by very specific exposures. For example, it is plausible to surmise that aspirin-induced asthma may be associated with a specific set of genetic variants that control its expression, but it is also true that these variants will have very little influence on the risk for asthma in the population as a whole. At the other end of the spectrum it is likely that each of a large number of variants associated with the more common forms of asthma will have a small influence on the risk for the disease, although the population risk associated with them may be larger simply because they are present in a larger number of subjects with the disease.

The above considerations have very important consequences for researchers involved in studies of the genetics of asthma: there is no doubt that special attention needs to be paid to refining as much as possible the definition of asthma used in such studies. A more specific definition of the phenotype will move the study toward the right in the spectrum shown in Figure 4.2, and thus will make the finding of variants associated with asthma more likely. But, at the same time, as the definition of asthma becomes more specific, the genetic influences detected will also become more specific to the asthma phenotype selected, and the conclusions of the study will become less relevant to all asthmatics. Based on these considerations, Collins et al[12] have concluded that, for a phenotype like asthma, probably thousands of sib pairs would be needed to detect, with sufficient power, a large proportion of the genetic variants responsible for the expression of asthma, that is, most of those present on the left side of the distribution in Figure 4.2.

To attempt to circumvent some of these problems, researchers have identified so-called intermediate phenotypes for asthma, that is, traits that are known to be associated with the risk to develop asthma. Some of these phenotypes (i.e. total serum IgE levels or sensitization to specific aeroallergens) have been shown to be controlled by major genes in segregation analyses or in association studies.[13-16] The assumption is that, by identifying genes that control the expression of these intermediate phenotypes it will be possible to understand better the genetic determination of the disease. However, the relation between these phenotypes and asthma is complex[10] and cannot be reduced to a simple cause-and-effect paradigm. This will be discussed at more length below, but it is clear that

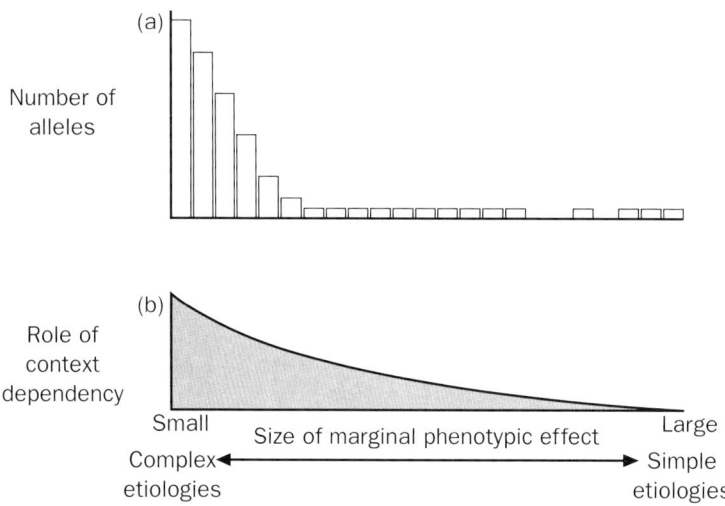

Figure 4.2 (a) The relationship between the expected frequency distribution of disease susceptibility alleles and their expected marginal phenotypic effects. (b) The relationship between context dependency and expected marginal phenotypic effect.

genes associated with serum IgE levels, bronchial hyperresponsiveness, or eosinophilia cannot simply be considered 'asthma genes', and their role will become more apparent only when functional studies are available.

These complex methodological issues are very important to consider here because they shed light on the studies of the genetics of asthma already available which will be discussed in the following paragraphs.

Strategies to identify asthma-related genes

The main objectives of genetic studies of asthma are to identify variations in genes that increase the risk of asthma and to determine the way in which these variations affect gene expression or the function of the protein that the gene codes for. The traditional steps to identify these genes have been to perform either genome-wide searches or candidate gene approaches. In the former, no knowledge of the potential disease mechanisms is needed, and linkage hits are blindly searched in all chromosomes. When a linkage 'hit' is clearly identified, the gene responsible is identified by a complex strategy that combines searches for polymorphisms in all known genes in the chromosomal region that may be relevant for asthma with identification of genetic markers within the area of interest which may allow for more accurate localization of the disease gene. Candidate gene approaches, on the other hand, aim directly at genes or chromosomal regions that can be surmised to be important for the disease, based on the researcher's knowledge of disease mechanisms. Once the genetic variant directly associated with the disease is identified, functional studies are needed to determine how the polymorphism affects the gene. A basic tenet of modern genetics is that this will allow us to understand better what causes the disease process.

Linkage studies

The conclusion that asthma is genetically heterogeneous has been confirmed by several genome-wide searches that have been published during the late 1990s.[17-21] These studies are usually performed in pairs of siblings in which both members of the pair are affected with the disease. Although a detailed explanation of linkage theory goes beyond the scope of this chapter, the statistical reasoning behind these studies is straightforward: for any particular genetic locus, children of the same parents inherit one allele from the father and one from the mother. Since each parent has two copies of the gene, the children have a 25% chance of sharing the same allele from both parents, 50% chance of sharing one but not the other, and 25% chance of not sharing either. In other words, full siblings share, as a mean, 50% of the genetic material transmitted by their parents in any particular chromosomal location. If for a particular genetic location pairs of siblings affected by the same disease share significantly more than 50% of the genetic material, then the conclusion has to be that in that region of the genome a genetic variant is present that increases the risk for the development of asthma. The strategy used by most genome-wide searches is therefore to genotype both members of sibling pairs with asthma and their parents for markers 'strategically' located all along the genome. These markers are chosen because they have high heterozygocity, in other words they usually have many alleles and at least 70–80% of the population has different alleles on each member of the chromosome pair. This facilitates estimation of the proportion of alleles truly shared by the two siblings from their parents (also called 'identity by descent' or 'ibd'). Obviously, many comparisons are made in the same subjects when a genome-wide search using 250–300 markers is performed, and therefore a correction needs to be made in the calculation of the null hypothesis, because apparent deviations from the expected 50% allele-sharing ibd could simply owe to chance.

The results of the genome-wide searches have been reviewed[22,23] and have not revealed any particular locus that indicates the presence of a major gene for asthma: no single chromosomal region has been linked to asthma in all searches. As discussed earlier, this was to be expected: most studies included a rather small number of sibpairs (<200), and the definition of asthma was usually not very stringent. In addition, no single genome-wide search has identified linkage 'hits' with a statistical significance that reaches the accepted threshold (after correction for multiple comparisons). However, a pattern emerges suggesting that certain areas of the genome may have genes associated with asthma. A recent meta-analysis by Collins and co-workers[12] identified candidate regions for asthma and asthma-related traits on chromosomes 6, 5, 16, 11, 12, 13, 14, 7, 20, and 10, in rank order from strongest to weakest evidence.

The problem that we now face is the large number of potential candidate genes present in most of these regions. Chromosome 6, for example, contains the genes for the HLA system, a large array of loci arranged in complex haplotypes that influence many diseases and disease processes. Chromosome 5q contains the so-called cytokine cluster, with at least eight known genes directly involved in the allergic response (IL-4, IL-9, IL-5, IL-13, IL-3, IL-12B, GMCSF, and IRF-1) and many others known to be potentially important in the expression of the disease (glucocorticosteroid receptor, β_2-adrenergic receptor, CD14, etc.). The relative role of genetic variants in any of these genes in determining asthma will be very difficult to elucidate, because small effects could be expected from many of them. Similar considerations can be made for any of the other regions identified by Collins et al.[12] In addition, there may be genes still to be identified that may play a role beyond that of known genes, and this possibility cannot be overlooked. The task is clearly daunting. However, the advances made in the Human Genome Project aimed at identifying all human genes and the parallel effort underway to catalog most of the genetic polymorphisms present in the genome may offer important tools to facilitate this task.

Association studies

Faced with these complexities, many researchers have attempted a different strategy, which consists of first identifying proteins that are known to be involved in the pathogenesis of asthma and then searching for polymorphisms in the genes that code for these proteins. The assumption is that these polymorphisms may change either the structure of the protein or the expression of the gene, thus influencing asthma risk. The frequency of asthma or other asthma-related phenotypes is then studied in the different genotypes or, when several polymorphisms occur in the same gene, in the haplotypes, that is, in the combinations of alleles within the same chromosome.

Detailed discussion of the difficulties that researchers have to face in association studies is beyond the scope of this chapter. However, the reader needs to be aware of the fact that these studies should be interpreted with caution, and that cross-validation and replication are always needed to determine if the apparent association does not owe to chance or to factors other than a true causal relation between polymorphism and phenotype. Among these factors, two will be addressed here: population stratification and linkage disequilibrium.

Population stratification
Given the fact that the epidemiologic design of genetic association studies is usually that of a comparison between cases and controls, these studies are prone to the same biases of any case–control study. Specifically, cases may be different from controls not only in the variable of interest (in this case, asthma), but also in other variables that remain uncontrolled and that may confound the results. For example, if asthma is more abundant in a certain ethnic group and cases are not matched with controls for ethnicity, all genes that determine specific ethnic traits will be spuriously associated with asthma. Unfortunately, it is not always possible to foresee all possible confounders and thus to control for them in association studies. For this reason, replication of the results of association studies in different populations is always necessary. New tests based not on comparing the frequency of certain alleles in cases and controls but on the likelihood of parents transmitting or not transmitting an allele to an affected individual (the transmission disequilibrium test or TDT) have been proposed.

Linkage disequilibrium
Even if a certain genetic polymorphism is associated with asthma or other traits and this association does not owe to confounding factors, it is not possible to say a priori that the specific polymorphism is biologically related to the trait under study. It is possible that the polymorphism may be located in close proximity to another one that is the true determinant of the trait. Polymorphisms that are very close to each other in a chromosome may have alleles that are transmitted together more often than what would be expected by chance, such that one acts as a marker for the other. Thus, whenever an association is reported and confirmed not to owe to chance or confounding, it is important to search for polymorphisms in the same gene or in flaking genes and, at the same time, to determine if the polymorphism is associated with functional changes in gene function or protein function which may explain its association with asthma or asthma-related traits.

These complexities notwithstanding, it is clear that association studies will play a crucial role in identifying genetic polymorphisms associated with asthma in the future. The availability of high-throughput sequencing and genotyping techniques will allow us to study scores of polymorphisms simultaneously in different populations, thus markedly increasing power and decreasing the potential influence of biases like those described above. The fact that certain polymorphisms may be transmitted together with others within a chromosome more often than expected may allow us to use tens of thousands of these polymorphisms, regularly distributed in the whole genome, for genome-wide searches, in a manner similar to that of linkage studies using sibpairs, as described earlier. Clearly, significant advances in our understanding of the genetics of asthma can be expected in the near future.

GENDER

The relation between asthma and gender is complex. Up to the age of puberty, asthma is almost twice as frequent in males as in females.[24] Over 60% of all prepubertal asthmatics are males, and the distinction is observed from the very first years of life.[4] The factors that determine this increased risk of asthma in males are not well understood. Boys tend to have more skin test reactivity to aeroallergens than females.[25] Males are also more likely to have bronchial hyperresponsiveness than females, independent of their atopic status.[26] Airway size is apparently also a factor. Males have significantly lower maximal expiratory flows at given lung volumes than girls both early in life[27] and later during their prepubertal years.[28] Therefore, both immune factors and lung-specific factors seem to be important.

However, the relative prevalence of asthma in boys and girls changes quite dramatically during puberty.[29] More boys than girls show remission of asthma during puberty, and incidence of new cases of asthma during puberty is much more likely to happen in girls than in boys.[30] Neither of these two intriguing phenomena is clearly understood. However, airway size increases more rapidly, relative to lung size, in boys than in girls.[31] It is thus possible that airway structure may protect boys against airway obstruction during the prepubertal years.

Recent observations by our own group and others suggest that hormonal factors may be important in the increased risk of asthma observed in girls during adolescence. It has been reported that increased incidence of asthma among prepubertal girls is mainly observed among those who become obese during their prepubertal years.[32,33] Since girls who become obese during their prepubertal years are also more likely to have early menarche, it is plausible to surmise that a common factor determines the likelihood of developing asthma on the one hand and both early menarche[34] and obesity on the other hand. It is also possible that obesity itself may influence the hormonal balance that determines the timing of menarche and, by this mechanism, may predispose prepubertal girls to the development of asthma. The connections between obesity, hormonal regulation, and asthma are indeed complex and will require further elucidation.

MATERNAL EFFECTS

Several epidemiologic studies have reported that a history of asthma in the mother is associated with a larger increase in asthma risk than a history of asthma in the father.[35] Although it is possible that these findings may owe at least in part to preferential reporting of their own symptoms by mothers, the consistency of the finding makes it unlikely that all the effect is explained by reporting bias. It has been suggested that maternal effects may owe to direct influences of the atopic/asthmatic mother on the development of the immune system in the fetus.[36] Recent evidence from at least two studies suggests that breastfeeding may be protective against virus-triggered asthma in early life, but may be associated with increased risk of atopy-related asthma during the school years.[37,38] It is thus possible that maternal effects on the developing immune system may not be confined to the fetal period but could also act through breast milk. More work needs to be done in this complex area.

ATOPY

There is little doubt that by the late school years, most asthmatic subjects, independent of gender, become sensitized to the allergens to which they are exposed in their local environment.[39] When this phenomenon is analyzed in more detail, it becomes apparent that the development of asthma is more strongly associated with sensitization to certain allergens and not others. In coastal regions, for example, the prevalence of asthma is almost invariably associated with sensitization to house dust mites.[25] Because many of the initial studies of the association between allergic sensitization and asthma were done in such coastal regions, the strong association between sensitization to house dust mites and asthma suggested the possibility that the former could be the cause of the latter.[40] The logical corollary of these assumption was that reducing the prevalence of sensitization to house dust mites could be a potential strategy for the reduction of asthma prevalence.

Studies performed in areas of the world where the house dust mite is not prevalent have challenged this contention. In desert regions in inland Australia[41] and in the southwest of the United States[42] children are much less exposed to house dust mites than they are in coastal regions. As a consequence, sensitization to house dust mites in these regions is much less likely to occur, especially among subjects born and raised in these areas. However, in spite of much lower rates of sensitization to house dust mites, asthma is as frequent or even more frequent in these areas than it is in coastal regions of the same countries.[41] The mold *Alternaria* seems to take the place of house dust mites as the main allergen to which subjects who will develop asthma become sensitized.

Perhaps the most intriguing findings in this area are those reported from the northernmost province of Sweden, Norrbotten.[43,44] Studies performed in schools and houses showed complete absence of dust mite allergens. Moreover, most members of the genus *Alternaria* seem to be very unusual in this part of the world. It was therefore interesting to determine the prevalence of asthma in this area, because one would have expected that, if sensitization to either or both of these allergens was somehow causally related to the development of asthma, asthma should be infrequent where exposure to these allergens is almost non-existent. However, the prevalence of asthma in this part of the world is not low and recently has been rising to estimates of 6–8%.[44] Allergic sensitization in 110 asthmatic children living in this area was compared with that of 63 controlled children, all studied subjects being 7–8 years of age. The authors reported that 43% of asthmatics were sensitized to local allergens, compared with only 11% of controlled children. Among asthmatics, 30% were sensitized to cat epithelium, 25% to birch, and 15% to dog. Among controls these sensitization rates were 3.2%, 1.6%, and 4.8%, respectively. These very high levels of sensitization to cat and dog occurred in spite of levels of exposure that were not significantly higher than those observed in Charlottesville, Virginia, where the main allergen associated with asthma is house dust mites but where sensitization to cat allergen was lower among asthmatics than that observed among asthmatics in northern Sweden.

The finding that asthma is quite prevalent in an area of the world where exposure to and sensitization to *Alternaria*, house dust mites, and cockroaches is almost completely absent seriously questions the assumption that sensitization to these allergens is causally related to asthma. Of great interest is the fact that in northern Sweden there was a strong association between asthma risk and sensitization to birch. In areas of high exposure to house dust mites, children are often exposed to and become sensitized to pollen, but sensitization to pollen is not significantly related to asthma risk once sensitization to house dust mites is taken into account.[45] In conjunction with the above-reported observation that predominant allergens associated with asthma vary by locale, these data suggest that in most cases of childhood asthma, sensitization to specific, ubiquitous allergens is not causally related to the development of asthma. More likely, the data suggest that individuals who are susceptible to the development of asthma tend to become sensitized to the allergens that are predominant in the locale where they live. It is still possible that the severity of the disease may be related to the specific allergen to which the subject is exposed. However, the data are not compatible with the idea that developing asthma is the consequence of having become sensitized to one specific allergen, because one would expect large differences in asthma prevalence depending on patterns of exposure, which clearly is not the case.

What determines that individuals who will go on to develop asthma are more prone to becoming sensitized to certain allergens is not well understood. Further epidemiologic insights come from comparisons of the association between allergic sensitization and asthma on the one hand and allergic rhinitis on the other. Sears and co-workers[39] observed that the prevalence of diagnosed asthma in a large population sample was strongly correlated with the number of positive skin test to local aeroallergens, but hay fever without asthma did not show such an association. The risk of asthma was related to the magnitude of the skin test response to house dust mites and cats, whereas the risk of hay fever was primarily associated with grass pollen sensitivity. Peat and co-workers[46] studied the relation between allergic sensitization and persistent asthma symptoms and persistent allergic rhinitis in children tested by skin prick test at ages 8 and 12 years. They found that persistent asthma symptoms and bronchial hyperresponsiveness were mainly present among children who were already sensitized by the age of 8 years. Children who were sensitized after the age of 8 years were not more likely to have significant bronchial hyperresponsiveness and persistent asthma symptoms than those who were never sensitized. However, children who were sensitized after the age of 8 years were more likely to have allergic rhinitis than children who were never sensitized.[46]

These findings suggest that the patterns of allergic sensitization to ubiquitous aeroallergens are different for children with asthma than for those with allergic rhinitis but no asthma. Asthma seems to be associated with early allergic sensitization and with sensitization to perennial allergens such as animal dander, house dust mites, *Alternaria*, cockroaches, etc. Allergic rhinitis, on the other hand, may be associated with either early or late sensitization, and is more likely to be associated with skin test reactivity against seasonal allergens such as pollen.

The factors that determine these different patterns of allergic sensitization are not well understood. It is possible that the immune mechanisms that determine sensitization to asthma-related allergens may be different from those that determine sensitization to those allergens that are not related to asthma in a specific community. Support for these notions comes from studies in which sensitization to asthma-related allergens was related to patterns of immune response during the first years of life.[47] In Tucson, Arizona, where *Alternaria* is the major allergen related to childhood asthma,[42] children who became sensitized to *Alternaria* by the age of 6 years showed very poor interferon gamma (IFN-γ) responses by peripheral blood mononuclear cells stimulated nonspecifically during the first year of life. No such association was found between sensitization to pollen by age 6 years and cellular responses during the first year of life. These results thus suggest the possibility that sensitization to asthma-related allergens may be the consequence of alterations in the development of the immune system either shortly after birth or during the first years of life. Indeed, children of atopic/asthmatic parents, who are known to be at higher risk for the development of asthma than those of non-atopic/non-asthmatic parents, were more likely to have lower IFN-γ responses by their peripheral blood mononuclear cells than their peers.[47] It is thus likely that diminished IFN-γ responses, by predisposing to early allergic sensitization to a wide variety of allergens present in the environment, including those more strongly associated with asthma risk, may be a key factor explaining the association between sensitization to ubiquitous aeroallergens and the development of asthma.

RESPIRATORY INFECTIONS AS RISK FACTORS FOR ASTHMA

The association between respiratory infections in early life and the subsequent development of asthma has been the matter of much controversy. For years it was known that children who had LRIs due to respiratory syncytial virus (RSV) in early life were more likely to show subsequent episodes of recurrent wheezing than those who did not have such LRIs.[48] The factors that determine this association, however, were not well understood. Since almost all children develop respiratory infection with RSV during the first two years of life,[49] it was unlikely that RSV by itself was responsible for the association. More likely, some specific characteristic of the subjects who develop RSV LRIs could determine both the first episode of wheezing and the subsequent persistent wheezing in individuals with RSV LRIs. Alternatively, it has been proposed that the interaction between the immune system and RSV in susceptible individuals may prime either the lungs or the immune system or both in a way that may increase the risk for the development of asthma.

Results of recent longitudinal studies have demonstrated that the association between RSV infection in early life and subsequent persistent wheezing is a complex one. Although a small proportion of children who have RSV LRIs go on to have persistent episodes of wheezing, the majority have only one or a few episodes, but their symptoms remit and rarely show further relapses. Most of these children have their wheezing episodes during the first year of life[4] and seldom have episodes beyond the second year. However, other children do continue to have wheezing episodes, but until recently the factors determining which children with RSV LRIs would have transient episodes and which would go on to have persistent wheezing were not understood.

Several observations suggest that immune responses to viruses in children with persistent wheezing are different from those of children with transient wheezing. Welliver and co-workers[50] first reported that, in children with confirmed RSV LRIs during the first 6 months of life, persistence of wheeze up to 4 years of age was directly related to the level of RSV-specific IgE in nasopharyngeal secretions during bronchiolitis. Martinez et al[51] showed that children who had persistent episodes of wheezing up to the age of 6 years and who had a history of LRIs owing to RSV and other viruses showed significant increases in total IgE during the initial acute episodes. No such total serum IgE responses were observed in children who had LRIs owing to the same viruses in early life but who did not go on to have persistent wheezing. Moreover, when eosinophil counts at the time of the initial LRI (which occurred at a mean age of 11 months in both persistent wheezers and transient wheezers) were assessed, persistent wheezers had significantly higher eosinophil counts in circulation when compared with transient wheezers. Very similar results were recently published by Welliver et al.[52] In other studies, it has been shown that children who show high levels of eosinophilic cationic protein (ECP) at the time of their first acute lower respiratory illnesses were more likely to show three or more episodes of wheezing subsequently than children who did not show high ECP levels.[53] These findings suggest that the nature of the immune response to the virus is a marker of subsequent persistent wheezing. Children who show responses that are biased toward the production of IgE and toward higher levels of circulating eosinophils are at higher risk of subsequent persistent wheezing. It thus appears that already at the time of their first encounter with viruses (usually RSV during the first year of life), subjects who will go on to develop asthma show the type of immune responses that are characteristic of asthma itself: IgE mediated and eosinophil mediated. It is not yet understood whether the nature of the immune response to the virus determines the bronchial obstruction observed in these children at the time of that episode, but it is tempting to speculate that it is the persistence of this form or immune response into the school years which determines the development of asthma in susceptible individuals.

The above explanation notwithstanding, factors other than IgE mediated and eosinophil mediated responses must be involved in determining risk for wheezing during RSV LRI. When risk factors for allergic asthma such as family history of asthma, eczema, etc. are controlled for, there remains a residual increased risk of subsequent persistent episodes of wheezing in children who had RSV LRIs during the first 3 years of life.[54] Several studies published in the late 1990s provide important new clues for the understanding of the pathogenesis of persistent wheezing in children who had RSV LRIs as infants. In some of these studies, levels of lung function were measured, using various techniques, in infants before they developed any lower respiratory illness.[27,55,56] These studies have invariably reported that lower levels of lung function are present shortly after birth in children who go on to have wheezing LRIs during the first years of life. These lower levels of lung function persist beyond the early years, and are at least partially reversible after the administration of inhaled bronchodilators.[54] It is thus plausible to surmise that either the structure of the lungs, the control of airway smooth muscle tone, or both may be congenitally abnormal in children who will have episodes of bronchial obstruction associated with RSV. However, these data do not allow us to exclude the possibility that RSV infection itself may alter lung structure or the regulation of airway tone, as suggested by some animal models of RSV infection.[57]

More recently, studies of acute immune responses in children with RSV bronchiolitis suggest an additional mechanism that may be involved in determining persistent wheezing in children with RSV LRIs. Bont et al observed that children who had RSV bronchiolitis and went on to have recurrent wheezing episodes during the following year had enhanced IL-10 responses by peripheral blood mononuclear cells during the convalescent phase of the initial acute disease.[58] IL-10 is a cytokine produced both by antigen presenting cells and by Th1-like and Th2-like cells in humans.[59] IL-10 downregulates the immune response by acting both on macrophages and on T-helper cells.[59] It is thus possible that individuals who respond to viral infections with strong IL-10 responses may have a decreased capacity to eliminate the virus and/or to limit its capacity to invade lung tissues.

These studies have enhanced our understanding of the role of viral infections associated with wheezing in early life in the inception of asthma. Different mechanisms related both to the immune response to the virus and to the structure and function of the lung play a role in different asthma phenotypes.

MICROBIAL BURDEN IN EARLY LIFE AS A PROTECTIVE FACTOR AGAINST ATOPIC ASTHMA

As explained at the beginning of this chapter, the prevalence of asthma is clearly on the rise in developed countries, and the factors that have determined these increases are not understood. Many hypotheses have been proposed[60] and no single explanation is available that can explain the increases in asthma occurring in very different communities and countries. However, several recent empirical observations suggest that atopic asthma and allergic disease in general are less frequent during the school years in children who have a history of more frequent contacts with other children in early life and thus presumably had a higher overall burden of infection.[61] This burden does not refer to any specific infection, although some studies have studied markers of single infections such as hepatitis A[62] or measles.[63] It is important here to make a distinction between *infection* and *illness* associated with it. For RSV, for example, there is clear evidence indicating that all children have at least one infection with this virus during the first 2 years of life (see above). Thus, the associations discussed in the previous section refer to those between illnesses owing to RSV and subsequent wheezing. The discussion in this section refers, on the contrary, to microbial burden, and here both illnesses-associated microbial encounters as well as those that remain asymptomatic may be important.

The mechanisms by which exposure to other children may protect against the development of atopic asthma and allergies in general are beginning to be understood. Recent advances in the understanding of the early phases of the development of the immune system in general and of specific immune responses to environmental antigens in particular have provided a fresh approach to our understanding of the factors that determine the inception of asthma. It is now established that humans are born with immune responses that are clearly downregulated. Specifically, IFN-γ responses both by CD4-positive and CD8-positive cells are much lower in neonates than in older children and adults.[64] Moreover, natural killer (NK) cell responses also appear to be immature, and production of IFN-γ by NK cells is impaired in newborns.[65] The development of mature, balanced immune responses seems to be the result of complex interactions between environmental exposures and genetic background.

We[66] and others have postulated that it is the delay in the development of a mature immune response during the first years of life that fosters sensitization to local aeroallergens, and that this delay, and not exposure to aeroallergens per se, is an important determinant of asthma risk. Based on the observations of an inverse relation between indirect markers of frequent infections in early life and the subsequent development of atopic asthma, we also suggested that the development of mature balanced Th1/Th2 responses in early life is fostered by the microbial burden to which the individual is exposed during this period. Of particular interest are the studies in which direct or indirect markers of endotoxin exposure during childhood were related to the development of asthma and allergies. Various studies have shown that individuals born and raised on farms, especially those in which animals are kept, have marked decreased risk of developing allergic sensitization and asthma during the school years.[67] Studies by von Ehrenstein and co-workers in Germany,[68] Riedler and co-workers in Austria,[69] and Braun-Fahrlander and co-workers in Switzerland[70] consistently showed that children living in small rural communities and not exposed to animal farms had significantly more skin test reactivity, bronchial hyperresponsiveness, diagnosed asthma, and allergy symptoms than children living on small farms, especially animal farms. In subsequent studies, these authors showed that one characteristic that distinguished individuals living on animal farms with respect to those living in the same rural setting but away from animal farms was the degree of exposure to endotoxin, which was much higher in the former than in the latter. This suggested the hypothesis that endotoxin exposure could somehow influence the development of the immune system in early life by stimulating antigen presenting cells to produce IL-12 and other cytokines that direct the immune response away from a Th-2-type, thus decreasing the likelihood of IgE-mediated sensitization and, as a consequence, decreasing the risk for the development of asthma.

Strong support for this hypothesis was provided by Gereda and co-workers.[71] These authors studied concentrations of house dust endotoxin in the homes of 61 infants aged 9–24 months. They showed that the homes of children who became sensitized to a panel of common inhalant and food allergens contained significantly lower concentrations of house dust endotoxin than those of non-sensitized infants. Increased house dust endotoxin concentrations also correlated with increased proportions of IFN-γ producing CD4 T-cells in circulation.[71] This landmark study thus suggested that exposure to endotoxin may increase IFN-γ production and by this mechanism deviate immune responses away from the Th2-like type in early life. The importance of this finding cannot be overstated, because several studies have shown that one of the strongest risk factors for the subsequent development of asthma is early IgE-mediated sensitization to aeroallergens[46] or sensitization to food allergens followed by subsequent sensitization to aeroallergens in the same individuals.[72] Thus, by enhancing the maturation of immune responses early in life, endotoxin exposure may prevent the development of asthma.

These results appear in contradiction with other studies showing that lipopolysaccharide (LPS), a component of endotoxin, upregulates IgE-mediated responses[73] and may exacerbate asthma in individuals who already have the disease.[74] This complex relation between endotoxin exposure and IgE-mediated responses has recently been explored in an experimental model by Tulic et al.[75] These authors exposed rats to a single aerosol of LPS 1 day before or 1, 2, 4, 6, 8, or 10 days after sensitization with ovalbumin. These experiments showed that a single exposure to LPS 1 day before and up to 4 days after intraperitoneal injection of ovalbumin protected against the development of ovalbumin-specific IgE. LPS exposure 6, 8, or 10 days after sensitization, on the contrary, further exacerbated the ovalbumin-induced cellular influx. Therefore, the timing of exposure to LPS with respect to the development of specific immune responses may be crucial. If the exposure occurs before or during the process of development of the primary immune response, IgE-mediated responses may be prevented. On the contrary, if the exposure occurs when the primary immune response has already been established and is already deviated toward a Th-2-like response, IgE-mediated responses may be exacerbated by LPS.

We reasoned that exposure to endotoxin/LPS offered a cogent model for the study of gene–environment interactions in the development of early allergic sensitization and consequently of asthma. It has been well established that cytokine responses by human peripheral blood cells stimulated with LPS show large individual variations. In the case of one specific cytokine, IL-10, such individual variation has been shown to have a genetic component of over 70%.[76] We thus surmised that polymorphisms in the genes that code for the receptor system for LPS could determine levels of these receptor components both in their soluble and non-soluble forms. At the same time, these polymorphisms could influence cytokine responses at the time of antigen presentation by making cells more sensitive to the influence of LPS, and thus could influence the type of immune response occurring after antigen presentation.[77] Indeed, we screened the gene for CD14, the main component of the receptor system for LPS. This gene is located in chromosome 5q31, an area that several groups (including our own) have shown to be linked with asthma-related phenotypes.[19,78,79] We discovered and were the first to report a polymorphism in the promoter region of CD14.[80] This polymorphism, CD14/-159, consisted of a C-to-T transition, and we showed that carriers of the T allele had significantly higher levels of sCD14, the soluble form of the receptor present in circulation. Other authors more recently have shown that the T allele is also associated with higher levels of expression of the membrane-bound form of CD14.[81] Subsequent work by our group has clearly established that CD14/-159 is located within a consensus sequence that binds proteins of the SP family of transcription factors, and that the T allele of CD14/-159 is associated with increased rates of CD14 gene transcription.

Our group also showed that carriers of the T allele have significantly lower levels of circulating IgE.[80] We subsequently showed that the association between IgE levels and CD14/-159 was not observed either at birth or at the age of 9 months and only became apparent during the school years (unpublished observations). Preliminary observations from different longitudinal studies in Australia[82] and in Vancouver[83] showed very similar results, with no association being observed in newborns and significant associations being observed later in life between the T allele and lower levels of IgE in circulation. Two other studies, one in The Netherlands (Postma, personal communication) and one among British individuals, showed similar results.[84] We postulated that individuals with a higher expression of CD14 could be more sensitive to the influence of LPS in early life, and that this influence could act by deviating the immune responses away from those mediated by IgE.

Studies of the potential role of early microbial burden and endotoxin exposure as preventive factors for the development of asthma offer a new approach to the understanding of asthma causation and may allow us to develop new strategies for the primary prevention of the disease in the future.

REFERENCES

1. Carman PG, Landau LI. Increased paediatric admissions with asthma in Western Australia—a problem of diagnosis? *Med J Aust* 1990; **152:** 23–6.
2. Yuninger J, Reed CE, O'Connell EJ et al. A community-based study of the epidemiology of asthma. Incidence rates, 1964–1983. *Am Rev Respir Dis* 1992; **146:** 888–94.
3. Barbee RA, Dodge R, Lebowitz ML et al. The epidemiology of asthma. *Chest* 1985; **87:** 21S–25S.
4. Martinez FD, Wright AL, Taussig LM et al. Asthma and wheezing in the first six years of life. *N Engl J Med* 1995; **332:** 133–8.
5. Anderson HR, Pottier AC, Strachan DP. Asthma from birth to age 23: incidence and relation to prior and concurrent atopic disease. *Thorax* 1992; **47:** 537–42.
6. Skadhauge LR, Christensen K, Kyvik KO et al. Genetic and environmental influence on asthma: a population-based study of 11,688 Danish twin pairs. *Eur Respir J* 1999; **13:** 8–14.
7. Duffy DL, Martin NG, Battistutta D et al. Genetics of asthma and hay fever in Australian twins. *Am Rev Respir Dis* 1990; **142:** 1351–8.
8. Holberg CJ, Elston RC, Halonen M et al. Segregation analysis of physician-diagnosed

asthma in Hispanic and non-Hispanic white families. A recessive component? *Am J Respir Crit Care Med* 1996; **154:** 144–50.
9. Wang TN, Ko YC, Wang TH et al. Segregation analysis of asthma: recessive major gene component for asthma in relation to history of atopic diseases. *Am J Med Genet* 2000; **93:** 373–80.
10. Martinez FD. Complexities of the genetics of asthma. *Am J Respir Crit Care Med* 1997; **156:** S117–S122.
11. Sing CF, Haviland MB, Reilly SL. Genetic architecture of common multifactorial diseases. In: Chadwick D, Cardew G, eds. *Variation in the Human Genome*, Vol 197. Chichester: John Wiley, 1996.
12. Collins A, Ennis S, Tapper W et al. Mapping oligogenes for atopy and asthma by meta-analysis. *Genet Molec Biol* 2000; **23:** 1–10.
13. Holberg CJ, Halonen M, Wright AL et al. Familial aggregation and segregation analysis of eosinophil levels. *Am J Respir Crit Care Med* 1999; **160:** 1604–10.
14. Townley RG, Bewtra A, Wilson AF et al. Segregation analysis of bronchial response to methacholine inhalation challenge in families with and without asthma. *J Allergy Clin Immunol* 1986; **77:** 101–7.
15. Sampogna F, Demenais F, Hochez J et al. Segregation analysis of IgE levels in 335 French families (EGEA) using different strategies to correct for the ascertainment through a correlated trait (asthma). *Genet Epidemiol* 2000; **18**: 128–42.
16. Martinez FD, Holberg CJ, Halonen M et al. Evidence for Mendelian inheritance of serum IgE levels in Hispanic and non-Hispanic white families. *Am J Hum Genet* 1994; **55:** 555–65.
17. Daniels SE, Bhattacharrya S, James A et al. A genome-wide search for quantitative trait loci underlying asthma. *Nature* 1996; **383:** 247–50.
18. The Collaborative Study on the Genetics of Asthma. A genome-wide search for asthma susceptibility loci in ethnically diverse populations. *Nat Genet* 1997; **15:** 389–92.
19. Ober C, Cox NJ, Abney M et al. Genome-wide search for asthma susceptibility loci in a founder population. The Collaborative Study on the Genetics of Asthma. *Hum Mol Genet* 1998; **7:** 1393–8.
20. Wjst M, Fischer G, Immervoll T et al. A genome-wide search for linkage to asthma. *Genomics* 1999; **58:** 1–8.
21. Dizier MH, Besse-Schmittler C, Guiloud-Bataille M et al. Genome screen for asthma and related phenotypes in the French Egea Study. *Am J Resp Crit Care Med* 1999; **159:** A649.
22. Ober C, Moffatt MF. The pathobiology of asthma: implications for treatment. *Clin Chest Med* 2000; **21:** 1–18.
23. Cookson WOC, Moffatt MF. Genetics of asthma and allergic disease. *Hum Molec Genet* 2000; **9:** 2359–64.
24. Sears MR. Evolution of asthma through childhood. *Clin Exp Allergy* 1998; **28** (suppl 5): 82–9.
25. Sears MR, Burrows B, Herbison GP et al. Atopy in childhood. II. Relationship to airway responsiveness, hay fever and asthma. *Clin Exp Allergy* 1993; **23:** 949–56.
26. Burrows B, Sears MR, Flannery EM et al. Relations of bronchial responsiveness to allergy skin test reactivity, lung function, respiratory symptoms, and diagnoses in thirteen-year-old New Zealand children. *J Allergy Clin Immunol* 1995; **95:** 548–56.
27. Martinez FD, Morgan WJ, Wright AL et al. Diminished lung function as a predisposing factor for wheezing respiratory illness in infants. *N Engl J Med* 1988; **319:** 1112–17.
28. Knudson RJ, Burrows B, Lebowitz MD. The maximal expiratory flow-volume curve: its use in the detection of ventilatory abnormalities in a population study. *Am Rev Respir Dis* 1976; **114:** 871–9.
29. Von Mutius E. Progression of allergy and asthma through childhood to adolescence. *Thorax* 1996; **51** (suppl 1): S3–S6.
30. Strachan DP, Butland BK, Anderson HR. Incidence and prognosis of asthma and wheezing illness from early childhood to age 33 in a national British cohort. *BMJ* 1996; **312:** 1195–9.
31. Pagtakhan RD, Bjelland JC, Landau LI et al. Sex differences in growth patterns of the airways and lung parenchyma in children. *J Appl Physiol* 1984; **56:** 1204–10.
32. Castro-Rodriguez JA, Holberg CJ, Morgan WJ et al. Increased incidence of asthma-like symptoms in girls who become overweight or obese during the school years. *Am J Resp Crit Care Med* 2000: in press.
33. Chen Y, Dales R, Krewski D et al. Increased effects of smoking and obesity on asthma among female Canadians: the National Population Health Survey, 1994–1995. *Am J Epidemiol* 1999; **150:** 255–62.
34. Wattigney WA, Srinivasan SR, Chen W et al. Secular trend of earlier onset of menarche with increasing obesity in black and white girls: the Bogalusa Heart Study. *Ethn Dis* 1999; **9:** 181–9.

35. Martinez FD. Maternal risk factors in asthma. *Ciba Found Symp* 1997; **206:** 233–9.
36. Brown MA, Halonen MJ, Martinez FD. Cutting the cord: is birth already too late for primary prevention of allergy? *Clin Exp Allergy* 1997; **27:** 4–6.
37. Rusconi F, Galassi C, Corbo GM et al. Risk factors for early, persistent, and late-onset wheezing in young children. SIDRIA Collaborative Group. *Am J Respir Crit Care Med* 1999; **160:** 1617–22.
38. Wright AL, Holberg CJ, Taussig LM et al. Maternal asthma status alters the relation of infant feeding to asthma and recurrent wheeze in childhood. *Thorax* 2000: in press.
39. Sears MR, Herbison GP, Holdaway MD et al. The relative risks of sensitivity to grass pollen, house dust mite and cat dander in the development of childhood asthma. *Clin Exp Allergy* 1989; **19:** 419–24.
40. Peat JK, Tovey E, Toelle BG et al. House dust mite allergens. A major risk factor for childhood asthma in Australia. *Am J Respir Crit Care Med* 1996; **153:** 141–6.
41. Peat JK, Tovey E, Mellis CM et al. Importance of house dust mite and Alternaria allergens in childhood asthma: an epidemiological study in two climatic regions of Australia. *Clin Exp Allergy* 1993; **23:** 812–20.
42. Halonen M, Stern DA, Wright AL et al. Alternaria as a major allergen for asthma in children raised in a desert environment. *Am J Respir Crit Care Med* 1997; **155:** 1356–61.
43. Ronmark E, Lundback B, Jonsson E et al. Asthma, type-1 allergy and related conditions in 7- and 8-year-old children in northern Sweden: prevalence rates and risk factor pattern. *Respir Med* 1998; **92:** 316–24.
44. Perzanowski MS, Ronmark E, Nold B et al. Relevance of allergens from cats and dogs to asthma in the northernmost province of Sweden: schools as a major site of exposure. *J Allergy Clin Immunol* 1999; **103:** 1018–24.
45. Sears MR, Burrows B, Flannery EM et al. Atopy in childhood. I. Gender and allergen related risks for development of hay fever and asthma. *Clin Exp Allergy* 1993; **23:** 941–8.
46. Peat JK, Salome CM, Woolcock AJ. Longitudinal changes in atopy during a 4-year period: relation to bronchial hyperresponsiveness and respiratory symptoms in a population sample of Australian schoolchildren. *J Allergy Clin Immunol* 1990; **85:** 65–74.
47. Martinez FD, Stern DA, Wright AL et al. Association of interleukin-2 and interferon-gamma production by blood mononuclear cells in infancy with parental allergy skin tests and with subsequent development of atopy. *J Allergy Clin Immunol* 1995; **96:** 652–60.
48. Pullen C, Hey E. Wheezing, asthma, and pulmonary dysfunction 10 years after infection with respiratory syncytial virus in infancy. *BMJ* 1982; **5:** 1665–9.
49. Glezen P, Denny FW. Epidemiology of acute lower respiratory disease in children. *N Engl J Med* 1973; **288:** 498–505.
50. Welliver RC, Sun M, Rinaldo D et al. Predictive value of respiratory syncytial virus-specific IgE responses for recurrent wheezing following bronchiolitis. *J Pediatr* 1986; **109:** 776–80.
51. Martinez FD, Stern DA, Wright AL et al. Differential immune responses to acute lower respiratory illness in early life by subsequent development of persistent wheezing and asthma. *J Allergy Clin Immunol* 1998; **102:** 915–20.
52. Welliver RC. Immunology of respiratory syncytial virus infection: eosinophils, cytokines, chemokines and asthma. *Pediatr Infect Dis J* 2000; **19:** 780–3.
53. Koller DY, Wojnarowski C, Herkner KR et al. High levels of eosinophil cationic protein in wheezing infants predict the development of asthma. *J Allergy Clin Immunol* 1997; **99:** 752–6.
54. Stein RT, Sherrill D, Morgan WJ et al. Respiratory syncytial virus in early life and risk of wheeze and allergy by age 13 years. *Lancet* 1999; **353:** 541–5.
55. Young S, Arnott J, O'Keeffe PT et al. The association between early life lung function and wheezing during the first 2 yrs of life. *Eur Respir J* 2000; **15:** 151–7.
56. Adler A, Tager IB, Brown RW et al. Relationship between an index of tidal flow and lower respiratory illness in the first year of life. *Pediatr Pulmonol* 1995; **20:** 137–44.
57. Colasurdo GN, Hemming VG, Prince GA et al. Human respiratory syncytial virus produces prolonged alterations of neural control in airways of developing ferrets. *Am J Respir Crit Care Med* 1998; **157:** 1506–11.
58. Bont L, Heijnen CJ, Kavelaars A et al. Monocyte IL-10 production during respiratory syncytial virus bronchiolitis is associated with recurrent wheezing in a one-year follow-up study. *Am J Resp Crit Care Med* 2000; **161:** 1518–23.
59. Borish L. IL-10: evolving concepts. *J Allergy Clin Immunol* 1998; **101:** 293–7.

60. Woolcock AJ, Peat JK. Evidence for the increase in asthma worldwide. *Ciba Found Symp* 1997; **206:** 122–34.
61. Ball TM, Castro-Rodriguez JA, Griffith KA et al. Siblings, day-care attendance, and the risk of asthma and wheezing during childhood. *N Engl J Med* 2000; **348:** 538–43.
62. Matricardi PM, Rosmini F, Riondino S et al. Exposure to foodborne and orofecal microbes versus airborne viruses in relation to atopy and allergic asthma: epidemiological study. *BMJ* 2000; **320:** 412–17.
63. Shaheen SO, Aaby P, Hall AJ et al. Measles and atopy in Guinea-Bissau. *Lancet* 1996; **347:** 1792–6.
64. Prescott SL, Macaubas C, Smallacombe T et al. Development of allergen-specific T-cell memory in atopic and normal children. *Lancet* 1999; **353:** 196–200.
65. Uksila J, Lassila O, Hirvonen T. Natural killer cell function of human neonatal lymphocytes. *Clin Exp Immunol* 1982; **48:** 649–54.
66. Martinez FD, Holt PG. Role of microbial burden in aetiology of allergy and asthma. *Lancet* 1999; **354** (suppl 2): 12–15.
67. Ernst P, Cormier Y. Relative scarcity of asthma and atopy among rural adolescents raised on a farm. *Am J Respir Crit Care Med* 2000; **161:** 1563–6.
68. Von Ehrenstein OS, von Mutius E, Illi S et al. Reduced risk of hay fever and asthma among children of farmers. *Clin Exp Allergy* 2000; **30:** 187–93.
69. Riedler J, Eder W, Oberfeld G et al. Austrian children living on a farm have less hay fever, asthma and allergic sensitization. *Clin Exp Allergy* 2000; **30:** 194–200.
70. Braun-Fahrlander C, Gassner M, Grize L et al. Prevalence of hay fever and allergic sensitization in farmer's children and their peers living in the same rural community. SCARPOL team. Swiss Study on Childhood Allergy and Respiratory Symptoms with Respect to Air Pollution. *Clin Exp Allergy* 1999; **29:** 28–34.
71. Gereda JE, Leung DYM, Thatayatikon A et al. Relation between house-dust endotoxin exposure, type 1 T-cell development, and allergen sensitization in infants at high risk of asthma. *Lancet* 2000; **355:** 1680–3.
72. Zeiger RS, Heller S. The development and prediction of atopy in high-risk children: follow-up at age seven years in a prospective randomized study of combined maternal and infant food allergen avoidance. *J Allergy Clin Immunol* 1995; **95:** 1179–90.
73. Nakamura M, Nagata T, Xavier M et al. Ubiquitin-like polypeptide inhibits the IgE response of lipopolysaccharide-activated B cells. *Int Immunol* 1996; **8:** 1659–65.
74. Michel O, Kips J, Duchateau J et al. Severity of asthma is related to endotoxin in house dust. *Am J Respir Crit Care Med* 1996; **154:** 1641–6.
75. Tulic MK, Wale JL, Holt PG et al. Modification of the inflammatory response to allergen challenge after exposure to bacterial lipopolysaccharide. *Am J Respir Cell Mol Biol* 2000; **22:** 604–12.
76. Westendorp RG, Langermans JA, Huizinga TW et al. Genetic influence on cytokine production and fatal meningococcal disease. *Lancet* 1997; **349:** 170–3.
77. Gagro A, Gordon J. The interplay between T helper subset cytokines and IL-12 in directing human B lymphocyte differentiation. *Eur J Immunol* 1999; **29:** 3369–79.
78. Martinez FD, Solomon S, Holberg CJ et al. Linkage of circulating eosinophils to markers in chromosome 5q. *Am J Respir Crit Care Med* 1998; **158:** 1739–44.
79. Marsh DG, Neely JD, Breazeale DR et al. Linkage analysis of IL4 and other chromosome 5q31.1 markers and total serum immunoglobulin E concentrations. *Science* 1994; **264:** 1152–6.
80. Baldini M, Lohman IC, Halonen M et al. A polymorphism in the 5'-flanking region of the CD14 gene is associated with circulating soluble CD14 levels and with total serum IgE. *Am J Resp Cell Mol Biol* 1999; **20:** 976–83.
81. Hubacek JA, Pit'ha J, Skodova Z et al. C(-260)→T polymorphism in the promoter of the CD14 monocyte receptor gene as a risk factor for myocardial infarction. *Circulation* 1999; **99:** 3218–20.
82. O'Donnell AR, Hayden CM, Laing IA et al. Association study of CC16 and CD14 polymorphisms in an unselected population assessed at age 8 and 25. *Am J Resp Crit Care Med* 2000; **161:** A928.
83. Joos L, Zhu S, Becker A et al. Polymorphisms of the CD14 and TGFB1 genes in a cohort of infants at high risk of allergic disorders. *Am J Resp Crit Care Med* 2000; **161:** A928.
84. Gao PS, Mao XQ, Baldini M et al. Serum total IgE levels and CD14 on chromosome 5q31. *Clin Genet* 1999; **56:** 164–5.

5

Relationship of viral and bacterial infections to the development and course of asthma

Amjad Tuffaha, William W Busse

Introduction • Epidemiology of viral infections and asthma • Epidemiology of bacterial infections and asthma • Respiratory viruses' interactions with immunoinflammatory mechanisms involved in asthma • Mechanisms of viral-induced airway obstruction and asthma • Effects of respiratory viruses on airway inflammation • Summary

INTRODUCTION

Viral respiratory tract infections are the major cause of asthma exacerbations in children and adults. Up to 85% of asthma exacerbations in children[1] and 44% in adults[2] are associated with viral upper respiratory tract infections. These observations suggest that respiratory viruses are a major factor in provoking existing asthma and may accomplish this by enhancing existing airway inflammation. Furthermore, there is evidence that respiratory tract infections cause frequent episodes of wheezing in infants and may even be a factor in causing expression of asthma. Thus, respiratory infections can have two major effects on asthma: (1) a 'possible' etiological role in initiating asthma in infants and (2) the major cause of asthma exacerbations in patients who already have the disease. The evidence for a role of bacterial respiratory infection in either the initiation or promotion of asthma is not as well understood or established as in the case of viral respiratory infections. In this chapter, we will focus mainly on the role and contribution of viral respiratory infections to asthma. We will present a review of the epidemiology of viral/bacterial infection and asthma, the interactions between respiratory viruses and other risk factors for asthma, and the possible mechanisms of virus-induced asthma exacerbations.

EPIDEMIOLOGY OF VIRAL INFECTIONS AND ASTHMA

Respiratory virus infections are associated with the onset of asthma in some children and are the major cause of asthma exacerbations in those with existing disease. A group of respiratory viruses have been implicated as being potentially responsible for the onset of the asthmatic phenotype in the first years of life (Table 5.1). Respiratory syncytial virus (RSV) and parainfluenza virus (PIV) are the major causes of bronchiolitis, which can cause symptoms that mimic asthma. These features include cold-like symptoms and a low-grade fever which is followed 1–2 days later by tachypnea, chest retractions, and wheezing.[3,4] Respiratory syncytial virus is responsible for most bronchiolitis episodes (up to 70%[5]) and is the most common cause of bronchiolitis and pneumonia in infants requiring hospitalization.[6] The peak incidence

Table 5.1 Sequelae of respiratory viral infections

Age group	Virus	Risk factors	Outcomes
Infants	RSV, PIV	None	URI
		↓ PFT, Passive smoking	Bronchiolitis
	Measles	Active immunization	↓ risk of allergen Sensitization
Children & adults	RV & others	None	URI
		Asthma	Wheezing

of RSV infection is between 6 weeks and 6 months of age;[7] infants in this age range are also most prone to develop lower respiratory tract symptoms, but only a subset of those who wheeze subsequently develop persistent asthma.

Viral infections in early childhood may also interact with the immune system to modify the subsequent risk of allergen sensitization and/or asthma.[8] For example, several studies have shown that the possibility of allergen sensitization is inversely related to the number of older siblings in the family, a reflection of exposure to viral respiratory infections in early childhood.[9-11] In contrast, data also indicate that severe RSV infection may enhance allergen sensitization and the risk of developing asthma;[12] however, not all studies have found an increase in the risk of allergy following RSV infections.[13-15]

The relationship between bronchiolitis and the development of the asthmatic phenotype remains controversial. Diagnosis of asthma, recurrent wheezing, or increase in airway hyperresponsiveness, as long-term outcome parameters after bronchiolitis infection, has been influenced by study design, study population, the severity of bronchiolitis symptoms, age at the time of the infection, and the type of virus associated with the symptoms (RSV, PIV, influenza, or coronavirus). These findings indicate the need for prospective controlled studies to determine more precisely the long-term effects of childhood infection on the immune system, the subsequent risk for allergy and asthma, and the likely complexity of this interaction.

A recent 11 year prospective study, involving 880 children who were enrolled at birth, evaluated selected interrelationships between early respiratory viral infection and later development of asthma.[16] The identified children were followed over the first 3 years of life for the development of lower respiratory tract illnesses and the presence of physician-diagnosed asthma and/or recurrent wheezing at ages 6 and 11 years. Lung functions were measured in the first few months of life, before the development of lower respiratory tract infections (LRI) and provided important baseline values. At 6 years of age, physician-diagnosed asthma was present in 13.6%, 10.2%, and 4.6% of the children with pneumonia, LRI, and no LRI, respectively. By 11 years of age, these values had increased to 25.9%, 16.1% and 11%, respectively. Moreover, V_{max} and functional residual capacity (FRC) at baseline, before any LRI were lower in the children with pneumonia and LRI than in children with no LRI. These measurements of lung functions continued to be lower at age 6 years, and by 11 years of age similar differences in the various groups persisted. In spite of the persistence of lower baseline lung functions in both the pneumonia and LRI groups, many of the markers of airflow limitation showed significant reversibility following administration of β_2-adrenergic receptor agonists. The finding of reversible airflow obstruction to a beta-agonist further supports the possibility that an earlier LRI is an important risk factor for asthma.

In addition to the effect of baseline lung functions on these interactions, the influence of atopy on the development of asthma phenotype in relationship with viral infections has been of interest. Atopy, itself a risk factor for the development of childhood asthma, can also influence the lower airway response to viral infections.[17] Viral infections, on the other hand, can influence the development of allergen sensitization with subsequent development of elevated levels of total and allergen specific IgE.[17] This interaction seems to be a dynamic but complex relationship and continues to be a focus of increasing interest and importance. For example, Laing et al.[18] found that children who were most likely to have persistent wheezing after viral respiratory infections were those infants born to an atopic parent. Pullan and Hey,[19] however, did not find this relationship. In the same context, Castro-Rodríguez et al.[16] found that personal atopy is not increased in symptomatic children after documented bronchiolitis; others have found that RSV bronchiolitis significantly increases the chances for subsequently developing IgE antibody to both food and aeroallergens.

For those with existing allergic disease, the presence of an atopic status may define a host susceptibility to wheezing with a respiratory infection. For example, Duff et al.[20] studied children above 2 years of age who presented to an emergency room department with wheezing. Children over 2 years of age were more likely to have respiratory allergies and a confirmed respiratory viral infection when compared with children with no wheezing. Children with the highest risk for wheezing were those who had respiratory allergies and respiratory viral infection, which implies that respiratory viral infections and respiratory allergies may have synergistic effects on lower airway physiology and enhance the likelihood of wheezing with respiratory infection. In children less than 2 years of age, wheezing was also noted but risk factors for wheezing were quite different. These infants were not allergic, had RSV as the major virus isolate, and had passive cigarette smoke as a major risk factor for wheezing. These data suggest that wheezing in children less than 2 years old is associated with RSV infection, and factors other than allergy appear to determine or influence this outcome. In contrast, children greater than 2 years of age are more likely to wheeze with rhinovirus (RV) infection and to be atopic (positive radioallergosorbent test (RAST)).

Respiratory viruses are common causes of asthma exacerbations in asthmatic subjects of different age groups.[1,2,21,22] Serology and/or culture detection methods for viruses initially indicated an association with these respiratory infections and asthma exacerbations.[22,23] These methods of detection are relatively insensitive for viruses like rhinovirus. Consequently, the use of reverse transcription polymerase chain reaction (RT-PCR) assays has proven more sensitive to detect rhinoviruses, which are difficult to detect using standard virologic methods.[24,25] In this regard, Johnston et al.[1] found that 80–85% of school-aged children with acute wheezing episodes tested positive for a virus using RT-PCR and other standard virologic techniques. The most common virus detected was RV. Similar studies were done in adults by Nicholson et al.[2] using RT-PCR virus-detecting methods and found that about one-half of the asthma exacerbations in adults were associated with RV infection. Seasonal patterns of upper respiratory virus infections correlate closely with hospital admissions for asthma, particularly in pediatric age groups.[26] These studies indicate that RV infections are the most common cause of asthma exacerbations in children.

EPIDEMIOLOGY OF BACTERIAL INFECTIONS AND ASTHMA

The role of bacterial infection in the initiation or promotion of asthma is not as prominent as has been the association with viral respiratory infections. Nonetheless, it has been noted that certain antibiotics (such as erythromycin) can reduce the severity of airway hyperresponsiveness in some asthma patients and thus reduce their symptoms, though this might be secondary to the general effect of antibiotics.[27]

It has been shown as well that asthma patients have increased concentrations of IgA and IgM in bronchoalveolar lavage.[28] Recent research has suggested that atypical bacterial infections may play a role in asthma pathogenesis. For example, one-third of children having neonatal chlamydia trachomatis developed asthma before school age.[29] Hahn et al. found that 47% of adults with acute *Chlamydia pneumoniae* had asthmatic symptoms, and that the presence of asthmatic bronchitis correlated with *C. pneumoniae* antibody titer 6 months after respiratory illness.[30] Similar studies showed that acute *C. pneumoniae* infections can also trigger exacerbations of asthma in children,[31,32] and that anti-chlamydial antibiotic therapy can help to improve or bring about a total remission of asthma.[33,34] Thus far, there is no evidence that *C. pneumoniae* or any other atypical bacterial infection may be responsible for the increase in asthma prevalence during recent decades.

RESPIRATORY VIRUSES' INTERACTIONS WITH IMMUNOINFLAMMATORY MECHANISMS INVOLVED IN ASTHMA
(Figure 5.1)

Respiratory viruses, and RSV in particular, can infect the lower airway epithelium. Infection of the epithelium may alter lower airway integrity and thus enhance absorption of aeroallergens across the airway barrier, leading to allergen sensitization. In addition, infection of local airway inflammatory cells can generate several cytokines (TNF-α, IL-1β, IL-1α, IL-6, IL-8) and chemokines (MIP-1α, MCP-1, RANTES), and increased expression of adhesion molecules (ICAM-1) to modulate or augment the ongoing inflammatory response. It has also been suggested that RSV antigen presentation to subpopulations of lymphocytes may lead to a series of interactions to enhance TH$_2$-like responses. In infants 1–15 months of age with acute bronchiolitis caused by RSV, IFN-γ production was

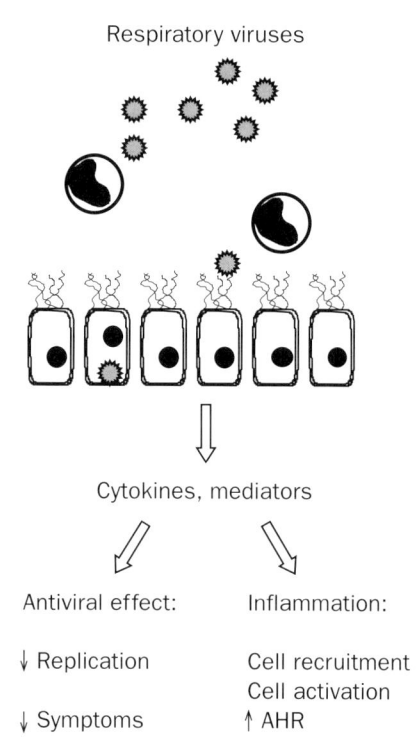

Figure 5.1 Respiratory virus interaction with immunoinflammatory mechanisms in asthma.

suppressed, and IL-4/IFN-γ ratio was significantly increased. In a similar study[35] blood samples from infants hospitalized with acute bronchiolitis were obtained at the time of acute infection and 5 months later. An increased percentage of CD4+, CD25+, and CD23+ lymphocytes at the 5 months follow-up was noticed. Plasma IL-4 levels, which were not significantly different from those in control subjects initially, increased significantly in the infected patients when measured 5 months later. In addition, peripheral blood lymphocytes produced less IFN-γ in response to IL-12 at the time of infection in the children who developed symptoms of recurrent wheezing after the acute infection was over. Peripheral blood lymphocytes from infants who continued to have persistent wheezing produced more IL-4 in response to *Dermatophagoides farinae* antigen. The investigators concluded that a lower production of IFN-γ at the time of bronchiolitis infection was associated with reduced pulmonary function and increased airway hyperresponsiveness to histamine 5 months after acute infection. This study provided evidence for an association of diminished IFN-γ generation and/or increased IL-4 production with bronchial hyperresponsiveness and recurrent wheezing.

T-cell responses to viral infection are mainly involved in the induction of antigen-specific cytotoxic CD8+ T-cells which can lyse target cells sharing MHC class 1 molecules complexed with viral peptides. CD4+ T-cells divide into TH_1 and TH_2 subsets depending on the cytokine profile produced by each subset. CD8+ T-cells induce IFN-γ and IFN-β, both of which are considered TH_1 markers. CD8+ T-cells may also produce TH_2-type cytokine via a subset of CD8+ T-cells referred to as 'Tc_2'; this property enhances the ability of CD8+ T-cells to regulate several immune inflammatory processes. The cytokines, present in the local environment where inflammatory processes are active, are important as well in giving these inflammatory processes a TH_1 versus TH_2 identity. For example, IL-4 may switch CD8+ T-cells to a predominant Tc_2 type. In a transgenic murine model used to evaluate the interactions between atopy and viral infection, local TH_2 responses, which were mediated by CD4+ T-helper cells that had been induced by allergen exposure, influenced virus-specific CD8+ T-cells to produce IL-5.[36] When these IL-5-producing cells were subsequently challenged with a virus peptide, pulmonary eosinophilic infiltration occurred. This suggests that a tissue with a background rich in TH_2 cytokines, as might occur in an atopic individual, for example, can influence the T-cell cytokine response that may occur following viral infection. A bias towards a TH_2 response could then significantly affect the features of the immunoinflammatory airway response and ultimately lead to persistent airway inflammation and, possibly, the induction of the asthmatic phenotype.

In this respect, a rat model of virus-induced airway dysfunction has been developed to evaluate the relationships between viral infection, atopy (as a marker of TH_1/TH_2 imbalance), and immune system and/or lung development components.[37] Compared with a low IgE antibody producing Fischer 344 (F344) strain, the Brown Norway (BN) strain is a high IgE antibody producer. When both strains are infected with a parainfluenza 1 virus at 3–4 weeks of age, the F344 rats recover completely whereas the BN rats go on to develop chronic episodic reversible airway obstruction associated with airway inflammation, characteristics of remodeling, and evidence of airway hyperresponsiveness that can persist for up to 8–12 weeks following the infection.[38] The progression of this asthma-like syndrome in the BN strain is associated with a TH_1/TH_2 cytokine imbalance in the lung and increased expression of TH_2 cytokines; its development can be significantly attenuated by treatment with exogenous IFN-γ just before and during the viral infection.[39] This model in the rat presents evidence that not only are genetic (atopy, cytokine dysregulation) and environmental (virus infection) factors important in the initiation of the asthmatic phenotype, but also the immune response to the infection appears to be a contributing factor as well.

MECHANISMS OF VIRAL-INDUCED AIRWAY OBSTRUCTION AND ASTHMA (Table 5.2)

Increased bronchial hyperresponsiveness

Increased bronchial responsiveness has been found in normal and asthmatic subjects following infections with RV[40] and influenza A.[41–45] In a study by Cheung et al.[46] 14 subjects with mild asthma were inoculated with RV16 or placebo. The maximal contractile response to inhaled methacholine was significantly greater during the RV16 infection and remained enhanced for up to 15 days after the acute infection. This study indicates that an upper respiratory viral infection can enhance the reactivity of the lower airway and the magnitude of bronchoconstriction, both of which can persist for weeks after acute infection.

Respiratory viral infection effects on lower airway responses are also influenced by host

Table 5.2 Mechanisms of viral-induced airway obstruction

↑ **Airway responsiveness**
Increased sensitivity
Increased maximal response

Altered neural control mechanisms
Enhanced parasympathetic efferent signal
- ↓ M_2 receptor function
- M_2 independent factors

Sensory C fibers
- ↑ Neuropeptide release
- Loss of neutral endopeptidase

Defective NANC responses
- ↓ NO production

Altered small airway geometry
Airway wall thickening
Plugging of the lumen
- Mucus secretions
- Cellular debris

---

factors. In particular, allergic subjects experience greater changes in airway responsiveness after viral infection than do nonallergic control subjects.[47,48] Furthermore, subjects with lower FEV_1 values tend to have greater changes in airway responsiveness during viral infection.[48] These studies suggest that pre-existing conditions such as allergy and the intrinsic lower airway functions are likely to promote airway hyperresponsiveness during respiratory viral infection and to raise the possibility that patients prone to virus-induced asthma exacerbations are at increased risk for such problems with colds.

Neural control of the airways

Potential neuromechanisms by which viral infections cause bronchoconstriction and increased airway responsiveness include:

(a) enhanced parasympathetic bronchoconstrictive responses;
(b) airway sensory nerve stimulation;
(c) interference with the bronchodilatory functions of the nonadrenergic, noncholinergic neurons.

Parasympathetic effects

Increases in bronchial responsiveness with a viral respiratory infection can be induced via cholinergic overactivity. For example, Empey et al. showed that bronchial hyperresponsiveness associated with a respiratory infection can be blocked by atropine and reversed by isoproterenol.[49] Buckner et al. investigated this hypothesis further in guinea pigs and showed that overactivity of the efferent cholinergic nerves after viral infection augments the bronchoconstriction caused by electrical stimulation of the vagus nerve.[50] Subsequent work has suggested that viruses may cause M_2 muscarinic receptors dysfunction. When Fryer et al.[51] treated uninfected control guinea pigs with gallamine, an M_2 muscarinic receptor blocker, it was found that an increase in airway response to vagal stimulation occurred. Much less response was noticed in guinea pigs infected with parainfluenza virus. The effect on M_2 receptors by respiratory infections could increase the cholinergic responsiveness, since M_2 receptors are inhibitory neural autoreceptors; therefore, blockade of their activity would remove the negative feedback loop that normally limits acetylcholine release from cholinergic nerves.

Viral illness may also cause M_2 receptor dysfunction through the effects of virus-generated neuraminidase[52] or by inducing the release of inflammatory cell products like eosinophil cationic proteins, which can then block this neuroregulatory response.[53] It is also possible that mechanisms independent of M_2 receptors may contribute to cholinergic overactivity. For example, in rats infected with parainfluenza type I (Sendai), the inhibitory M_2 function is restored shortly after the virus is cleared from the airways; although the M_2 receptor function has normalized by this time, the bronchoconstrictor response to parasympathetic nerve stimulation continues to be enhanced for at least 2 weeks.[54] This observation raises the possibility that factors in addition to M_2 receptor dysfunction contribute to alterations in airway function during a respiratory infection.

Sensory C fibers

C fibers in the airway can initiate bronchoconstriction by release of neuropeptides like substance P and neurokinin A,[55,56] both of which have a direct stimulatory effect on airway smooth muscles. Neuropeptides can in addition increase leukotriene synthesis,[57] mast cell mediator release,[52] and airway mucous secretion,[58] which can contribute to airway obstruction and hyperresponsiveness. Viral infection can potentiate the release and/or the effect of neuropeptides in animal models. An increased airway contractile response to neuropeptides has also been observed in PIV-infected guinea pigs[59–62] and influenza A infected ferret tracheas. The enhanced effects of neuropeptides on infected airways can be explained by damage to airway epithelium caused by the viral infection exposing sensory nerves, which then are more easily stimulated by inflammatory mediators.

The contribution of the sensory C fibers and tachykinins to virus-induced asthma exacerbations in humans is not well established despite the information obtained from animal model experiments.

Nonadrenergic, noncholinergic effects

Nonadrenergic, noncholinergic neurons serve to oppose airway smooth muscle contraction. The nonadrenergic inhibitory neural response is not detected in tracheal smooth muscle from RSV-infected cotton rats.[63] In addition, release of nitric oxide, a potent bronchodilator putative mediator, is decreased in hyperresponsive tracheas from infected guinea pigs.

Structural effects on the small airways

Changes in small airways structure and function may also contribute significantly to the severity of hyperinflation and gas exchange abnormalities noted in acute asthma exacerbations. The maximal airway contractile response to methacholine in mild asthmatic subjects is increased during a cold, which is probably secondary to excessive airway narrowing due to airway wall thickening, airway parenchymal uncoupling, or abnormalities in smooth muscle contraction.[46] Significant changes in airway morphology are noticed in animals with acute viral respiratory illness, which may then lead to marked bronchiolar narrowing and plugging with mucus. These changes include bronchiolar airway edema and cell infiltration, epithelial hyperplasia, folding, and sloughing of airway epithelial surfaces. In addition, rats with a mild increase in pulmonary resistance and methacholine sensitivity during acute viral respiratory illness show evidence of air trapping and ventilation–perfusion mismatches,[54] indicating that viruses can induce significant changes in the peripheral airways which have significant functional outcomes in the absence of marked changes in airway obstruction and responsiveness measures.

EFFECTS OF RESPIRATORY VIRUSES ON AIRWAY INFLAMMATION (Table 5.3)

Respiratory viruses can cause inflammation and injury to healthy airways and worsen airway injury already involved in an inflammatory

Table 5.3 Effect of respiratory viruses on airway inflammation

Nonspecific immune responses
Epithelial cells
Endothelial cells
Macrophages and monocytes
Granulocytes

T-cell responses to viral infection
Antigen independent
Antigen specific

Interaction with pre-existing airway inflammation

process like in asthma. Respiratory viruses can induce an inflammatory process by direct cytopathic effect on the airway epithelium (e.g. RSV bronchiolitis), and can induce an immune response that can be responsible for triggering an asthma exacerbation without significant direct cytopathic effect on the respiratory mucosa (e.g. rhinovirus).

The virus-induced immune response can contribute to airway inflammation and asthma by:

(a) nonspecific responses to viral infection which may be mediated by epithelial cells, granulocytes, mononuclear cells, and phagocytes;
(b) adaptive immune response mediated by T-lymphocytes.

Effect on epithelial cells (Figure 5.2)

Upper respiratory tract viruses first target and interact with airway epithelium. Rhinovirus has the ability to infect epithelium and to upregulate the surface expression of intercellular adhesion molecule (ICAM-1),[64] which is the receptor for the major group of rhinoviruses.[65,66] This enhanced expression of adhesion proteins may explain the persistence and severity of inflammation in asthmatic subjects and possibly the greater susceptibility of asthmatic children to colds compared with non-asthmatic children.[67] Bronchial epithelial lines have been used to study the effects of virus infection on epithelial cytokine production. Generation of IL-6 and IL-8 has been reported following RSV and RV infection of epithelial cell lines,[68-70] RANTES and macrophage inflammatory protein (MIP)-1α following RSV infection,[71] granulocyte macrophage colony stimulating factor (GM-CSF) following RV infection,[72] and IL-11 following RSV, parainfluenza 3, and RV infection.[73]

IL-8, a potent neutrophil chemoattractant, is found in high concentrations in nasal secretions of children with virus-induced asthma. IL-8 levels in nasal secretions correlate with neutrophil myeloperoxidase values, suggesting an involvement with neutrophil activation.[74] RANTES is a chemoattractant for eosinophils,[75] and GM-CSF is a potent activator of eosinophil survival, adhesion molecule expression, and eosinophil degranulation and superoxide production.[76-78] In addition, RV and RSV can induce production of high IL-11 levels from infected epithelial cells in vitro; IL-11 may have direct effects on bronchial hyper-responsiveness.[73,79]

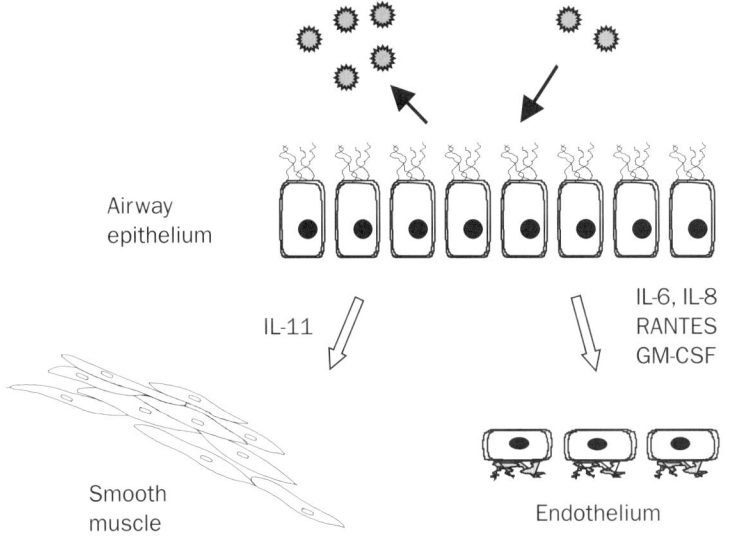

Figure 5.2 Airway epithelium activation by viral replication.

Mechanisms for the activation of the cytokine gene in epithelial cells are under investigation. It is known that nuclear factor kappa B (NF-κB) activation is important in virus-induced transcriptional regulation of IL-6[80] and is possibly a key transcription factor for the synthesis of a variety of other inflammatory cytokines.[81]

Effect on inflammatory cells (Figure 5.3)

Effect on granulocytes

IL-6 and leukotriene B_4 (LTB_4) can contribute to the recruitment of neutrophils to the airway during the acute stages of viral respiratory infection.[82–84] Respiratory viruses can activate neutrophil inflammatory functions, and complexes of RSV and antibody can induce IL-6 and IL-8 secretions from neutrophils which can then further enhance neutrophil and eosinophil recruitment to the lung, thus establishing a vicious cycle. Neutrophils seem to have an important role in the pathogenesis of virus-induced asthma exacerbations. Grünberg et al.[85] experimentally inoculated 35 atopic asthma subjects with either RV16 or placebo and found that neutrophil counts in the peripheral blood correlated with the cold and asthma symptom scores and cold-induced changes in airway hyperresponsiveness.

There is evidence that some respiratory viral infections can activate eosinophils. Eosinophil granular proteins and leukotriene C_4 (LTC_4) have been detected in the nasal secretions of infants and children, presumably with RSV wheezing illnesses.[86–89] Increased concentrations of sputum eosinophil cationic protein (ECP) found during the acute phase of RV infection correlated with increases in airway responsiveness in a group of adults with asthma after experimental inoculation with RV16.[90] In vitro experiments indicate that RV does not activate eosinophils directly, but inflammatory mediators and cytokines secreted by virus-activated cells in the lung contribute to eosinophil activation.[91] Finally, guinea pigs infected with PIV develop airway eosinophils and airway hyperresponsiveness,[92] and this outcome is blocked if the guinea pigs are pretreated with IL-5-neutralizing antibody.[93]

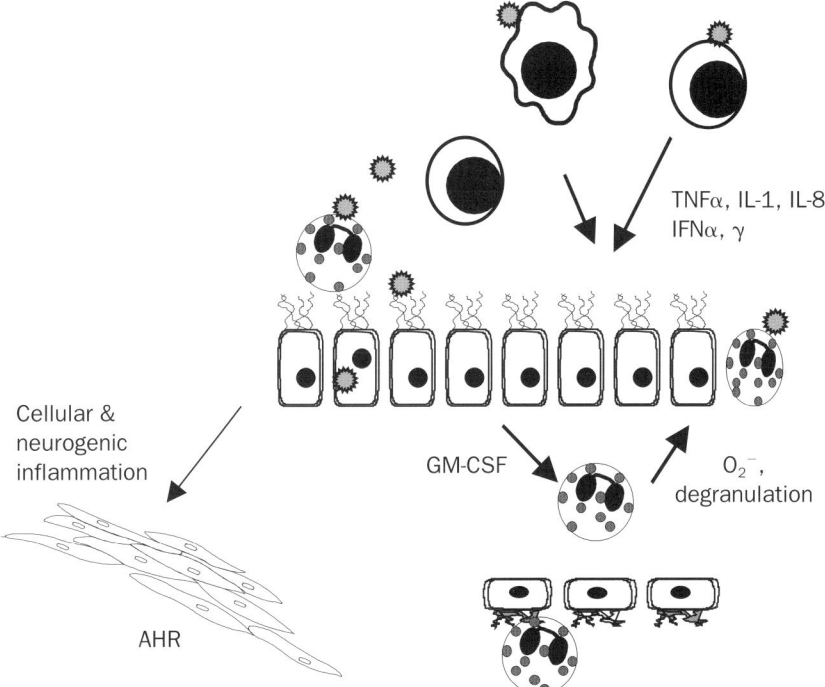

Figure 5.3 Immune cell influx and activation.

Effect on monocytes and macrophages

Monocytes and macrophages express high levels of ICAM-1[94] and act as important cells in the early response to respiratory viruses. In vitro infection of human monocytes with respiratory viruses leads to a potent proinflammatory cytokine response characterized by the release of IL-8, IL-1, and TNF-α.[95–97] IL-1 and TNF-α can also increase cell recruitment into the airway through effects on ICAM-1 expression on endothelial cells. In addition, TNF-α has been associated with wheezing illnesses in infancy[98] and the development of late phase allergic reaction and asthma.[99,100] Monocytes and macrophages produce interferon that can be measured in nasal secretions and coincides with the onset of the recovery process.

In addition to cytokine production, macrophages incubated with RSV or PIV produce lipid mediators like prostaglandin E_2, platelet-activating factor, and thromboxane B_2,[101–103] which also can augment airway inflammation. On the other hand, viral infections can interfere with antigen presentation by macrophages. Influenza, RV, and RSV inhibit T-cell proliferation in vitro[104–107] possibly owing to effects on antigen processing by macrophages.

Effect on T-cells

Respiratory viral infections can activate T-cells and induce specific or nonspecific T-cell responses which may determine the severity of asthma. Rhinovirus infections are usually associated with peripheral lymphopenia and an increase in nasal secretions and lower airway epithelium lymphocyte infiltration. The degree of peripheral blood lymphopenia and lymphocytic infiltration of the airway epithelium has been correlated with increases in airway responsiveness.[46,108]

As discussed above, T-cells are involved in antiviral immune responses which require the involvement of natural killer cells, CD8+ cytotoxic T-cells, and CD4+ T-cells. CD8+ T-cells have the ability to produce IFN-γ during the viral infection which can lyse virus-infected cells. CD4+ T-cells help in the recovery from the infection by directing the immune response through the secretions of cytokines in response to the viral infection. These cytokines can commit T-helper cells toward TH_1 versus TH_2 immune responses that are important in coordinating both cytotoxic and antibody responses to viral infection.

Several studies have shown that viral infections activate a wide range of T-cells. Evidence for this comes from experiments in mice in which most of the T-cells found in the lung after an acute viral infection are not virus specific.[109] Taking into consideration the large number of cytokines and inflammatory mediators present in the lung during viral infection, it is likely that local T-cells are activated in an antigen-independent manner and activated early in the process of viral infection. Experiments in which peripheral blood cells were incubated with RV found that 25–50% of T-cells were expressing the early activation marker CD69. In addition, IFN-γ mRNA and protein were induced.[110] RANTES, induced by respiratory viruses, at high concentrations can also induce antigen-independent T-cell activation.[111] These studies suggest that respiratory viruses can induce early nonspecific T-cell activation and recruitment and this can significantly increase the intensity of airway inflammation, which translates into more airway dysfunction and respiratory symptoms.

SUMMARY

Respiratory infections commonly precipitate wheezing symptoms. RV appears to be the most important virus in producing exacerbations of asthma in the older child who already has established the disease. One of the mechanisms by which this occurs is through the virus's ability to interact with immune cells such as lymphocytes, eosinophils, neutrophils, and macrophages and then to cause airway inflammation over a prolonged period of time. Furthermore, for reasons that are not well defined, the upregulation of inflammation by the viral respiratory infection persists long beyond the acute viral respiratory infection. It is important not only to understand the frequency of this problem, but also to consider that airway inflammation may be the major cause of symptomatology in these asthmatic children. Current and future treatments need to be directed toward this airway inflammation rather than the symptomatic relief of airflow obstruction.

REFERENCES

1. Johnston SL, Pattemore PK, Sanderson G, Smith S, Campbell MJ, Josephs LK. Community study of role of viral infections in exacerbations of asthma in 9–11 year old children. *BMJ* 1995; **310**: 1225–9.
2. Nicholson KG, Kent J, Ireland DC. Respiratory viruses and exacerbations of asthma in adults. *BMJ* 1993; **307**: 982–6.
3. McConnochie KM. Bronchiolitis: what's in the name? *Am J Dis Child* 1983; **137**: 11–13.
4. Whol MEB. Bronchiolitis. In: Chernick V, Kendig EL Jr, eds. *Disorders of the Respiratory Tract in Children*, 5th edn. Philadelphia: WB Saunders, 1990, 360–70.
5. McKenzie S. Respiratory tract infection. In: Campbell AGM, McIntosh N, eds. *Forfar and Arneil's Textbook of Paediatrics.* Edinburgh: Churchill Livingstone, 1992, 633–44.
6. Hoberg CJ, Wright AL, Martinez FD. Risk factors for respiratory syncytial virus-associated lower airway illness in the first year of life. *Am J Epidemiol* 1991; **133**: 1135–51.
7. Parrott RH, Kim KW, Arrobio JO, Hodes DS, Murphy BR, Brandt CD et al. Epidemiology of respiratory syncytial virus infection in Washington DC. II. Infection and disease with respect to age, immunologic status, race and sex. *Am J Epidemiol* 1973; **98**: 289–300.
8. Shaheen SO. Changing patterns of childhood infection and the rise in allergic disease. *Clin Exp Allergy* 1995; **25**: 1034–7.
9. von Mutius E, Martinez FD, Fritzsch C, Nicolai T, Reitmeir P, Thiemann JJ. Skin test reactivity and number of siblings. *BMJ* 1994; **308**: 692–5.
10. Strachan DP. Hay fever, hygiene, and household size. *BMJ* 1989; **299**: 1529–60.
11. Strachan DP, Harkins LS, Johnston IDA, Anderson HR. Childhood antecedents of allergic sensitization in young British adults. *J Allergy Clin Immunol* 1997; **99**: 6–12.
12. Sigurs N, Njarnason R, Sigurbergsson F, Kjellman B, Bjorksten B. Asthma and immunoglobulin E antibodies after respiratory syncytial virus bronchiolitis: a prospective cohort study with matched controls. *Pediatrics* 1995; **95**: 500–5.
13. Cogswell JJ, Halliday DF, Alexander JR. Respiratory infections in the first year of life in children at risk of developing atopy. *BMJ* 1982; **284**: 1011–13.
14. Welliver RC. RSV and chronic asthma. *Lancet* 1995; **364**: 789–90.
15. Pullan CR, Hey EN. Wheezing, asthma, and pulmonary dysfunction 10 years after infection with respiratory syncytial virus in infancy. *BMJ* 1982; **284**: 1665–9.
16. Castro-Rodríguez JA, Holberg CJ, Wright AL, Halonen M, Taussig LM, Morgan WJ et al. Association of radiologically ascertained pneumonia before age 3 yr with asthma like symptoms and pulmonary function during childhood. A prospective study. *Am J Respir Crit Care Med* 1999; **159**: 1891–7.
17. Martinez FD, Wright AL, Taussig LM, Holberg CJ, Halonen M, Morgan WJ et al. Asthma and wheezing in the first six years of life. *N Engl J Med* 1995; **332**: 133–8.
18. Laing I, Riedel F, Yap PL, Simpson J. Atopy predisposing to acute bronchiolitis during an epidemic of respiratory syncytial virus. *BMJ* 1982; **284**: 1070–2.
19. Pullan CR, Hey EN. Wheezing, asthma, and pulmonary dysfunction 10 years after infection with respiratory syncytial virus in infancy. *BMJ* 1982; **284**: 1665–9.
20. Duff AL, Pomeranz ES, Gelber LE, Price HW, Farris H, Hayden FG et al. Risk factors for acute wheezing in infants and children: viruses, passive smoke, and IgE antibodies to inhalant allergens. *Pediatrics* 1993; **92**: 535–40.
21. Cypacar D, Busse WW. Role of viral infections in asthma. *Immunol Allergy Clin North Am* 1993; **13**: 745–66.
22. Pattemore PK, Johnston SL, Bardin PG. Virus are precipitants of asthma symptoms, I: epidemiology. *Clin Exp Allergy* 1992; **22**: 325–36.
23. Dick EC, Inhorn SL. Rhinoviruses. In: Feigin RD, Cherry JD, eds. *Textbook of Pediatric Infectious Diseases.* Philadelphia: WB Saunders, 1992, 1507–32.
24. Gama RE, Horsnell PR, Hughes PJ, North C, Bruce CB, al-Nakib W et al. Amplification of

25. Johnston SL, Xie P, Johnson W. Comparison of standard virology and PCR in diagnosis of rhinovirus and respiratory syncytial virus infections in nasal aspirates from children hospitalized with wheezing illness and bronchiolitis. *Am J Respir Crit Care Med* 1996; **153:** A503.
26. Johnston SL, Pattemore PK, Sanderson G, Smith S, Campbell MJ, Josephs LK et al. The relationship between upper respiratory infections and hospital admissions for asthma: a time trend analysis. *Am J Respir Crit Care Med* 1996; **154:** 654–60.
27. Miyataka H, Taki F, Taniguchi H, Suzuki R, Tagaki K, Satake T. Erythromycin reduces the severity of hyperresponsiveness in asthma. *Chest* 1991; **99:** 670–3.
28. Peebles RS, Liu MC, Lichtenstein LM, Hamilton RG. IgA, IgG, and IgM quantification in bronchoalveolar lavage fluids from allergic rhinitis, allergic asthmatics, and normal subjects by monoclonal antibody-based immunoenzymetric assays. *J Immunol Methods* 1995; **179:** 77–86.
29. Weiss S, Newcomb R, Beem M. Pulmonary assessment of children after chlamydia pneumonia in infancy. *J Pediatr* 1986; **108:** 659–64.
30. Hahn DL, Dodge R, Golubjantnikov R. Association of Chlamydia pneumoniae (strain TWAR) infection with wheezing, asthmatic bronchitis, and adult-onset asthma. *JAMA* 1991; **226:** 225–30.
31. Emre U, Roblin PM, Gelling M, Dumornay W, Rao M, Hammershchlag MR et al. The association of Chlamydia pneumoniae infection and reactive airway disease in children. *Arch Pediatr Adolesc Med* 1994; **148:** 727–32.
32. Kroppi M, Leinonen M, Saikku P. Chlamydial infection and reactive airway disease. *Arch Pediatr Adolesc Med* 1994; **149:** 341–2.
33. Hahn DL. Clinical experience with antichlamydial therapy for adult-onset asthma. *Am Rev Respir Dis* 1993; **147:** 297A.
34. Kawane H. Chlamydia pneumoniae. *Thorax* 1995; **48:** 871.
35. Renzi PM, Turgeon JP, Marcotte JE, Drblik SP, Bérubé D, Gagnon MF et al. Reduced interferon-γ production in infants with bronchiolitis and asthma. *Am J Respir Crit Care Med* 1999; **159:** 1417–22.
36. Coyle AJ, Erard F, Bertrand C, Walti S, Pircher H, Le Gros G. Virus specific CD8+ cells can switch to interleukin 5 production and induce airway eosinophilia. *J Exp Med* 1995; **181:** 1229–33.
37. Uhl EW, Castleman WL, Sorkness RL, Busse WW, Lemanske RF Jr, Mcallister PK. Parainfluenza virus-induced persistence of airway inflammation, fibrosis, and dysfunction associated with TGF-$β_1$ expression in brown Norway rats. *Am J Respir Crit Care Med* 1996; **154:** 1834–42.
38. Kumar A, Sorkness R, Kaplan MR, Castleman WL, Lemanske RF Jr. Chronic, episodic, reversible airway obstruction after viral bronchitis in rats. *Am J Respir Crit Care Med* 1997; **155:** 130–4.
39. Sorkness RL, Castleman WL, Kumar A, Kaplan MR, Lemanske RF Jr. Prevention of chronic post-bronchiolitis airway sequelae with interferon-γ treatment in rats. *Am J Respir Crit Care Med* 1999; **160:** 705–10.
40. Ward BJ, Griffin DE. Changes in cytokine production after measles virus vaccination: predominant production of IL-4 suggests induction of a Th$_2$ response. *Clin Immunol Immunopathol* 1993; **67:** 171–7.
41. Laitinen LA, Elkin RB, Empey DW, Jacobs L, Mills J, Nadel JA. Bronchial hyperresponsiveness in normal subjects during attenuated influenza virus infection. *Am Rev Respir Dis* 1991; **143:** 358–61.
42. Laitinen LA, Kava T. Bronchial reactivity following uncomplicated influenza A infection in healthy subjects and asthmatic patients. *Eur J Respir Dis* 1980; **106:** 51–8.
43. Little JW, Hall WJ, Douglas G Jr, Mudholkur GJ, Speers DM, Patel K et al. Airway hyperreactivity and peripheral airway dysfunction in influenza A infection. *Am Rev Respir Dis* 1978; **118:** 295–303.
44. Anand SC, Itkin IH, Kind LS. Effect of influenza vaccine on methacholine sensitivity in patients with asthma of known and unknown origin. *J Allergy* 1968; **42:** 87–91.
45. Ouellete JJ, Reed CE. Increased response of asthmatic subjects to methacholine after influenza vaccine. *J Allergy* 1965; **36:** 558–63.
46. Cheung D, Dick EC, Timmers MC, De Klerk EPA, Spaan WJM, Sterk PJ. Rhinovirus inhalation causes long lasting excessive airway narrowing in response to methacholine in asthmatic subjects in vivo. *Am J Respir Crit Care Med* 1995; **152:** 1490–6.
47. Bardin PG, Sanderson G, Robinson BS, Holgate

ST, Tyrell DAJ. Experimental rhinovirus infection in volunteers. *Eur Respir J* 1996; **9**: 2250–5.
48. Gern JE, Calhoun WJ, Swenson C, Shen G, Busse WW. Rhinovirus infection preferentially increases lower airway responsiveness in allergic subjects. *Am J Respir Crit Care Med* 1997; **155**: 1872–6.
49. Empey DW, Laitnen LA, Jacobs L, Gold WM, Nadel JA. Mechanisms of bronchial hyperreactivity in normal subjects after upper respiratory tract infection. *Am Rev Respir Dis* 1976; **113**: 131–9.
50. Buckner CK, Songsiridej V, Dick EC, Busse WW. In vivo and in vitro studies on the use of the guinea pig as a model for virus-provoked airway hyperreactivity. *Am Rev Respir Dis* 1985; **132**: 305–10.
51. Fryer A, Jacoby D. Parainfluenza virus infection damages inhibitory M_2 muscarinic receptors on pulmonary parasympathetic nerves in the guinea pig. *Br J Pharmacol* 1991; **102**: 267–71.
52. Fryer AD, El-Fakahany EE, Jacoby DB. Parainfluenza virus type 1 reduces the affinity of agonists for muscarinic receptors in guinea-pig lung and heart. *Eur J Pharmacol* 1990; **181**: 51–8.
53. Akira S, Taga T, Kishimoto T. Interleukin-6 in biology and medicine. *Adv Immunol* 1993; **54**: 1–78.
54. Sorkness R, Clough JJ, Castleman WL, Lemanske RF Jr. Virus-induced airway obstruction and parasympathetic hyperresponsiveness in adult rats. *Am J Respir Crit Care Med* 1994; **150**: 28–34.
55. Kowalski ML, Didier A, Kaliner MA. Neurogenic inflammation in the airways, I: neurogenic stimulation induces plasma protein extravasation into the rat airway lumen. *Am Rev Respir Dis* 1989; **140**: 101–9.
56. Piedimonte G, Hoffman JIE, Husseini WK, Snider RM, Desai MC, Nadel JA. NK1 receptors mediate neurogenic inflammatory increase in blood flow in rat airways. *J Appl Physiol* 1993; **74**: 2462–8.
57. Yang XX, Powell WS, Hojo M, Martin JG. Hyperpnea-induced bronchoconstriction is dependent on tachykinin-induced cysteinyl leukotriene synthesis. *J Appl Physiol* 1997; **82**: 538–44.
58. Coles SJ, Neill KH, Reid LM. Potent stimulation of glycoprotein secretion in canine trachea by substance P. *J Appl Physiol* 1984; **57**: 1323–7.
59. Ladenius ARC, Folkerts G, van der Linde HJ, Nijkamp FP. Potentiation by viral respiratory infection of ovalbumin-induced guinea pig tracheal hyperresponsiveness: role for tachykinins. *Br J Pharmacol* 1995; **115**: 1048–52.
60. Dusser DJ, Jacoby DB, Djokic TD, Rubinstein I, Borson DB, Nadel JA. Virus induces airway hyperresponsiveness to tachykinins: role of neutrol endopeptidase. *J Appl Physiol* 1989; **67**: 1504–11.
61. Saban R, Dick EC, Fishleder RI, Buckner CK. Enhancement by parainfluenza 3 infection of contactile responses to substance P and capsiacin in airway smooth muscle from the guinea pig. *Am Rev Respir Dis* 1987; **136**: 586–91.
62. Jacoby DB, Tamaoki J, Borson DB, Nadel JA. Influenza infection causes airway hyperresponsiveness by decreasing enkephalinase. *J Appl Physiol* 1988; **64**: 2635–8.
63. Colasurdo GN, Hemming VG, Prince GA, Loader JE, Graves JP, Larsen GL. Human respiratory syncytial virus affects nonadrenergic noncholinergic inhibition in cotton rat airways. *Am J Physiol* 1995; **12**: L1006–11.
64. Papi A, Wilson S, Johnston S. Rhinoviruses increase production of cell adhesion molecules (CAM) and NF-κB. *Am J Respir Crit Care Med* 1996; **153**: A866.
65. Staunton D, Merluzzi V, Rothlein R, Barton R, Marlin S, Springer T. A cell adhesion molecule, ICAM-1, is the major surface receptor for rhinovirus. *Cell* 1989; **56**: 849–53.
66. Greve JM, Davis L, Meyer AM, Forte CP, Yost S, Marlow CW et al. The major human rhinovirus receptor is ICAM-1. *Cell* 1989; **56**: 839–47.
67. Johnston S, Pattemore P, Lampe F, Holgate S. The role of asthma and atopy in the susceptibility to respiratory viral infection in children. *Am J Respir Crit Care Med* 1994; **149**: A50.
68. Noah TL, Becher S. Respiratory syncytial virus-induced cytokine production by a human bronchial epithelial cell line. *Am J Physiol* 1993; **265**: L472–8.
69. Becker S, Koren H, Henke D. Interleukin-8 expression in normal nasal epithelium and its modulation by infection with respiratory syncytial virus and cytokines tumor necrosis factor, interleukin-1, and interleukin-6. *Am J Respir Cell Mol Biol* 1993; **8**: 20–7.
70. Elias J, Zheng T, Einarsson O, Landry M, Trow T, Revert N et al. Epithelial interleukin-11: regulation by cytokines, respiratory syncytial virus and retinoic acid. *J Biol Chem* 1994; **269**: 22261–8.

71. Siddiqi A, Peeples M, Brees B, Moy J. Respiratory syncytial virus-induced release of RANTES and MIP-1 by bronchial epithelial and peripheral mononuclear cells. *J Allergy Clin Immunol* 1996; **37**: 305–9.
72. Subauste M, Jacoby D, Richards S, Proud D. Infection of a human respiratory epithelial cell line with rhinovirus. *J Clin Invest* 1995; **96**: 549–57.
73. Einarsson O, Geba G, Zhu Z, Landry M, Elias J. Interleukin-11: stimulation in vivo and in vitro by respiratory viruses and induction of airway hyperresponsiveness. *J Clin Invest* 1996; **97**: 915–24.
74. Teran LM, Johnston SL, Schroder JM, Church MK, Holgate ST. Role of nasal interleukin-8 in neutrophil recruitment and activation in children with virus-induced asthma. *Am J Respir Crit Care Med* 1997; **155**: 1362–6.
75. Kameyoshi Y, Dorschner A, Mallet AI, Christopher E, Schroder JM. Cytokine RANTES released by thrombin-stimulated platelets is a potent attractant for human eosinophils. *J Exp Med* 1992; **176**: 587–92.
76. Nagata M, Sedgwick JB, Kita H, Busse WW. Adhesion to VCAM-1 and exposure to GM-CSF synergistically activate eosinophil superoxide anion (O_2^-) generation and degranulation. *Am J Respir Crit Care Med* 1995; **151**: A240.
77. Lopez AF, Williamson DJ, Gamble JR, Begley CG, Harlan JM, Klebanoff SJ et al. Recombinant human granulocyte-macrophage colony-stimulating factor stimulates in vitro mature human neutrophil and eosinophil function, surface receptor expression, and survival. *J Clin Invest* 1986; **78**: 1220–8.
78. Sedgwick JB, Quan SF, Calhoun WJ, Busse WW. Effect of interleukin-5 and granulocyte-macrophage colony stimulating factor on in vitro eosinophil function: comparison with airway eosinophils. *J Allergy Clin Immunol* 1995; **96**: 375–85.
79. Tang W, Geba GP, Zheng T, Ray P, Homer RJ, Kuhn C et al. Targeted expression of Il-11 in the murine airway causes lymphocytic inflammation, bronchial remodeling, and airways obstruction. *J Clin Invest* 1996; **98**: 2845–53.
80. Ichinose M, Barnes P. Bradykinin-induced airway microvascular leakage and bronchoconstriction are mediated via a bradykinin B_2 receptor. *Am Rev Respir Dis* 1990; **142**: 1104–7.
81. Baraniuk J, Lundgren J, Mizpgwhi H, Peden D, Gawin A, Merida A et al. Bradykinin and respiratory mucous membranes. Analysis of bradykinin binding sites distribution and secretory responses in vitro and in vivo. *Am Rev Respir Dis* 1990; **141**: 706–14.
82. Turner RB. The role of neutrophils in the pathogenesis of rhinovirus infections. *Pediatr Infect Dis J* 1990; **9**: 832–5.
83. Levandowski RA, Weaver CW, Jackson GG. Nasal secretion leukocyte populations determined by flow cytometry during acute rhinovirus infection. *J Med Virol* 1988; **25**: 423–32.
84. Everard ML, Swarbrick A, Wrightham M, Mcintyre J, Dunkley C, James PD et al. Analysis of cells obtained by bronchial lavage of infants with respiratory syncytial virus infection. *Arch Dis Child* 1994; **71**: 428–32.
85. Grünberg K, Timmers MC, Smits JJ, de Klerk EPA, Dick EC, Spaan WJM et al. Effect of experimental rhinovirus 16 colds on airway hyperresponsiveness to histamine and interleukin-8 in nasal lavage in asthmatic subjects in vivo. *Clin Exp Allergy* 1997; **27**: 36–45.
86. Garofalo R, Kimpen JL, Welliver RC, Ogra PL. Eosinophil degranulation in the respiratory tract during naturally acquired respiratory syncytial virus infection. *J Pediatr* 1992; **120**: 28–32.
87. Rakes GP, Arruda E, Ingram JM, Joover GE, Hayden FG, Platts-Mills TE et al. Assessment of viral pathogens and eosinophilic cationic protein in nasal washes from wheezing infants and children. *Am J Respir Crit Care Med* 1995; **151**: A362.
88. Seminario MC, Squillace C, Bardin PG, Fraenkel DJ, Gleich GJ, Johnston SL. Increased levels of eosinophil major basic protein in nasal secretions in rhinovirus infection. *J Allergy Clin Immunol* 1995; **95**: 259.
89. Volvovitz B, Welliver RC, De Castro G, Krystofik DA, Ogra PL. The release of leukotrienes in the respiratory tract during infection with respiratory syncytial virus: role in obstructive airway disease. *Pediatr Res* 1988; **24**: 504–7.
90. Grünberg K, Smits HH, Timmers MC, de Klerk EPA, Dolhain RJEM, Dick EC et al. Experimental rhinovirus 16 infection: effects on cell differentials and soluble markers in sputum in asthmatic subjects. *Am J Respir Crit Care Med* 1997; **156**: 609–16.
91. Handzel ZT, Busse WW, Sedgwik JB, Vrtis R, Lee WM, Kelly EA et al. Eosinophils bind rhinovirus and activate virus-specific T cells. *J*

Immunol 1998; **160**: 1279–84.
92. Folkerts G, Esch BV, Janssen M, Nijkamp FP. Virus-induced airway hyperresponsiveness in guinea pigs in vivo: study of bronchoalveolar cell number and activity. *Eur J Pharmacol* 1992; **228**: 219–27.
93. van Oosterhout AJ, van Ark I, Folkerts G, van der Linde HJ, Savelkoul HF, Verheyen AK et al. Antibody to interleukin-5 inhibits virus-induced airway hyperresponsiveness to histamine in guinea pigs. *Am J Respir Crit Care Med* 1995; **151**: 177–83.
94. Kamp S, Kreff B, Braun J, Dalhoff K. A rapid semiautomatic enzyme linked immunoassay identifying intercellular adhesion molecule-1 (ICAM-1) on the alveolar macrophage surface. *Eur J Clin Chem Clin Biochem* 1994; **32**: 455–60.
95. Gern JE, Dick EC, Lee WM, Murray S, Meyer K, Handzel ZT et al. Rhinovirus enters but does not replicate inside monocytes and airway macrophages. *J Immunol* 1996; **156**: 621–7.
96. Roberts NJ, Prill AH, Mann TN. Interleukin 1 and interleukin 1 inhibitor production by human macrophages exposed to influenza virus or respiratory syncytial virus. *J Exp Med* 1986; **163**: 511–19.
97. Johnston SL, Papi A, Monick MM, Hunninghake GW. Rhinoviruses induce interleukin-8 mRNA and protein production in human monocytes. *J Infect Dis* 1997; **175**: 323–9.
98. Balfour-Lynn IM, Valman HB, Wellings R, Webster ADB, Taylor GW, Silverman M. Tumour necrosis factor-alpha and leukotriene E_4 production in wheezy infants. *Clin Exp Allergy* 1994; **24**: 121–6.
99. Anticevich SZ, Hughes JM, Black JL, Armour CL. Induction of human airway hyperresponsiveness by tumour necrosis factor-alpha. *Eur J Pharmacol* 1995; **284**: 221–5.
100. Gosset P, Tsicopoulos A, Wallaert B, Vannimenus C, Joseph M, Tonnel AB et al. Increased secretion of tumor necrosis factor α and interleukin-6 by alveolar macrophages consecutive to the development of the late asthmatic reaction. *J Allergy Clin Immunol* 1991; **88**: 561–71.
101. Panuska JR, Midulla F, Cirino NM, Villani A, Gilbert IA, McFadden ER Jr et al. Virus-induced alterations in macrophage production of tumor necrosis factor and prostaglandin E2. *Am J Physiol* 1990; **259**: L396–402.
102. Villani A, Cirino NM, Baldi E, Kester M, McFadden ER Jr, Panuska JR. Respiratory syncytial virus infection of human mononuclear phagocytes stimulates synthesis of platelet-activating factor. *J Biol Chem* 1991; **266**: 5472–9.
103. Henricks PAJ, Van Esch B, Engels F, Nijkamp FP. Effects of parainfluenza type 3 virus on guinea pig pulmonary alveolar macrophage functions in vitro. *Inflammation* 1993; **17**: 663–75.
104. Salkind AR, McCarthy DO, Nichols JE, Donnelly SC, Walsh EE, Roberts NJ. Interleukin-1-inhibitor activity induced by respiratory syncytial virus: abrogation of virus-specific and alternate human lymphocyte proliferative responses. *J Infect Dis* 1991; **163**: 71–7.
105. Roberts NJ. Different effects of influenza virus, respiratory syncytial virus, and sendai virus on human lymphocytes and macrophages. *Infect Immun* 1982; **35**: 1142–6.
106. Gern JE, Joseph B, Galagan DM, Dick EC. Rhinovirus inhibits antigen-specific T cell proliferation through an intracellular adhesion molecule-1-dependent mechanism. *J Infect Dis* 1996; **174**: 1143–50.
107. Toth T, Hesse RA. Replication of five bovine respiratory viruses in cultured bovine alveolar macrophages. *Arch Virol* 1983; **75**: 219–24.
108. Faenkel DJ, Bardin PG, Sanderson G, Lampe F, Johnston SL, Holgate ST. Lower airway inflammation during rhinovirus colds in normal and in asthmatic subjects. *Am J Respir Crit Care Med* 1995; **151**: 879–86.
109. Doherty PC, Hou S, Tripp RA. CD8+ T-cell memory to viruses. *Curr Opin Immunol* 1994; **6**: 545–52.
110. Gern JE, Vrtis R, Kelly EAB, Dick EC, Busse WW. Rhinovirus produces nonspecific activation of lymphocytes through a monocyte-dependent mechanism. *J Immunol* 1996; **157**: 1605–12.
111. Bacon KB, Premack BA, Gardner P, Schall TJ. Activation of dual T cell signaling pathways by the chemokine RANTES. *Science* 1995; **269**: 1727–30.

6

Chronic cough and/or wheezing in infants and children less than 5 years old: diagnostic approaches

Andrew Bush

Definition • Nomenclature • Clinical approach to the child with excessive cough and/or wheeze • Does the child have a serious underlying condition? • Useful ancillary investigations in the child with excessive wheeze and/or cough • Is it asthma, doctor? • Does cough-variant asthma exist? • When symptoms seem to be exaggerated • Summary

DEFINITION

The child with recurrent cough and/or wheeze must be placed into one of three diagnostic categories, usually on the basis of the history and physical examination. These categories are:

(a) normal child
(b) one of the variants of the asthma spectrum (see Table 6.1 and below)
(c) serious underlying condition needing a specific diagnosis and treatment.

The diagnosis of 'normal child' is perhaps the most difficult in the whole of paediatrics, and requires the most clinical experience. With regard to asthma, the International Consensus Group[1] proposed the excellent definition of asthma as 'cough and/or wheeze in a setting where asthma is likely, and other rare causes have been excluded'. The great merit of this definition is that it makes no assumptions about underlying pathology and therefore the most appropriate treatment. Not being based on assumptions about pathology it is likely to stand the test of time, and is not vulnerable to being overturned by new insights into pathophysiology. Furthermore, it is the definition we have to use for most clinical purposes in children too young for us to perform lung function tests. Whenever the term 'asthma' is used in this chapter, this clinical definition is what is meant.

Three elements to this apparently simple definition need close attention, and form the bulk of this chapter:

(a) what is meant by wheeze?
(b) what is excessive cough?
(c) how in practice should other conditions be ruled out, given that most children cough and/or wheeze at some time?

Furthermore, even if the child is given a clinical diagnosis of asthma, the pathological phenotype should be determined as far as possible (Table 6.1).[2,3] The key clinical question is: does the child have Th_2-driven, eosinophil-mediated airway inflammation,[4-6] or is the main problem one of developmental reduction in baseline airway calibre, which may be associated with parental atopy, parental smoking in pregnancy,

Table 6.1 Components of the asthma phenotype	
Problem	**Manifestation**
1. Symptoms	Cough, wheeze, breathlessness
2. Child/family perceptions	Objective measurements and subjective perception do not correlate
3. Bronchial hyperreactivity	Abnormal bronchoconstriction in response to histamine, methacholine, exercise challenges; peak flow lability
4. Baseline airway calibre	Fixed narrowing; developmental or secondary to airway remodelling
5. Airway inflammation	Release of locally active mediators; cell recruitment by cytokines and chemokines; neurogenic inflammation

Note: The diagnosis of asthma always requires symptoms to be present; the relative contributions of 4 and 5 should be assessed in each individual case.

or maternal hypertension of pregnancy.[7–9] This may be very difficult to answer, but is fundamental to the choice of treatment, in particular whether inhaled corticosteroids are to be used.

NOMENCLATURE

Wheezing due to airway narrowing sounds like a high-pitched, musical whistle, akin to organ music or the wind whistling in chimneys. However, many parents in England at least will use the same word to describe many other different noises, for example a palpable crackling in the chest, a noise as if the child needs to clear his or her throat, or even nasal snufflings. The significance of these sounds is very different, and time must be spent on the history to determine exactly what is meant. In some languages (e.g. German) there is no word for 'wheeze'. This does call into question the validity of large epidemiological studies which may uncritically rely on the assumption that everyone means the same by 'wheeze'. It is also important to realize that differentiating stridor from wheeze in the tachypnoeic child may be difficult for parents. Sometimes it may help if the doctor tries to mimic some of these different noises (if Thespian talents permit).

Coughing is universal in childhood at least at the time of viral upper respiratory infections. The assessment of cough is notoriously unreliable by both subjects and observers, with poor correlation between diary cards or tape recorders and perception of severity.[10,11] Cough monitoring using a specially designed recorder[12,13] or a modified Holter monitor[14] has been used predominantly in older children to document how much coughing is normal, but these are not routinely available in clinical practice. Even if cough frequency is greater than normal, its significance and its relationship to asthma are controversial. This point is discussed in more detail below.

CLINICAL APPROACH TO THE CHILD WITH EXCESSIVE COUGH AND/OR WHEEZE

The differential diagnosis of cough and wheeze in the young child is very wide, and it is impracticable to carry out every possible test on every child; indeed most will be managed correctly with no investigations at all. When considering the history, it is wise to remember conditions other than asthma which may present with cough and wheeze. The first step in the assessment of the child is always a detailed and focused history and physical examination.

History taking

Having established whether the child truly wheezes, and as far as possible whether there is excessive cough, the next step is to identify the pattern and severity of symptoms. The key distinction in the pattern of symptoms is whether the child has symptoms solely at the time of a viral cold (VAW), or additional symptoms in between colds. If the latter, symptom frequency and triggers should be determined. Specific triggers may include exercise, excited emotional behaviour including laughing or crying, dust, exposure to furry pets (the English disease), weather or environmental temperature change, strong perfumes or aerosol sprays, and smoke from cigarettes or open fires. The investigation and treatment approach to VAW is likely to be completely different to that for the child with chronic symptoms in between viral colds.

The severity of symptoms should next be determined, both in terms of the disruption to the child and also to the family, in order to ensure that treatment is appropriately focused. The family of a child who coughs intermittently but is not particularly breathless may merely be seeking reassurance that there is no serious underlying disease, rather than seeking a prescription for regular inhaled medication. Conversely, the family of a child who is a so-called 'fat, happy wheezer' may be well aware that their child is not in danger of death, but are very eager for some treatment to try to ensure a good night's sleep. Other factors that may influence treatment decisions are a history of atopy in the child or first-degree relatives. Particularly in the child with symptoms between colds, there are questions that should be asked which may give important diagnostic clues (summarised in Table 6.2).

The upper airway can be the forgotten area of paediatric respirology.[15] Much the common-

Table 6.2 Points to seek in the history which suggest an underlying serious diagnosis

Are the child/family really describing wheeze?
Upper airway symptoms: snoring, rhinitis, sinusitis
Symptoms from the first day of life
Very sudden onset of symptoms
Chronic moist cough/sputum production
Worse wheeze or irritable after feed, worse when lying down, vomiting, choking on feeds
Any feature of a systemic immunodeficiency
Continuous, unremitting or worsening symptoms

Note: A detailed history targeted towards other respiratory conditions is an essential first step in the child with recurrent cough and wheeze.

est cause of chronic cough is the catarrhal child with postnasal drip. Symptoms suggestive of obstructive sleep apnoea (OSA) should be sought, including snoring, apnoeic pauses, restlessness, daytime somnolence and poor concentration. Adenotonsillectomy may be completely curative of the chronic cough, and prevent the (rare) dangers of night-time respiratory failure. In general, the earlier the onset of symptoms, the more likely that an important diagnosis will be found. Symptoms from the first day of life should always be investigated; they must be distinguished from symptoms starting at a few weeks of age, which may be due to asthma. The mother should be asked whether the problem started literally from day one of life. If this is the case, structural abnormalities of the airway should be excluded. If there is prominent and persistent rhinitis from birth (almost inevitably and fatuously diagnosed as the baby being born with a viral cold), then primary ciliary dyskinesia (PCD, Kartagener's syndrome) should be considered (Figure 6.1).[16] The very sudden onset of symptoms is strongly suggestive of endobronchial foreign body (Figure 6.2). Parents may not volunteer the history, and should be asked specifically whether choking on a foreign body is a possibility.[17] Note that

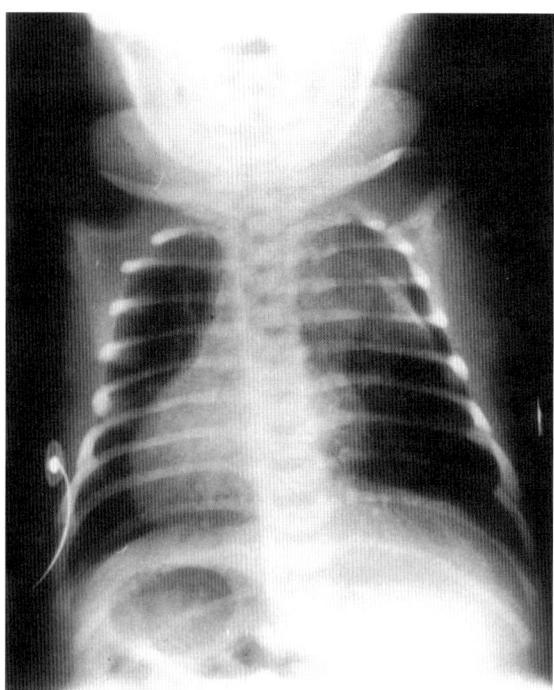

Figure 6.1 CXR of a newborn infant with respiratory distress. There is mirror image arrangement, a shallow left-sided pneumothorax and an infiltrate in the left-sided upper lobe. The diagnosis is primary ciliary dyskinesia.

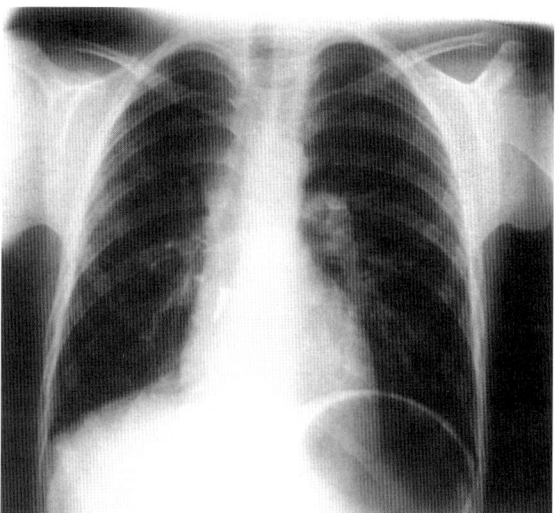

Figure 6.2 This child had cough and wheeze for 5 years. There is a screw in the right intermediate bronchus. He was asymptomatic after it was removed at rigid bronchoscopy.

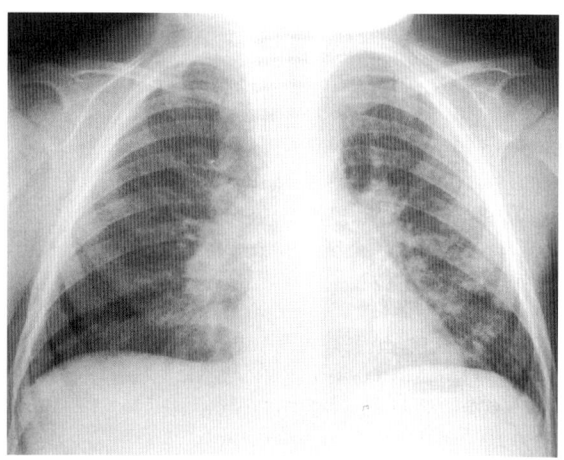

Figure 6.3 CXR showing bronchial wall thickening and patchy consolidation in an infant recently diagnosed with cystic fibrosis.

even babies too young to bring their own hands to their mouth may have older siblings who may have pressed small objects onto their face. Chronic sputum production or a moist cough when the child does not have a viral cold should always be a cause for concern. Although it may be due to postnasal drip or asthma, causes of chronic pulmonary sepsis (below) such as cystic fibrosis (CF) (Figure 6.3), PCD and agammaglobulinaemia should always be considered.

The thorax contains two organs of interest—the right lung and the left lung. A third, more minor organ of note is the oesophagus, which may be a factor in the production of chronic respiratory symptoms. Gastro-oesophageal reflux is suspected in an infant who is worse after feeds, is an irritable feeder and vomits or possets easily. Choking on feeds, particularly in a child with known neurodevelopmental handicap or neuromuscular disease, suggests that incoordinate swallowing due to bulbar or pseudo-bulbar palsy may be the cause of symptoms (Figure 6.4). Laryngeal cleft or H-type tracheo-oesophageal fistula may present with symptoms at the time of feeding.

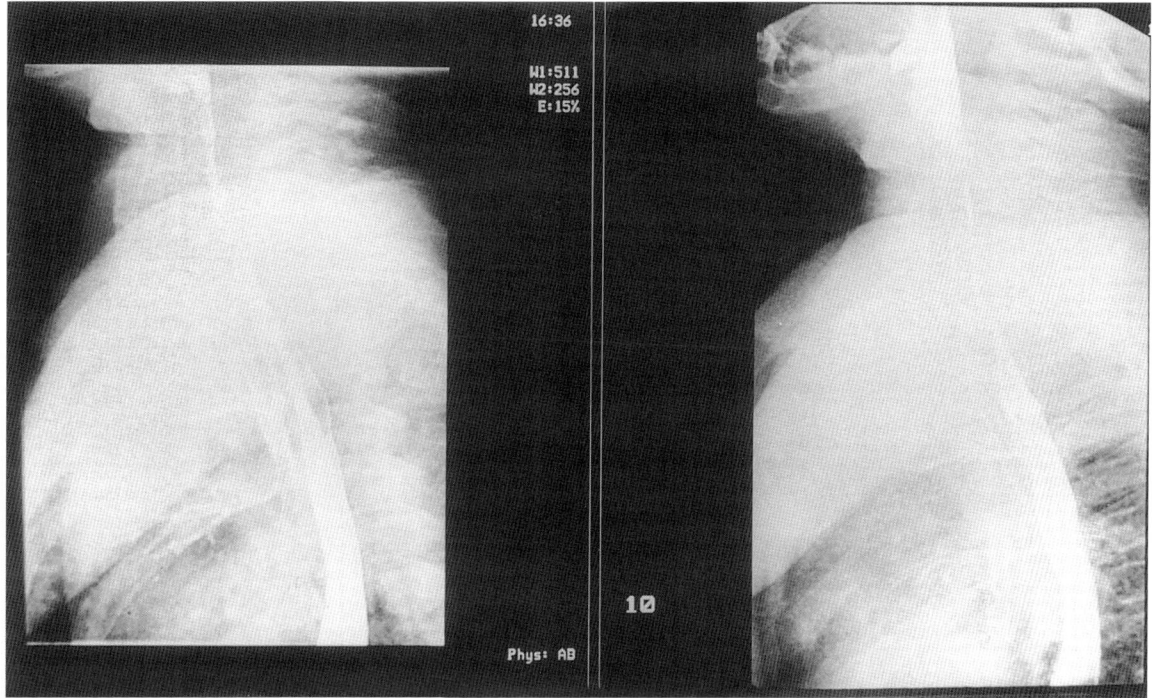

Figure 6.4 Cine-swallow showing direct aspiration of barium into the bronchial tree in an infant with neurodevelopmental handicap secondary to congenital cytomegalovirus infection.

Another pointer to the need to investigate further is whether there are any periods of remission. Although symptom-free periods do not exclude the possibility of a serious underlying disease, the child who has no days free of symptoms certainly merits critical consideration of alternative diagnoses. Finally, a history of systemic infections or poor weight gain in the context of chronic respiratory disease should never be dismissed lightly.

Physical examination

This section concentrates in particular on physical signs that are commonly missed, or the significance of which may be underestimated (see Table 6.3). Most often there will be no physical signs in the child with asthma. Digital clubbing is an obvious and important sign, but will not be found if not actively sought. My experience has been that children are not uncommonly referred with obvious chronic clubbing that has never been noticed. The upper airway should be inspected for rhinitis, and nasal polyps (Figure 6.5); the latter are virtually pathognomonic of CF in this age group. The nature and severity of any chest deformity should be noted; although a severe Harrison's sulcus and pectus carinatum can be due to uncontrolled asthma, the more severe the deformity, the greater the likelihood of another diagnosis. Palpation of the chest with the palms of the hands during quiet breathing or, in an older child, during blowing or huffing may be a better way of detecting airway secretions than auscultation. Careful auscultation may, however, elicit unexpected findings such as crackles, fixed monophonic wheeze, asymmetric signs or stridor, all of which mandate a further diagnostic work-up. Finally, signs of cardiac and systemic disease should be sought. At the end of the history and physical examination, the paediatrician must have determined the nature of

104 TEXTBOOK OF PEDIATRIC ASTHMA: AN INTERNATIONAL PERSPECTIVE

Table 6.3 Points to seek on examination which suggest an underlying serious diagnosis

Digital clubbing, signs of weight loss, failure to thrive
Upper airway disease: enlarged tonsils and adenoids, prominent rhinitis, nasal polyps
Unusually severe chest deformity (Harrison's sulcus, barrel chest)
Fixed monophonic wheeze
Stridor (monophasic or biphasic)
Asymmetric wheeze
Signs of cardiac or systemic disease

Note: Most children with cough and wheeze will have no physical signs; however, none will ever be found unless they are actively sought.

Table 6.4 Disease that presents as recurrent cough and wheeze

Upper airway disease: adenotonsillar hypertrophy, rhinosinusitis, postnasal drip
Congenital structural bronchial disease: complete cartilage rings, cysts, webs
Bronchial/tracheal compression: vascular rings and sling, enlarged cardiac chamber, lymph nodes enlarged by tuberculosis or lymphoma
Endobronchial disease: foreign body, tumour
Oesophageal/swallowing problems: reflux, incoordinate swallow, laryngeal cleft or tracheo-oesophageal fistula
Causes of pulmonary suppuration: cystic fibrosis, primary ciliary dyskinesia, any systemic immunodeficiency including agammaglobulinaemia, severe combined immunodeficiency
Miscellaneous: bronchopulmonary dysplasia, congenital or acquired tracheomalacia, pulmonary oedema

Note: These conditions need to be considered and excluded before escalating therapy.

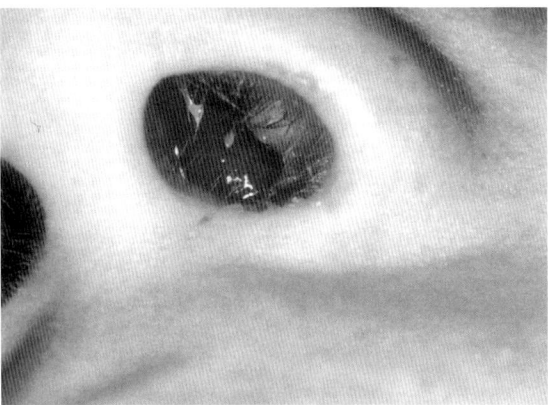

Figure 6.5 Nasal polyps, which are virtually diagnostic of cystic fibrosis in children.

the complaint, and the need (if any) for further investigation. Further testing is often wise in the young child, especially with any atypical features, and especially if symptoms are present when the child does not have a viral cold.

DOES THE CHILD HAVE A SERIOUS UNDERLYING CONDITION?

The major serious diagnoses that should be considered are listed in Table 6.4. Some specific pointers in the history and physical examination are discussed above. Details of some of the more important conditions are given below.

Congenital abnormalities

Airway abnormalities commonly present at or soon after birth, often with stridor rather than wheeze; the differentiation may be difficult in practice. The commonest abnormality is laryngomalacia, usually an uncomplicated clinical diagnosis, settling with observation, and, in typical cases, requiring no investigation. A variant of this condition, presenting with coarser upper airway rumbling noises rather than true stridor, is 'pharyngomalacia', in which at bronchoscopy the soft tissues of the pharynx collapse markedly causing respiratory obstruction,

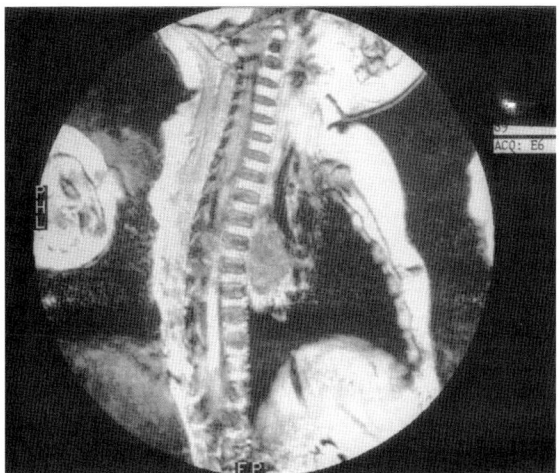

Figure 6.6 MRI scan showing compression of the lower trachea by a bronchogenic cyst, in an atopic child presenting with chronic wheeze.

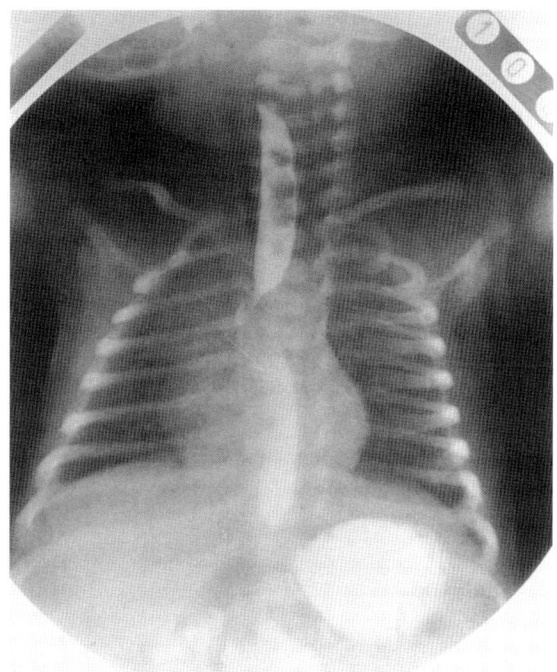

Figure 6.7 A barium swallow showing compression of the oesophagus by a double aortic arch.

in the absence of any other lesion. If, as in two of the cases we have seen,[124] there is marked obstructive sleep apnoea, the treatment is with a nasopharyngeal prong until the child outgrows the condition. Marked pharyngeal collapse may also be seen secondary to an obstructive lesion lower in the respiratory tract, including severe laryngomalacia. Other conditions presenting with stridor in the newborn period include congenital webs or cysts of the larynx, laryngeal haemangioma, and compression of the bronchial tree by cystic malformations (Figure 6.6).

A very important group of congenital anomalies is abnormalities of the mediastinal vasculature, comprising vascular ring (double aortic arch, and other aberrant vessels) and pulmonary artery sling (origin of left pulmonary artery from the right pulmonary artery, which then runs back across the mediastinum between the trachea and oesophagus, compressing the former in particular).[18,19] These may present with stridor or wheeze in the newborn period, but late diagnosis is common.

There are a considerable number of possible investigations that may be considered, but the definitive test in the stridulous child is fibreoptic bronchoscopy (FOB). We carry this out using a light general anaesthetic with the child breathing spontaneously, so airway dynamics can be appreciated. The bronchoscope is passed through the nose via a facemask held in position by the anaesthetist. Skilled and experienced anaesthetic assistance is essential in small, stridulous or wheezy infants. Technical points of importance include a careful inspection of the subglottic region from above the vocal cords before attempting to pass the bronchoscope, in case a friable haemorrhagic lesion is traumatized and this causes complete respiratory obstruction. Fibreoptic bronchoscopy allows inspection of the whole of the respiratory tract; multiple lesions are common in the stridulous child.[20] It also allows the assessment of the importance of an aberrant left subclavian artery, which may be a normal variant, or may form part of a vascular ring. My own practice if a vascular compression is seen is to confirm the finding with a barium swallow (Figure 6.7) and an echocardiogram before referral for surgery, but not to use these tests as a routine before bronchoscopy. If a pulmonary artery sling is diagnosed, then an angiogram should be performed to exclude origin of the right upper lobe artery from the left pulmonary artery; if this variant is not diagnosed, then right upper lobe infarction is a risk at surgery.

The treatment of anatomical lesions such as cysts or vascular rings is clearly surgical; postoperative airway malacia, particularly if the diagnosis has been delayed, is common. If the obstruction is functional (e.g. severe laryngomalacia or bronchomalacia) then it is prudent to carry out a sleep study to rule out obstructive sleep apnoea, and to arrange that the child be followed up to ensure he or she thrives.

CF and other suppurative and infective lung disease

Immunodeficiency frequently presents as recurrent respiratory infections, which undiagnosed can lead on to bronchiectasis. CF in its classical form with diarrhoea and failure to thrive should not present a diagnostic problem, but atypical forms, particularly with normal pancreatic function, may present late, even well on into adult life.[21-23] If doubt exists at all in the minds of either doctor of family, it is wise to perform a sweat test, which reveals a chloride concentration >60 mmol/l in 98% of cases of CF.[23] Rare atypical cases of CF need further diagnostic evaluation, including CF genotype.[24] Management should involve a centre with special expertise in CF.

Kartagener originally described a syndrome mirror image arrangement, bronchiectasis and sinusitis.[25] The underlying problem is immotile or dysmotile respiratory cilia. Subsequently it was realized that 50% of these patients had normal organ arrangement. Rare associated features include complex congenital heart disease often with disorders of laterality,[26] severe oesophageal disease,[26] biliary atresia[27] and hydrocephalus.[28] Diagnosis is by direct examination of ciliary beat frequency and pattern, usually on a nasal brush biopsy. Ciliary ultrastructure is determined by electron microscopy

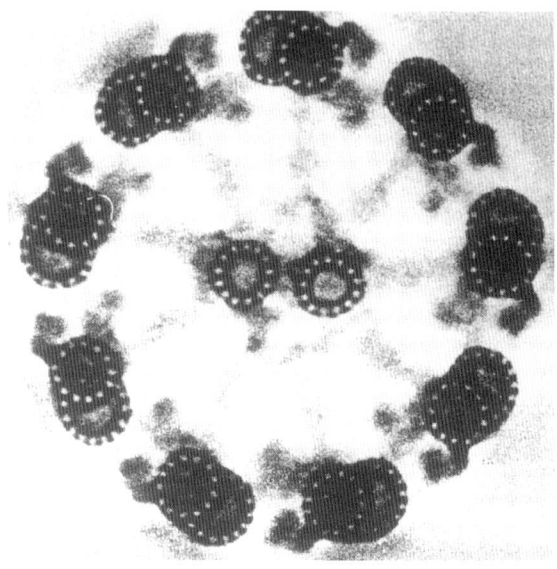

(a)

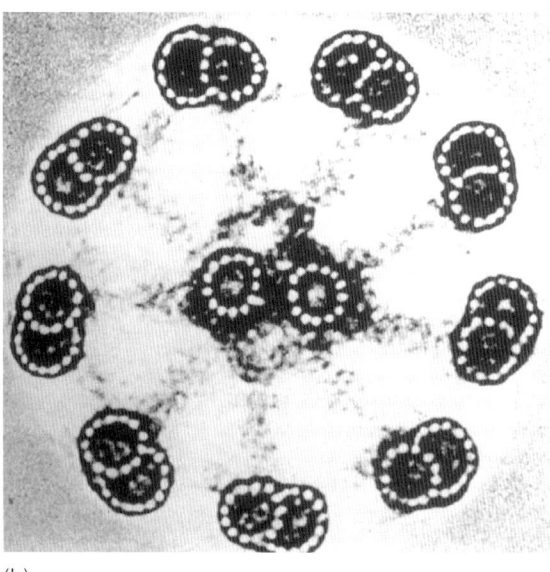

(b)

Figure 6.8 **(a)** Normal ciliary morphology demonstrated on electron microscopy. **(b)** Electron microscopy of nasal cilia showing absent dynein arms in a child with primary ciliary dyskinesia.

(Figure 6.8).[16] In older children, other helpful investigations include the saccharine test[29] and measurement of nasal nitric oxide.[30] Management is with aggressive use of chest physiotherapy and antibiotics, and avoiding where possible tympanostomy tube placement for treatment of chronic secretory otitis media with effusion.[31]

A wide range of systemic immunodeficiencies may present with recurrent bacterial infection, particularly those diseases affecting the B-cell axis such as agammaglobuminaemia. A diagnostic clue to the presence of severe combined immunodeficiency which is often missed is lymphopaenia on the full blood count.[32] If immune deficiency is strongly suspected and simple investigations such as immunoglobulins, subclasses and the response to vaccine antibodies are unrevealing, it is wise to seek the advice of a paediatric immunologist.

Oesophageal disease (reflux, fistula, dyscoordinate swallow)

Gastro-oesophageal reflux bears a complex relation to respiratory disease; it may:

(a) be an irrelevant, chance finding;
(b) whether or not there is direct aspiration into the airway, be a primary cause of respiratory problems;
(c) arise secondary to an underlying respiratory disorder, in which case it may either exacerbate the underlying disorder or be an irrelevant chance finding.

This differentiation may be hard to make. One pointer is that symptoms that disappear with a climate change, for example on holiday, are highly unlikely to be due to reflux.[33] However, an empirical trial of anti-reflux medication may be fully justified. My own choice would be to use feed-thickening agents in non-breast-fed babies, and, in an otherwise healthy infant, add in domperidone 0.2 mg/kg three times per day, preferably before feeds. Note that this is an unlicensed use of this medication. If there is no response to this approach, and there is a strong clinical suspicion of reflux, further investigation, which may include a pH probe, milkscan and bronchoalveolar lavage for fat-laden macrophages, is essential.

Incoordinate swallowing may be central (cerebral damage due to cerebral palsy, congenital infection or metabolic disease) or peripheral (neuromuscular). The history is of choking on feeds, and detailed investigation with a cine swallow using feeds of various textures and the help of a skilled speech therapist may be necessary. If the underlying cause is not treatable, management is to give all nutrition via a gastrostomy (and performing a fundoplication if there is associated gastro-oesophageal reflux, common if the child is hypotonic), and to give glycopyrrhalate patches to dry up saliva. The differential diagnosis includes a laryngeal cleft, which may require a careful upper airway examination with a rigid endoscope and may be very difficult to detect.[34]

Finally, an H-type tracheo-oesophageal fistula may present with recurrent respiratory symptoms, often with associated abdominal distension from passage of inspired air through the fistula into the stomach. Barium swallow is often not diagnostic, and a pressure injection of barium into the oesophagus (tube oesophagram) is needed to delineate the fistula. A rigid bronchoscopy can be used to demonstrate the tracheal opening of the fistula. Treatment is surgical repair.

Endobronchial foreign body

Suspicion of this diagnosis mandates urgent referral. If the suspected foreign body is radio-opaque, then diagnosis is easy from the plain radiograph. There is little point in trying to obtain inspiratory and expiratory chest X-rays (CXRs) in an infant under age 5 years; although fluoroscopy may be helpful, the definitive investigation is bronchoscopy, which should be performed if there is any doubt about the diagnosis.

Most if not all foreign bodies should be removed with a rigid endoscope. Some units advocate a preliminary flexible bronchoscopy to confirm the diagnosis and locate the foreign body to guide the thoracic surgeon; our own practice in suspicious cases is to proceed straight to a rigid bronchoscopy, performed by an experienced thoracic surgeon. The consequences of missing the diagnosis, which include recurrent pneumonia, bronchiectasis and lung abscess, are so grave and the diagnostic procedure so safe that there should always be a low threshold for bronchoscopy; there is no discredit to a negative examination.

Organic foreign bodies such as nuts are particularly prone to setting up an inflammatory reaction in the airways, and careful follow-up is essential to ensure that there is no secondary damage. Problems are commoner on the left rather than the right side, and if there was initial consolidation on the CXR.[35] One group recommends follow-up with an isotope ventilation scan a few weeks after bronchoscopy, with further investigation only if the scan is abnormal.[35]

Upper airway disease

Rhinitis from very early in life may be a sign of PCD, particularly if it is persistent.[16] The relationship between allergic rhinitis, postnasal drip and lower respiratory symptoms is hotly debated; however, in a child with prominent upper airway symptoms, an attempt to identify allergic factors (below) should be undertaken, and a trial of oral antihistamines and nasal steroids considered. Symptoms suggestive of obstructive sleep apnoea should be sought, and adenotonsillectomy considered if there are recurrent bouts of debilitating tonsillitis, significant nocturnal desaturation, or nasal obstruction with marked symptomatic disturbance resistant to medical management. It should also be remembered that obstructive sleep apnoea may cause failure to thrive, pulmonary hypertension and congestive cardiac failure if severe. The lymphoid tissue of the upper airway may not always be a benign structure.

Other conditions

Virtually any respiratory diagnosis may present as cough and/or wheeze in this age group. Diagnostic traps include pulmonary oedema, early onset interstitial lung disease and tracheobronchomalacia. Chronic lung disease of prematurity is not a diagnostic trap, but may pose many therapeutic problems; its management is outside the scope of this chapter. The commonest cause of recurrent pulmonary oedema presenting as wheeze is occult congenital cardiac disease with left to right shunt, usually a patent arterial duct, and ventricular and atrial septal defects. The enlarged left atrium may compress in particular the left main bronchus, causing lobar or segmental collapse. An echocardiogram should always be performed if this diagnosis is in question.

Interstitial lung disease is very rare in this age group, and presents with nonspecific symptoms such as cough, tachypnoea and failure to thrive.[36] Numerous specific and nonspecific diagnoses enter the clinical picture. Specific diagnostic considerations include surfactant protein B deficiency,[37] congenital infections such as cytomegalovirus,[38] congenital lymphangiectasia,[39] pulmonary vascular diseases such as pulmonary veno-occlusive disease[40] and arteriovenous malformation,[41] and idiopathic pulmonary haemosiderosis.[42] Nonspecific entities include the recently described chronic pneumonitis of infancy and nonspecific interstitial pneumonitis.[43] Full details of the investigation and management of these rare conditions can be found elsewhere;[36,43,44] in general, a high resolution CT scan should be performed to confirm that an interstitial process is present, even if the CXR is normal, and most will subsequently require histological diagnosis. Although techniques for transbronchial and transthoracic needle biopsy have been described in this age group, our own preference is for an open surgical procedure.

Bronchomalacia may be congenital or acquired. Congenital bronchomalacia may be isolated, with generally a good prognosis, at least in the short term;[45] and has been described in association with other congenital abnormalities,[46] including connective tissue disorders, and Larsen[47] and Fryn's[48] syndrome. Acquired bronchomalacia may be iatrogenic after treatment of neonatal respiratory distress,[49] secondary to extrinsic compression by cysts[50] or the vasculature,[51] complicating obliterative bronchiolitis after lung transplantation,[52] and after surgery for tracheo-oesophageal fistula. Williams and Campbell described a syndrome of diffuse bronchomalacia affecting the second to the seventh generations of the bronchial tree.[53] Occurrence in two siblings[54] and very early onset of symptoms suggest a congenital aetiology. The recently described association of bronchomalacia with an exceptionally rare triad (normal atrial arrangement, left bronchial isomerism, normal abdominal viscera) seems very unlikely by chance and suggests that this is a truly new syndrome.[55]

Diagnosis of bronchomalacia relies first on a high index of suspicion. If the diagnosis is suspected, it may be confirmed by fibreoptic bronchoscopy, bronchography or ultrafast computed tomography.[56] Treatment includes removal of any predisposing factors if practical. Medical treatment may be expectant, with consideration of respiratory support such as nasal continuous positive airway pressure or ventilation, particularly at night.[57,58] Surgical options include airway stenting if there is a localized area of disease,[59,60] or aortopexy for tracheomalacia or central bronchomalacia.[61]

Finally, in some parts of the world, compression of the airway by tuberculous lymph nodes is a common cause of infant wheeze. If tuberculosis (TB) is suspected, then Mantoux testing and a CXR are essential. Other investigations that may be considered include early morning gastric aspirates and bronchoscopy and bronchoalveolar lavage (BAL). A rapid answer can often be obtained by polymerase chain reaction of the samples for TB RNA or DNA.[62] Guidelines for treatment and prophylaxis have been issued;[63] the younger the child the more urgent the need for a rapid diagnosis. Energetic attempts should be made to detect and treat the adult contact from whom the child has contracted the disease.

USEFUL ANCILLARY INVESTIGATIONS IN THE CHILD WITH EXCESSIVE WHEEZE AND/OR COUGH

In most children, history and physical examination will rule out serious conditions and the child will be deemed to be normal or have a variant of asthma (below). Problematic cases will require further investigation. Table 6.5 contains a summary of the investigations to be considered to exclude particular conditions.

Chest radiograph

A full review of the interpretation of the CXR is beyond the scope of this chapter; clearly a wide knowledge of normal variants and disease is needed. If there is an abnormality, then it is

Table 6.5 Investigations to be considered in the child with recurrent cough and wheeze

Suspected oesophageal disease: pH probe, barium swallow, tube oesophogram, oesophagoscopy

Suspected upper airway disease: polysomnography, RAST tests (radiograph of postnasal space is rarely useful)

Suspected cystic fibrosis: sweat test, nasal potentials, genotype, stool elastase, faecal fat

Suspected primary ciliary dyskinesia: saccharine test, nasal ciliary motility, electron microscopy including orientation studies, nasal and exhaled nitric oxide

Suspected systemic immunodeficiency: immunoglobulins and subclasses; vaccine antibodies; lymphocyte subsets; lymphocyte and neutrophil function tests; HIV test

Suspected structural airway disease: fibreoptic bronchoscopy

Suspected tuberculosis: Heaf test, fibreoptic bronchoscopy and/or gastric lavage, combined with culture and PCR

Suspected cardiovascular disease: echocardiogram, barium swallow to exclude a vascular ring or pulmonary artery sling, angiography

Suspected bronchiectasis: high resolution CT scan, investigations for local or systemic immunodeficiency

Note: A selective approach is necessary, depending on what clues have been elicited from history, examination and simple investigations.

important to try to obtain previous films. If the child has had previous episodes of 'pneumonia' I always try to obtain the previous films. I would only investigate someone for immunodeficiency because of recurrent lower respiratory infections if there has been radiological confirmation. Too many children with a viral cold and a moist cough are (wrongly) labelled as 'chest infection' when any CXR performed would in fact be normal.

The remainder of this section concentrates on particular diagnostic clues that may be missed if not specifically sought. Particular attention should be paid to the large airway. Although the CXR cannot rule out a compressive lesion, evidence of one may be seen if the tracheal shadow is carefully studied. This includes checking the side of the aortic arch (Figure 6.9)—although a right-sided arch can be a normal variant, it may also be part of a vascular ring,[64] and its presence at least in a symptomatic child should prompt investigation to exclude this diagnosis (Figure 6.10). The airway branching pattern should be studied to exclude in particular left bronchial isomerism (bilateral bilobed lungs with a long main bronchus), which may be associated with bronchomalacia.[55] Left lower lobe collapse may be missed if the typical sail-shaped shadow behind the heart with loss of the crisp edge of the left hemidiaphragm is not specifically sought. Finally, the ribs and vertebral bodies should be studied; vertebral body abnormalities may provide a clue to concomitant oesophageal disease as part of the VATER/VACTERLS spectrum.[65]

Allergy testing

In this age group, allergy testing (usually either skin prick testing, total IgE or specific RAST tests) can be used (a) to determine if the child is atopic, (b) to guide environmental manipulations, and (c) possibly to predict prognosis in the wheezy child. Both methods have the disadvantage of a high false negative rate particularly under age 3 years. However, if positive, they are likely to be significant.

Atopic status may be clinically obvious in a

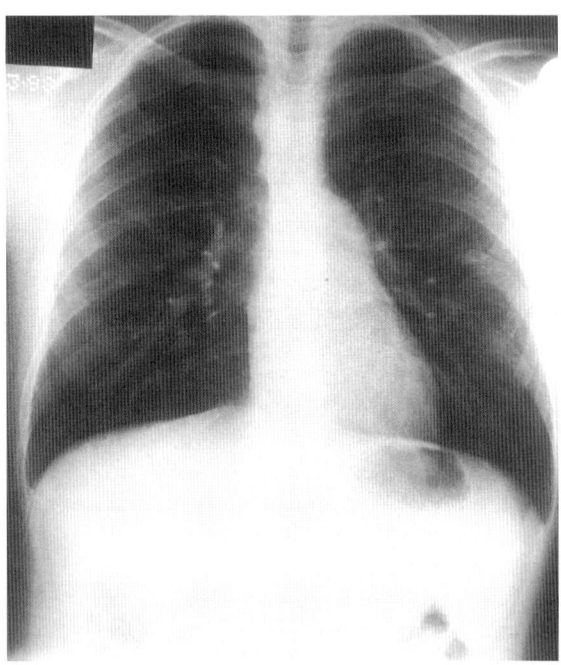

Figure 6.9 CXR showing a right-sided aortic arch with tracheal compression. The child had a vascular ring, completed by an aberrant left subclavian artery and a left-sided ligamentum arteriosum.

child with typical flexural eczema. If there is no skin disease, then testing to determine the presence of atopy may be a guide to treatment; most would be more ready to treat an atopic wheezy child with inhaled steroids, although many atopic children will not have airway eosinophilia and will outgrow their symptoms within 2 years even in the absence of anti-inflammatory treatment.[66]

Environmental manipulation is covered in more detail elsewhere in this volume. The important allergens will vary in different regions and under different environmental conditions.[67,68] House dust mite allergy should be sought in particular if there is prominent perennial rhinitis, with sneezing and irritation of the nose on waking. My own view is that furry pets should not be allowed in any house with any infant, let alone one who has respiratory symptoms; skin prick or RAST testing may help to

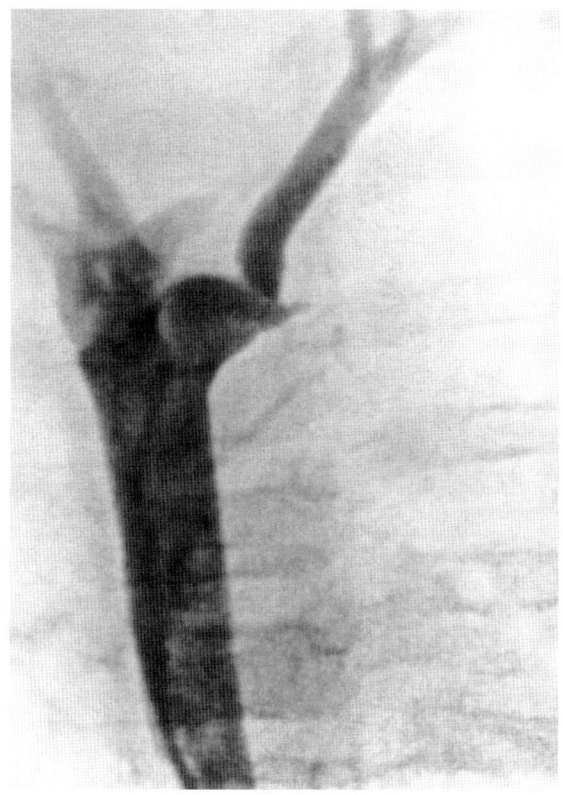

Figure 6.10 Angiogram using digital subtraction technique demonstrating a right-sided aortic arch, a diverticulum of Kommerel and an aberrant subclavian artery.

convince the family to ban the pet. The exception is in English practice, where the family is more likely to get rid of the children.

A more novel use of allergy testing is to try to predict long-term outlook. The Tucson study group[69] have shown that high total IgE at less than 1 year of age (but not at birth) were predictive of a sustained elevation of IgE at age 6 and 11 years, and were associated with prolonged wheezing, whereas children who wheezed in the first year of life but had a normal IgE outgrew their symptoms. However, as with many measurements, total IgE may be more useful to study groups rather than as a guide to individual management. Specific allergy testing may be of more use in individuals than total IgE. The recent ETAC (Early Treatment of the Atopic Child) trial[70] was a double-blind, placebo-controlled study of the effect of oral cetirizine in infants with atopic dermatitis, with the aim of determining whether cetirizine prevented the development of wheeze. For the group as a whole, there was no difference between cetirizine and placebo. A positive RAST to grass, house dust mite and cat allergen was predictive of wheezing in a cohort of children with atopic dermatitis. For the subgroups who were RAST positive to either house dust mite or grass pollen (20% of the total group), there was about a 50% reduction in wheezing with cetirizine treatment. The findings conflicted with those of another group who found that a positive RAST to egg was predictive of long-term wheeze.[71] Further prospective studies are needed to clarify this.

The role of inflammatory markers (eosinophil products, blood cytokine measurements and nitric oxide)

The chief aim of these measurements is to try to determine whether airway inflammation is present, thus justifying inhaled corticosteroid treatment. There is most experience with eosinophil products, usually serum eosinophilic cationic protein (ECP). This marker has been of dubious value. Firstly, it is elevated in atopics whether they wheeze or not;[72] and follow-up studies show that up to half of even atopic wheezers are asymptomatic within 2–4 years.[66] One study suggested that an elevation of ECP in non-atopic wheezers between wheezing episodes was predictive of ongoing symptoms, but there was considerable overlap between groups, making ECP useful only if it was very high.[73] A more promising study showed that a raised ECP at the time of the first wheezing episode was predictive of subsequent wheezing episodes.[74] Neither study looked at whether the outcome was affected by treatment. At the present time, a high serum ECP in a wheezing, non-atopic infant might be considered an indirect marker for airway inflammation, and be a pointer towards early treatment with inhaled steroids. However, even this view is controversial, and, if a therapeutic trial showed no symptomatic benefit for inhaled steroids, then I would not persist with them, whatever the level of ECP.

The use of ECP has been extended by some groups into nasal lavage, using the nasal mucosa as a model for the lower airway.[75] A dilution marker such as inulin should be added to the fluid before the lavage.[76] Increases in lavage ECP, cytokines and neutrophils have been found in different groups of wheezing infants.[76,77] Whether any or all of these measurements can predict either response to treatment or prognosis is not known, and the relation of upper airway lavage cytology to bronchial wall inflammation is also not clear.

In studies of older asthmatics, elevated interleukin-4 (IL-4), interleukin-5 (IL-5) and activated T-lymphocytes are found in peripheral blood, and levels fall with inhaled corticosteroid therapy.[78,79] Most patients studied have been over age 5 years, and again there is overlap between groups. These sophisticated measurements are not yet part of routine clinical practice, but may in the future provide useful diagnostic and therapeutic information.

Nitric oxide (NO) has been measured many times in older children and adults.[80–82] Studies in babies are limited, and their place in the diagnostic process is unclear. By analogy with older children, nasal NO may be useful in the diagnosis of PCD,[30] provided the undoubted technical problems can be overcome. One small study showed that NO is elevated in some babies with wheeze, and falls in association with oral steroid therapy.[83] Nitric oxide levels in exhaled gas collected during tidal breathing correlated with levels taken from endotracheal samples obtained after intubation for elective surgery. The fact that the paranasal sinuses are relatively underdeveloped in this age group suggests that upper airway contamination may be less important than in older children and adults. By analogy with studies in older age groups, elevated NO may be a marker of eosinophilic inflammation.[84] The non-invasive nature of NO measurements makes them an appealing tool, but more research is needed before they come into clinical practice in this age group.

Overall, there is unfortunately no reliable inflammatory marker that can currently be used to guide clinical practice in children under 5 years. There is a clear need for further research in this area.

The role of fibreoptic bronchoscopy

The most direct way of determining whether the airway is inflamed is by fibreoptic bronchoscopy, with BAL and bronchial biopsy. Transbronchial biopsy (TBB), although a diagnostic tool,[36] has not been studied in asthmatic children, and there is only limited experience of this technique in asthma research even in adults.[85] Owing to the invasive nature of FOB, there is very little published in the field of paediatric asthma. One study, published in abstract, looked at bronchial wall histology in 27 children with nonspecific respiratory symptoms, following them up 22–80 months later.[86] Those who at review had developed clinical asthma had more activated eosinophils and tryptase-positive mast cells, and a greater thickness of the subepithelial lamina reticularis in their bronchial biopsies. The data were significant for the groups, but with sufficient overlap between the groups that the technique may not be useful as a diagnostic tool in the individual. Conversely, a second study, also published in abstract, found no evidence of correlation between basement membrane thickness and subsequent outcome.[87]

Blind[88] and bronchoscopic[89] lavage studies have demonstrated clearly *for different populations* that airway cytology is very different; atopic wheezers as a group have an eosinophilic lavage fluid, whereas normals and those with virus-associated wheeze do not; many infant wheezers in fact have a neutrophilic lavage. However, there is considerable overlap between individuals, and the key evidence missing is whether BAL is predictive of response to treatment or subsequent outlook.

What then is the role of bronchoscopy in the diagnosis and management of the wheezy infant? The technique is clearly indicated to exclude other diagnoses (see above). It may come to be used to determine in doubtful cases whether there is truly airway inflammation and hence a need for inhaled corticosteroid therapy, but at the moment more data are needed on its utility *in individuals* before it can be widely recommended. In terms of predicting outcome, it remains a fascinating research tool only.

Pulmonary function testing

Many elegant techniques including squeeze and raised volume squeeze, plethysmography and gas dilution have contributed to studies fundamental to our understanding of infant wheeze,[7–9,90–92] but they are rarely available as a clinical tool. Tidal volume indices are easy to perform and require relatively simple apparatus,[93] but they are dependent on factors such as respiratory rate, and, although they may be used to follow response to treatment, they should be used with caution in individuals. As with more sophisticated methods, they have been of greater use in large epidemiological studies than to guide clinical decision making in infants. Measurements of transcutaneous oxygen and carbon dioxide tensions have been used both to follow response to treatment with bronchodilators and for challenge testing,[94] although not all groups have found it useful.[95] As with older age groups, histamine and methacholine challenge give useful data in studies of groups but are not of much value to determine whether an individual has asthma or not. Indeed, individuals with virus-associated wheeze do not have bronchial hyperreactivity.[96,97]

A relatively new indirect test which has been used as a clinical tool is the interrupter technique.[98] In principle, the child breathes through a mouthpiece, and expiratory or inspiratory flow is transiently interrupted by a shutter. Airway resistance is estimated by dividing the flow rate by the equilibrium pressure immediately after occlusion. It is a deceptively simple technique, which hides many assumptions about the behaviour of the respiratory system. It gives at best an estimate of a property of the respiratory system which is related to airway resistance, but has the merit of being simple to use. It has also been applied in clinical practice to measure baseline resistance and acute bronchodilator responsiveness.[99] It may find its real use in measuring change with therapy, rather than as an absolute guide to airway resistance. Other techniques such as forced oscillation may find a role in the future.[100,101] Overall, however, most children under 5 years have to be managed in clinical practice without recourse to lung function testing.

IS IT ASTHMA, DOCTOR?

The key question parents want answered is whether their child will continue with symptoms and be asthmatic requiring medication in mid-childhood. At the moment, there are no tests that can answer this question. Even in the high risk group, atopic wheezers, nearly half will be symptom free by age 5 years.[66] Allergy and immunology testing may act as a guide to further management (e.g. removing a source of allergen from the environment of the child) and have some predictive value; a major goal of future research is to try to answer this question. This is brought into sharp focus by evidence that delayed treatment of airway inflammation may prejudice later lung function,[102,103] but that overtreatment of children who do not really need it may result in growth retardation with no catch-up after stopping therapy.[104,105] There are also worries from animal work that steroids may interfere with secondary septation during alveolar development, reducing the size of the alveolar-capillary membrane.[106] The period in humans when this is important is the first 18 months of life;[107] whether the animal studies are relevant is as yet unknown.

Ultimately, after a detailed evaluation, diagnostic doubt may remain and the question of a therapeutic trial is raised. If the main problem is cough and wheeze at the time of viral colds, and the investigator is satisfied that the symptoms are sufficiently outside the normal range such that treatment is indicated, then intermittent bronchodilator therapy with either an anticholinergic or beta-2 agonist is suggested. Usually the paediatrician will have to rely upon clinical impression as to response. Both medications may be tried; despite popular belief that there are no beta receptors in the airway under 1 year of age, there is definite physiological evidence that at least some children respond favourably to inhaled beta agonists.[108] The drug delivery device should be a mask and spacer, with appropriate instruction in use, usually from a respiratory nurse. In older children there is ample evidence that this is at least as effective as a nebulizer.[109–111] Nebulizers are expensive and take longer to use; often the mask is removed and the nebulizer itself is held next to the face of a fractious child, thus ensuring inefficient drug delivery.

If intermittent therapy is unavailing, a trial with an anti-inflammatory medication should be considered. It may seem illogical to use an inhaled steroid in virus-associated wheeze because the evidence is that the main problem is due to *in utero* airway maldevelopment,[7–9] with lung function being abnormal before the first episode of wheeze,[90–92] the absence of any evidence of bronchial hyperresponsiveness in VAW,[96,97] the generally poor response of VAW to inhaled steroids,[112] the absence of eosinophils in BAL,[88,89] and the clear evidence that long-term prognosis is unaffected by this therapy.[113] Nevertheless, occasionally a trial of inhaled steroids may be merited under carefully circumscribed conditions even in children with VAW; occasionally, there is a dramatically beneficial effect, and the family realize that in fact the child had interval symptoms that were not appreciated until they were treated.

The other circumstance under which I would consider a therapeutic trial is in the child with nonspecific chronic symptoms, especially if atopic. The choices would appear to be either inhaled bronchodilators, inhaled corticosteroids or cromoglycate, or oral steroid. There are no evidence-based data to guide the clinician in this dilemma; my own practice is to use moderately high dose inhaled steroids (for example, budesonide 800 mcg/day) via a spacer, with a mask if age appropriate. If the child does not show any response, then asthma is a highly unlikely diagnosis. The alternative choices for a therapeutic trial would be high dose beta-2 agonists, cromoglycate, or oral prednisolone. It is true that asthmatics should show some response to bronchodilators, but it is likely that if they fail, a trial of a more potent medication is likely to be performed to ensure that asthma can be ruled out, and the beta-2 agonist trial only delays matters. Cromoglycate has been shown to be largely ineffective in children of this age.[114] Oral steroids are effective in asthmatics, but also treat allergic rhinitis and temporarily reduce the size of the adenoids, and so are not specific for lower airway inflammation, as well as having greater potential for side-effects.

If the symptoms disappear after 3 months on inhaled steroids, the treatment must be stopped to ensure that the child has not improved coincidentally, after for example prolonged post-mycoplasma or post-viral cough. Only if symptoms recur on stopping inhaled steroids can the diagnosis of asthma be said to be established, and long-term treatment be instituted according to established guidelines. If there is no response to therapeutic trials, a detailed re-evaluation of other diagnostic possibilities along the lines discussed above is mandated. Referral to a paediatrician with special expertise in respiratory medicine should be considered.

DOES COUGH-VARIANT ASTHMA EXIST?

Cough is undoubtedly a common symptom of asthma. Can it be the only symptom, and, if so, how commonly? The answer will be different, depending on the setting in which the question is posed. There is no doubt that large epidemiological studies show that *in a community setting*, where by definition the vast majority of children are well, isolated cough is rarely due to asthma and rarely responds to asthma medications.[115,116] There is no doubt that isolated cough may frequently be overdiagnosed as asthma.[117] Chronic nonspecific cough frequently improves with time and without treatment.[118,119]

However, in a specialist clinic, where a highly selected group of children are seen, children who cough in response to typical asthma triggers and improve when treated with asthma medications are not uncommonly seen.[120] My diagnostic criteria are:

(a) abnormally increased cough, with no evidence of any non-asthma diagnosis
(b) clearcut response to asthma medications
(c) relapse on stopping medications with second response to recommencing them.

Many children with chronic cough in fact have only a nonspecific problem, and have been shown on bronchoscopic and blind lavage studies to have no evidence of eosinophilic airway inflammation.[89,121] Follow-up studies show that most will get better over 1–2 years. Others, however, will show evidence of deterioration of BHR over time, wheeze, and develop the symptoms of classical asthma.[122] If coughing is troublesome and the precautions outlined above are followed, then there is little to be lost in attempting a brief therapeutic trial. The only danger is that ineffectual and potentially harmful medication may be continued long term unless a trial off therapy is rigorous. In older children who can perform lung function, there is no justification for a therapeutic trial without making every attempt to document variable airflow obstruction.

WHEN SYMPTOMS SEEM TO BE EXAGGERATED

Usually, the mother's assessment of symptom severity is accurate, and certainly much better than that of the physician. Just occasionally, a child is brought to the hospital with complaints of multiple symptoms who seems to be very well. Such infants rush energetically around the room without coughing, wheezing or breathlessness, and may never have been admitted to hospital with objective evidence of respiratory distress (tachypnoea, recession, desaturation). In such cases, an admission to hospital for observation by experienced paediatric nurses may clarify the position. More rarely still, extreme anxiety may merge into the picture of Munchausen's syndrome by proxy.[123] These difficult cases require sensitive exploration and help for the family.

SUMMARY

The vast majority of infants with cough and wheeze are allocated to the appropriate diagnostic group merely by taking a history and performing a good physical examination. The occasional child requires detailed specialist investigation if an important diagnosis is not to be missed. The key skill is to learn how to separate out this small group, and carry out the appropriate investigations to ensure correct management.

REFERENCES

1. Warner JO, Gotz M, Landau L et al. Management of asthma: a consensus statement. *Arch Dis Child* 1989; **64**: 1065–79.
2. Crimi E, Spanevello A, Neri M et al. Dissociation between airway inflammation and airway hyperresponsiveness in allergic asthma. *Am J Respir Crit Care Med* 1998; **157**: 4–9.
3. Rosi E, Ronchi MC, Grazzini M, Duranti R, Scano G. Sputum analysis, bronchial hyperresponsiveness, and airway function in asthma. Results of a factor analysis. *J Allergy Clin Immunol* 1999; **103**: 232–7.
4. Wardlaw AJ, Dunnette S, Gleich GJ, Collins JV, Kay AB. Eosinophils and mast cells in bronchoalveolar lavage in subjects with mild asthma: relationship to bronchial hyperreactivity. *Am Rev Respir Dis* 1988; **137**: 62–9.
5. Bradley LB, Azzawi M, Jacobson M et al. Eosinophils, T-lymphocytes, mast cells, neutrophils, and macrophages in bronchial biopsy specimens from atopic subjects with asthma: comparison with biopsy specimens from atopic subjects without asthma and normal control subjects and relationship to bronchial hyperresponsiveness. *J Allergy Clin Immunol* 1991; **88**: 661–74.
6. Djukanovic R, Wilson JM, Britten KM et al. Effect of inhaled corticosteroid on airway inflammation and symptoms in asthma. *Am Rev Respir Dis* 1992; **145**: 669–74.

7. Lodrup-Carlsen KC, Jaakkola JJ, Nafstad P, Carlsen KH. In utero exposure to cigarette smoking influences lung function at birth. *Eur Respir J* 1997; **10:** 1774–9.
8. Stick SM, Burton PR, Gurrin L, Sly PD, LeSouef PN. Effects of maternal smoking during pregnancy and a family history of asthma on respiratory function in newborn infants. *Lancet* 1996; **348:** 1060–4.
9. Young S, LeSouef PN, Geelhoed GC et al. The influence of a family history of asthma and parental smoking on airway responsiveness in early infancy. *N Engl J Med* 1991; **324:** 1166–73.
10. Archer LNJ, Simpson H. Night cough counts and diary card scores in asthma. *Arch Dis Child* 1985; **60:** 473–4.
11. Falconer A, Oldman C, Helms P. Poor agreement between reported and recorded nocturnal cough in asthma. *Pediatr Pulmonol* 1993; **15:** 209–11.
12. Munyard P, Busst C, Logan-Sinclair R, Bush A. A new device for ambulatory cough recording. *Pediatr Pulmonol* 1994; **18:** 178–86.
13. Munyard P, Bush A. How much coughing is normal? *Arch Dis Child* 1996; **74:** 531–4.
14. Chang AB, Newman R, Phelan PD, Robertson CF. 24-hour continuous ambulatory cough meter: a new use for an old Holter monitor. *Am J Respir Crit Care Med* 1996; **153:** A501.
15. de Benedictis FM, Bush A. Hypothesis paper: rhinosinusitis and asthma—epiphenomenon or causal association? *Chest* 1999; **115:** 550–6.
16. Bush A, Cole P, Hariri M et al. Primary ciliary dyskinesia: diagnosis and standards of care. *Eur Respir J* 1998; **12:** 982–8.
17. Puterman M, Gorodischer R, Lieberman A. Tracheobronchial foreign bodies: the impact of a postgraduate educational program on diagnosis, morbidity and treatment. *Pediatrics* 1982; **70:** 96–8.
18. Burch M, Balaji S, Deanfield JE et al. Investigation of vascular compression of the trachea: the complementary roles of barium swallow and echocardiography. *Arch Dis Child* 1993; **68:** 171–6.
19. Gikonyo BM, Jue KL, Edwards JE. Pulmonary vascular sling: report of seven cases and review of the literature. *Pediatr Cardiol* 1989; **10:** 81–9.
20. Wood RE. Spelunking in the pediatric airways: explorations with the flexible bronchoscope. *Pediatr Clin North Am* 1984; **31:** 785–99.
21. van Biezen P, Overbeek SE, Hilvering C. Cystic fibrosis in a 70 year old woman. *Thorax* 1992; **47:** 202–3.
22. Gan K-H, Geus WP, Bakker W, Lamers CBHW, Heijerman HGM. Genetic and clinical features of patients with cystic fibrosis diagnosed after the age of 16 years. *Thorax* 1995; **50:** 1301–4.
23. Cystic Fibrosis Foundation, Patient Registry 1996 Annual Data Report. Bethesda, MD: 1997.
24. Rosenstein BJ, Cutting GR, for the Cystic Fibrosis Foundation Consensus Panel. The diagnosis of cystic fibrosis: a consensus statement. *J Pediatr* 1998; **132:** 589–95.
25. Kartagener M. Zur pathogenede der bronkiektasin bei situs viscerum inversus. *Britage zur Klinik und Erforshung der Tuberkulose ond der lungen krankheiten* 1933; **83:** 489–501.
26. Gemou-Engesaeth V, Warner JO, Bush A. New associations of primary ciliary dyskinesia syndrome. *Pediatr Pulmonol* 1993; **16:** 9–12.
27. Baruch GR, Gottfried E, Pery M, Sahin A, Etzioni A. Immotole cilia syndrome including polysplenia, situs inversus and extrahepatic biliary atresia. *Am J Med Genet* 1989; **33:** 390–3.
28. Greenstone MA, Jones RWA, Dewar A, Neville BGR, Cole PJ. Hydrocephalus and primary ciliary dyskinesia. *Arch Dis Child* 1984; **59:** 481–2.
29. Stanley P, MacWilliam L, Greenstone M, Mackay I, Cole P. Efficacy of a saccharin test for screening to detect abnormal mucociliary clearance. *Br J Dis Chest* 1984; **78:** 62–5.
30. Karadag B, James AJ, Gultekin E, Wilson NM, Bush A. Nasal and lower airway level of nitric oxide in children with primary ciliary dyskinesia. *Eur Respir J* 1999; **13:** 1402–6.
31. Hadfield PJ, Rowe-Jones JM, Bush A, Mackay IS. Treatment of otitis media with effusion in children with primary ciliary dyskinesia. *Clin Otolaryngol* 1997; **22:** 302–6.
32. Hague RA, Rassam S, Morgan G, Cant AJ. Early diagnosis of severe combined immunodeficiency syndrome. *Arch Dis Child* 1994; **70:** 260–3.
33. Sheikh S, Stephen T, Howell L, Eid N. Gastroesophageal reflux in infants with wheezing. *Pediatr Pulmonol* 1999; **28:** 181–6.
34. Moungthong G, Holinger LD. Laryngotracheo-esophageal clefts. *Annals Otol Rhinol Laryngol* 1997; **106:** 1002–11.
35. Davies H, Gordon I, Matthew DJ et al. Long term follow up after inhalation of foreign bodies. *Arch Dis Child* 1990; **65:** 619–21.
36. Bush A, du Bois R. Congenital and pediatric interstitial lung disease. *Current Opinion Pulmonary Med* 1996; **2:** 347–56.

37. Chetcuti PAJ, Ball RJ. Surfactant apoprotein B deficiency. *Arch Dis Child* 1995; **73:** F125–7.
38. Schwebke K, Henry K, Balfour HH, Olson D, Crane RT, Jordan MC. Congenital cytomegalovirus infection as a result of nonprimary cytomegalovirus disease in a mother with acquired immunodeficiency syndrome. *J Pediatr* 1995; **126:** 293–5.
39. Gardner TW, Domm AC, Brock CE, Pruitt AW. Congenital pulmonary lymphangiectasis. *Clin Pediatr* 1983; **22:** 75–8.
40. Sondheimer HM, Lung MC, Brugman SM, Ikle DN, Fan LL, White CW. Pulmonary vascular disorders masquerading as interstitial lung disease. *Pediatr Pulmonol* 1995; **20:** 284–8.
41. Knight WB, Bush A, Busst CM et al. Multiple pulmonary arteriovenous fistulas in childhood. *Int J Cardiol* 1989; **23:** 105–16.
42. Blanco A, Solis P, Gomez Z, Valbuena C, Telleria JJ. Antineutrophil cytoplasmic antibodies (ANCA) in idiopathic pulmonary hemosiderosis. *Pediatr Allergy Immunol* 1994; **5:** 235–9.
43. Katzenstein AA, Gordon LP, Oliphant M, Swender PT. Chronic pneumonitis of infancy. A unique form of interstitial lung disease occurring in early childhood. *Am J Surg Pathol* 1995; **19:** 439–47.
44. Bush A. Diagnosis of interstitial lung disease. *Pediatr Pulmonol* 1996; **22:** 81–2.
45. Finder JD. Primary bronchomalacia of infants and children. *J Pediatr* 1997; **130:** 59–66.
46. Godfrey S. Association between pectus excavatum and segmental bronchomalacia. *J Pediatr* 1980; **96:** 649–52.
47. Rock MJ, Green CG, Pauli RM, Peters ME. Tracheomalacia and bronchomalacia associated with Larsen syndrome. *Pediatr Pulmonol* 1988; **5:** 55–9.
48. Strattion RF, Young RS, Heiman HS, Carter JM. Fryn's syndrome. *Am J Med Genet* 1993; **45:** 562–4.
49. Miller RW, Woo P, Kellman RK, Slagle TS. Tracheobronchial abnormalities in infants with bronchopulmonary dysplasia. *J Pediatr* 1987; **111:** 779–82.
50. Kosloske AM. Left mainstem bronchopexy for severe bronchomalacia. *J Pediatr Surg* 1991; **26:** 260–2.
51. Robotin MC, Bruniaux J, Serraf A et al. Unusual forms of tracheobronchial compression in infants with congenital heart disease. *J Thorac Cardiovasc Surg* 1996; **112:** 415–23.
52. Novick RJ, Ahmad D, Menkis AH et al. The importance of acquired diffuse bronchomalacia in heart–lung transplant recipients with obliterative bronchiolitis. *J Thorac Cardiovasc Surg* 1991; **101:** 643–8.
53. Williams H, Campbell P. Generalised bronchiectasis associated with deficiency of cartilage in the bronchial tree. *Arch Dis Child* 1960; **35:** 182–91.
54. Wayne KS, Taussig LM. Probable familial congenital bronchiectasis due to cartilage deficiency (Williams Campbell syndrome). *Am Rev Respir Dis* 1976; **114:** 15–22.
55. Bush A. Left bronchial isomerism, normal atrial arrangement and bronchomalacia mimicking asthma: a new syndrome? *Eur Respir J* 1999; **14:** 475–7.
56. Kao SC, Smith WL, Sato Y, Franken EA Jr, Kimura K, Soper RT. Ultrafast CT of laryngeal and tracheobronchial obstruction in symptomatic postoperative infants with esophageal atresia and tracheoesophageal fistula. *Am J Roentgenol* 1990; **154:** 345–50.
57. Neijens HJ, Kerrebijn KF, Smalhout B. Successful treatment with CPAP of two infants with bronchomalacia. *Acta Paediatr Scand* 1978; **67:** 293–6.
58. Miller RW, Pollack MM, Murphy TM, Fink RJ. Effectiveness of continuous positive pressure in the treatment of bronchomalacia in infants: a bronchoscopic documentation. *Crit Care Med* 1986; **14:** 125–7.
59. Vinograd I, Filler RM, Bahoric A. Long-term functional results of prosthetic airway splinting in tracheomalacia and bronchomalacia. *J Pediatr Surg* 1987; **22:** 38–41.
60. Filler RM, Forte V, Fraga JC, Matute J. The use of expandable metallic airway stents for tracheobronchial obstruction in children. *J Pediatr Surg* 1995; **30:** 1050–5.
61. Corbally MT, Spitz L, Kiely E, Brereton RJ, Drake DP. Aortopexy for tracheomalacia in oesophageal anomalies. *Eur J Pediatr Surg* 1993; **3:** 264–6.
62. Gomez-Pastrana D, Torronteras R, Caro P et al. Diagnosis of tuberculosis in children using a polymerase chain reaction. *Pediatr Pulmonol* 1999; **28:** 344–51.
63. Joint Tuberculosis Committee of the British Thoracic Society. Chemotherapy and management of tuberculosis in the United Kingdom: recommendations. *Thorax* 1998; **53:** 536–48.
64. Payne DNR, Lincoln C, Bush A. Right sided aortic arch in children with persistent respiratory symptoms. *BMJ* 2000; **321:** 687–8.

65. Temtamy SA, Miller JD. Extending the scope of the VATER association: definition of a VATER syndrome. *J Pediatr* 1974; **85:** 345.
66. Brooke AM, Lambert PC, Burton PR, Clarke C, Luyt DK, Simpson H. The natural history of respiratory symptoms in preschool children. *Am J Resp Crit Care Med* 1995; **152:** 1872–8.
67. ETAC study group. Determinants of total and specific IgE in infants with atopic dermatitis. *Pediatr Allergy Immunol* 1997; **8:** 177–84.
68. Wilson NW, Robinson NP, Hogan MB. Cockroach and other inhalant allergies in infantile asthma. *Annals Allergy* 1999; **83:** 27–30.
69. Sherrill DL, Stein R, Halonen M, Holberg CJ, Wright A, Martinez FD. Total serum IgE and its association with asthma symptoms and allergic sensitisation among children. *J Allergy Clin Immunol* 1999; **104:** 28–36.
70. ETAC study group. Allergic factors associated with the development of asthma and the influence of cetirizine in a double-blind, randomised, placebo controlled trial. *Pediatr Allergy Immunol* 1998; **9:** 116–24.
71. Burr ML, Merrett TG, Dunstan FD, Maguire MJ. The development of allergy in high-risk children. *Clin Exp Allergy* 1997; **27:** 1247–53.
72. Lanz MJ, Leung DYM, McCormick DR et al. Comparison of exhaled nitric oxide, serum eosinophilic cationic protein, and soluble interleukin-2 receptor in exacerbations of pediatric asthma. *Pediatr Pulmonol* 1997; **24:** 305–11.
73. Villa JR, Garcia G, Rueda S, Nogales A. Serum eosinophilic cationic protein may predict clinical course of wheezing in young children. *Arch Dis Child* 1998; **78:** 448–52.
74. Koller DY, Wojnarowski C, Herkner KR et al. High levels of eosinophilic cationic protein in wheezing infants predict the development of asthma. *J Allergy Clin Immunol* 1997; **99:** 752–6.
75. Ingram JM, Rakes GP, Hoover GE, Platts-Mills TAE, Heymann PW. Eosinophil cationic protein in serum and nasal washes from wheezing infants and children. *J Pediatr* 1995; **127:** 558–64.
76. Balfour-Lynn IM, Valman B, Silverman M, Webster ADB. Nasal IgA response in wheezy infants. *Arch Dis Child* 1993; **68:** 472–6.
77. Balfour-Lynn IM, Valman B, Wellings R, Webster ADB, Silverman M. Tumour necrosis factor α and leukotriene E4 production in wheezy infants. *Clin Exp Allergy* 1993; **24:** 121–6.
78. Gemou-Engesaeth V, Kay AB, Bush A, Corrigan CJ. Activated peripheral blood CD4 and CD8 T-lymphocytes in child asthma: correlation with eosinophilia and disease severity. *Pediatr Allergy Immunol* 1994; **5:** 170–7.
79. Gemou-Engesaeth V, Bush A, Kay AB, Hamid Q, Corrigan C. Inhaled glucocorticoid therapy of childhood asthma is associated with reduced peripheral blood T cell activation and 'Th2-type' cytokine mRNA expression. *Pediatrics* 1997; **99:** 695–703.
80. Kharitonov SA, Yates D, Robbins RA et al. Increased nitric oxide in exhaled air of asthmatic patients. *Lancet* 1994; **343:** 133–5.
81. Byrnes CA, Dinarevic S, Shinebourne EA, Barnes PJ, Bush A. Exhaled nitric oxide measurements in normal and asthmatic children. *Pediatr Pulmonol* 1997; **24:** 312–18.
82. Kharitonov S, Alving K, Barnes PJ. Exhaled and nasal nitric oxide: recommendations. *Eur Respir J* 1997; **10:** 1683–93.
83. Baraldi E, Dario C, Ongaro R et al. Exhaled nitric oxide concentrations during treatment of wheezing exacerbation in infants and young children. *Am J Respir Crit Care Med* 1999; **159:** 1284–8.
84. Payne D, Adcock IM, Oates T et al. Airway inflammation in children with difficult asthma. *Am J Respir Crit Care Med* 1999; **159:** A122.
85. Kraft M, Djukanovic R, Wilson S, Holgate ST, Martin RJ. Alveolar tissue inflammation in asthma. *Am J Respir Crit Care Med* 1996; **154:** 1505–10.
86. Pohunek P, Roche WR, Turzikova J, Kudmann J, Warner JO. Eosinophilic inflammation in the bronchial mucosa of children with bronchial asthma. *Eur Respir J* 1997; **10**(suppl 25): 160S.
87. Teig N, Philippou S, Wagner C, Beck T, Schauer U, Rieger C. Subepithelial basement membrane thickness in wheezy infants and development of asthma at an age of 5 years. *Eur Respir J* 1999; **14**(suppl 30): 281S.
88. Stevenson EC, Turner G, Heaney LG et al. Bronchoalveolar lavage findings suggest two different forms of childhood asthma. *Clin Exp Allergy* 1997; **27:** 1027–35.
89. Marguet C, Jouen-Bodes F, Dean TP, Warner JO. Bronchoalveolar cell profiles in children with asthma, infantile wheeze, chronic cough, or cystic fibrosis. *Am J Respir Crit Care Med* 1999; **159:** 1533–40.
90. Martinez FD, Morgan WJ, Wright AL et al. Diminished lung function as a predisposing factor for wheezing respiratory illness in infants. *N Engl J Med* 1988; **319:** 1112–17.
91. Tager IB, Hanrahan JP, Tostesan TD et al. Lung

function, pre- and post-natal smoke exposure, and wheezing in the first year of life. *Am Rev Respir Dis* 1993; **147**: 811–17.
92. Young S, O'Keeffe PT, Arnot J, Landau L. Lung function, airway responsiveness, and respiratory symptoms before and after bronchiolitis. *Arch Dis Child* 1995; **72**: 16–24.
93. Rusconi F, Gagliardi L, Aston H, Silverman M. Changes in respiratory rate affect tidal expiratory flow indices in infants. *Pediatr Pulmonol* 1996; **21**: 236–40.
94. Wilson NM, Bridge P, Phagoo SB, Silverman M. The measurement of methacholine responsiveness in 5 year old children: three methods compared. *Eur Respir J* 1995; **8**: 364–70.
95. Yong SC, Smith CM, Wach R, Kurian M, Primhak RA. Methacholine challenge in preschool children: methacholine-induced wheeze versus transcutaneous oximetry. *Eur Respir J* 1999; **14**: 1175–8.
96. Clarke JR, Reese A, Silverman M. Bronchial responsiveness and lung function in infants with lower respiratory tract illness over the first six months of life. *Arch Dis Child* 1992; **67**: 1454–8.
97. Stick S, Arnott J, Landau LI, Turner D, Sy S, LeSoeuf P. Bronchial responsiveness and lung function in recurrently wheezy infants. *Am Rev Respir Dis* 1991; **144**: 1012–15.
98. Phagoo SB, Wilson NM, Silverman M. Evaluation of a new interrupter device for measuring the bronchial response to bronchodilator in 3 year old children. *Eur Respir J* 1996; **9**: 1374–80.
99. Bridge PD, Ranganathan S, McKenzie SA. Measurement of airway resistance using the interrupter technique in preschool children in the ambulatory setting. *Eur Respir J* 1999; **13**: 792–6.
100. Bisgaard H, Klug B. Lung function measurement in awake young children. *Eur Respir J* 1995; **8**: 2067–75.
101. Klug B, Bisgaard H. Measurement of lung function in awake 2–4 yr-old asthmatic children during methacholine challenge and acute asthma: a comparison of the impulse oscillation technique, the interruptor technique, and transcutaneous measurement of oxygen versus whole body plethysmography. *Pediatr Pulmonol* 1998; **25**: 322–31.
102. Agertoft L, Pedersen S. Effects of long-term treatment with an inhaled steroid on growth and lung function in asthmatic children. *Respir Med* 1994; **88**: 373–81.
103. Haahtela T, Jarvinen K, Kava T et al. Effects of discontinuing inhaled budesonide in patients with mild asthma. *N Engl J Med* 1994; **331**: 700–5.
104. Doull IJ, Freezer N, Holgate ST. Growth of children with mild asthma treated with inhaled beclomethasone dipropionate. *Am J Respir Crit Care Med* 1995; **151**: 1715–19.
105. Doull IJ, Campbell MJ, Holgate ST. Duration of growth suppressive effects of regular inhaled corticosteroids. *Arch Dis Child* 1998; **78**: 172–3.
106. Thibeault DW, Heimes B, Rezaiekhaligh M, Mabry S. Chronic modifications of lung and heart development in glucocorticoid-treated newborn rats exposed to hyperoxia or room air. *Pediatr Pulmonol* 1993; **16**: 81–8.
107. Burri PH. Structural aspects of prenatal and postnatal development and growth of the lung. In: McDonald JA, ed. *Lung Growth and Development*. New York: Marcel Dekker, 1997.
108. Kraemer R, Bigler UJ, Casaulta-Aebischer C, Weder M, Birrer P. Clinical and physiological improvement after inhalation of low-dose beclomethasone dipropionate and salbutamol in wheezy infants. *Respiration* 1997; **64**: 342–9.
109. Parkin PC, Saunders NR, Diamond SA, Winders PM, Macarthur C. Randomised trial spacer v nebuliser for acute asthma. *Arch Dis Child* 1995; **72**: 239–40.
110. Kerem E, Levison H, Schuh S et al. Efficacy of albuterol administered by nebuliser versus spacer device in children with acute asthma. *J Pediatr* 1993; **123**: 313–17.
111. Dewar AL, Stewart A, Cogswell JJ, Connett GJ. A randomised controlled trial to assess the relative benefits of large volume spacers and nebulisers to treat acute asthma in hospital. *Arch Dis Child* 1999; **80**: 421–3.
112. Wilson N, Sloper K, Silverman M. Effects of continuous treatment with topical corticosteroids on episodic viral wheeze in preschool children. *Arch Dis Child* 1995; **72**: 317–20.
113. Oswald H, Phelan PD, Lanigan A et al. Childhood asthma and lung function in mid-adult life. *Pediatr Pulmonol* 1997; **23**: 14–20.
114. Tasche MJA, van der Wouden JC, Uijen JHJM et al. Randomised placebo-controlled trial of inhaled sodium cromoglycate in 1–4 year old children with moderate asthma. *Lancet* 1997; **350**: 1060–4.
115. McKenzie S. Cough—but is it asthma? *Arch Dis Child* 1994; **70**: 1–3.

116. Chang AB. Isolated cough—probably not asthma? *Arch Dis Child* 1999; **80:** 211–13.
117. Kelly YJ, Brabin BJ, Milligan PJM, Reid JA, Heaf D, Pearson MG. Clinical significance of cough and wheeze in the diagnosis of asthma. *Arch Dis Child* 1996; **75:** 489–93.
118. Powell CVE, Primhak RA. Stability of respiratory symptoms in unlabelled wheezy illness and nocturnal cough. *Arch Dis Child* 1996; **75:** 549–54.
119. Brooke AM, Lambert PC, Burton PR, Clarke C, Luyt DK, Simpson H. Night cough in a population-based sample of children: characteristics, relation to symptoms and associations with measures of asthma severity. *Eur Respir J* 1996; **9:** 65–71.
120. Cloutier MM, Loughlin GM. Chronic cough in children: a manifestation of airway hyperreactivity. *Pediatrics* 1981; **67:** 6–12.
121. Forsythe P, McGarvey PA, Heaney LG, MacMahon J, Elborn JS. Neurotrophin levels in BAL fluid from patients with asthma and non-asthmatic cough. *Eur Respir J* 1999; **14**(suppl 30): 470S.
122. Koh YY, Jeong JY, Park Y, Kim CK. Development of wheezing in patients with cough variant asthma during an increase in airway responsiveness. *Eur Respir J* 1999; **14:** 302–8.
123. Meadow R. What is, and what is not, 'Munchausen syndrome by proxy'? *Arch Dis Child* 1995; **72:** 534–8.
124. Crowley S, Balfour-Lynn I, Rosenthal M, Bush A. Pharyngomalacia causing upper airway obstruction. *Am J Respir Crit Care Med* 2000; **161:** A26.

7

Pharmacologic management of asthma in infants and small children

Joseph D Spahn, Ronina A Covar, Melanie C Gleason, David G Tinkelman, Stanley J Szefler

Introduction • Issues in the management of asthma in small children • Pharmacologic therapy • Summary

INTRODUCTION

Asthma remains the number one cause of admission to the hospital, and the most common cause of missed time from school.[1] Hospital admission rates for acute asthma exacerbations have increased,[2] and although the annual rate of asthma mortality has stabilized, it is still significantly higher than in the past.[3] Infants and young children are at particular risk for asthma morbidity. The rates of admission for asthmatic children less than 4 years of age are greater than those for all other age groups.[4] Several studies have found a bimodal age distribution of exacerbations requiring intubation and assisted ventilation, with the largest peak occurring in children ~2 years of age and a second smaller peak in adolescents.[5,6] Not only are young asthmatic children at greater risk for hospitalization, they are also more likely to require readmission to a hospital for repeated acute exacerbations.[7] In this observational study of over 1000 children admitted to a large hospital in Australia for acute asthma, the investigators found readmission to the hospital to be a common occurrence with over 50% of children being readmitted with acute asthma over a 2 year period. Young age (<5 years) was one of the risk factors, with a relative risk (RR) of 1.71. Other risk factors included female sex, number of previous admissions (RR increased with increasing numbers of previous hospitalizations), and need for intravenous medications. Thus, asthma is a major childhood disease that affects society greatly. Given the scope of this disease, a significant effort has been made to better understand and manage this chronic disease, with several guidelines developed in recent years.

Our understanding of the pathogenesis of this disease has evolved over time. We now know that asthma (in adults) is a disease characterized by chronic airway inflammation.[8,9] As a result, the emphasis has shifted from viewing asthma as a bronchospastic disease treated primarily with bronchodilator medications to viewing it as an inflammatory disease with a bronchospastic component. Thus, for all but the mildest asthmatics, routinely administered anti-inflammatory medications are now recommended. Bronchodilators are used primarily as needed, as rescue medications for significant asthma exacerbations and acute episodes of bronchospasm. They are also recommended before exercise with the purpose of preventing exercise-induced asthma. This review will attempt to provide a comprehensive evaluation of therapies available to infants and young children with asthma.

We will begin with a discussion of the many issues that make treating this group of children unique and, in many ways, more difficult. Issues such as who and when to treat, with what medications, how the medications are delivered, how one monitors the response to treatment, and the many confounding factors that make the definitive diagnosis hard to attain. Next, we will discuss the two major categories of asthma medications—the quick-relief and the long-term control medications—including a discussion of the appropriate use of these medications.

ISSUES IN THE MANAGEMENT OF ASTHMA IN SMALL CHILDREN

Who should be treated and when?

We now know that not every infant and small child who wheezes in the first few years of life will go on to develop asthma. In a landmark study by Martinez and associates,[10] over 1200 newborns were prospectively enrolled to evaluate factors involved in early-onset wheezing in relationship to persistent wheezing at 6 years of age. At 6 years of age, 52% of the children had never wheezed; 20% had had at least one episode of wheezing associated with a respiratory tract infection during the first 3 years of life but had no wheezing at 6 years; 15% had not wheezed during the first 3 years of life but had wheezing at 6 years; and 14% had wheezing both before 3 years and at 6 years of age. Those children who had early-onset but transient wheezing were more likely to have premorbid diminished airway function and a history of maternal smoking. They were also less likely to be atopic. In contrast, those children who had early onset wheezing that persisted at 6 years of age were more likely to have a positive maternal history of asthma, elevated IgE levels with normal lung function at 1 year, and diminished lung function with elevated IgE levels at 6 years. Thus, only a minority of children who wheezed with viral respiratory tract infections during the first 3 years went on to develop asthma. A genetic predisposition for the asthma phenotype appears to be a prerequisite for persistent wheezing later in life.[10]

This finding has obvious clinical relevance. Not all children who wheeze early in life will go on to develop asthma. Thus, only children with persistent wheezing should be targeted for long-term asthma therapy. Unfortunately, we have no way of knowing prospectively who will go on to develop asthma. If we did, we could begin anti-inflammatory therapy early in the course of the disease and, by doing so, potentially alter the subsequent course of the disease. Alternatively, one could treat all children early on. There are two major weaknesses with that approach. First, since many of the children will not develop persistent wheezing, it will be difficult to determine the effectiveness of the therapy used. Second, and more clinically important, are the issues of cost, effort, and safety related to long-term anti-inflammatory treatment especially as it pertains to inhaled corticosteroid (ICS) therapy.

The available control medications are limited

The range of control medications available for use in children less than 6 years of age is extremely limited. First, most of the medications used to treat asthma are not labeled for use with children less than 6 years of age, forcing health care professionals to use many medications off label in young asthmatics. Second, the only available control medication in the United States for use in a nebulizer is cromolyn. As will be discussed in a subsequent section, cromolyn's effectiveness is limited. A nebulizable suspension of budesonide has been available for use in much of the world, with much clinical experience gained, but it has only recently been approved by the Food and Drug Administration in the United States. Once available, it should offer a significant advance in the treatment of small children with moderate and severe persistent asthma. Third, worldwide, the use of oral anti-inflammatory compounds such as the leukotriene receptor antagonists in infants and very young children is not yet approved. Oral medications are easier to administer, more consistently delivered, and more likely to be adhered to than inhaled medications. Montelukast is the only leukotriene-modifying agent approved for use in children. It is presently available for use in children 6 years of age or older. Clinical studies using a 4 mg chewable tablet in children 2 years of age and older have been completed and the product has been recently approved for use in the United States.

How to treat: medication delivery devices

Treating the infant and young child with aerosol therapy presents unique challenges. The preferential nasal breathing, small airways, low tidal volume, and high respiratory frequency of the neonate and infant markedly increase the difficulty of drug targeting to the pulmonary airways.[11] Young children are incapable of reliably performing the maneuvers specified for optimal delivery of aerosol therapy. Specifically, slow inhalation through the mouth with a period of breath holding for pressurized metered-dose inhalers (pMDIs) or the rapid and forceful inhalation required in the case of dry powder inhalers is not possible. For these reasons, medication delivery devices suitable for the young child are limited to those that require a minimum of skills and cooperation from the child. At present there are two basic delivery systems that are frequently used in this age group: the nebulizer and the pMDI with spacing/holding chamber and facemask.

Within these two general types of delivery systems numerous products are available, which vary widely in performance. Clinical efficacy in infants and young children has been demonstrated with both the nebulizer and the pMDI with spacing/holding chamber, but there is no clear evidence that either system is superior to the other for the treatment of asthma in young children. Unfortunately, there is a paucity of well-designed in vivo studies comparing the two methods and more research in this area is greatly needed. The available published data have been reviewed in depth and a summary comparing the findings follows.

There are diverging trends with respect to the preferred medication delivery device in infants and young children. The National Heart, Lung, and Blood Institute (NHBLI) guidelines prefer the use of a nebulizer for the delivery of cromolyn and high dose short-acting β-agonist.[12] Budesonide for use with a nebulizer has only recently become available in the United States. Inhalation of steroids via a pMDI with spacing/holding device and facemask is considered acceptable though perhaps not the preferred means of administering topical steroids to young children and infants. In contrast, the International Pediatric Consensus statement[13] and the British guidelines[14] recommend the use of pMDI with spacing/holding device and facemask as the preferred method.

Nebulizers

Over the past century, jet nebulizers have been the mainstay of aerosol treatment[15] and remain the first choice of delivery system for the treatment of infants and young children incapable of using other devices. A major advantage of the nebulizer is the simple technique required of relaxed tidal breathing. This feature makes the nebulizer a logical choice for the delivery of inhaled medications to infants and young children. However, there is a huge variation in the output from the various devices and this in turn affects drug delivery and therapeutic response. Drug deposition is variable and ranges from less than 1% to over 20% of the nominal dose. See Chapter 17 for a more thorough review of this topic.

In a small study of males aged 9 to 36 months, the amount of cromolyn deposited into the lungs was accessed via measurement of urinary sodium cromoglycate.[16] In this study, two methods of administration—jet nebulizer and metered dose inhaler with a valved spacer device—were compared. A significantly greater cumulative urinary excretion of sodium cromoglycate was observed when the children were treated with nebulizer than with a pMDI and spacer. Only a fraction of drug was absorbed with 0.76% of the nominal dose of sodium cromoglycate via the nebulizer, versus 0.30% for the pMDI and spacer. It was concluded that the nebulizer delivered more drug than the spacer, but that this may be clinically insignificant, since the dose delivered by either method was poor. The authors proposed that some of the problems of treatment in young children are the result of inadequate medication reaching the lungs. Nasal breathing reduces the pulmonary deposition to about one-quarter of the value obtained during mouth breathing. In a report assessing the amount of nebulized budesonide delivered to infants of similar age (4–30 months) a significantly higher percentage of medication was delivered as measured via filters attached to the facemask. An average of 14% (range 9–19%, increasing with age) of the nominal dose of budesonide was found in the inhalation filter.[17] A much greater amount delivered was recently reported by Wennergren et al,[18] who found deposition of 21–27% of the nominal dose. The filter test reflects the amount of aerosol available to the patient but is clearly an overestimation of the dose delivered to the lower respiratory tract. Various studies in school-aged children report lung doses of 3–6%. It is expected that the lung dose to infants and small children would be considerably less than this given the large proportion of aerosol loss in the upper airway as a consequence of nasal breathing. Despite the relatively small amount of nebulized medication reaching the lower airway, efficacy studies and response to clinical treatment support the use of this delivery device. Furthermore, efficacy studies of nebulized budesonide performed in steroid-dependent preschool-aged children[19] and infants with severe asthma[20] noted significant improvements with a high acceptance rate. Thus, these studies show that despite low lung deposition by nebulized treatment, at least with budesonide suspension, this delivery system is efficacious in young children. There are several disadvantages of this system, including the obvious: expense, cumbersome equipment, inefficiency (medication waste), need for a power source, time-consuming treatments, and potential for bacterial contamination. Perhaps less obvious, but more important, is the highly variable drug output from the different devices. Owing to the heightened awareness of cost-effectiveness and failure of adherence to burdensome treatment plans there is a gradual move to other delivery devices, namely, the pMDI with spacing/holding chamber and facemask.[13]

Metered dose inhalers and spacing/holding chamber with facemask

The advancement of valved holding chambers and spacing devices has revolutionized aerosol delivery to school-aged children and adults. As a result, the use of these devices has been extended to infants and young children. The British guidelines recommend the spacing/holding chamber with facemask as the first

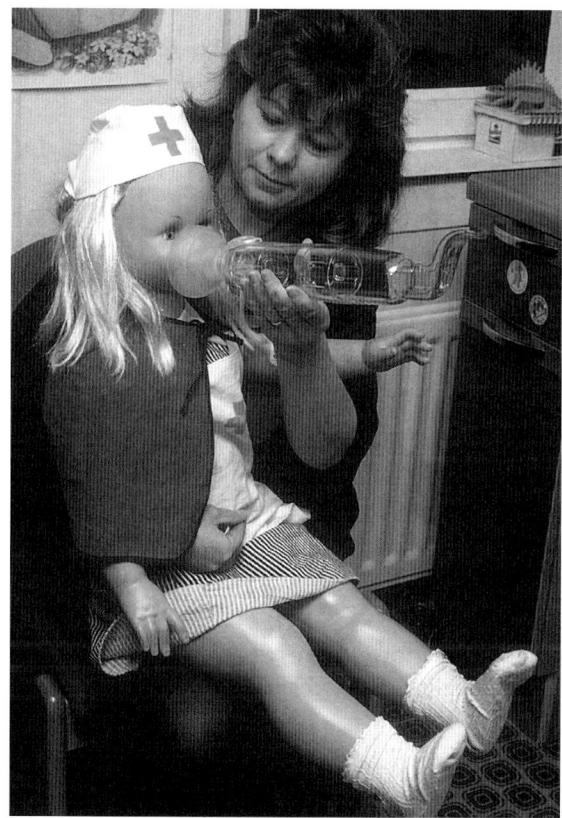

Figure 7.1 The use of a Babyhaler (low volume valved spacer) demonstrated on a mannequin.

choice for delivery of inhaled medications to neonates and young infants. Even in the United States, there has been a gradual shift to the preferential use of the pMDI and holding chambers with facemask.

Recent studies comparing delivery of short-acting β-agonist via pMDI with the nebulizer have been equivocal in most cases. This includes the emergency setting when comparable doses of medication are administered to infants and young children.[21,22] Parkin et al,[21] found albuterol/salbutamol delivered via pMDI to be as effective as the same drug delivered via a nebulizer in 60 preschool children who were hospitalized with acute asthma. However, nearly one-third of the subjects randomized to pMDI eventually required nebulized β-agonist. To our knowledge, there is only one published study[23] that evaluated lower respiratory tract deposition of a radiolabeled drug given by a pMDI with a spacer and facemask to children less than 5 years old. The results of this study documented that on average less than 2% of the nominal dose was deposited in the lower respiratory tract. Even less is known about the adequacy of inhaled corticosteroids delivery in infants and young children using a pMDI with spacer and mask. There have been two placebo-controlled trials of budesonide administered via metered dose inhaler and holding chamber with attached facemask which demonstrated efficacy compared with placebo.[24,25] The patients in these studies had milder asthma compared with those enrolled in studies evaluating the efficacy of nebulized budesonide, and neither study attempted to measure the amount of inhaled steroid delivered in this fashion.

It is not advisable to extrapolate the experience of pMDIs and spacing/holding chambers used in the above studies (Nebuhaler and Babyhaler) to the devices currently available in the United States, since aerosol delivery is significantly different for the various devices. The Aerochamber with facemask is a valved holding chamber commonly used in the United States. This device performed significantly poorer than either the Nebuhaler or the Babyhaler in a comparison study in children aged 10–25 months.[26]

In summary, there is a tremendous gap in our knowledge of the efficiency of the various delivery devices available for administration of inhaled therapies to infants and young children. In part, this may owe to the difficulty in evaluating lung deposition, since it may require radiolabeled material and or invasive techniques (serial venipuncture) for pharmacokinetic analysis. Current practice in infants and young children is more an art than a science. Silverman in a commentary cited in an article by Agertoft and Pedersen[26] eloquently summarized the problem in this area: 'When one considers the huge effort that has gone into the development and marketing of topical asthma drugs, the trivial investment that has gone into the development of therapeutic devices for preschool children seems almost negligible.'

Monitoring response to therapy

Once therapy is initiated, it is difficult to objectively assess response. Measures of efficacy in terms of clinical scores, pulmonary function testing, and degree of airway hyperresponsiveness are difficult to standardize in such a young population.[27] Lung function measurements, which serve as the gold standard in adults and older children, are, at best, difficult to perform in young children and are limited to a handful of sites across the world which have particular expertise with infant pulmonary function studies.[28] Thus, we are left with subjective measures, including asthma symptom scoring systems,[29] need for rescue bronchodilator or oral corticosteroid (CS) therapy, and emergent care visits/hospitalizations, with which to judge efficacy. At present there are no non-invasive, easily measured markers of airway inflammation which might help not only in making the diagnosis of asthma but also in guiding response to therapy. A number of candidates, including circulating eosinophils, serum eosinophil cationic protein (ECP), exhaled nitric oxide, urinary LTE4, and induced sputum for eosinophils, have been studied but at present all have significant limitations, and very few have specifically been evaluated in children less than 5 years old. In one of the few studies designed to specifically address the role of ECP in recurrently wheezing children less than 2 years old, Carlsen et al found a strong correlation between serum ECP and response to albuterol/salbutamol using the tidal flow volume loop technique in children 0–2 years of age.[30] These investigators suggested that ECP may be measuring airway inflammation and that it may have some prognostic value in diagnosing asthma in infants and toddlers with recurrent wheezing.

Adherence

Because asthma is a chronic relapsing disease that often requires long-term medication use even during times of good clinical control, adherence can be a major issue. A recent study by Milgrom et al, which evaluated adherence in a group of asthmatic children requiring chronically administered ICS therapy, illustrates this point nicely.[31] They found that adherence to ICS therapy was only 40%. Individuals who required an oral CS burst owing to an acute asthma exacerbation were those who had used their ICS the least (less than 15% of the time!).

The issue of adherence in infants and small children is even more complicated, since the child is entirely dependent on the care giver to administer the medication. Thus, when discussing adherence in this age group, one is really evaluating the ability of the care giver to administer the medication as directed. In an observational study of preschool children, Gibson et al sought to evaluate adherence with inhaled prophylactic medications delivered through a large volume spacer using an electronic timer.[32] These investigators found adherence to be only 50% with a range of 0–94%. Only 42% of the subjects received the prescribed medication on each study day. Interestingly, reporting of symptoms in the diary cards did not correlate with good compliance with the prophylactic medication, nor was a correlation found between frequency of administration and adherence. In another study by the same investigators, parental reporting of symptom scores correlated with measured bronchodilator use in only 63% of preschool children.[33] In this study, enrollment in day care was associated with poorer adherence even though the prophylactic medications were not administered while in day care. The authors speculated that parents who utilize day care may be too busy to ensure adequate adherence with prescribed therapy. Only a few studies have attempted to address why care givers are unable to administer medications as prescribed. Lim et al sought to address this issue by asking parents why they were reluctant to administer prophylactic medications (ICS) to their young children with asthma.[34] Several reasons were cited including hesitancy to use medications for fear of dependence, side effects, and overdosage. Fortunately, patient education programs developed for parents of small children with asthma have been demonstrated to improve asthma morbidity and self-management outcome.[35,36] Although Gibson et al[32] found no relationship between frequency of administration and adherence with prescribed therapy, other studies in older children have shown compliance rates to be inversely proportional to the frequency of medication administration.[37] Thus, treatment strategies must be designed to minimize the frequency with which medications are administered. Few, if any, studies have sought to address adherence with nebulized medications in small children.

Confounding factors

Inherent to this age group are a number of factors that can not only mimic asthma, but also contribute to poor asthma control. Consequently, the diagnosis and assessment of asthma severity can be more difficult. Although small airways, as discussed above, and asthma account for the majority of cases, several other disease processes can manifest as wheezing. In addition, infants and small children have a greater degree of bronchial hyperresponsiveness, which may predispose them to wheeze. Drugs that rely on hepatic metabolism are more difficult to use in infants and small children owing to the wide fluctuations in clearance as a consequence of maturation changes and the effect certain viral infections associated with fever have on the liver's ability to metabolize drugs (see section on theophylline below). The differential diagnosis of wheezing includes conditions such as foreign body aspiration, congenital airway anomalies, abnormalities of the great vessels, occult cardiac disease, cystic fibrosis, recurrent aspiration, immunodeficiency, tuberculosis, and mediastinal masses. Clearly, making the correct diagnosis is essential, since the treatment for the above conditions can vary drastically. For example, in children with significant gastroesophageal reflux, improvement in asthma symptoms with concomitant reduction in asthma medication use occurred after a prokinetic agent was instituted.[38] A separate chapter gives a more comprehensive approach to the diagnosis and management of these disorders (Chapter 7).

PHARMACOLOGIC THERAPY

The NHLBI EPR-2 guidelines[12] have a specific section devoted to the management of children 5 years of age and less. In general, the approach to asthma control in small children is similar to that in older children and adults; the same classification system is used for determining level of severity. Since small children cannot perform lung function measurements, symptoms are used primarily in assessing severity. The NHLBI EPR-2 guidelines have categorized asthma medications into two general classes: long-term control medications (controllers) and quick-relief medications (relievers). The controllers are used to achieve and maintain control of persistent asthma, whereas the relievers are used to alleviate acute asthma symptoms and exacerbations.

At about the same time the revised NHBLI recommendations were released, the British Thoracic Society published their guidelines. This set of guidelines also has a section on asthma management in children less than 5 years of age,[14] which provides a more thorough discussion of both chronic and acute management than the NHLBI EPR-2 guidelines.

Long-term-control medications

Inhaled anti-inflammatory agents
General comments
Cromolyn and nedocromil are related compounds having similar effects on inhibiting mediator release from mast cells. Administered prophylactically, they inhibit both the early and late phase pulmonary components of the allergic response following inhalation of an allergen in sensitized subjects.[39] They are also effective at inhibiting exercise-induced bronchospasm (EIB)[40] and are often used in conjunction with a β-agonist where EIB is refractory to β-agonist treatment alone. Both medications are indicated for mild to moderate asthma, and are considered first-line anti-inflammatory drugs for children with mild persistent asthma, according to the NHLBI EPR-2 guidelines and the International Pediatric Consensus statement.[12,13] These medications are not as potent in terms of their anti-inflammatory effects as the ICS, but they have few adverse effects.

Safety and efficacy of cromolyn
Nebulized cromolyn has been used extensively for over 20 years in young children, with several controlled studies since the mid 1970s evaluating its efficacy and safety. Table 7.1 summarizes many of the controlled studies utilizing cromolyn in children with asthma 6 years of age and less.[41-49] Most have been randomized, placebo-controlled, crossover studies employing small numbers of patients, and many were published before 1990. Two large randomized, placebo-controlled, parallel design studies have been published since 1990. The following discussion will highlight the results of some of the more illustrative studies published to date.

Hiller et al, in 1977, found nebulized cromolyn to be effective in improving both daytime and night-time cough in 17 asthmatic children with a mean age of 41 months (range 27–54 months).[41] All of the children had 'troublesome' asthma with 16/17 having required hospitalization for acute asthma at least once in the past. The study was a placebo-controlled, crossover trial in which the subjects received

Table 7.1 Summary of efficacy and safety of cromolyn in small children with asthma

Study	Methodology	Delivery/dose	Number and age of subjects	Asthma severity of subjects	Efficacy	Adverse effects
Ref. 41	16 weeks DB, PC, crossover trial	Nebulized solution 20 mg tid	17 subjects ma = 41 months r = 27–54 months	16/17 previously hospitalized	Less cough (day and night), no difference in PEFR	None
Ref. 44	DB, PC crossover, placebo vs. water vs. cromolyn	Nebulized solution 20 mg 5 min before run	14 subjects ma = 48 months r = 38–61 months	6/14 on maintenance cromolyn	Blocked exercise-induced asthma vs. water and placebo	None
Ref. 42	24 weeks DB, PC crossover trial of placebo, theophylline, or cromolyn	Nebulized solution 20 mg qid	16 subjects ma = 41 months r = 21–53 months	15/16 had received GCs in past, all had ~2 attacks in past 6 weeks	No difference in symptom scores; cromolyn better than placebo in maintaining daily activities	None
Ref. 43	12 months DB, PC crossover trial	Nebulized solution 20 mg qid	27 subjects ma = 33 months r = 14–49 months	All ~1 previous hospitalization; 7/27 were atopic	Improved daily activities, overall severity, cough; no reduction in rate of hospitalizations or need for IV therapy	No mention of adverse effects
Ref. 45	6 weeks DB, PC crossover trial ex-premature infants with wheezing	pMDI 1 puff (5 mg) qid	16 subjects (ex 29 weeks EGA); ma = 15 months postnatal age r = 4–31 months	Symptoms 3–4 times/week; 10/16 hospitalized with wheezing, all on intermittent medications	Symptom scores reduced 49%; reduced β-agonist use; FRC increased 10/16 while on cromolyn vs. 2/16 while on placebo	No mention of adverse effects

Ref. 46	6 months DB, PC crossover of cromolyn, ipratropium, or placebo	Cromolyn 20 mg, ipratropium 250 µg, or water tid	23 subjects ma = 11.8 months r = 4–24 months	'Troublesome asthma', 10/23 previously hospitalized with bronchiolitis	No difference in daily symptom scores between 3 groups; parents reported cromolyn and ipratropium superior to placebo	No mention of adverse effects
Ref. 47	10 weeks DB, PC parallel group preceded by 4–8 weeks baseline period	Nebulized cromolyn 20 mg tid	54 subjects ma = 25 months r = 1–4 years	Attacks ~1 time/month; 184 previous hospitalizations (3.4 per patient)	Cromolyn no more effective than placebo in reducing symptoms, sleep disturbance, β-agonist use, acute MD visits or hospitalizations	Mouth eczema in 1 patient on cromolyn
Ref. 48	6 weeks DB, PC parallel group	Nebulized cromolyn 40 mg tid	31 subjects ma = 7.8 months r = 4–12 months	Symptoms ~1 per month; wheezing ~2 times/week, cough 5 times/week MD documented wheezing	Both groups significantly improved, no difference in symptom scores, or lung function between cromolyn and placebo	No mention of adverse effects
Ref. 49	20 weeks DB, PC parallel group preceded by 4 weeks baseline period	pMDI cromolyn 10 mg tid	218 subjects ma = 30 months r = 1–4 years	Moderate asthma symptoms >1 per week, interference with daily activities, sleep	No difference between cromolyn and placebo in % symptom-free days, or any other outcome measure	Facial eczema, cough with cromolyn

Abbreviations: DB = double-blind, PC = placebo-controlled, ma = mean age, r = range, tid = three times daily, qid = four times daily, EGA = estimated gestational age, pMDI = pressurized metered dose inhaler.

cromolyn 20 mg three times daily or placebo for 2 months with a crossover to the alternative therapy for another 2 months. Cromolyn significantly reduced nocturnal and daytime cough, while having no effect on reported wheeze or peak expiratory flow (PEF) rates. Specifically, night-time cough score was 100 for cromolyn versus 90 for placebo, the higher the score the fewer the symptoms. A less pronounced difference was seen with daytime cough with scores of 98 and 93 for cromolyn and placebo, respectively. Glass et al, in a double-blind, crossover trial, evaluated the effectiveness of 8 weeks each of nebulized cromolyn (20 mg four times daily), theophylline (6.7 mg/kg four times daily), or placebo in 16 asthmatic children with a mean age of 51 months.[42] Neither theophylline nor cromolyn was more effective than placebo in reducing symptom scores for sleep disturbance, cough, and wheeze, but cromolyn was more effective than placebo in maintaining daily activities. In a longer study (12 months), with a slightly younger group of children (mean age 33 months, range 14–49 months), Cogswell and Simpkiss found cromolyn 20 mg administered four times daily to be statistically superior to placebo in terms of reducing the night-time cough score (0.77 versus 1.16), improving the daily activity score (0.44 versus 0.82), increasing the percentage of symptom-free days (60% versus 50%), and improving the asthma overall severity score (0.53 versus 0.92).[43] The scale for symptom scores ranged from 0 for no symptoms to 10 for very severe symptoms. The above findings warrant further comment. As a group, the children were not very symptomatic during the study, with symptom scores of less than 2. Because the children were not symptomatic, it may have been difficult to detect significant differences between the two groups. Second, although significant differences were detected in some parameters between the two groups, it is unlikely that the differences were clinically significant, especially when one considers the fact that no difference in the rate of hospitalization or need for intravenous medications as detected between cromolyn and placebo. Unfortunately, cromolyn neither prevented nor modified acute severe asthma attacks requiring hospitalization. The authors concluded that nebulized cromolyn 'is a tedious prophylactic treatment for the young asthmatic, but it is useful when other treatments fail.'

Cromolyn has also been shown to be effective in reducing exercise-induced bronchospasm in preschool children with asthma.[44] It has also been shown to be effective in the treatment of ex-premature infants with recurrent episodes of wheezing.[45] In this double-blind, placebo-controlled, crossover study by Yuskel et al, 16 ex-premature infants with recurrent respiratory symptoms received cromolyn, 5 mg four times daily, via pMDI and spacer or placebo for 6 weeks.[45] Cromolyn therapy resulted in a 49% reduction in symptom scores, and a significant reduction in number of days requiring use of a β-agonist (2.9 versus 7.9 days). In addition, while on cromolyn, lung function as measured by an increase in functional residual capacity (FRC) improved in 11/16 subjects whereas only 2/16 subjects demonstrated improvement while on placebo. In all of the above studies, cromolyn was well tolerated with no adverse effects noted.

Unfortunately, not all studies have demonstrated cromolyn to be effective in young children with asthma. Bertelsen and colleagues evaluated the effectiveness of 10 weeks of cromolyn or placebo in 54 toddlers (mean age 25 months, range 12–48 months) with recurrent 'wheezy bronchitis' preceded by a 4–8 week baseline period.[47] Before entry into the study, the total number of hospitalizations within the group was 184 for acute severe wheezing episodes, with a mean of 3.4 hospitalizations per subject. In addition, all had recurrent episodes of wheezing which required treatment more than once a month. The symptoms were scored on a 0–3 scale of increasing symptoms. The investigators found both treatment groups to be associated with fewer symptoms during the treatment period compared with the pre-treatment baseline period. The daytime cough symptom score while on cromolyn fell from 0.73 to 0.63 compared with a reduction from 0.89 to 0.72 during therapy with placebo. Similar reductions in both treatment groups were noted for daytime wheezing and sleep disturbance. Cromolyn was no more effective than placebo in reducing daytime wheezing and cough or reducing night-time symptoms. There was also no difference in β-agonist use, physician visits for acute episodes of wheezing, and parental preference between placebo and cromolyn. When the investigators analyzed the subgroup of patients who were atopic, they again found no difference in efficacy between cromolyn and placebo.

Similar findings were reported by Furfaro et al, who studied the efficacy of cromolyn in infants with persistent wheezing.[48] Thirty one persistently wheezing infants with a mean age of 8 months were randomized to receive either nebulized cromolyn (40 mg three times daily) or placebo for 6 weeks. No difference in symptom scores, or lung function ($V_{max}FRC$) was found between the cromolyn and placebo treated groups. The authors concluded that cromolyn was ineffective in infants less than 1 year old. They also stated that there were many potential factors that could contribute to its lack of efficacy in infants, including poor topical delivery, method of delivery, nasal breathing (which could act as a filter and reduce drug delivery to the lung), and duration of administration. It should also be noted that the pathogenesis of persistent wheezing in children less than 1 year old may be quite different than that of wheezing in older children and adults, with inflammation playing less of a prominent role. Unfortunately, we badly lack studies that have attempted to understand the pathogenesis of recurrent wheezing in children less than 2 years of age.

The largest and most recently published study evaluating the efficacy of cromolyn in young children is by Tasche et al.[49] In this randomized, placebo-controlled study, 218 children 1–4 years old, with a mean age of 2.6 years, were enrolled to receive cromolyn 10 mg three times daily via pMDI with a spacer or placebo for 5 months preceded by a 1 month baseline period. As had been noted in the Bertelsen study, both cromolyn and placebo treated groups improved during treatment compared with the baseline period.[47] However, there were no differences between the cromolyn and placebo groups in terms of symptom-free days or any other outcome measure. The authors concluded that in the majority of small children inhalation therapy with an MDI and spacer is feasible, but that long-term prophylactic cromolyn therapy is no more effective than placebo. This is by far the largest study published to date. A better study would have been to perform this clinical trial with nebulized cromolyn. It is likely that lung deposition in small children is greater following administration of a solution of cromolyn via the nebulizer compared with administration of the drug via an MDI and spacer. If this is indeed the case, then it is important to know, in a large placebo-controlled study, whether cromolyn is indeed effective as a long-term control medication in small children with persistent asthma. All one can take from this study is that cromolyn administered via an MDI and spacer device in children aged 1–4 years is not an effective therapy.

Summary

Despite widespread use for over 20 years, it remains to be determined how effective cromolyn is in young children with asthma. Roughly equal numbers of controlled studies have reported diametrically opposing outcomes. Half have reported cromolyn to be effective in reducing symptoms while the other half have reported cromolyn to be no better than placebo (see Table 7.1). Among the studies that showed cromolyn to be effective, the improvements in symptoms were at best modest. Complicating the issue of efficacy further is the age of the studies. The majority of the studies were performed over 15 years ago, before recent advances in our understanding of the pathogenesis of this disease. In addition, the measures used to evaluate efficacy have changed, as has the depth of data presented in current clinical research papers. For example, Cogswell and Simpkiss state in their discussion that cromolyn had no effect in reducing 'devastatingly severe attacks of asthma' which require hospitalization.[43] Unfortunately, they do not provide specifics. How many children had acute exacerbations during the study and, of those who did, how many required hospitalization? Without that information one cannot draw much from the authors' conclusions. Another problem with the above studies arises from the apparently mild nature of the disease studied. Did many of the studies enroll children that would presently be considered mild intermittent asthmatics who only had symptoms with respiratory tract infections? Data that would indirectly support this point come from an analysis of the age of patients studied. The mean age of the participants of the five studies that demonstrated efficacy was 35.6 months (see Table 7.1), whereas the mean age of the participants from the studies that failed to demonstrate efficacy was only 18.7 months. Do infants and toddlers who wheeze with viral infections have the same disease as older children with established asthma? If not, it may be that all of the available anti-inflammatory medications used to treat asthma will be found less effective in this subgroup of patients. Since cromolyn is the only controller medication approved for use in young children and given its excellent safety profile, it should still be attempted as first-line therapy as recommended by the NHLBI EPR-2 guidelines and the International Pediatric Consensus statement.[12,13] If a child fails to respond to cromolyn, both guidelines recommend treatment with low dose ICS therapy.

Inhaled corticosteroids
General comments
Corticosteroids are available for use in parenteral, oral, and inhaled forms. They are the most potent and effective medications used to treat both acute and chronic asthma.[50,51] Inhaled CS are used in the long-term control of persistent asthma whereas systemic CS are used either to optimize asthma control or to manage persistent asthma. The development of MDIs that can effectively deliver potent CS directly into the airway has revolutionized asthma therapy in both adults and older children. ICS therapy has been shown to reduce asthma symptoms, improve baseline pulmonary function, and reduce BHR in both adults and older children with asthma.[52,53] In addition, since small quantities are delivered topically, the incidence of adverse effects is greatly diminished compared with chronically administered oral CS therapy.[53] Although ICS are widely used in adult asthmatics, their use in pediatric asthma has lagged behind. The reluctance to use ICS in childhood asthma is related to concern about the risk of adrenal suppression, growth suppression, and osteoporosis. Few long-term studies have attempted to address these concerns.

The NHLBI EPR-2 guidelines recommend a stepwise approach to asthma pharmacotherapy as summarized in Table 7.2.[12] The first two steps encompass mild asthma, with step 1 being mild intermittent and step 2 mild persistent asthma. The guidelines recommend cromolyn or nedocromil for young children (~5 years) with mild persistent asthma. ICS therapy is recommended in increasing doses as preferred therapy for steps 3 and 4, which encompass moderate and severe asthma, respectively. It should be stressed that the published information on use of ICS in the young child with persistent wheezing is extremely limited. Many clinicians attempt to administer the available ICS formulations utilizing a spacer and facemask. Unfortunately, no studies have attempted to quantify the delivery of the drug utilizing a spacer and facemask to the lower airway. No studies show efficacy and safety of ICS therapy administered via a pMDI with spacer and with or without a mask. Therefore, the following discussion will focus primarily on budesonide, the only CS for use in a nebulizable form. Nebulized budesonide has been widely available throughout the world, but has only recently been approved for use in the United States. As will be discussed several studies have evaluated the efficacy and safety of budesonide, and others have focused on the delivery and pharmacokinetics of budesonide in the young child with asthma.

Efficacy/safety of nebulized budesonide
Nebulized budesonide has been studied extensively since the early 1990s. Table 7.3 summarizes many of the controlled studies utilizing

Table 7.2 Stepwise approach for managing infants and young children (~5 years old) with acute or chronic asthma symptoms

Asthma severity	Long-term control medication	Quick relief medication
Step 4 severe persistent	Daily anti-inflammatory medication: • high-dose inhaled CS with spacer and facemask; • if needed, add systemic CS 2 mg/kg per day and reduce to lowest daily or alternate-day dose that stabilizes symptoms	Bronchodilator as needed for symptoms (see step 1) up to 3 times a day
Step 3 moderate persistent	Daily anti-inflammatory medication. Either: • medium-dose inhaled CS with spacer and facemask; OR, once control is established: • medium-dose inhaled CS plus nedocromil; OR: • medium-dose inhaled CS plus long-acting bronchodilator (theophylline).	Bronchodilator as needed for symptoms (see step 1) up to 3 times a day
Step 2 mild persistent	Daily anti-inflammatory medication. Either: • cromolyn (nebulizer is preferred; or MDI) or nedocromil (MDI only) tid to qid; • infants and young children usually begin with trial of cromolyn or nedocromil; OR: • low-dose inhaled CS with spacer and face mask.	Bronchodilator as needed for symptoms (see step 1)
Step 1 mild intermittent	No daily medication needed.	Bronchodilator as needed for symptoms <2 times/week. Intensity of treatment depends on severity of exacerbation. Either: • inhaled short-acting β-agonist by nebulizer or spacer and facemask. OR with viral respiratory tract infection: • Bronchodilator every 4–6 hours up to 24 hours (longer with physician consultation) • Consider systemic GC if exacerbation is severe or patient has history of previous severe attacks

Abbreviations: CS = corticosteroid, MDI = metered dose inhaler, tid = three times daily, qid = four times daily.
Modified from reference 12.

nebulized budesonide in children with asthma 6 years of age and less. Most have been randomized, placebo-controlled, parallel studies from Europe employing relatively small numbers of patients (25–102 subjects per study). In the past year, three large studies (178–480 subjects) from the United States have also been published. The following discussion will highlight the results of some of the more illustrative studies published to date.

Most of the early studies on nebulized budesonide in young children were performed in patients with moderate to severe persistent asthma. The three studies that evaluated budesonide in children with severe persistent and/or steroid-dependent asthma all documented budesonide to be superior to placebo in improving symptoms, reducing prednisone use, and/or improving overall asthma control.[19–20,55] De Blic et al, in a double-blind, placebo-controlled, parallel study, evaluated the efficacy of nebulized budesonide 1 mg twice daily or placebo for 12 weeks in 40 toddlers (mean age 17 months) with severe asthma.[20] Budesonide therapy resulted in fewer exacerbations (40% versus 83%), less prednisone use (0% versus 14.5% of days), less wheezing (day and night), and improved asthma control (89% versus 44%) compared with placebo. Ilangovan et al enrolled a slightly older and more severe group of asthmatic children in their study of budesonide 1 mg twice daily or placebo for 8 weeks in 36 children with a mean age of 27 months (range 10–60 months) who were dependent on oral CS.[19] After 8 weeks of budesonide therapy, there was an 80% reduction in the mean oral CS requirement in the budesonide-treated group versus a 41% reduction in the placebo-treated group ($p < 0.05$). Five of the eight children under 2 years who were randomized to budesonide were able to discontinue oral CS completely versus only one-eighth randomized to placebo. Budesonide also significantly improved symptoms scores (0–3) with a reduction in daytime score from 1.3 to 0.4 versus 1.5 to 2.0 for placebo, and overall health status compared with placebo.

Three large and recently published studies from the United States have evaluated the efficacy and safety of nebulized budesonide in children with mild to moderate persistent asthma. Both studies employed older children and evaluated multiple budesonide dosages. Shapiro et al studied the efficacy and safety of three doses of budesonide (0.25 mg, 0.5 mg, and 1 mg bid) over a 12 week period in a randomized, placebo-controlled, double-blind, parallel group study of 178 children, 4–8 years old, on chronic ICS therapy.[56] All doses of budesonide were superior to placebo in reducing daytime symptoms, with changes from baseline to treatment of −0.11, −0.45, −0.53, −0.55 for placebo, 0.25, 0.50, and 1.0 mg budesonide bid, respectively, and night-time asthma symptoms (−0.08, −0.36, −0.37, −0.36 for placebo, 0.25, 0.50, 1.0 mg bid budesonide, respectively). In addition, budesonide resulted in significant improvements in am PEF rates (−1.3, 15.3, 11.8, 10.4 litres/min for placebo, 0.25, 0.50, 1.0 mg budesonide bid, respectively), and fewer withdrawals from the study secondary to poorly controlled asthma (36% for placebo versus 9% for budesonide; $p < 0.02$). Although this was a short-term study, budesonide therapy did not result in any linear growth suppression, nor was it associated with basal or ACTH-stimulated cortisol suppression. No dose-dependent effects were noted with any of the efficacy parameters studied. In other words, all of the doses of budesonide were equally effective. This would suggest that in mild to moderate childhood asthma, 0.5 mg/day of nebulized budesonide appears to be an effective and safe starting dose, with subsequent dose adjustments based on clinical need and assessment of response. This has clear clinical implications in that the lower the ICS used, the smaller the potential for systemic absorption, and the less likely that clinically significant adverse effects will occur with long-term treatment.

Kemp et al sought to evaluate the efficacy of nebulized budesonide administered once daily (0.25, 0.5, or 1.0 mg) in a 12 week randomized, double-blind, placebo-controlled study of 359 children, 6 months to 8 years old (mean age 4.7 years), with mild persistent asthma who were not already on ICS.[57] All doses of budesonide were superior to placebo in reducing night-time asthma symptoms, with mean changes in symptom scores from baseline of −0.16, −0.49, −0.42, −0.42 in the placebo, 0.25, 0.50, 1.0 mg QD budesonide, respectively. Similar reductions in the daytime asthma symptom scores were also noted. Nebulized budesonide also resulted in fewer days of rescue β-agonist use compared with placebo. Specifically, the mean reduction in the number of days rescue medication required per 2 week period was 4.19, 6.26, 6.31, and 5.98 for placebo, 0.25, 0.50, and 1.0 mg budesonide groups, respectively. Lastly, am PEFR (55% of patients could adequately perform the procedure) increased from baseline by 7.1, 14.4, 6.5, and 10.9 litres/min in the placebo, 0.25, 0.50, and 1.0 mg budesonide groups, respectively. Budesonide was no more effective than placebo in improving PEF rates. In the 36% of randomized children who could consistently perform spirometry, 0.5 mg ($p < 0.04$) and 1.0 mg ($p < 0.03$) budesonide were more effective than placebo in terms of improving baseline FEV1, although the absolute change of 0.03 litre for both groups is of little clinical significance.

In an even larger study, Baker et al studied several different doses and frequency of doses of budesonide (0.25 mg or 1 mg once daily, 0.25 mg or 0.5 mg twice daily) versus placebo in 480 children, aged 6 months to 8 years (mean age 4.6 years), over a 12 week period.[58] The investigators found all dosing regimens to be more effective than placebo in improving symptom scores, improving lung function, and reducing rescue medication use. Improvement in symptom scores occurred as early as 2 weeks after starting budesonide. As was noted in the Shapiro study, dose-dependent effects were not apparent. Twice daily dosing of 0.5 mg appeared to be more effective than 1 mg administered once daily. The investigators found 0.5 mg per day of budesonide to be the minimal effective dose. They suggested that for mild asthma doses of 0.25 mg/day may be sufficient, whereas those with moderate asthma should be treated with 0.5–1.0 mg/day, and those with severe oral-steroid-dependent asthma should be treated with 1–2 mg/day. There were no differences in basal cortisol levels during the treatment period for any group. There was no difference in the ACTH-stimulated cortisol levels between any active treatment group and placebo.

Inhaled corticosteroids and growth in small children

In one of the few studies to assess linear growth of young children on long-term ICS therapy, Reid et al, in an open label study, measured linear growth velocity in 40 small children (mean age 1.4 years) before and during treatment with nebulized budesonide.[59] All of the children had 'troublesome' asthma despite treatment with an ICS (pMDI with spacer and mask) or nebulized cromolyn before entering the study. They were then administered 1–4 mg/day of nebulized budesonide depending on their asthma severity/control. The median interval of time for linear growth determinations during the run-in period was 6 months and during the treatment period it was 1 year. The height standard deviation scores (SDS) for the group during the run-in period was −0.21, at baseline −0.46, and after at least 6 months of nebulized budesonide −0.17. Note that an SDS of less than zero denotes impaired growth velocity or impaired growth. Thus, the subjects were growing at less than a normal rate prior to treatment and that nebulized budesonide did not result in further growth suppression. In fact, there was a trend toward improved growth velocity while on nebulized budesonide.

Similar results were reported by Ninan and Russell, who evaluated the growth of 58 older children (mean age 3.5 years for males, 4.4 years for females) with asthma over a 5 year period.[60] Each child's asthma was classified as being in good, moderate, and poor control according to asthma symptoms during a 2 year observational period before beginning ICS therapy. The study group as a whole had diminished growth velocity to start the study with a mean height velocity standard deviation (HVSD) score of −0.51. The children whose asthma was in good control had the least evidence for growth suppression before instituting ICS therapy, and continued to grow at the same rate while on therapy (HVSD score −0.01 before versus −0.07 during ICS treatment). In contrast, the subjects whose asthma was poorly controlled grew poorly regardless of whether or not they were receiving ICS (HVSD score −1.50 before versus −1.55 during). Those with moderately controlled asthma actually demonstrated improved growth velocity while on ICS therapy, with the HVSD score increasing from −0.83 to −0.49. These investigators concluded that poor asthma control, more than ICS therapy, significantly impacted growth. Both studies support the long-known but often overlooked fact that asthma can negatively influence growth.[61,62]

Pharmacokinetics of nebulized budesonide in small children

Little is known about the amount of drug delivered, by any inhaled device and with any drug, to infants and young children with asthma (for further information on this topic see Chapter 17). This issue is of great clinical importance especially as it pertains to ICS. As will be discussed in Chapter 9, ICS may have the potential for adverse effects such as growth suppression and effects on bone growth and development. Because of this, it is of critical importance to deliver the smallest amount of drug required for effectiveness. Concern has been raised regarding the doses of nebulized budesonide used in many of the previously discussed studies. Doses ranging from 0.5 to 2.0 mg/day are doses considered high even when administered to adults. Some have suggested that doses administered should be on a mg/kg basis. Agertoft et al sought to address this very issue by performing a series of studies designed to evaluate the systemic availability and pharmacokinetic parameters of nebulized budesonide in a group of preschool children with chronic asthma.[63] Ten children with a mean age of 4.7 years underwent pharmacokinetic studies of both intravenously administered budesonide (125 µg) and budesonide administered via the nebulizer (1 mg). They calculated the mean amount of drug delivered to the patient by subtracting the amount of budesonide remaining in the nebulizer, the amount emitted into the ambient air, and the amount found in the mouth after rinsing from the initial amount of budesonide in the nebulizer (nominal dose). The mean dose to the subject was 23% of the nominal dose (231 µg) whereas the systemic availability was 6.1% (61 µg) of the nominal dose. The clearance of budesonide was calculated to be 0.54 liter/min with a $t_{\frac{1}{2}}$ of 2.3 hours, and V_{dss} of 55 liters. The systemic availability in these small children was approximately half that seen in adults. In addition, the clearance of budesonide in these children was 50% higher than in adults. Thus, the low systemic availability in combination with a higher clearance rate in young children allows for these younger age groups to use an adult dose without an increased risk of undesirable systemic effects. Dosing of nebulized budesonide by mg/kg of body weight to reduce the risk of adverse effects is not necessary.

Summary

In summary, according to the limited information available, nebulized budesonide is an effective therapeutic agent for young children with moderate and severe asthma. All of the studies published to date demonstrate budesonide to result in statistically significant improvement in asthma symptoms (Table 7.3). It appears to have oral CS-sparing effects in small children with steroid-dependent asthma. In the studies where lung function has been measured, nebulized budesonide does not appear to be as effective in small children compared with similar studies performed in older children using ICS delivered via the Turbuhaler or conventional MDIs. The etiology for this discrepancy is unknown. It may be that smaller children are unable to perform lung function procedures with sufficient consistency. Alternatively, there may be a difference in the amount of drug delivered to the lower airways between the delivery devices. Small children may not have the same degree of airflow obstruction given the relatively short duration of asthma, thus making the amount of reversibility less. Lastly, these children may have less of an inflammatory component to their disease, and if this were the case, they would be less likely to improve with ICS therapy. In the few studies that evaluated safety, budesonide therapy was not associated with significant adrenal suppression, nor was it associated with suppression of linear growth. Issues that at present remain unresolved include whether inhaled budesonide should be used as the preferred form of therapy in all levels of persistent asthma including mild, whether early intervention with budesonide will be associated with long-term disease modification, and whether long-term use of budesonide will be associated with normal linear growth and bone development.

Other controller medications
General comments
The British and NHLBI EPR-2 guidelines and the International Pediatric Consensus Statement[12–14] recommend use of other control medications for moderate to severe asthma in an attempt to limit the dose of ICS in moderate asthma, and oral CS in severe asthma. These medications include theophylline, long-acting β_2-agonists, and leukotriene-modifying agents. It should be noted that these recommendations are for older children and adults. The United States guidelines mention the addition of theophylline only in combination with medium dose ICS in small children with moderate asthma whereas the British guidelines recommend theophylline and long-acting β-agonists.

Theophylline
Theophylline is now used less frequently owing to concerns about potential toxicity, although because of its relatively lower cost it remains a popular drug in developing countries. Older studies in small children have demonstrated its efficacy.[64,65] More recent studies in adults with mild to severe asthma have demonstrated the immunomodulatory/anti-inflammatory effects of low dose theophylline. Sullivan et al, in a randomized, double-blind study in adults with mild asthma, found a significant reduction in the number of EG2-positive activated eosinophils and total eosinophils in bronchial biopsy specimens after an allergen challenge in those patients treated with low dose theophylline compared with those who received placebo.[66] However, these changes were not associated with differences in symptom scores, peak flow rates, or rescue medication use. In a study by Kidney et al in adults with severe asthma previously on theophylline and high dose ICS therapy, a randomized, placebo-controlled withdrawal of theophylline resulted in worsening of asthma control associated with increases in $CD4^+$ and $CD8^+$ cells and activation marker $CD25^+$ in the airway and a fall in the number of these cells in the peripheral blood.[67] However, despite the recent evidence suggestive of more than just bronchodilatory property, it is no longer considered a first-line agent. The NHLBI EPR-2 guidelines state that 'theophylline may have particular risks of adverse side effects in infants, and theophylline should only be considered if serum concentration levels will be carefully monitored.'[12] With increasing emphasis on inflammation playing a major role in the pathogenesis of asthma, there has been a trend away from using bronchodilators such as theophylline as monotherapy. Theophylline has a narrow therapeutic window and, consequently, levels need to be routinely monitored, especially if the child has a viral illness associated with a fever or is placed on a medication known to delay theophylline clearance, such as macrolide antibiotics (erythromycin and clarithromycin), cimetidine, antifungals, and ciprofloxacin.[68] Further complicating the use of theophylline in small children is the variability in theophylline metabolism from infancy through childhood, requiring frequent dose monitoring and dose adjustments. Lastly, sustained-release theophylline can be erratically absorbed.[69]

Long-acting inhaled β_2-agonists
Salmeterol is a long-acting inhaled β_2-agonist intended for maintenance therapy in the treatment of asthma in patients over 12 years of age. The British guidelines for small children recommend it as an alternative medication in children with moderate persistent asthma (step 3); it is not mentioned at all in the NHLBI EPR-2 guidelines. Salmeterol is not meant to be a rescue medication for acute episodes of bronchospasm, nor is it meant to replace inhaled anti-inflammatory agents. Salmeterol has a

Table 7.3 Summary of efficacy and safety of nebulized budesonide in small children with asthma

Study	Methodology	Delivery/dose	Number and age of subjects	Asthma severity of subjects	Efficacy	Adverse effects
Ref. 19	8 weeks DB, PC parallel group	Nebulized suspension; 1 mg bid	36 subjects ma = 26.7 months r = 10 months to 5 years	Severe, steroid-dependent (oral) asthma	Less need for oral GC; improved overall health	Facial rash in 2 BUD-treated children
Ref. 55	24 weeks DB, PC parallel group	pMDI spacer/mask 200 μg bid	40 subjects ma = 21.6 months r = 1–3 years	Severe; symptoms ~3 times per week	Decreased cough; increased % symptom-free days; fewer dropouts	Facial rash in 1 BUD patient; no growth suppression
Ref. 20	12 weeks DB, PC parallel group	Nebulized suspension 1 mg bid	40 subjects ma = 17.3 months r = 6–30 months	Severe; required oral GC at least monthly for 3 months	Fewer exacerbations, decreased wheezing and po GC use, greater % with improved asthma control	No growth suppression, no facial rash, 1 case of candidiasis
Ref. 56	12 weeks DB, PC parallel group	Nebulized suspension 0.25, 0.5, 1.0 mg bid	178 subjects ma = 80.6 months (6.7 years) r = 4–8 years	Inhaled GC-dependent asthma	Decreased am, pm symptoms, rescue medication use, and fewer dropouts	No change in basal and ACTH-stimulated cortisol levels
Ref. 57	12 weeks DB, PC parallel group	Nebulized suspension 0.25, 0.50, 1.0 mg qd	359 subjects ma = 56 months (4.7 years) r = 6 months to 8 years	Mild persistent asthma not on inhaled GCs	Decreased am, pm symptom scores, less rescue use, improved FEV_1 in 0.5, 1.0 mg groups	No difference in adverse effects, basal and ACTH-stimulated cortisol levels

Ref.	Study design	Treatment	Subjects	Asthma status	Outcomes	Adverse effects
Ref. 58	12 weeks DB, PC parallel group	Nebulized suspension 0.25, 1.0 qd, 0.25, 0.5 bid	480 subjects ma = 55.0 months (4.6 years) r = 6 months to 8 years	Persistent asthma on any controller medication	Minimal effective dose 0.5 mg/day; improved symptom scores, PEF, FEV_1, less rescue use	No difference in ACTH-stimulated cortisol levels
Ref. 103	DB, PC BUD vs. PLAC × 7 days at time of first URI symptoms	pMDI with spacer (800 µg) ± mask (1600 µg) bid	25 subjects with 28 treatment pairs; r = 1–5 years	Intermittent wheezing with URIs only, none on controller medications	8/10 po GC bursts associated with placebo; modest decrease in wheeze in first week with BUD	No assessment
Ref. 18	18 weeks DB, non-placebo-controlled	Nebulized 1 mg with every 3 weeks taper vs. 0.25 mg bid	102 subjects ma = 22 months r = 5–47 months	Not controlled, not on inhaled GC 42/102 on cromolyn	Control gained in 1 month control for both groups; 47% had good control on 0.25 mg bid	10% candidiasis; 10% facial rash; no loss of growth velocity during BUD therapy
Ref. 104	10 weeks DB, non-placebo controlled	Nebulized 1 mg tapered to 0.25 mg bid vs. 0.25 mg bid	42 subjects ma = 19.3 months r = 6 months to 3 years	~3 wheezing episodes + symptoms > 40% of days × 3 months	High initial dose (1 mg tapered to 0.25 bid in 7 day); more rapid improvement in wheezing and cough	No difference in am and post-ACTH stimulated cortisol levels between groups and baseline levels
Ref. 59	52 weeks open label, height SDS before and following ~6 months BUD	Nebulized 1–4 mg/day for a mean of 1 year	40 subjects ma = 17 months r = 0.3–2.8 years	Severe and uncontrolled on iGC via MDI spacer/facemask	Control in 45%; partial control 30%; uncontrolled 25%; 11–14% nominal dose delivered	SDS: pre-BUD −0.21 baseline −0.46 BUD × 6 months = −0.17

Abbreviations: ACTH = adrenocorticotropic hormone, DB = double-blind, PC = placebo-controlled, ma = mean age, r = range, BUD = budesonide, po = oral, qd = once daily, bid = twice daily, pMDI = pressurized metered dose inhaler, URI = upper respiratory tract infection, SDS = standard deviation score.

prolonged onset of action with maximal bronchodilation approximately 1 hour following administration, and a prolonged duration of action of at least 12 hours. Given its long duration of action, it is especially well suited for patients with nocturnal asthma,[70] and for individuals who require frequent use of short-acting β-agonist inhalations during the day to prevent exercise-induced asthma.[71] At the present time, no studies are available demonstrating salmeterol's efficacy and safety in children less than 5 years of age. A few studies have been performed among older children. These studies have found salmeterol to be effective in blocking exercise-induced asthma[71] and in improving lung function.[72] The addition of either salmeterol or more beclomethasone to a daily dose of 400 μg beclomethasone failed to result in any further benefit.[73] This is in marked contrast to several studies in adults.[74,75]

Leukotriene-modifying agents

Leukotrienes are potent pro-inflammatory mediators that induce bronchospasm, mucus secretion, and airway edema. In addition, they may be involved in eosinophil recruitment into the asthmatic airway.[76] Two classes of leukotriene modifiers have been developed: those that inhibit the production of leukotrienes (synthesis inhibitors) and those that block the binding of leukotrienes to their receptors (receptor antagonists). Leukotriene modifiers have beneficial effects in terms of reducing asthma symptoms, and supplemental β-agonist use while improving baseline pulmonary function.[77–79] Unfortunately, no studies have been published utilizing any of the available agents in children less than 6 years of age. Only montelukast is available for use in children as young as 2 years of age.

The receptor antagonists prevent the binding of LTD_4 to its receptor. These agents can also block both the early and late phase allergic response following allergen challenge. Zafirlukast and montelukast are the only members of this class of drugs currently approved for use in asthma. Zafirlukast is administered twice daily, and it too is not recommended for children under 7 years. Montelukast is the first leukotriene-modifying agent with a pediatric indication (i.e. approved for children above 2 years of age). Knorr et al were the first to evaluate a leukotriene-modifying agent in childhood asthma.[80] They evaluated the safety and effectiveness of 8 weeks of therapy with montelukast (5 mg once daily) or matching placebo in a large cohort of children 6–14 years old. The children had moderate airflow obstruction with a mean baseline FEV_1 of 72% predicted and roughly one-third of the children remained on an ICS during the study. The mean am FEV_1 for the children randomized to montelukast increased modestly by 8.23% compared with an increase of 3.6% in the placebo group for a difference of roughly 5% between the two groups. In addition, montelukast therapy was associated with significant decreases in $β_2$-agonist use and circulating eosinophils. There were no differences in patient-reported am or pm peak expiratory flows, nocturnal awakening, discontinuations owing to worsening asthma, or rescue prednisone use. The results of this study appear less impressive than those seen with ICS in children.[81] The results of Phase III clinical studies that have evaluated the safety and efficacy of a 4 mg chewable montelukast tablet in children with asthma aged 2–5 years are pending publication.[82]

Quick-relief medications

Short-acting $β_2$-agonists

Given their rapid onset of action, and fairly long duration of action (4–6 hours), these medications are the treatment of choice for significant asthma exacerbations and acute episodes of bronchospasm.[12] Their efficacy and safety even in children less than 2 years of age with recurrent wheezing have been documented.[83] In addition, they are the drugs of choice for preventing EIB in older children. β-Agonists are now considered rescue medications, and should only be used if symptomatic. Although controversial, there have been recent concerns regarding the regular use of inhaled $β_2$-agonists. Some studies have suggested that routine use of these medications can result in increased bronchial hyperresponsiveness (BHR) and worsening asthma control.[84,85] In contrast, a recent study found no change in either BHR or worsened asthma control in mild asthmatics randomized to albuterol/salbutamol administered four times a day compared with albuterol/salbutamol administered as needed for asthma symptoms.[86] These studies were performed on adults with asthma and the effect of regular β-agonists in young children with asthma is unknown.

Recommended inhaled doses for children ~5 years of age have varied from no dosage recommendations (NHLBI EPR-2 guidelines) to a fixed dose of albuterol/salbutamol 2.5–5 mg via a nebulizer.[13] In older children, the NHLBI EPR-2 recommends 0.05 mg/kg with a minimum dose of 1.25 mg and a maximum of 2.5 mg in 2–3 ml saline. An insightful study from Penna et al found young children (~5) to have lower plasma albuterol/salbutamol concentrations following multiple nebulized treatments despite having received a greater amount of albuterol/salbutamol (178.8 versus 137 µg/kg) than children aged over 5 years.[87] This finding was independent of the severity of the initial attack. The authors concluded that their finding of reduced serum albuterol/salbutamol levels in the younger children who had received greater doses was secondary to either enhanced clearance of the drug or less efficient delivery of the drug in this age group. These data suggest that smaller children require a larger amount of albuterol/salbutamol per kilogram, and that albuterol/salbutamol toxicity is less likely to occur owing to either enhanced clearance or ineffective delivery of the drug. Detailed pharmacokinetic studies would be required to fully answer this question.

Anticholinergic agents
The anticholinergic agent ipratropium bromide has recently become available for nebulizer administration. Its use as an adjunct therapy for acute exacerbations in childhood asthma has increased. Schuh et al were among the first to demonstrate the additive effect of nebulized ipratropium bromide combined with albuterol/salbutamol on lung function in children presenting to the emergency room with acute asthma.[88] Several subsequent studies that involved even children less than 5 years of age have confirmed and extended their results.[89] Quareshi et al, in a large randomized, double-blind, placebo-controlled study, evaluated whether the addition of ipratropium bromide to standard emergency department therapy for acute asthma in children 2–18 years of age would reduce hospitalization rates.[90] Over 400 children were randomized to receive nebulized albuterol/salbutamol every 20 minutes for 1 hour or nebulized albuterol/salbutamol three times plus the addition of ipratropium bromide with the second and third albuterol/salbutamol treatments plus prednisone. The overall rate of hospitalization was lower in the ipratropium group compared with the control group (27.4% versus 36.5%: $p < 0.05$). Although no difference in hospitalization rates was observed for patients with moderate exacerbations, patients with severe exacerbations (PEFR < 50%) were far less likely to be hospitalized if they received ipratropium compared with the control group (37.5% versus 52.6%; $p < 0.02$). Ipratropium was also effective in reducing the asthma symptom score and mildly improving the oxygen saturation but had no effect on improving PEF rates. This reduction in hospitalization is of clinical significance. The investigators stated that for every seven patients with severe acute asthma treated with ipratropium, one hospitalization could be prevented. In contrast, a more recent study failed to confirm the ability of ipratropium to result in fewer asthma hospitalizations.[91] Zorc et al[91] studied 427 children over 12 months of age (11% were <2 years old) with mild to severe attacks, and found no difference in the rates of hospital admission between the two treatment groups (22% in the control and 18% in the treatment groups; $p = 0.33$). However, of those discharged from the emergency room, ipratropium-treated patients had a shorter time till discharge by about 30 minutes ($p < 0.001$), with the effect most marked in children less than 5 years old. Moreover, fewer albuterol/salbutamol doses were delivered to the treatment group.

In conclusion, ipratropium bromide appears to be an effective adjunct therapy in acute childhood asthma. The combination of albuterol/salbutamol and ipratropium clearly results in greater improvement in lung function than that seen with either agent alone. Whether it is effective in reducing hospitalization rates for acute asthma remains to be more fully elucidated.

Short-course systemic corticosteroid therapy
Several studies have demonstrated clinical efficacy of CS therapy in the treatment of acute childhood asthma. Efficacy has been demonstrated in studies evaluating single doses of oral and parenteral CS administered in the emergency room,[92–93] short courses of oral CS in the clinic setting,[94] and both oral and intravenous (IV) CS therapy for children hospitalized with acute exacerbations of asthma.[95–98]

Studies have also demonstrated orally administered CS to be as effective as IV CS for most children admitted to the hospital with an acute asthma exacerbation. Since orally administered liquid CS preparations are rapidly absorbed (30 min to 1 hour) and are usually as effective as IV CS in the management of acute asthma in young children,[99] oral therapy can be used in many cases. The NHBLI EPR-2 guidelines suggest 1–2 mg/kg per day (maximum 60 mg/day) of prednisone or methylprednisolone in a single dose or two divided doses for 3–10 days' outpatient management of acute exacerbations whereas the British guidelines recommend initiating a short course of prednisolone for 1–3 days (1–2 mg/kg per day for age <1 year and 20 mg/day for 1–5 years) for children with mild/moderate episodes requiring 3–4 hourly bronchodilator treatments after 12 hours. However, the optimal dose and duration of treatment remain a matter of debate, and dosing strategies are empiric. In a randomized, double-blind study, 98 children aged 1–15 years admitted to the hospital were randomized to receive prednisolone 0.5, 1.0, or 2.0 mg/kg per day administered as a single daily dose.[100] Clinical measures of efficacy, such as symptom scores, oxygen saturation, heart rate, number of albuterol/salbutamol treatments required, and duration of hospitalization, were compared between the three groups. The investigators found no difference between the three groups in any of the clinical parameters studied. Combined cough and wheeze score and use of rescue bronchodilators within 2 weeks of discharge were also comparable between the groups. This study suggests that low dose prednisolone is as effective as high dose prednisolone. This is one of many studies that have failed to demonstrate a dose–response effect for systemically administered CS. As we have become more aware of the potential for adverse effects with CS therapy in general, it makes sense to use the lowest effective dose. This is especially important in children with moderately severe asthma, who often require frequent short courses of prednisone for acute asthma exacerbations. These children will often also be on moderate to high dose ICS therapy and an additive effect between intermittent oral and inhaled CS on adverse effects may occur.

The findings from this study should not be extrapolated to those patients admitted with severe asthma associated with respiratory distress. Hospitalized children who require high flow rates of oxygen to adequately treat hypoxemia are obvious candidates for IV CS therapy. The NHLBI guidelines for acute severe asthma recommend administering intravenous methylprednisolone at 1 mg/kg per dose every 6 hours for 48 hours, tapering to 1–2 mg/kg per day (maximum 60 mg/day) in two divided doses until the patient's PEFR reaches 70% of predicted or personal best.[12]

Theophylline in acute asthma
The routine use of theophylline in acute asthma has significantly declined over the past several years owing mainly to a series of studies that show theophylline provides no additive effect on top of frequently administered β_2-agonists in the majority of cases. A study by Strauss et al illustrates this point in older children.[101] These investigators found intravenous theophylline offered no additional benefit to frequently used inhaled β_2-agonists and parenteral CS in 31 children aged 5–18 years hospitalized with acute asthma. Specifically, it was no more

effective than placebo in improving pulmonary function, decreasing need for inhaled β_2-agonists, or shortening the length of hospitalization. The only statistically significant difference was in the incidence of adverse effects. Theophylline was associated with a greater incidence of headache, nausea, emesis, abdominal pain, and palpitations compared with placebo. It should be noted that these children had moderate asthma exacerbations, with none requiring admission to the intensive care unit. Theophylline may still play an important role in acute, life-threatening asthma, as demonstrated in a recent study by Yung et al.[102] These investigators, in a randomized, double-blind, placebo-controlled trial in 163 children (1–19 years old) with an acute severe asthma exacerbation, found intravenous theophylline to be an effective therapy. Specifically, those on theophylline showed greater improvement in lung function after 6 hours and oxygen saturation in the first 30 hours compared with placebo. In addition, fewer patients on theophylline required treatment with intravenous albuterol/salbutamol. All five patients that required intubation for respiratory failure had been randomized to the placebo group. This suggests that intravenous theophylline can be an important adjunctive therapy in young children with acute, life-threatening severe asthma requiring admission to the intensive care unit.

SUMMARY

The management of infants and small children with asthma remains problematic. Not only do we have few medications approved for use in this population, the few that are available are at best only modestly effective. It remains to be determined who should be treated and with what controller medication. There are many areas of need. Many of the studies performed before the 1990s studied older drugs such as cromolyn and theophylline, using the old paradigm of treatment, i.e. treating symptoms. The new paradigm stresses the role of inflammation in the pathogenesis of asthma; treatment strategies are aimed not only to treat symptoms but also to suppress the underlying inflammatory reaction. Long-term studies evaluating anti-inflammatory drugs such as ICS and the leukotriene-modifying agents need to be performed. In addition, large prospective studies need to be performed evaluating the impact of early pharmacologic intervention on the natural history of infantile asthma. Fortunately, several industry and government sponsored studies are underway or will soon be underway which will begin to fill in the void in our knowledge. The National Heart, Lung, and Blood Institute's Childhood Asthma Management Program (CAMP) study will provide valuable information on the long-term efficacy and safety of two controller medications, nedocromil and budesonide compared with albuterol/salbutamol alone in a large cohort of older children (5–12 years old at entry and over 1000 enrolled in eight sites across the United States and Canada) over a 4–5 year period. The National Institute of Child Health and Human Development's Pediatric Pharmacology Research Unit (PPRU) is a consortium of centers participating with the Food and Drug Administration (FDA) and the pharmaceutical industry in an attempt to gain medical labeling in small children. A cooperative effort must be undertaken between government and industry in designing and sponsoring studies that will fill the gaps in our understanding and treatment of this group of patients.

Acknowledgment
The research reported here was funded in part by NICHHD Pediatric Pharmacology Research Unit Network HD 37237-02.

REFERENCES

1. Larsen GL. Asthma in children. *N Engl J Med* 1992; **326:** 1540–5.
2. Gergen PJ, Weiss KB. Changing patterns of asthma hospitalization among children: 1979–1987. *JAMA* 1990; **264:** 1688–92.
3. Sly RM, O'Donnell R. Stabilization of asthma mortality. *Ann Allergy Asthma Immunol* 1997; **78:** 347–54.
4. *Morbidity and Mortality Weekly Report* 1996; **45:** 350–3.

5. Seddon PC, Heaf DP. Long term outcome of ventilated asthmatics. *Arch Dis Child* 1990; **65:** 1324–27.
6. Paret G, Kornecki A, Szeinberg A et al. Severe acute asthma in a community hospital pediatric intensive care unit: a ten years' experience. *Ann Allergy Asthma Immunol* 1998; **80:** 339–44.
7. Mitchell EA, Bland JM, Thompson JMD. Risk factors for readmission to hospital for asthma in childhood. *Thorax* 1994; **49:** 33–6.
8. Wenzel SE. Asthma as an inflammatory disease. *Ann Allergy* 1994; **72:** 261–71.
9. Hegele RG, Hogg JC. The pathology of asthma: an inflammatory disorder. In: Szeffer SJ, Leung DYM, eds. *Severe Asthma: Pathogenesis and Clinical Management*. New York: Marcel Dekker, 1995, 61–76.
10. Martinez FD, Wright AL, Taussig LM et al. Asthma and wheezing in the first six years of life. *N Engl J Med* 1995; **332:** 133–8.
11. Newhouse MT. Pulmonary drug targeting with aerosols: principles and clinical applications in adults and children. *Amer J Asthma Allergy Pediatr* 1993; **7:** 23–35.
12. *Expert Panel Report II: Guidelines for the Diagnosis and Management of Asthma.* Bethesda, MD: National Institutes of Health, National Heart, Lung, and Blood Institute, 1997.
13. Warner JO, Naspitz CK, Cropp GJA. Third International Pediatric Consensus Statement on the Management of Childhood Asthma. *Pediatric Pulmonology* 1998; **25:** 1–17.
14. British Thoracic Society, British Paediatric Association, Royal College of Physicians of London et al. Asthma in children under five years of age. *Thorax* 1997; **52**(suppl 1): S9–21.
15. Bisgaard H. Delivery of inhaled medication to children. *J Asthma* 1997; **34:** 443–67.
16. Salmon B, Wilson NM, Silverman M. How much aerosol reaches the lungs of wheezy infants and toddlers? *Arch Dis Child* 1990; **65:** 401–3.
17. Carlsen KCL, Nikander K, Carlsen KH. How much nebulized budesonide reaches infants and toddlers. *Arch Dis Child* 1992; **67:** 1077–9.
18. Wennergren G, Nordvall SL, Hedlin G et al. Nebulized budesonide for the treatment of moderate to severe asthma in infants and toddlers. *Acta Paediatr* 1996; **85:** 183–9.
19. Ilangovan P, Pedersen S, Godfrey S et al. Treatment of severe steroid dependent preschool asthma with nebulized budesonide suspension. *Arch Dis Child* 1993; **68:** 356–9.
20. De Blic J, Delacourt C, Le Bourgeois M et al. Efficacy of nebulized budesonide in treatment of severe infantile asthma: a double blind study. *J Allergy Clin Immunol* 1996; **98:** 14–20.
21. Parkin PC, Saunders NR, Diamond SA et al. Randomized trial spacer vs nebuliser for acute asthma. *Arch Dis Child* 1995; **72:** 239–40.
22. O'Callaghan C, Milner AD, Swarbick A. Spacer device with face mask attachment for giving bronchodilators to infants with asthma. *BMJ* 1989; **298:** 160–1.
23. Tal A, Golan H, Grauer N et al. Deposition pattern of radiolabeled salbutamol inhaled from a metered-dose inhaler by means of a spacer with mask in young children with airway obstruction. *J Pediatr* 1996; **128:** 479–84.
24. Noble V, Ruggins NR, Everard ML et al. Inhaled budesonide for chronic wheezing under 18 months of age. *Arch Dis Child* 1992; **67:** 285–8.
25. Gleeson JGA, Price JF. Controlled trial of budesonide given by the nebuhaler in preschool children with asthma. *BMJ* 1988; **297:** 161–3.
26. Agertoft L, Pedersen S. Influence of spacer device on drug delivery to young children with asthma. *Arch Dis Child* 1994; **71:** 217–220.
27. American Thoracic Society, European Respiratory Society. Respiratory mechanics in infants: physiologic evaluation in health and disease. *Am Rev Respir Dis* 1993; **147:** 474–96.
28. Stocks J, Sly PD, Tepper RS et al. *Infant Respiratory Function Testing*. New York: Wiley-Liss, 1996.
29. Wilson N, van Bever H. Overall symptom measurement: which approach? *Eur Resp J* 1996; **S9:** 8s–11s.
30. Carlsen KCL, Halvorsen R, Ahlstedt S et al. Eosinophil cationic protein and tidal flow volume loops in children 0–2 years of age. *Eur Resp J* 1995; **8:** 1148–54.
31. Milgrom H, Bender B, Ackerson L et al. Noncompliance and treatment failure in children with asthma. *J Allergy Clin Immunol* 1996; **98:** 1051–7.
32. Gibson NA, Ferguson AE, Aitchison TC et al. Compliance with inhaled asthma medication in preschool children. *Thorax* 1995; **50:** 1274–9.
33. Ferguson AE, Gibson NA, Aitchison TC et al. Measured bronchodilator use in preschool children with asthma. *BMJ* 1995; **310:** 1161–4.
34. Lim SH, Goh DYT, Tan AYS et al. Parents' perceptions towards their child's use of inhaled

medications for asthma therapy. *J Paediatr Child Health* 1996; **32:** 306–9.
35. Mesters I, Meertens R, Kok G et al. Effectiveness of a multidisciplinary education protocol in children with asthma (0–4 years) in primary health care. *J Asthma* 1994; **31:** 347–59.
36. Wilson SR, Latini D, Starr NJ et al. Education of parents of infants and very young children with asthma: a developmental evaluation of the Wee Wheezers program. *J Asthma* 1996; **33:** 239–54.
37. Coutts JA, Gibson NA, Paton JY. Measuring compliance with inhaled medication in asthma. *Arch Dis Child* 1992; **67:** 332–3.
38. Ibero M, Ridao M, Artigas R et al. Cisapride treatment changes the evolution of infant asthma with gastroesophageal reflux. *Invest Allergol Clin Immunol* 1998; **8:** 176–9.
39. Dahl R, Pedersen B. Influence of nedocromil sodium on the dual asthmatic reaction after antigen challenge: a double blind, placebo controlled study. *Eur J Respir Dis* 1986; **69**(suppl 147): 263–7.
40. Muittari A, Kreus KE. Disodium cromoglycate in exercise-induced asthma. *Br J Med* 1969; **4:** 170.
41. Hiller EJ, Milner AD, Lenney W. Nebulized sodium cromoglycate in young asthmatic children: double-blind trial. *Arch Dis Child* 1977; **52:** 875–6.
42. Glass J, Archer LNJ, Adams W et al. Nebulized cromoglycate, theophylline, and placebo in preschool asthmatic children. *Arch Dis Child* 1981; **56:** 648–51.
43. Cogswell JJ, Simpkiss MJ. Nebulized sodium cromoglycate in recurrently wheezy preschool children. *Arch Dis Child* 1985; **60:** 736–8.
44. Lenney W, Milner D. Nebulized sodium cromoglycate in the preschool wheezy child. *Arch Dis Child* 1978; **53:** 474–6.
45. Yuskel B, Greenough A. Inhaled sodium cromoglycate for pre-term children with respiratory symptoms at follow-up. *Respir Med* 1992; **86:** 131–4.
46. Henry RL, Hiller EJ, Milner AD et al. Nebulised ipratropium bromide and sodium cromoglycate in the first two years of life. *Arch Dis Child* 1984; **59:** 54–7.
47. Bertelsen A, Andersen JB, Busch P et al. Nebulized sodium cromoglycate in the treatment of wheezy bronchitis. *Allergy* 1986; **41:** 266–70.
48. Furfaro S, Spier S, Drblik SP et al. Efficacy of cromoglycate in persistently wheezing infants. *Arch Dis Child* 1994; **71:** 331–4.
49. Tasche MJA, Van Der Wouden, Uijen JHJM et al. Randomized placebo-controlled trial of inhaled sodium cromoglycate in 1–4 year old children with moderate asthma. *Lancet* 1997; **350:** 1060–4.
50. Szefler SJ. Glucocorticoid therapy for asthma: clinical pharmacology. *J Allergy Clin Immunol* 1991; **88:** 147–64.
51. Spahn JD, Leung DYM. The role of glucocorticoids in the management of asthma. *Allergy & Asthma Proc* 1996; **17:** 341–50.
52. van Essen-Zandvliet EE, Hughes MD, Waalkens HJ et al. Effects of 22 months of treatment with inhaled corticosteroids and/or beta-agonists on lung function, airway responsiveness, and symptoms in children with asthma. *Am Rev Respir Dis* 1992; **146:** 547–54.
53. Haahtela T, Jarvinen M, Kava T et al. Comparison of a β$_2$-agonist, terbutaline, with an inhaled corticosteroid, budesonide, in newly detected asthma. *N Engl J Med* 1991; **325:** 388–92.
54. Barnes PJ, Pedersen S. Efficacy and safety of inhaled corticosteroids in asthma. *Am Rev Respir Dis* 1993; **148:** S1–26.
55. Connett GC, Warde C, Wooler E et al. Use of budesonide in severe asthmatics aged 1 to 3 years. *Arch Dis Child* 1993; **69:** 351–5.
56. Shapiro G, Mendelson L, Kraemer MJ et al. Efficacy and safety of budesonide inhalation suspension (Pulmicort Respules) in young children with inhaled steroid-dependant, persistent asthma. *J Allergy Clin Immunol* 1998; **102:** 789–96.
57. Kemp JP, Skoner DP, Szefler SJ et al. Once-daily budesonide inhalation suspension for the treatment of persistent asthma in infants and young children. *Ann Allergy Asthma Immunol* 1999; **83:** 231–9.
58. Baker JW, Mellon M, Wald J et al. A multiple-dosing, placebo-controlled study of budesonide inhalation suspension given once or twice daily for treatment of persistent asthma in young children and infants. *Pediatrics* 1999; **103:** 414–21.
59. Reid A, Murphy C, Steen HJ et al. Linear growth of very young asthmatic children treated with high-dose nebulized budesonide. *Acta Paediatr* 1996; **85:** 421–4.
60. Nina TK, Russell G. Asthma, inhaled cortico-

steroid treatment, and growth. *Arch Dis Child* 1992; **67:** 703–5.
61. Reimer LG, Morris HG, Ellis EF. Growth of asthmatic children during treatment with alternate-day steroids. *J Allergy Clin Immunol* 1975; **55:** 224–31.
62. Russell G. Asthma and growth. *Arch Dis Child* 1993; **69:** 695–8.
63. Agertoft L, Andersen A, Weibull E et al. Systemic availability and pharmacokinetics of nebulized budesonide in preschool children. *Arch Dis Child* 1999; **80:** 241–7.
64. Neijens HJ, Duiverman EJ, Graatsma BH et al. Clinical and bronchodilating efficacy of controlled-release theophylline as a function of its serum concentrations in preschool children. *J Pediatr* 1985; **107:** 811–15.
65. Stratton D, Carswell F, Hughes AO et al. Double-blind comparisons of slow-release theophylline, ketotifen, and placebo for prophylaxis of asthma in young children. *Br J Dis Chest* 1984; **78:** 163–7.
66. Sullivan P, Bekir S, Jaffar Z et al. Anti-inflammatory effects of low-dose oral theophylline in atopic asthma. *Lancet* 1994; **343:** 1006–8.
67. Kidney J, Dominguez M, Taylor PM et al. Immunomodulation by theophylline in asthma. *Am J Respir Crit Care Med* 1995; **151:** 1907–14.
68. Hendeles L, Weinberger M, Szefler SJ et al. Safety and efficacy of theophylline in children with asthma. *J Pediatrics* 1992; **120:** 177–83.
69. Haltom JR, Szefler SJ. Theophylline absorption in young asthmatic children receiving sustained-release formulation. *J Pediatr* 1985; **107:** 805–10.
70. Fitzpatrick MF, Mackay T, Driver H et al. Salmeterol in nocturnal asthma: a double-blind, placebo controlled trial of a long-acting inhaled β_2 agonist. *BMJ* 1990; **301:** 1365–8.
71. Green CP, Price JF. Prevention of exercise induced asthma by inhaled salmeterol xinafoate. *Arch Dis Child* 1992; **67:** 1014–17.
72. Von Berg A, De Blic J, La Rosa M et al. A comparison of regular salmeterol vs. 'as required' salbutamol in asthmatic children. *Respir Med* 1998; **92:** 292–9.
73. Verberne AA, Frost C, Duiverman EJ et al. Addition of salmeterol versus doubling the dose of beclomethasone in children with asthma. The Dutch Asthma Study Group. *Am J Respir Crit Care Med* 1998; **158:** 213–19.
74. Greening AP, Ind PW, Northfield M et al. Added salmeterol versus higher-dose corticosteroid in asthma patients with symptoms on existing inhaled corticosteroid. *Lancet* 1994; **344:** 219–24.
75. Woolcock A, Lundback B, Ringdal N et al. Comparison of addition of salmeterol to inhaled steroids with doubling the dose of inhaled steroids. *Am J Respir Crit Care Med* 1996; **153:** 1481–1488.
76. Chung KF. Leukotriene receptor antagonists and biosynthesis inhibitors: potential breakthrough in asthma therapy. *Eur Respir J* 1995; **8:** 1203–13.
77. Israel E, Rubin P, Kemp JP et al. The effect of inhibition of 5-lipoxygenase by zileuton in mild-to-moderate asthma. *Ann Int Med* 1993; **119:** 1059–66.
78. Liu MC, Dube LM, Lancaster J. Acute and chronic effects of a 5-lipoxygenase inhibitor in asthma: a 6-month randomized multicenter trial. Zileuton Study Group. *J Allergy Clin Immunol* 1996; **98:** 859–71.
79. Spector SL, Smith LJ, Glass M. Effects of 6 weeks of therapy with oral doses of ICI 204,219, a leukotriene D4 receptor antagonist, in subjects with bronchial asthma. ACCOLATE Asthma Trialists Group. *Am J Respir Crit Care Med* 1994; **150:** 618–23.
80. Knorr B, Matz J, Bernstein JA et al. Montelukast for chronic asthma in 6- to 14-year-old children. *JAMA* 1998; **279:** 1181–6.
81. Van Essen-Zandvliet EE, Hughes MD, Waalkens HJ et al. Effects of 22 months of treatment with inhaled corticosteroids and/or beta-2-agonists on lung function, airway responsiveness, and symptoms in children with asthma. *Am Rev Respir Dis* 1992; **146:** 547–54.
82. Knorr B, Larson P, Chervinsky P. Selection of a montelukast dose in 2- to 5-year-olds by a comparison of pediatric and adult single-dose pharmacokinetic profiles. *Clin Pharmacol Ther* 1998; **63:** 191.
83. Bentur I, Kerem E, Canny G et al. Response of acute asthma to a beta2 agonist in children less than two years of age. *Annals of Allergy* 1990; **65:** 122–6.
84. Spitzer WO, Suissa S, Horowitz RI et al. The use of beta-agonists and the risk of death and near death from asthma. *N Engl J Med* 1972; **326:** 501–6.
85. Sears MR, Taylor DR, Print CG et al. Regular inhaled beta-agonist treatment in bronchial

asthma. *Lancet* 1990; **336:** 1391–6.
86. Drazen JM, Israel E, Boushey HA et al. Comparison of regularly scheduled with as-needed use of albuterol in mild asthma. *N Engl J Med* 1996; **335:** 841–7.
87. Penna AC, Dawson KP, Manglick P et al. Systemic absorption of salbutamol following nebulizer delivery in acute asthma. *Acta Paediatr* 1993; **82:** 963–6.
88. Schuh S, Johnson DW, Callahan S et al. Efficacy of frequent nebulized ipratropium bromide added to frequent high dose albuterol in the treatment of severe childhood asthma. *J Pediatr* 1995; **126:** 639–45.
89. Plotnick LH, Ducharme FM. Should inhaled anticholinergics be added to β_2 agonists for treating acute childhood and adolescent asthma? A systemic review. *BMJ* 1998; **317:** 971–7.
90. Quareshi F, Pestian J, Davis P et al. Effect of nebulized ipratropium on the hospitalization rates of children with asthma. *N Engl J Med* 1998; **339:** 1030–5.
91. Zorc JJ, Pusic MV, Ogborn CJ et al. Ipratropium bromide added to asthma treatment in the pediatric emergency department. *Pediatrics* 1999; **103:** 728–52.
92. Scarfone RJ, Fuchs SM, Nager AL et al. Controlled trial of oral prednisone in the emergency department treatment of children with acute asthma. *Pediatrics* 1993; **92:** 513–18.
93. Tal A, Levy N, Bearman J. Methylprednisolone therapy for acute asthma in infants and toddlers: a controlled clinical trial. *Pediatrics* 1990; **86:** 350–6.
94. Harris JB, Weinberger MM, Nassif E et al. Early intervention with short courses of prednisone to prevent progression of asthma in ambulatory patients incompletely responsive to bronchodilators. *J Pediatr* 1987; **110:** 627–33.
95. Pierson WE, Bierman W, Kelley VC. A double-blind trial of corticosteroid therapy in status asthmaticus. *Pediatrics* 1974; **54:** 282–8.
96. Younger RE, Gerber PS, Herrod HG et al. Intravenous methylprednisolone efficacy in status asthmaticus of childhood. *Pediatrics* 1987; **80:** 225–30.
97. Ratto D, Alfaro C, Sipsey J et al. Are intravenous corticosteroids required in status asthmaticus? *JAMA* 1988; **260:** 527–9.
98. Connett GJ, Warde C, Wooler E et al. Prednisolone and salbutamol in the hospital treatment of acute asthma. *Arch Dis Child* 1994; **70:** 170–3.
99. Barnett PLJ, Caputo GL, Baskin M et al. Intravenous versus oral corticosteroids in the management of acute asthma in children. *Ann Emergency Med* 1997; **29:** 212–17.
100. Hewer SL, Hobbs J, Reid F et al. Prednisolone in acute childhood asthma: clinical response to three dosages. *Respir Med* 1998; **92:** 541–6.
101. Strauss RE, Wertheim DL, Bonagura VR et al. Aminophylline therapy does not improve outcome and increase adverse effects in children hospitalized with acute asthmatic exacerbations. *Pediatrics* 1994; **93:** 205–210.
102. Yung M, South M. Randomised controlled trial of aminophylline for severe acute asthma. *Arch Dis Child* 1998; **79:** 405–10.
103. Connett G, Lenney W. Prevention of viral induced asthma attacks using inhaled budesonide. *Arch Dis Child* 1993; **68:** 85–7.
104. Volovitz B, Soferman R, Blau H et al. Rapid induction of clinical response with a short-term high-dose starting schedule of budesonide nebulizing suspension in young children with recurrent wheezing episodes. *J Allergy Clin Immunol* 1998; **101:** 464–9.

8

Management of chronic asthma in children between 5 and 18 years of age

John O Warner, Charles K Naspitz, Maria C Rizzo

Introduction • Paediatric asthma guidelines • Therapeutic algorithms • The aims of management • Add-on therapy to achieve ICS-sparing • Strategies in relatively steroid-insensitive patients • Future perspectives on asthma management • Mucolytics and expectorants • Muscarinic receptor antagonists • Complementary and alternative medicine • Summary

INTRODUCTION

Asthma in childhood is an eminently controllable, though not a curable condition in the vast majority of cases. Sadly, however, in many parts of the world it remains under-diagnosed and under-treated. Conversely, in some parts of the developed world, mild infrequent episodic disease is over-treated. In the twelfth century, Moses Maimonides, a Jewish physician and philosopher, wrote in his handbook for his patient, the Sultan Saladin's son, 'I have no magic cure to report. Asthma has many aetiological aspects and should be treated according to the various causes that bring it about.'[1] While there have been considerable advances in the development of palliative therapies for asthma, particularly in the last 30 years, we still do not have a cure. Thus, the approach is multidisciplinary for this multifactorial condition and will involve consideration of avoidance of precipitants, attention to psychosocial factors and pharmacotherapy.

Given the wide spectrum and manifestation of the disease, management must be tailored to the individual's requirements. To some extent, the ideal recipe is achieved by a process of trial and error, using a rational sequence of therapeutic approaches. This has been the basis of the overwhelming majority of therapeutic guidelines that have been published on this topic. However, with experience it becomes clear that by assessing severity, it is possible to identify the therapeutic strategy immediately without need to resort to a series of therapeutic trials. A prerequisite in administering therapy is assessment of response which must include objective measurement. The goal of treatment is to return the child to a normal existence, allowing participation in all the usual childhood activities, which is possible in all but a minority of cases.

Therapy must be based on a thorough knowledge of anatomical and physiological, as well as immunopathological, issues that relate to the disease. There needs to be a full understanding of the pharmacokinetics of the drugs being administered which, of course, varies with age. There should be an understanding of the natural history of the disease and its various manifestations. Finally, the physician involved must have appropriate paediatric training to understand the complexities of the child within their environment and how to give appropriate patient family guidance and education.

Many of the issues are clearly addressed in other chapters and the reader is referred to Chapters 1, 2, 3, 4 and 5 on understanding of all the basic mechanisms and natural history of the disease, and the diagnosis and management of the infant in Chapters 6 and 7. Issues related to non-pharmacological approaches, such as allergen avoidance and psychosocial issues, are addressed in Chapters 12–16. This chapter, therefore, focuses exclusively on pharmacotherapy.

PAEDIATRIC ASTHMA GUIDELINES

Hitherto, there has only been one exclusive paediatric guidelines consensus group that has published on three successive occasions on management of childhood asthma worldwide.[2–4] However, the recommendations are very much in keeping with those of Global Initiative for Asthma (GINA)[5] and national guidelines in the USA[6] and Great Britain.[7] For the latter, paediatric recommendations are merged in with recommendations for all other age groups. There have been some concerns expressed by paediatricians that extrapolation from studies of adult asthma has been inappropriate when applied to childhood asthmatics, and particularly to wheezing and coughing younger children. However, with diminishing age, the evidence base on which to make any therapeutic recommendations diminishes such that in infancy, there is very little accumulated evidence and much practice is dictated by personal experience using drugs outside their standard labelling age limits.

In generating guidelines, there has been an effort to develop them against an evidence base but, where this is not available, lesser grades of evidence have been used. Thus, the types of evidence may be classified in the following order:[8]

1. Evidence obtained from meta-analysis of randomised controlled trials.
2. Evidence obtained from at least one large randomised controlled trial.
3. Evidence obtained from at least one large well-designed controlled study without randomisation.
4. Evidence obtained from at least one other type of well-designed quasi-experimental study.
5. Evidence obtained from well-designed non-experimental descriptive studies such as comparative studies, correlation studies and case control studies.
6. Evidence obtained from expert committee reports or opinions and/or clinical experience of respected authorities.

Sadly, all too frequently, guidelines are based on the least weight of evidence in category 6. However, it should be emphasised that the application of evidence-based medicine, taken just on the basis of controlled trials, does not take into account clinical judgement and experience, qualitative factors, attitudes of patients and their carers, and demands related to the individual clinical consultation. Furthermore, there is a need to account for potential publication bias with negative controlled randomised studies being less likely to be published.

Recommendations are based on gold standard management in developed countries where even expensive medications can be obtained. However, there is a need to adapt these guidelines for circumstances where many medications may not be available and the costs too high for the majority (see Chapter 20). It is important, also, to be aware that the guidelines are not written in 'tablets of stone', demanding adherence from all clinicians. The use of the word 'guidelines' indicates that they are to be viewed as an aid to clinical practice and to be interpreted in the light of individual clinical situations and the individual clinician's judgement.

Over the last 10–15 years, the generation of guidelines has achieved considerable uniformity in approach to management. Thus, the health-related professions now have a clear view of asthma management in which the primary focus is on controlling airway inflammation supplemented by symptomatic relief where required. However, where guidelines have totally failed, is in delivering the message to patients and their families. Maybe this is because the patients and families were not involved in the generation of the guidelines. Physicians tend to give patients what they believe is required rather than listening to the patients' wishes. Older children, who are able to express themselves about what they feel is appropriate to do and, more importantly what they will not do, often focus on inhaler usage, concerns about side-effects of drugs and the adverse effects of peer influence and image. These issues are addressed in Chapters 15 and 16.

There is also a paradigm underlying asthma management which requires some thought, namely that uncontrolled airway inflammation produces progressively increasing remodelling, which, in turn, leads to an irreversible component to airflow limitation. The natural conclusion from this assertion, based predominantly on adult studies, is that the earlier effective therapeutic control of the inflammation is introduced, the fewer the chronic irreversible changes. One uncontrolled observational study from a specialist paediatric clinic has suggested that the later inhaled corticosteroids are introduced to a childhood asthmatic after the onset of their symptoms, the less the increase in lung function in successive years during growth.[9] However, the paradigm does need to be further investigated because evidence from long-term cohort studies would suggest that infrequent episodic asthma in childhood untreated with inhaled steroids remains a mild problem, with no abnormality in lung function after 28 years of follow-up.[10] Conversely, ongoing asthma in early childhood was associated with abnormal lung function and bronchial hyperresponsiveness at presentation.[11] In other words, severe and persistent disease, at its outset, already has features of significant airway abnormality. This is discussed in greater detail in Chapter 2. There is a suggestion that the so-called remodelling process occurs very early, if not before the first symptoms appear, and is not the consequence of long-standing inflammation, but occurs in parallel with it. Thus, the implications are that the only way in which the natural history of this disease might be truly modified is by pre-symptomatic preventive strategies, and these are discussed in Chapter 19.

THERAPEUTIC ALGORITHMS (Figure 8.1)

All guidelines present the pharmacological treatment strategy in the form of an algorithm. Thus, there is stepwise approach of increasing therapy dependent on frequency and severity of the disease. The latest paediatric consensus statement[4] suggests that asthma can be divided into infrequent episodic disease where there is normal spirometry between episodes which may be treated with intermittent short-acting beta-agonist inhalations alone. With more frequent episodic disease occurring more often than once every four weeks, there is a suggestion that prophylaxis may be employed even if spirometry is relatively normal between episodes. The first prophylactic compound recommended is either cromolyn sodium or low-dose inhaled corticosteroid (ICS) (less than 400 µg per day of beclomethasone dipropionate (BDP) or equivalent) (Table 8.1). For any patients with abnormal spirometry between episodes, the classification is of persistent asthma where ICS are considered mandatory. Once beta-agonists are needed more frequently than three times per week, in addition to low dose ICS, then the guidelines recommend considering the use of long-acting beta-agonists, slow-release theophylline or, based on more recent published evidence, leukotriene antagonists. As the disease becomes progressively more severe with poor response to ICS, patients are often classified as steroid-insensitive or steroid-resistant. Alternative strategies to be considered then include the use of a range of speculative treatments, including intravenous immunoglobulin, methotrexate, cyclosporin and troleandomycin. Each of these drugs will be discussed in turn.

152 TEXTBOOK OF PEDIATRIC ASTHMA: AN INTERNATIONAL PERSPECTIVE

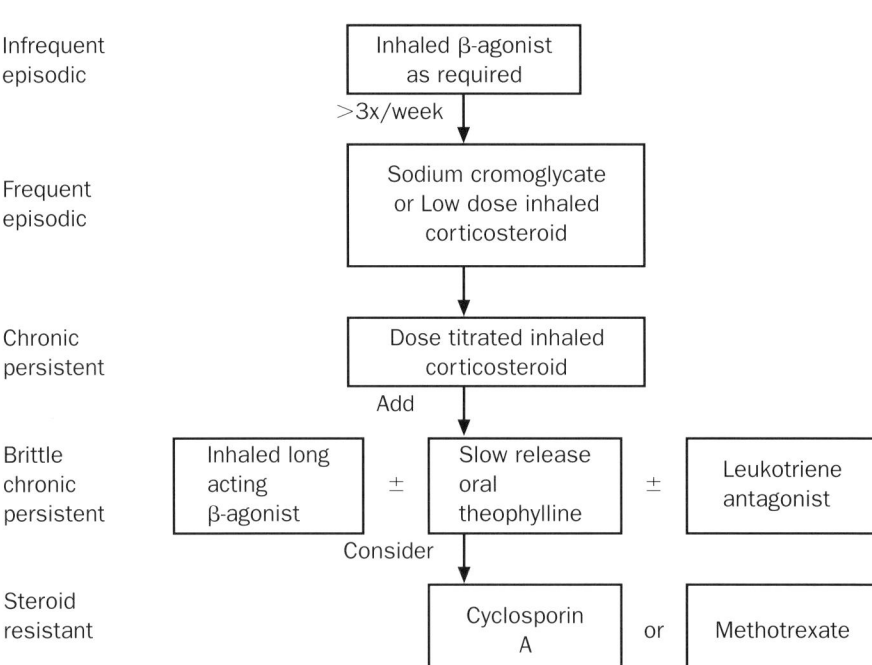

Figure 8.1 The therapeutic algorithm for the management of chronic asthma in school age children demonstrating a stepwise approach where episodic disease may be treated with reliever medications alone but once it becomes more severe or there is evidence of persistent lung function deficit, preventive therapies become mandatory. All alternatives are shown as add-on therapy where inhaled corticosteroid requirements increase.

Table 8.1 Inhaled steroid dose equivalence by comparison with beclomethasone dipropionate (BDP) with CFC propellant. Equivalence is based on approximations from efficacy/systemic activity profiles

	BDP		
CFC propellant	HFA 134a propellant	Budesonide	Fluticasone propionate
1	2*	1†	2†

*The equivalence ratios for ICS in new propellants may vary dependent on the manufacturer.
† These ratios are based on pMDI delivery and will differ if attached to spacers or delivered by dry powder inhaler (see Chapter 17).

THE AIMS OF MANAGEMENT (Figure 8.2)

The aims of management should be to enable patients to enjoy a normal life comparable with non-asthmatic individuals, which will include participation in energetic exercise. School absence should not be excessive. Symptoms should not occur either by day or night. Lung function should be normalised with no excessive diurnal variation, and there should be little need to resort to relieving doses of short-acting beta-agonists, which preferably should be less than once every 2–3 days. Clearly, this goal must be achieved without undue side-effects from administration of medications, which must particularly focus on the maintenance of normal growth and development. For the overwhelming majority of children, it should be possible to normalize lifestyle. However, for some, this is not possible. Such children continue frequently to resort to inhaled beta-agonists and in such cases, great care is required to balance the potential adverse effects of the interventions against the risks from the disease.[12]

Routes of administration

Anti-asthma medications can theoretically be administered by many different routes, including inhalation, ingestion or parenteral by subcutaneous, intramuscular, or intravenous injection. There is a considerable advantage to the inhaled route because this delivers the drug directly to the airway in concentrations that are likely to be effective, while systemic side-effects are minimized or even avoided.[13] Furthermore, there are some medications which are only effective by inhalation because of inadequate absorption by the oral route. The additional bonus for the inhaled route is the rapidity of onset of action, particularly when using beta-agonists for bronchodilatation.

There are a wide range of inhalation devices available and these are discussed in Chapter 17 and will not, therefore, be elaborated upon further in this chapter other than when it is relevant to a specific medication. However, it must be emphasised that one of the commonest reasons why inhaled medications appear to fail to control disease is either because an inappropriate device has been prescribed for the age and capacity of the child, or inadequate training and education have been given to enable the child to use the device effectively. One of the single, most important components of a management programme, therefore, is adequate education and training, particularly in the appropriate use of the medications. This can often be most effectively achieved either by an asthma nurse specialist or by a physiotherapist.

Optimal disease control

Normal lung function
No exercise limitation
No nocturnal symptoms
Little or no need for 'relievers'
Normal growth and development

Avoidance of adverse effects of medication

Normal growth and development
Normal bone accretion
No short-term side-effects

Figure 8.2 A diagrammatic representation of the balance between optimal disease control and avoidance of adverse effects of medication.

Classes of medications (Table 8.2)

There has been a fashion in guidelines to describe medications in two groups, namely *controllers* and *relievers*. The former are taken regularly on a long-term basis to achieve and maintain control of persistent asthma. In general, these are considered to be synonymous with medications that have been demonstrated to have some form of anti-inflammatory effect, and most would focus almost exclusively on ICS. The second category of drugs – relievers – predominantly alleviate bronchospasm associated with acute wheezing and sometimes also relieve other associated symptoms, such as cough and chest tightness. In general, this focuses predominantly on short-acting bronchodilating medications.

Latterly, a number of medications have been identified that do not quite fit into either of the two above groups. Indeed, even the old group of medications, theophyllines, has recently been shown to have some degree of anti-inflammatory, as well as bronchodilating effect.[14] The new leukotriene antagonist drugs both achieve bronchodilatation and have some degree of

Table 8.2 The three groups of asthma medications for use in children

Group	Specific drugs	Administration	Potential problems	Comments
Relievers	Short-acting beta-agonists	Inhaled preferred	Sub-sensitization of receptors	Best used as needed
	Muscarinic receptor antagonists	Inhaled only	Less effective than beta-agonists	May be additive to beta-agonists
Preventers	Sodium cromoglycate	Inhaled only	Less effective than ICS	Safe, irritant
	Inhaled corticosteroid (ICS)	Inhaled	In high doses affects growth	Mandatory use for persistent asthma
Controllers (added-on therapy)	Long-acting beta-agonists	Formoterol – inhaled Salmeterol – inhaled Bambuterol – oral	Sub-sensitization	No anti-inflammatory effects
	Slow-release theophylline	Oral	Narrow therapeutic window	May have anti-inflammatory effects
	Leukotriene antagonists	Oral	Good safety profile but relatively recent introduction	Anti-inflammatory as well as bronchodilator

anti-inflammatory effect.[15] Furthermore, while long-acting beta-agonists do not have any clear-cut anti-inflammatory effects, they certainly can improve long-term control of more difficult asthma not being controlled on low-dose ICS.[16]

Thus, in this chapter the drugs will be considered in the order in which they are likely to be employed, as described in all the guidelines.

Short-acting beta-adrenergic agonists
(Table 8.3)

The beta-adrenergic agonists have been a fundamental part of asthma treatment for several decades. Today, they are still the most effective bronchodilators available and are the treatment of choice for acute asthmatic episodes. They work much more rapidly by inhalation than orally, in very much smaller doses, and yet have the same duration of action.

The beta-adrenergic agonists act through G protein-linked beta-adrenoceptors in cell membranes. Stimulation of the receptor produces activation of adenylate cyclase, which leads to the production of cyclic adenosine monophosphate; this, in turn produces relaxation of smooth muscle in the airways, thereby achieving bronchodilatation. In addition, there is enhanced muco-ciliary clearance, decreased vascular permeability and some modulation of release of mediators from mast cells.[17] There are two beta-adrenoceptors labelled β_1 and β_2. β_1-receptors are located mainly in the heart, while β_2 are in the airways, heart, blood vessels, muscles and inflammatory cells. Adrenaline (epinephrine) was the first adrenoceptor agonist used in the treatment of asthma but had effects on both α- and β_1-, as well as β_2-receptors, thereby producing unacceptable side-effects, including anxiety, tremor, tachycardia and cardiac arrhythmias. Nevertheless, its vasoconstrictor effect has been of enormous importance in the treatment of anaphylactic shock. Subsequent drug development focused on isolating beta from alpha adrenergic activity and subsequently to focus entirely on β_2-specific agonists. Thus isoprenaline (isoproterenol) had both β_1 and β_2 effects. The newer short acting β_2 specific antagonists, salbutamol (albuterol), terbutaline, rimiterol and isoeffrine, have equivalent β_2 specificity, while orciprenaline and fenoterol are somewhat less β_2-selective.[18-20]

The median duration of action of the most frequently used short-acting β_2-agonists, salbutamol (albuterol) and terbutaline is four hours, with a range of 1–6, with the protection against exercise-induced asthma, if taken prior to exercise, having a shorter duration than that of bronchodilatation.[21] The onset of action is within one minute and near-maximal response is achieved within ten minutes of the dose.[22]

There are innumerable trials, providing

Table 8.3 Adrenoceptor agonists. Tabulation of the relative efficacy of bronchodilators by β_2 activity in relation to adrenoceptor agonist selectivity based on inhaled use of the drugs

	Beta-2	Beta-1	Alpha
Epinephrine	+++	+++	+++
Isoprenaline	+++	+++	–
Orciprenaline	+++	++	–
Fenoterol	++++	++	–
Salbutamol	+++	+	–
Terbutaline	+++	+	–

grade 1 evidence that inhaled β_2-agonists are most appropriate for the treatment of acute wheezing episodes and also effective in protecting or diminishing exercise-induced asthma.[23]

Side-effects
Side-effects on the whole are directly related to the concentration of drug getting into the systemic circulation. Thus in high doses, skeletal muscle tremor, headache, a feeling of agitation and palpitations can occur. However, there is a tendency for tolerance to systemic side-effects to develop fairly rapidly.[24] High doses can also produce hyperglycaemia, hypokalaemia and increase circulating fatty acids.[24] At high doses, there will be some effect on the β_2 receptors in the heart, which could produce a ventilation/perfusion imbalance. In severe acute asthma with hypoventilation, high-dose β_2-specific agonists might increase shunting of blood through under-ventilated lung and thereby produce hypoxaemia.

Tolerance
The main concern, and indeed controversy, about β_2-agonists is the question of so-called tolerance or tachyphylaxis. This has been demonstrated for the systemic effects of the drug when administered in high doses long term.[24] Some, but not all, studies have suggested that there is reduced protection against induced bronchoconstriction. The variability in this phenomenon has now been explained by molecular genetics. A particular polymorphism in the β_2-adrenoceptor gene is associated with a higher probability of the development of tolerance but this is not a uniform phenomenon.[25]

One alternative explanation for the apparent deterioration that occurs with continuous beta-agonist usage may be a facilitative effect on the development of inflammation. At a simplistic level, bronchodilatation might increase inhalation of allergen and irritants. There is also a potential for beta-agonists to interfere with the anti-inflammatory effects of corticosteroids. A study by Aldridge et al. has investigated this proposal and demonstrated adverse effects of continuous high-dose beta-agonist on bronchial hyperresponsiveness and the percentage of eosinophils in induced sputum. When high-dose beta-agonists were used together with ICS, there was a less satisfactory improvement in bronchial hyperresponsiveness than on ICS alone, though with no different effects on eosinophils.[26] A previous study perhaps provides some explanation for the observations in demonstrating an adverse interaction between continuous inhaled β_2-agonists and ICS on airway responsiveness to allergen as well as metacholine.[27]

Bound up with the concept of tolerance or beta-adrenoceptor subsensitization has been the concern that chronic long-term dosing with beta-agonists might actually induce a deterioration of asthma control.[28] There have also been suggestions that such treatment will increase bronchial hyperresponsiveness[29] and even increase the risk of asthma death.[30,31] A meta-analysis of various case controlled studies of beta-agonist use and death from asthma has suggested that the main effect was related to the use of the drug in high doses through nebulizers, mainly in adults with severe asthma.[32]

Against the background of concerns about the use of continuous short-acting β_2-agonists, all guidelines have emphasised that such drugs should only be used on an 'as needed' basis. Increased use of the drug more frequently than daily is indicative of a deterioration in asthma and the need to institute additional disease modifying therapy. Furthermore, failure to achieve rapid and sustained improvement in bronchospasm after an adequate dose, indicates a severe acute attack mandating the use of corticosteroids.

In general, therefore, short acting β_2-agonists are reserved as sole treatment for children with infrequent episodic asthma who have absolutely normal lung function, including spirometry between episodes. There is good evidence that such approaches do not compromise long-term management in very mild patients who retain normal lung function even after 28 years of follow-up.[10] Once inhaled, short acting β_2-agonists are required more frequently than three times a week; the Pediatric Asthma Consensus states that children should be considered to have frequent episodic asthma where the use of disease-modifying (anti-inflammatory therapy) is indicated.[4] Furthermore, in order to detect when it is necessary to effect the step-up in therapy, it is most appropriate only to prescribe only short acting β_2-agonists on an 'as needed' basis. Thus, monitoring of dose frequency gives an indication of the need for alternative strategies.

Sodium cromoglycate (cromolyn sodium)

Disodium (usually known as 'sodium') cromoglycate was developed in the 1970s as a derivative of a plant extract that was known to have some smooth-muscle relaxant activity. However, the effect on humans in studies conducted by Altounyan in experiments on himself, identified it to have a prophylactic effect. Indeed, Altounyan must be credited as the first person to identify the importance of attempting to modify the disease process rather than treat symptoms.[33] Despite 30 years in use, the mode of action of sodium cromoglycate is not fully understood. It has a non-steroidal, anti-inflammatory effect, partly mediated by inhibition of IgE-induced mediator release from mast cells and some suppressive effect on other inflammatory cells, such as macrophages, eosinophils and monocytes. There is some evidence that this drug and a related compound, nedocromil sodium, inhibit a chloride channel on inflammatory cells.[34]

Provided it is administered before allergen exposure, to a greater or lesser extent, it inhibits early- and late-phase allergen induced airflow limitation and also has an inhibitory effect on reactions to exercise, cold dry air and sulphur dioxide, but not pharmacological bronchoconstrictors such as histamine or metacholine.[35] Despite being classified as an anti-inflammatory drug, there is only one clinical study demonstrating that prolonged treatment is associated with a reduction in a pivotal inflammatory cell in the bronchoalveolar lavage in asthma, namely the eosinophil.[36] The drug is only effective by inhalation. Despite extensive absorption making it systemically bio-available, it is remarkably safe by comparison with any other anti-asthma drug and is predominantly excreted unmetabolised in the urine.[37] It is the remarkable safety record of this compound together with evidence of efficacy as a prophylactic compound that has led successive paediatric asthma consensus groups suggesting that this should be considered as the first preventer for infrequent episodic disease.[2–4]

Clinical, grade 2, studies in school-age children consistently showed significant advantages compared with placebo in reducing symptoms, frequency of exacerbation, improving lung function and reducing the need for concomitant bronchodilators.[38–40]

Despite the overwhelming majority of trials in school-age children showing beneficial effects, there has been a general scepticism about the place for this drug, and certainly its use has diminished progressively over the last 20 years.[12] Much of the judgement about this compound has been coloured by recent published large randomised controlled trials of the use of sodium cromoglycate in pre-school children, where almost uniformly the trials have been negative.[41] Indeed, a recent review attempting to perform a meta-analysis on sodium cromoglycate trials came to the conclusion that there was insufficient evidence for a beneficial effect of the drug.[42] Remarkably, however, this review fails to quote important controlled trials which clearly showed efficacy.[39,40] Indeed, one of these studies was conducted in 397 patients.[39]

Perhaps far more important criticisms may be levelled at the compound because of the need to administer doses four times daily for optimal effect, which is extremely difficult to sustain. Cough and throat irritation are relatively common minor side-effects occurring for a short period immediately after administration, particularly with the powder formulation. Furthermore, it is clear that ICS are far more potent disease-modifying anti-inflammatory compounds, which has led many to propose that ICS should always be preferred.[43] In the last International Pediatric Consensus,[4] several participants suggested that low-dose steroids should be the first prophylactic drug to be used, particularly in poorly compliant families. However, it is the balance of potential side-effects against benefits and the clinical evaluation of each individual patient that still suggests sodium cromoglycate should be used as a controller drug in episodic disease.

Nedocromil sodium

It has been difficult to incorporate nedocromil sodium into the pediatric asthma guidelines. While it has been shown to be significantly more potent than sodium cromoglycate in preventing induced bronchoconstriction, there are no head-to-head clinical comparisons.[44] Trials have demonstrated efficacy compared with placebo in childhood asthma.[45]

As with sodium cromoglycate, it is only efficacious by inhalation. While some trials have suggested that twice daily therapy may be effective, most demonstrating efficacy have used a four times daily schedule.[45] The Childhood Asthma Management Program (CAMP) showed that nedocromil twice daily reduced urgent care visits and courses of prednisolone compared with placebo in a 4–6-year double-blind trial. However, though not a double-blind comparison, budesonide (an ICS) was more efficacious.[46] It is not clear whether the children who fail to respond to sodium cromoglycate do or do not have any response to nedocromil. Based on the much greater published experience with cromoglycate and the lack of studies comparing the clinical response of sodium cromoglycate to nedocromil in the long-term treatment of asthmatic children, nedocromil sodium is not usually included in guideline recommendations.

Inhaled corticosteroids (ICS)

Corticosteroids are clearly anti-inflammatory in effect in switching off multiple inflammatory genes, thereby inhibiting production of cytokines, a range of pro-inflammatory mediators and adhesion molecules, which are important for inflammatory cell migration. Many human studies have been able to show that ICS reduce airway inflammation in asthma with a consequent long-term down-grading of airway hyperresponsiveness.[47,48] Clinical studies have demonstrated that ICS improve symptoms, frequency and severity of exacerbations, quality of life, lung function and decreased airway hyperresponsiveness.[49] While all corticosteroids share their anti-inflammatory effect, the essence of the inhaled preparations is their high topical potency associated with diminished systemic bio-availability. This latter property has been achieved by structural changes to the basic corticosteroid molecule. Each formulation has somewhat different dose response and pharmacokinetic profiles (see Table 8.1).[50]

Trials in children provide grade 1 evidence being consistent in demonstrating efficacy in virtually all age groups with improvements occurring within 1–2 weeks of onset and sustained over long periods with progressive improvement in bronchial reactivity.[29,46,51–53] Most importantly, long-term use of ICS reduces the need for oral corticosteroid and, indeed, is able to replace the equivalent of between 7.5 and 10 mg of prednisone or prednisolone per day, while clearly having immensely fewer side-effects.[54] It has been suggested that the earlier ICS are introduced, the less the influence of the chronic asthmatic inflammation on attenuating lung growth.[9] However, the same effect may be achieved by the use of sodium cromoglycate, at least in those who have a clinical response to this latter compound.[55] Furthermore, CAMP was unable to show any post-bronchodilator difference in FEV_1 between children treated with budesonide, nedocromil or placebo over 4–6 years,[46] raising doubts on a long-term and anti-inflammatory action of these drugs. Nevertheless, at the present time, ICS are still considered as the gold standard for anti-inflammatory drugs.

Efficacy versus safety

The key issue in positioning the use of ICS in childhood asthma is to understand the comparative efficacy/safety ratios.[50] Local adverse effects include increased predisposition to oropharyngeal candidiasis and a hoarse voice (dysphonia). Mouth-rinsing after use will decrease the former, and the latter is reversible if the treatment is stopped.[56] However, the important side-effects relate to systemic bio-availability and activity. This, in turn, is dictated by absorption from the gut, the degree of first-pass metabolism in the liver and the systemic half-life. This is affected not only by the activity of the individual compounds, but also by their particle size and the delivery system employed. Dependent on the experimental models used, budesonide and beclomethasone dipropionate (BDP), dose for dose, are equivalent, while fluticasone propionate is pharmacologically twice as potent.[57] Using the new hydro-fluoro alkane propellant rather than chloro-fluoro-carbon for BDP leads to reduced particle size of the aerosol with improved efficiency of delivery to smaller airway. This doubles its efficacy and, to a certain extent, increases systemic bio-activity profiles.[58] Using equi-efficacious doses of separate ICS, there is dispute as to the balance against adverse effect with at least some suggestion that fluticasone propionate might have a greater propensity for blood and tissue accumulation and thereby side-effects.[59] At present, there is insufficient evidence to make a judgement on which ICS has the best efficacy/safety profile. The decision on which to use may, therefore, be dictated by cost (generic BDP being cheap), availability and the suitability of the accompanying inhalation devices.

Hypothalamic pituitary adrenal axis

Despite the high first-pass metabolism of the standard ICS employed, all will have some systemic absorption; indeed that accessing the airway has a higher bio-availability as it will be absorbed directly into the systemic circulation. Despite well over 30 years of clinical use and extensive study, there remains a controversy about the risk/benefit ratios for the treatment. Much confusion arises because some studies have investigated systemic effects but have not necessarily identified whether these have any clinical relevance. What is clear, however, is that systemic activity is present, and this has a subtle impact on hypothalamic-pituitary-adrenal axis (HPA) even in relatively low doses. Whether this has any consequences may only become apparent after decades of longitudinal observation.

Many studies have now carefully evaluated the effects of ICS on the HPA axis. Results are conflicting because of variations in study design, sensitivity of the tests employed, the individuals studied, the type of ICS and the delivery system employed. Thus, for instance, there has been a suggestion that employing spacer devices might reduce the risk of systemic side-effects.[60] However, this observation is not reconcilable with the fact that spacers increase airway delivery which, in turn, should increase bio-availability.

Using highly sensitive techniques of HPA axis function, such as low-dose synacthen stimulation,[61] integrated measurement of cortisol over 12–24 hour periods[62] and/or urinary-free cortisol,[63] has shown a clear linear dose–response effect with the higher the dose of ICS, the greater the degree of suppression.[62] However, none of the studies have ever demonstrated any significant effect with doses of BDP at 200 µg per day or less. The effect, though subtle, becomes evident between 200 and 400 µg per day. This is most obviously demonstrated as a mild suppression of basal-endogenous cortisol secretion in the early hours of the morning but with no significant effect on peak cortisol production later in the morning.[63] It has been shown that this is neither an effect of prior steroid therapy nor due to the asthma, as identical outcomes are seen when ICS are given to healthy non-asthmatic individuals, whether in a single dose in the evening or after sustained treatment.[64]

Comparative studies between different corticosteroids have been conducted with different outcomes. A number have suggested greater adrenal suppression with BDP than equipotent doses of budesonide[65] or fluticasone propionate.[66] However, one recent meta-analysis which included information from 27 randomised controlled trials, predominantly in adults, concluded that there was a steeper dose–response and greater potential for systemic effects on the HPA axis with fluticasone propionate, especially when given at high doses.[59]

While the above studies have demonstrated a systemic effect, none has been able to correlate this effect with any clinically relevant outcomes. Indeed, studies of fluticasone propionate have, if anything, suggested lesser effects on growth compared with BDP,[67] despite the Lipworth meta-analysis[59] showing a greater systemic effect of this drug. This highlights the importance of establishing whether demonstration of systemic effects is associated with any clinically relevant complication.

Growth
Asthma per se has an effect on growth. Asthmatics tend to have a slower pre-pubertal growth velocity and a delayed pubertal growth spurt associated with delayed bone maturation, irrespective of therapy. However, ultimate height, other than in those treated with high-dose oral steroids, has been of normal distribution.[68] The more severe the asthma and the more poorly it is controlled, the greater the effect on growth delay.[9]

Superimposed on the effects of the disease are the effects of treatment, and growth retardation can be exacerbated by the use of oral corticosteroid with influences of both dose and duration of treatment.[69] To what extent the steroid therapy has an effect on ultimate height has not been clearly elaborated. Furthermore, the meta-analysis of studies of growth in children has failed to show any effect of ICS.[70] However, this review did not include an important long-term controlled trial that showed growth suppression with BDP.[71] Much more work is necessary for evaluating the real impact of ICS on growth, since two studies measuring final height in adults treated with ICS compared with asthmatics not given such treatment showed no significant differences.[72,73]

The above rather favourable outcomes must be compared with studies of short-term growth, which have consistently shown an adverse effect. Very accurate measurements of growth of the leg using knemometry have demonstrated, in short placebo-controlled double-blind studies, a dose-dependent effect of BDP, budesonide and fluticasone with small differences between them in favour of budesonide over BDP.[74–76] However, it is difficult to relate the findings from knemometry to long-term growth, and long-term prospective studies should be performed to answer this important question.

Notwithstanding the meta-analysis on growth outcomes[70], a number of recent randomised double-blind controlled studies in children with mild-to-moderate asthma have shown clear-cut medium-term effects of slowed growth over periods of seven months to one year. The average slowing was around 1–1.5 cm per year for budesonide[46] and for BDP.[52,71,77] In these studies the ICS were compared with placebo or alternative treatment for asthma, such as nedocromil, theophylline or inhaled salmeterol.[46,52,71,77] Fewer data are available for budesonide but there is a suggestion of less effect on statural growth, at least from one randomised controlled study on asthmatic teenagers.[78] This, again, must be balanced against the systemic effect study showing no difference between equivalent doses of budesonide and beclomethasone.[63] The long-term observational study of budesonide showed that low-to-moderate doses had no effect on growth; however, above 800 μg per day, there was perhaps some degree of growth slowing.[9] CAMP, however, did show an effect of budesonide, 200 μg twice daily, on growth compared with placebo and nedocromil. The growth deficit of 1.1 cm was apparent in the first year of treatment and no greater after 4–6 years.[46]

For fluticasone propionate, trials with low doses up to 200 μg per day for one year in mild-to-moderate childhood asthmatics have been associated with no apparent effect on growth,[79] and one comparison between fluticasone and BDP showed better growth on the former than the latter.[67] Nevertheless, in higher doses of fluticasone (greater than 400 μg) there have been significant concerns expressed about the use of fluticasone[80] which appear more in keeping with the meta-analysis of systemic effects.[59] All these contradictory results reinforce the need for a careful and judicious decision on the use of ICS in asthmatic children.

Effects on bone
Systemic steroids clearly increase bone reabsorption and decrease bone formation – the

consequence being increased risk of fractures in later life.[81] The effects of ICS on bone is not as well studied. Recent publications, however, have highlighted the potential for long-term therapy to have an effect on fracture risk[82] and bone mineral density.[83] The latter study[83] in 196 adults with asthma aged between 20 and 40 years who had taken ICS for a median of six years with very little systemic steroids, showed a clear negative correlation between total cumulative dose and bone mineral density.

Smaller cross-sectional and relatively short longitudinal studies, however, have tended to show no adverse effects of ICS on bone mineral density in children treated for up to six years.[67,84,85] However, studies do demonstrate some effects on biochemical markers of bone and collagen turnover in children receiving high doses of ICS, though again the clinical significance of these observations is unknown.[66,86]

Arguably, the long-term attrition on bone over decades of use of ICS potentially is the greatest concern about the use of these highly effective anti-asthma medications. The lack of very long-term prospective studies makes it impossible to judge the potential risks. Under such circumstances, a careful course must be steered between achieving good control of the asthma and using the lowest dose of treatment.

Local effects
Local effects of ICS include oropharyngeal candidiasis, hoarseness of voice (dysphonia) and cough during inhalation owing to direct irritant effects. There is a suggestion that this can be reduced by the use of large-volume spacers, mouth rinsing and gargling after inhalation.[56] Other concerns have included the potential for posterior subcapsular cataracts and bruising but observational studies on large numbers of children have failed to show an effect.[87] High doses, however, may be associated with skin thinning and easy bruising,[88] and either cataracts[89] or glaucoma.[90,91] There is one final concern about the use of high-dose ICS in infants under 2 years of age. At this age, new alveolus formation is still occurring and there is at least the potential for steroids to inhibit this normal development. As much wheezing in early infancy may be due to geometric problems in the airway rather than true asthma, there is the potential that inhaled steroids will increase the risk of chronic obstructive pulmonary disease in late adult life in such children (see Figure 8.3).[92]

The place of ICS in the therapeutic algorithm
Despite the undoubted consistent efficacy of ICS, which exceeds that of any other asthma prophylaxis, the lingering concerns about systemic effects, influences on growth and long-term effects on bone density and perhaps lung growth, dictate that the minimum dose to achieve control should be employed. The balance of evidence suggests that very low doses at 200 µg per day of BDP or equivalent are safe and may be employed as an alternative to cromones in frequent episodic asthma. However, treatment with ICS is mandatory for persistent asthma with titration of the dose initially to gain control as quickly as possible and then to reduce it to the minimum, which maintains good control. Once the dose required to achieve control creeps above 400 µg per day of BDP or equivalent, then thought must be given to the use of alternative strategies that might achieve control without raising the dose of ICS further.

Steroid insensitivity
Fortunately, the overwhelming majority of children have consistent good responses to ICS therapy. However, a small percentage of individuals even in childhood become relatively steroid-insensitive. Progressively increasing doses produce diminishing benefits. The exact mechanisms which are associated with this phenomenon are not well understood. Patients with this problem must be classified as a fatality-prone group.[93] There are a number of potential immunological mechanisms whereby steroid responsiveness can be compromised with high levels of interleukin-2 (IL-2) and IL-4 being particularly involved.[94] If a compliant patient is receiving high doses of ICS without clinical improvement, he/she must be sent to a specialist.

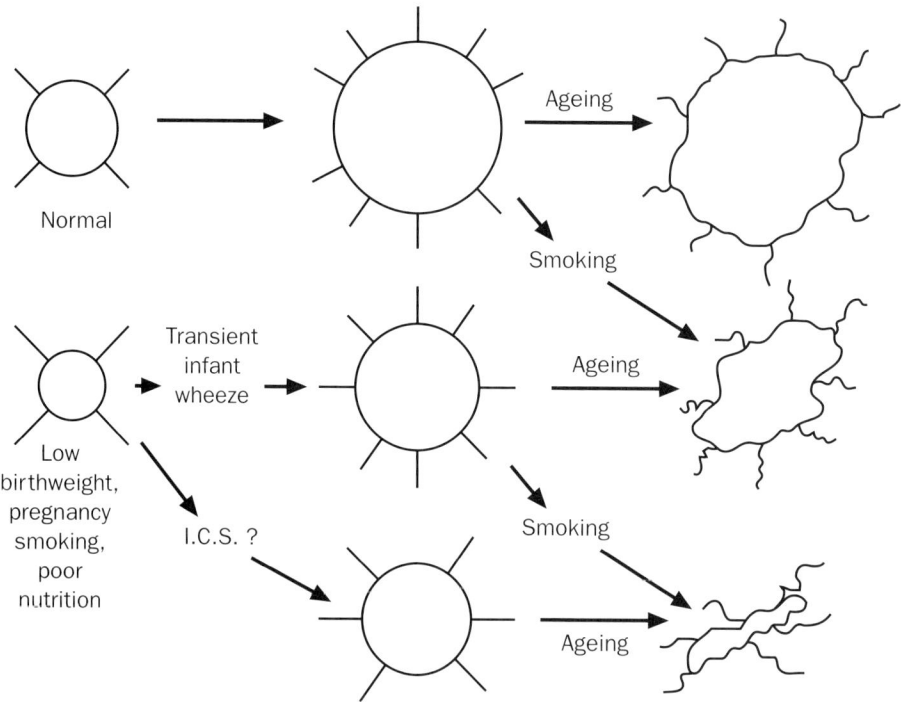

Figure 8.3 A diagrammatic representation of airway growth and new alveolus formation from infancy to mid-life and the effects of ageing with loss of elastic recoil, therefore reducing airway support. The potential for inhaled corticosteroids to interrupt new alveolus formation might have the consequence of increasing the risks of chronic obstructive pulmonary disease in late life due to reduced airway support from reduced alveolar number and loss of elastic recoil.

ADD-ON THERAPY TO ACHIEVE ICS-SPARING

Theophylline

Theophylline and its salts are frequently used in the treatment of chronic asthma. Because the bronchodilator effect of theophylline is less than that of β_2-agonists, theophylline is less prescribed for acute asthma therapy. The main indication for chronic asthma control is with sustained-release formulations as add-on therapy with low-dose ICS. Theophylline is especially useful for the control of nocturnal asthma symptoms, as well as day-time symptoms in patients with persistent asthma.[95] One of benefits of theophylline in children is that because it is orally active, compliance is improved. Kelloway et al.[96] showed 73% compliance with theophylline versus 30% with ICS in children. However, there is a generalised corticophobia among parents, which could have influenced the results. Theophylline also has beneficial extrapulmonary effects in increasing diaphragmatic muscle contractility[97] and strength.[98] The relevance of these effects to the clinical response in asthma is unknown.

Mechanisms of action
The mechanisms through which theophylline is presumed to exert its actions as bronchodilator are through phosphodiesterase (PDE) inhibition and adenosine receptor antagonism. The antagonism of adenosine receptors (A_1 and A_2) is achieved at low serum levels.[99] PDE inhibition, in contrast, is only reached at much higher concentrations.

The basis for its efficacy in the treatment of asthma remains unknown. More recently, theophylline has been shown to have anti-inflammatory activity that may be more important in its effectiveness in asthma.[100] Theophylline has the ability to inhibit T-cell proliferation (in vitro) within the therapeutic range of serum levels[101] and inhibits the migration of monocytes into tissues.[102] Very low concentrations of theophylline are able to suppress endotoxin-induced production of tumor necrosis factor α (TNF-α) by monocytes, in vivo.[103] Therapeutic concentrations of theophylline inhibit immunoglobulin-induced eosinophil degranulation and the release of basic proteins, in vitro.[104] The anti-inflammatory effects of theophylline may be present at lower serum concentrations than are typically the target for bronchodilation (10–20 µg/ml).[105] This may in part explain the efficacy of 'subtherapeutic' doses of theophylline.

Efficacy
There are recent studies with theophylline, indicating that its use especially in low doses has beneficial effects on chronic asthma management in adults.[106]

Dusdieker et al.[107] compared sustained-release theophylline with the oral preparation of β$_2$-agonist metaproterenol in 34 children with chronic asthma. The patients receiving theophylline had significantly fewer asthmatic symptoms, better pulmonary function, improved exercise tolerance and lower need of oral corticosteroid bursts. Hambleton et al.[108] performed a crossover study comparing three treatments – cromolyn, theophylline and the combination of both drugs in children with chronic asthma. Theophylline alone and theophylline plus cromolyn were significantly superior to cromolyn in terms of symptom-free days. Furukawa et al[109] compared cromolyn sodium and sustained-release theophylline in 46 children aged 5–15 years with daily symptoms of asthma. After three months of therapy, they concluded that cromolyn was as effective as theophylline. Nassif et al.,[110] in a study enrolling 33 chronic steroid-dependent asthmatic children, found that theophylline had corticosteroid-sparing potential. Similar data were found by Brenner et al,[111] studying five severe steroid-dependent children.

In a one-year-long study conducted by the American Academy of Allergy, Asthma and Immunology, comparing the clinical effectiveness of theophylline with inhaled BDP as a first-line agent for the treatment of mild-to-moderate asthma, there was good evidence that theophylline controlled the symptoms of most children.[71] Comparisons of addition of theophylline to low-dose ICS (BDP or budesonide) with high-dose of the same ICS, showed that low-dose ICS plus theophylline and high-dose ICS produced similar benefits. The above combination of the two drugs may, therefore, be preferable and cheaper than increasing the dose of ICS.[112,113] In a study with asthmatic children living in the inner city, a cross-sectional questionnaire survey was completed by 392 families (508 children with asthma). In children living in poor urban areas, theophylline was more frequently used than anti-inflammatory medications. Interestingly, more than half of children aged 9 years or over supervised their own medication.[114]

Administration
For children over 1 year of age, the initial dose recommendation has been 16 mg/kg/day, up to a maximum of 400 mg per day. After three days, if tolerated, the dose can be increased to 20 mg/kg/day up to a maximum of 600 mg/day, and a serum concentration measured after three days of this dose. These dosage recommendations have a target serum level of 5–15 µg/ml. However, as lower doses may have therapeutic efficacy, a more circumspect approach to increasing the dose is appropriate.

Adverse reactions
Theophylline toxicity is closely related to serum levels.[115] When the serum concentration is less than 15 µg/ml, most patients tolerate the drug quite well. Concentrations greater than 20 µg/ml may result in adverse effects such as nausea, vomiting, diarrhoea, tremors and mild central nervous system effects. However, the

presence of adverse reactions is very variable between individuals.

Monitoring of serum levels should be done. The interpretation of a serum level must take into consideration the preparation administered, its time to peak and trough, its time of administration, time and nature of last meal, other concomitant medications and intercurrent illnesses.

Interactions
Serum levels of theophylline, owing to liver metabolism, may be markedly affected by a number of variables, including age, diet, disease states and drug interactions, all of which contribute to the complexity of using this medication. Theophylline clearance is significantly lower in undernourished patients, necessitating lower doses for maintenance therapy.[116] Tobacco smoking increases theophylline metabolism, and febrile illnesses and high-carbohydrate diets significantly decrease theophylline metabolism. In addition, drug interactions must be considered and the theophylline dose adjusted accordingly. Phenytoin, phenobarbital, carbamazepine and rifampicin increase theophylline clearance by more than 25%, whereas macrolide antibiotics, cimetidine hydrochloride, ciprofloxacin hydrochloride and oral contraceptives decrease theophylline clearance by 10–25%.[115,117]

The place of theophyllines in the therapeutic algorithm
Theophyllines have had a renaissance in the last two years because of observed anti-inflammatory effects in low doses. While we now face questions regarding chronic administration of beta-agonists by inhalation or oral routes, the potential for growth suppression with chronic administration of ICS, and limited effectiveness of cromolyn in many children with moderate-to-severe asthma, the use of theophylline must be considered in children who have chronic asthma requiring daily medication.[118] In developing countries, the low cost of theophylline, compared to ICS and cromolyn, allows the recommendation that in non-affluent populations with limited access to inhaled drugs, the early introduction of oral theophylline in the therapeutic algorithm could be beneficial to many asthmatic patients, as prophylactic therapy.[4] However, owing to the potential serious side-effects of theophylline, all efforts should be made to provide asthmatic children with ICS. Theophylline may be regarded as an immunomodulator as well as a bronchodilator. This effect is exerted at plasma concentrations that are not associated with undesirable side-effects. In regions with important financial constraints (see Chapter 20), the cost and/or availability of serum assays of theophylline may not be possible for the majority of asthmatic children. The determination of serum levels of theophylline (additional cost) may not be necessary if low doses are used. Faced with the possibility of not having any other therapeutic alternative, a paediatrician can use careful observation of the patient's clinical state to guide dosage starting with 10 mg/kg/day and if necessary, increasing slowly up to 16 mg/kg/day). In this situation, the paediatrician must be always aware of illnesses and drugs that interfere with theophylline metabolism. In the developed world, slow-release theophyllines still have a place as add-on therapy to low-dose ICS, though other less risky alternatives such as long acting beta-agonists and leukotriene modifiers should also be considered.[4]

Leukotriene modifiers

Leukotriene modifiers, including both receptor antagonists (LTRAs) and synthesis inhibitors, are a newly developed class of anti-asthma medication.[119] Clinical studies have suggested that leukotriene modifiers can be defined as a controller medication in the treatment of asthma.

Mechanisms of action (Figure 8.4)
Following an inflammatory stimulus, there is cell activation with concomitant release of arachidonic acid from cell and perinuclear membrane phospholipids, by the action of phospholipase A2. The released arachidonic acid is converted by 5-lipoxygenase in the presence of FLAP (5-lipoxygenase activating

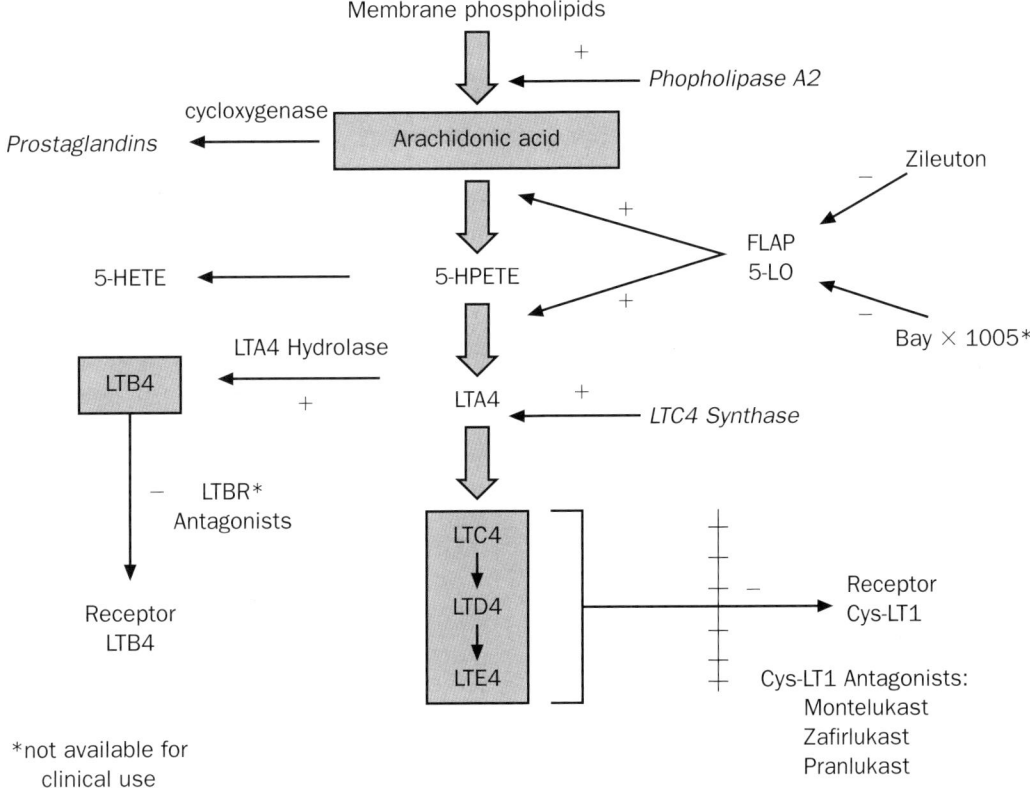

Figure 8.4 The leukotriene synthesis pathway with an indication where antagonists have their mechanism of action.
Flap = 5-lipoxygenase-activating protein
5-LO = 5-lipoxygenase
5-HPETE = 5-hydroxyperoxy-eicosatetraenoic acid
LTC4, LTD4, LTE4 = cysteinyl leukotrienes

protein) to the unstable intermediate, 5-hydroperoxy-eicosatetraenoic acid (5-HPETE) and then the epoxide intermediate, LTA4.[120]

LTA4 is unstable and may be hydrolyzed to the dihydroxy acid LTB4 by LTA4-hydrolase, or the tripeptide glutathione is incorporated to form the cysteinyl leukotriene (cysLT), LTC4, by the enzyme LTC4-synthase. The subsequent conversion of LTC4 to LTD4 is via the action of γ-glutamyl transpeptidase. LTD4 is further metabolized to the cysteinyl derivative LTE4 by the action of a dispeptidase. LTE4 is the most important urinary metabolite, the level of which has been used extensively to monitor in vivo cysteinyl leukotriene production in humans. An increased urinary excretion of LTE4 has been demonstrated after challenge with allergen, exercise and aspirin in sensitive subjects, as well as during the early asthmatic response.[121, 122] The concentration in urine correlates directly with the magnitude of this response.[123]

Bronchoalveolar lavage studies have shown increased levels of leukotrienes in asthmatic subjects with further increases after allergen challenge, demonstrating increased local production of leukotrienes in the lung.[124]

Cysteinyl leukotrienes (C4, D4, and E4) are produced by many types of inflammatory cells, especially mast cells, eosinophils, macrophages and basophils.[125] As the leukotrienes bind to their receptors, they are able to induce airway smooth-muscle contraction,[126] microvascular hyperpermeability and mucus hypersecretion,[127] decrease ciliary activity,[128] and promote eosinophil migration into airways mucosa.[129]

LTD4 has 1000 and 10 000 times more contractile potency in normal human bronchi than histamine and acetylcholine, respectively.[130]

Cysteinyl leukotrienes produce their effects by binding to and activating specific receptors. Three types of leukotriene receptors have been identified: one for LTB4 and two for the cysteinyl leukotrienes.

The receptor for LTB4 is designated the BLT-receptor. Two cysLT receptors (1 and 2 subtypes) are recognized. The CysLT1 receptor binds LTC4, LTD4 and LTF4. The molecular and pharmacological characterization of the cloned human CysLT1 receptor was recently described. CysLT1-receptor messenger RNA was detected in spleen, peripheral-blood leukocytes and lung. In normal human lung, expression of the CysLT1-receptor RNA was confined to smooth-muscle cells and tissue macrophages.[131] The CysLT2 receptor has been pharmacologically documented to be expressed in human pulmonary vein preparations. The human CysLT2 receptor has very recently been cloned and characterized, as a 346-amino acid protein with 38% amino acid identity to the CysLT1 receptor.[132] CysLT2 receptor mRNA was detected in lung macrophages and airway smooth muscle, cardiac Purkinje cells, adrenal medulla cells, peripheral-blood lymphocytes and brain. The receptor gene was mapped to chromosome 13q14, a region linked to atopic asthma. The CysLT1 receptor is the molecular target of the leukotriene antagonists (montelukast, zafirlukast and pranlukast), that have both anti-bronchoconstrictive and anti-inflammatory actions. Although the role of the CysLT2 receptor has not yet been clarified in human asthma, the possible linkage of polymorphisms within the CysLT2 receptor gene to the asthmatic phenotype is under investigation.[132]

Cysteinyl leukotrienes are the most important leukotrienes in the pathogenesis of asthma,[122] and agents developed to specifically antagonize the actions of leukotrienes have been important tools in confirming the role of leukotrienes in asthma (see Table 8.4).

Zafirlukast, montelukast and pranlukast are potent and selective CysLT1 receptor antagonists that block the effects of CysLTs on target cells and tissues. Zileuton blocks the synthesis of leukotrienes by inhibiting the enzyme 5-lipoxygenase. BAY u9773 is a non-selective antagonist at CysLT1 and CysLT2 receptors.

The CysLTs are important in the pathophysiology of exercise-induced bronchoconstriction in asthmatics, as they are released in response to loss of heat or water from the airways. At the same time, there is a release of PGE2, which partially attenuates further exercise-induced bronchoconstriction, perhaps explaining exercise refractoriness.

Certain types of asthmatic patients may not respond to these more specific therapies. This was observed recently in clinical trials with leukotriene inhibitors. This lack of response may be due to DNA sequence variations in the 5-lipoxygenase (ALOX5) gene, with a consequent diminished clinical response to treatment with a drug targeting this pathway.[133]

Efficacy

The clinical benefits of zafirlukast have been reported broadly in adults, and one study was recently performed in asthmatic children. Pearlman et al. tested the effects of zafirlukast on exercise-induced bronchoconstriction (EIB) in a randomized, double-blind, three-way, crossover study of 39 asthmatic children aged 6–14 years. They observed a decrease in EIB four hours after ingestion of zafirlukast.[134]

Diamant et al.[135] showed the protection conferred by a LTRA (montelukast) against allergen-induced early and late airway asthmatic responses, suggesting their effective role in the treatment of allergic asthma. There are several studies with montelukast in asthmatic children since it was the first LTRA approved for use in paediatric patients, from 2 years of age.

As Kikawa et al. demonstrated an increase in urinary LTE4 after exercise-induced broncho-

Table 8.4 Leukotriene receptor antagonists – route and doses of administration

LRA	Route	Doses/Ages
Montelukast (at bedtime)	Oral	10 mg once daily/adults
		5 mg once daily/6–14 years
		4 mg once daily/2–6 years
Zafirlukast (1 hr before or 2 hr after a meal)	Oral	20 mg bid/adults
		10 mg bid/7–11 years

constriction, in asthmatic children,[136] LTRAs may be viewed as valuable medications to use in children with EIB. Kemp et al.[137] confirmed protection against exercise-induced bronchoconstriction (EIB) by montelukast in 6–14-year-olds with asthma. Exercise challenge was performed 20–24 hours after the last of two once-daily doses of therapy. The EIB protection observed in this study was consistent with previously reported studies in adults.[138,139]

A recent study in adolescents and adults with mild asthma, compared the efficacy of montelukast versus salmeterol in exercise-induced bronchoconstriction over an eight-week treatment period. Montelukast was superior to salmeterol for controlling chronic, exercise-induced bronchoconstriction; there was tolerance to the bronchoprotective effects induced by the chronic use of salmeterol.[140] Conversely, in patients with persistent asthma, the majority of whom were receiving regular ICS therapy, salmeterol was significantly more effective than zafirlukast in improving pulmonary function studies and symptom control, over the 4-week treatment period.[141]

Knorr et al.[142] in a multicentre, double-blind, randomized study, using montelukast for 8 weeks in 336 asthmatic children, demonstrated its therapeutic benefit in chronic asthma by improving on morning forced expiratory volume in 1 second (FEV_1), β-agonist use, quality of life and exacerbation rates.

Malmstrom et al.[143] compared the clinical benefit of montelukast and inhaled beclomethasone. They observed that although beclomethasone had a larger beneficial effect than montelukast, both drugs provided clinical benefit to patients with chronic asthma, compared with placebo. An interesting feature in this heterogeneous group of patients with mild intermittent or mild-to-moderate persistent asthma was the distribution of responses in the two treatment groups: among patients who received beclomethasone or montelukast, 22% and 34%, respectively, did not have improvements in FEV_1 during 12 weeks of therapy. The additional clinical benefit with the co-administration of montelukast and an ICS (beclomethasone) in adolescents and adults was recently reported by Laviolette et al.[144] Decreased nitric oxide in exhaled air in asthmatic children, treated with montelukast,[145,146] suggested an anti-inflammatory role for this LTRA in the treatment of children with mild-to-moderate asthma.

Bisgaard and Nielsen showed that montelukast provided clinically significant bronchoprotection against the effects of cold-air hyperventilation in asthmatic children aged 3–5 years.[147] It was demonstrated in asthmatics that zafirlukast[148] and montelukast[149] given concomitantly with loratadine, compared with each anti-leukotriene antagonist alone, caused significant improvement in FEV_1. Combination of leukotriene antagonists and antihistamines may represent a new approach for the management of asthma.

Administration

Montelukast, the first leukotriene receptor antagonist approved for use in young children, has been demonstrated to improve asthma.[150,151] Zafirlukast has recently been approved for the treatment of asthma in children from 7 years of age. The efficacy and tolerability of zafirlukast was evaluated in the recommended dose of 10 mg bid, in school-aged children (5–11 years) with mild-to-moderate asthma. The drug significantly improved all efficacy outcomes, was well tolerated and side-effects were indistinguishable from placebo.[152]

Leukotriene modifiers are used by oral route, resulting in greater adherence. Zafirlukast is administered twice daily (20 mg for adults and 10 mg for children), montelukast once daily at bedtime (10 mg for adults, 5 mg for children aged 6–14 years and 4 mg for children aged 2–6 years), and zileuton is given four times a day (600 mg only for adults).

Studies with 4 mg montelukast in 2–5-year-olds with asthma showed that it was well tolerated in long-term administration (up to 13 months).[153] In the same age period, a double-blind, placebo controlled, parallel-group, 12-week study administered montelukast (4 mg chewable tablets) to 461 children. The drug caused significant improvements in daytime and overtime asthma control; adverse effects were similar to placebo.[154]

Adverse reactions

Reports of adverse effects of leukotriene antagonists have been limited. The most frequently reported adverse effect has been headache, but the frequency has not been significantly different from that observed with placebo.[155]

Abnormalities in liver function with elevated serum transaminase levels have occasionally been reported. This happens more commonly at doses higher than those currently recommended for leukotriene modifiers. Zileuton has been associated with mild and transient elevation of liver enzymes. The recommendation of the Food and Drug Administration (FDA) for zileuton treatment is to monitor the liver enzymes monthly in the first months. More limited data are available in children, but the side-effect profile appears to be the same as in adults.[156]

There have been reports of patients (adults) receiving zafirlukast, montelukast or pranlukast who developed a systemic vasculitis, Churg–Strauss syndrome.[157] These individuals had required oral corticosteroids to control their asthma. Apparently, the effectiveness of the LTRAs enabled the dose of oral corticosteroid to be reduced or discontinued, and shortly thereafter vasculitis was diagnosed. Although a direct effect of these drugs cannot be totally disregarded, the most probable explanation for the unmasking of Churg–Strauss syndrome is the reduction in the high doses of oral corticosteroids, facilitated by the use of leukotriene modifiers.

Drug–drug interactions

Zafirlukast inhibits the cytochrome P450 (CYP1A2) enzyme system, accounting for many of its drug interactions. Co-administration of zafirlukast with erythromycin, terfenadine and theophylline – all agents believed to cause induction of cytocrome P450 enzyme system – results in decreased plasma concentration of zafirlukast (30–40%). Co-administration with aspirin increases zafirlukast concentrations by 45%. Pharmacokinetic studies have not demonstrated effects of montelukast on the metabolism of theophylline, warfarin, digoxin, terfenadine, prednisone and prednisolone. Phenobarbital reduced plasma concentrations of montelukast.[158]

Similar to zafirlukast, zileuton interferes in theophylline pharmacokinetics increasing its half-life by more than 1.5 hours.[159]

Food interactions

Because food high in protein or fat reduces the absorption of zafirlukast, it should be taken one hour before or two hours after a meal.[160] Food interactions have not been reported with montelukast or with zileuton.

Positioning in asthma treatment

The positive attributes of leukotriene antagonists include oral administration, once or twice daily dosing, both bronchodilator and anti-inflammatory properties, and an excellent safety profile in adults and children. Their main negative attribute is the lower efficacy compared with ICS. However, the results of the recent CAMP study[46] (the largest prospective therapeutic study in children) are disappointing in the sense that the main outcome (FEV_1 post-bronchodilator) was the same for budesonide, nedocromil and placebo. Although at the end of the five-year study the children treated with budesonide had a small reduction in growth, their symptoms were much better controlled. As the CAMP study suggested that the dose of ICS able to control symptoms is not able to control inflammation, perhaps by changing the concept of 'gold standard', other long-term therapeutic options should be considered, such as oral anti-leukotrienes.

Except for patients with aspirin-sensitive asthma who respond very well to the LTRAs, it is not possible to identify the patients most likely to benefit from them. The 1997 USA Guidelines for the Diagnosis and Management of Asthma[6] have positioned leukotriene receptor antagonists as an alternative to ICS for mild persistent asthma, in suggesting that either of these drugs can be used as first-line therapy. The basis of the physician's and patient's choice is the superior efficacy of ICS versus the expected superior compliance associated with oral leukotriene modifiers.[161] For patients with mild persistent asthma, leukotriene antagonists could be a good first choice on the basis of their bioavailability, compliance, symptom improvement and safety.[162] There is evidence to supporting the recommendation of the use of montelukast (long-lasting effect without the development of tolerance) as first-line monotherapy to children who present predominantly exercise-induced asthma. However, the greatest weight of evidence of efficacy is with the use of LTRAs as add-on therapy to ICS, and this is reflected in the European product labelling. The European and other guidelines have only endorsed the use of LTRAs as add-on therapy with ICS and not as monotherapy for milder disease.

In vitro studies showed that dexamethasone increases expression of 5-lipoxygenase in human monocytes[163] and does not inhibit release of lipoxygenase products from alveolar macrophages from wheezy infants.[164] The treatment of rats for ten days with dexamethasone stimulated in the brain an inflammatory 5-lipoxygenase gene expression.[165]

Lymphocytes, when stimulated by antigen or other agents release a variety of cytokines. GM-CSF, IL-13, and TGF-γ increase expression of 5-lipoxygenase and FLAP. Glucocorticoids induce expression of 5-lipoxygenase and FLAP independently and augment the effect of these cytokines without blocking their release from lymphocytes. The net effect is increased capacity for leukotriene synthesis.[163] These studies suggest that leukotriene modifiers are capable of controlling an important part of the asthma inflammatory process, not controlled by glucocorticoids. Subjects treated even with high doses of ICS excreted significant quantities of leukotrienes into the urine. The hypothesis that corticosteroids inhibit eicosanoid formation in vivo, cannot be sustained.[166] There is good evidence that leukotriene receptor antagonists have complementary action to ICS in asthma.[167]

Montelukast also provides additional asthma control to patients benefiting from, but incompletely controlled on ICS.[144] Therefore, in patients with moderate-to-severe persistent asthma, leukotriene modifiers can be combined with lower doses of ICS to maintain control of asthma or can be added to an existing regimen to achieve better control of asthma.[161]

Leukotriene modifiers, the first new class of anti-asthma drugs to become available in the past 25 years, act across the whole spectrum of asthma severity. Based on the published data and on the results of the CAMP study,[46] the leukotriene antagonists, montelukast and zafilukast may be recommended in children and adolescents as a first-line drug for patients with mild persistent asthma (as an option for low-dose ICS) and with asthma-induced by exercise. However, at present the European guidelines and indications for use do not include these drugs as first-line monotherapy.

Prospective, long-term trials with leukotriene modifiers, compared to well-established treatments in asthmatic children and adolescents, will be awaited with great interest, for more specific recommendations of their role and place in asthma treatment.

Long-acting inhaled β_2-agonists

Formoterol and salmeterol are long acting β_2-agonists when taken by inhalation with effects lasting for up to 12 hours, both in adults and children.[168] Like short acting β_2-agonists, their primary effect is on airway smooth-muscle relaxation. There is no evidence that they have any beneficial effect on chronic airway inflammation.[169] Again, like short acting β_2-agonists, there is concern that, used as sole treatment for asthma, tolerance may occur.[170] Whether or not ICS will prevent the development of tolerance is unresolved, with some studies suggesting the development of tolerance, irrespective of ICS usage.[171] Overall, side-effects are similar to those for short-acting beta-agonists.

Notwithstanding the potential for tolerance, clinical studies have shown that the addition of long-acting inhaled beta-agonists to ICS therapy is every bit as good, if not better, than merely increasing the dose of ICS.[172,173] Furthermore, it has been shown to be more efficacious as add-on therapy than theophylline.[174] Similar benefits were achieved with formoterol.[175] Formoterol, however, has a more rapid onset of action, though the duration of effect is similar.[176] As meta-analysis has shown conclusively that the combination of long acting β_2-agonists with ICS is efficacious and better than increasing ICS,[177] there has been an inevitable move to producing combined formulations. Several studies have now been conducted with the combination of salmeterol and fluticasone, showing efficacy with potential for improved compliance, compared with administration of the components separately.[178,179]

One study has compared the use of a long-acting β_2-agonist with a leukotriene antagonist as add-on to ICS for asthma control over a four-week trial, suggesting greater efficacy for the long acting beta agonist.[141] However, in a comparison of a leukotriene antagonist with a long-acting β_2-agonist in relation to protection against exercise-induced bronchoconstriction, the leukotriene antagonist had a sustained effect, compared with some loss of efficacy with continuing long-acting beta-agonist over eight weeks.[140,180]

Positioning in treatment algorithm

The decision on which add-on therapy to employ may be dictated by cost, availability and issues of compliance. Based on the higher compliance and facility of administration with oral drugs, anti-leukotrienes could be the first choice. However, if after 3–4 weeks there is no clinical improvement, they should be substituted by long-acting beta-agonists. For poor regions, as discussed above, slow-release theophyllines are the preferred alternative.

STRATEGIES IN RELATIVELY STEROID-INSENSITIVE PATIENTS

Alternative drugs in chronic asthma therapy

Patients with severe asthma often require chronically administered oral glucocorticoid (GC) therapy to control their disease. Unfortunately, long-term oral GC therapy is associated with multiple debilitating effects, and there is a small subset of severe asthmatics that continue to demonstrate poor disease control despite aggressive conventional therapy, including the use of oral GC.

There are several medications used in the treatment of asthma that may reduce the requirement of oral or inhaled steroids, and they are called steroid sparing agents.

Several therapies for asthma have been considered as steroid-sparing agents. Intravenous immunoglobulins (IVIG), methotrexate (MTX), gold, cyclosporin A and troleandomycin (TAO) and other macrolides are among the main agents which have been evaluated as anti-inflammatory alternatives in severe asthma. Owing to side-effects, these therapies are indicated only as an additional therapy to reduce the requirement of oral GC.

Intravenous immunoglobulins

Intravenous immunoglobulins (IVIG) are sterile solutions of pooled, polyspecific human IgG. IVIG preparations were initially used only in the therapy of immunodeficiency disorders.[181]

Over the past decade, however, IVIG has been increasingly used in the therapy of a variety of autoimmune diseases and as a GC-sparing agent in asthma.[182]

Mechanisms of action
The mechanisms involved in its GC-sparing effects are largely unknown but may involve immunomodulation. In this regard, IVIG has been shown to reduce immediate skin test reactivity to allergens, inhibit lymphocyte activation in vivo and limit cytokine production.[183]

Because IVIG may act in suppressing T-lymphocyte activation by inhibiting IL-2 and IL-4 production, Spahn et al. hypothesized that asthmatic subjects on IVIG therapy would become more sensitive to GCs as a consequence of diminution of the inflammatory response and improvement in GCR-binding affinity.[184]

There are a number of possible mechanisms by which IVIG may modulate IgE-mediated responses. IVIG may inhibit the differentiation of B-cells to antibody-secreting cells.[185] Allergen-specific IgG present in the IVIG may neutralize the allergen, preventing (blocking) the allergen interaction with cell-bound IgE. IVIG may also down-regulate allergen-specific IgE production through anti-idiotypic antibodies, which have been shown to be present in IVIG preparations.[186] Vrugt et al.,[187] reporting two patients with severe corticosteroid-insensitive asthma, showed that treatment with IVIG produced a reduction in markers of disease activity in peripheral blood as well as a decrease in numbers of all cell types on bronchial biopsies (CD3+, CD4+ and activated CD25+ T lymphocytes).

Efficacy
Page et al.[188] treated five children with asthma and IgG subclass deficiency. They received a dose of 100–300 mg/kg IVIG monthly. There were noticeable improvements in many disease aspects, including pulmonary function, hospital admission rates, school absenteeism, medication requirements, signs and symptoms of sinopulmonary infection and asthma. Mazer and Gelfand[189] reported on the efficacy of IVIG as a steroid-sparing agent in severe, steroid-dependent asthmatic children. Their patients received IVIG in a dose of 1 g/kg as a 6% solution on two consecutive days monthly, for a total of six months. Clinical symptom scores, frequency of asthma exacerbations and peak expiratory flow rates were improved. Landewehr et al.[190] determined the efficacy of IVIG in severe asthma to reduce steroid requirements in an adolescent group. This effect was observed without deterioration of lung function. In severe asthmatic patients, Salmun et al.[191] observed a significant reduction in oral steroid requirement in both the IVIG-treated ($n = 16$) and the placebo-treated ($n = 12$) groups. In a subgroup ($n = 9$) of patients requiring high doses of oral steroids (> 2000 mg in the year before the study), treatment with IVIG had a significant steroid-sparing effect, which was not observed in the placebo-treated subgroup ($n = 8$). However, two recent papers were disappointing in that no benefits were seen after treatment with IVIG. Niggemann et al.,[192] in a prospective, double-blind, placebo-controlled study, investigated 31 children and adolescents, with severe asthma. Patients were treated with high-dose IVIG (1 g/kg body weight) or identical doses of human serum albumin, as placebo. Treatment with IVIG did not show a significant reduction in the incidence of upper respiratory tract infections; neither asthma severity nor bronchial hyperreactivity were affected by the treatment. Kishiyama et al.[193] treated severe, steroid-dependent asthmatic patients, between 6 and 68 years of age, with IVIG, 1 or 2 g/kg/month. In this randomised, double-blind, placebo-controlled multicentre study, high doses of IVIG did not demonstrate a clinically or statistically significant advantage over albumin (placebo). In the high-dose IVIG-treated group, three patients were hospitalised with aseptic meningitis.

Adverse reactions
The most frequent side-effect observed with IVIG therapy in asthma is headache, often 24–72 hours after completion of the infusion.[194] Other several reactions to IVIG therapy have been described: acute 'phlogistic reactions', anaphylactic reactions, aseptic meningitis,

haemolytic anaemia and transmission of viral infections.[195] Despite all the advances that have been obtained on the role of fractionation technology in ensuring the viral safety of IVIG, several cases of hepatitis C virus infection have been reported in association to IVIG.[196] During the period June 1985–November 1998, the FDA received 120 reports worldwide of renal adverse effects (RAE) (i.e. acute renal failure or insufficiency). The exact pathophysiology of RAE development following administration of various IVIG preparations remains unclear.[197]

Thus the potential beneficial role of IVIG in patients with severe asthma on high doses of oral corticosteroids, must be confirmed in larger, long-term controlled trials. At present, it does not even reach level 6 in the evidence base and, therefore, cannot be recommended.

Methotrexate

Methotrexate (MTX) is a potent inhibitor of DNA synthesis and, at low doses, has several anti-inflammatory properties. In low doses, MTX does not affect T-cells, B-cells or NK-cell function nor does it suppress macrophage function or immunoglobulin levels. It can inhibit neutrophils chemotaxis and the activity of IL-1 and blocks the release of inflammatory mediators from basophils.[198,199]

Efficacy
Preliminary studies suggested that MTX might be useful in treating steroid-dependent bronchial asthma. Aaron et al.[200] by using a meta-analysis, showed a relatively small benefit with its use in adults with severe asthma. Marin,[201] in a more recent meta-analysis on MTX usage in steroid-dependent asthmatic adults, concluded that low-dose MTX has a significant steroid-sparing effect, mainly when used for a long period. Vrugt et al.,[202] studying peripheral blood and endobronchial biopsies in eight patients with severe steroid-dependent atopic asthma after an 8-week treatment period with MTX, suggested that the steroid-sparing effect originated from increased sensitivity of lymphocytes to the modulatory inhibitory effects of glucocorticoids. MTX treatment was also associated with a significant fall in serum levels of free IL-8.

There are few studies using MTX in asthmatic children and all of them enrolled only a small number of patients. Stempel et al.[203] used MTX in five teenagers with severe steroid-dependent asthma. With three of these patients, it was possible completely to withdraw the corticosteroid during the MTX period and with the others, the initial doses were reduced at least by 50%. Guss et al.[204] treated seven severe asthmatic children with MTX and observed a reducing need for systemic corticosteroids. They concluded that the benefits of MTX in this group of severe asthmatics appeared to justify the potential risks involved in its use. Solé et al.[205] evaluated the action of methotrexate in eight severely steroid-dependent asthmatic children. After the third month of treatment, they observed a reduction of 56% of the initial dose of prednisone.

Administration
The usual regimen for the treatment of asthma is 10 mg/m^2 body surface area as a single dose per week.

Adverse reactions
Nausea, vomiting and abdominal pain are the main side-effects with MTX use in low doses. Pancytopenia, liver fibrosis, cirrhosis and lung fibrosis are toxic effects that may occur with patients receiving long-term treatment with MTX.[206]

Foods and drugs interactions
After oral administration, MTX absorption is dose-dependent and is affected by food intake. MTX excretion is mainly renal, and around 90% is eliminated within 24 hours.[207]

Various drugs interfere in the clearance of MTX, increasing its half-life and the risk of side-effects. These drugs are: probenecid, diuretics, non-steroidal anti-inflammatories, salicylates and sulphonamides.[208]

Methotrexate should be used by experienced physicians only in patients with severe asthma on long-term oral steroids (significant side-effects) despite high-dose inhaled steroids. There is at least level 5 evidence to justify its use in children.

Gold

The anti-inflammatory properties of gold salts have made them potentially attractive agents for the treatment of chronic asthma, but their exact mechanism is unknown, although they do possess activity against T-cells. The first studies on gold therapy in the management of severe asthma were open trials. In 1994, Honma et al. performed a double-blind clinical trial in 19 adult asymptomatic asthmatic subjects to investigate the mechanism of action of oral gold, auranofin, 3 mg twice a day. They showed a decrease on non-specific bronchial hyper-responsiveness to methacoline.[209] A large well-controlled trial (eight months) in 279 adult steroid-dependent asthmatic patients showed that the proportion of patients in the auranofin group achieving therapeutic success (reduction of daily oral steroid use by 50% or more) was 41%, which was significantly higher than that in the placebo group (27%).[210] Gold salts are associated with side-effects; the incidence is less with the oral preparation (auranofin), compared to intramuscular gold. The adverse effects include dermatitis, gastrointestinal disturbances, stomatitis, blood dyscrasias and changes in liver function.[211]

There are no reported studies of gold therapy in the management of severe childhood asthma, although gold salts are used in childhood progressive rheumatoid arthritis.[212]

Cyclosporin-A

Cyclosporin-A (CsA) acts as an immunosuppressant by blocking an early phase of a developing immune response. The principal targets of this drug are the CD4+ helper T lymphocytes. It inhibits the production of the cytokines, IL-2, IL-4, IL-5 and TNFα.[211] Placebo-controlled studies showed contradictory results in the steroid-sparing effect of CsA in cortico-steroid-dependent adult asthmatics.[213,214] In a double-blind, placebo-controlled study on the effects of CsA on allergen-induced bronchoconstriction, only the late asthmatic response could be abrogated. These data would support the idea that CsA in asthma inhibits T-lymphocytes rather than mast cells.[215] Mori et al.,[216] studied the effects of dexamethasone, FK506, CsA and nonactin on the synthesis control of IL-5 by human helper T-cells and eosinophilic inflammation in a murine asthma model. Dexamethasone, FK506 and CsA suppressed the production of IL-2, IL-4 and IL-5, by human helper T-cells. CsA and dexamethasone inhibited airway eosinophilia in vivo. The evidence on the action of CsA on airway inflammation in asthma, may suggest its use as an effective alternative treatment in severe, steroid-dependent asthmatics.

The main adverse effect of low-dose CsA is decreased renal function. Other side-effects in adults include hirsutism, paraesthesia, mild hypertension, headaches and tremor.[217] There is only one report on the use of CsA (5 mg/kg daily) in five children with severe asthma, requiring at least 10 mg of prednisone daily. The study was conducted over a period of 18 months. Trough whole blood CsA concentration was measured every 2–3 weeks and the dose was titrated to maintain blood concentrations 80–150 mg/l. In the cases described, four patients were weaned from prednisolone, but one quickly relapsed. One patient did not respond. Three patients complained of hirsutism. None of the patients had any rise in creatinine, potassium, or blood pressure over baseline. In this open trial, the benefit of CsA was lost once treatment was stopped.[218] Thus at present, evidence is too flimsy to make any recommendations on the use of CsA.

Troleandomycin and other macrolide antibiotics

Macrolide antibiotics, especially troleandomycin (TAO)[219] and erythromycin,[220] are able to reduce the elimination of methylprednisolone (MPn). TAO permits a considerable reduction in steroid dose requirements and thus produces a steroid-sparing effect. This effect is observed only when TAO is associated to MPn, but not if associated with prednisone administration.[118] TAO and other macrolides provide a selective inhibition of MPn metabolism. The reason for the effectiveness of TAO plus MPn is unknown. Possibly these drugs work together to stabilize the human basophil membrane, with impaired release of histamine or another mediators.

Fost et al.[221] showed that clarithromycin reduced MPn clearance by 65%, with a concomitant significantly higher mean plasma MPn concentration. The interactions between these two drugs showed potential steroid-enhancing effects. Clarythromycin was used as a solo therapy in 17 adult asthmatics. After eight weeks of treatment, there was a significant decrease in symptoms, bronchial responsiveness to methacholine, blood and sputum eosinophil counts, and sputum ECP levels.[222] In 14 adult patients with aspirin-sensitive asthma, the administration of roxithromycin for eight weeks was able to decrease not only asthmatic symptoms, but also the numbers of eosinophils and the concentrations of ECP in blood and induced sputum. Roxithromycin did not affect excretion of urinary LTE4 after challenge with sulpyrine; these results suggest that not only leukotriene overproduction, but also eosinophil-mediated bronchial inflammation are involved in the pathogenesis of aspirin-sensitive asthma.[223]

There are few clinical trials in asthmatic children, using macrolides. Eitches et al.[224] treated 11 asthmatic steroid-dependent children with TAO in association to MPn. After 12–28 months, patients required fewer emergency visits and hospitalizations and missed fewer days of school. However, all patients remained on TAO and continued to be steroid-dependent, although at reduced dosages. The patients' pulmonary function test results improved rapidly during the first week of treatment and continued to improve throughout the year. There was a suggestion that TAO may decrease bronchial hyperresponsiveness to methacholine in severely asthmatic children.[225]

Flotte et al.[226] administered TAO plus MPn in nine children with steroid-dependent asthma. They obtained a significant decrease in requirement of corticosteroids and in the number of hospitalizations. However, the incidence of steroid side-effects increased, despite the decrease in the amount of steroid required. These authors concluded that although TAO appears to be efficacious, caution is warranted for its use in younger children with steroid-dependent asthma. Kamada et al. treated 18 children with severe, steroid-requiring asthma, with TAO, for 12 weeks. They suggested that TAO may be a reasonable alternative treatment in a limited trial for patients who are unable to tolerate tapering of their GC dosage.[227] In a double-blind, placebo-controlled study, 25 children with bronchiectasis and increased airway responsiveness to methacholine were treated with roxithromycin for 12 weeks. The use of this macrolide decreased the degree of airway responsiveness.[228]

The anti-inflammatory/immunomodulatory activities in vivo and in vitro seem to be limited to the 14-membered ring macrolides, such as erythromycin, roxithromycin and clarithromycin.[229–231] The mechanisms by which macrolides inhibit mucus production are not clear.[236] The anti-bacterial action of these antibiotics might be considered, since the airway inflammation of asthma may reflect, at least in some patients, an immune response to chronic infection such as with mycoplasma or chlamydia.[232]

Adverse reactions
Major side effects include elevated liver function tests, gastrointestinal tract symptoms, increased cushingoid effects and altered moods.[233]

Drugs interactions
TAO can interact with theophylline, MPn, oral contraceptives, and even anticonvulsant agents, such as carbamazepine and ergotamines.[234]

The combined therapy of macrolide antibiotics and MPn, or only macrolides, should be approached cautiously in children and reserved for children with severe steroid-dependent asthma, despite the use of other alternative strategies. Macrolide antibiotics must still be considered experimental therapy in children.

FUTURE PERSPECTIVES ON ASTHMA MANAGEMENT

For centuries, the initial treatment for asthma was directed towards relieving bronchoconstriction. Recent emphasis has been placed on the control of inflammation, especially using corticosteroids. The constant advances in unravelling the molecular mechanisms of atopy (asthma), are identifying new targets for novel therapies in the future.[235,236] The following section will focus upon novel approaches for the management of human asthma that may or may not become therapeutic options in the future.

Anti IL-5

IL-5 may be an important target in the cascade of allergic inflammation. This cytokine is important in eosinophil differentiation, survival, activation and chemotaxis. A humanized IL-5 monoclonal antibody, SB-240563,[237] was given to patients with asthma.[238] A single injection was well tolerated, reducing blood eosinophils for over three months and preventing eosinophil recruitment into the airways after allergen challenge. This treatment did not modify the early and late reactions or airway hyperresponsiveness to the allergen challenge. These observations cast doubtfulness on the role of eosinophils in these responses. Humanized monoclonal antibodies to IL-5, SB-240563 and CH5570 are now in phase II of clinical trials.[237]

Anti IL-4

IL-4 is pre-eminent in the induction of Th-2 responses with the consequent synthesis of IgE by B lymphocytes. Neutralization of IL-4 through the use of a humanized monoclonal antibody, SB-240683, is in phase II of clinical trials.[237] However, the inhibition of IL-4 by nebulized soluble IL-4 receptors.[238] was efficacious in patients with moderate asthma and, when given as a once weekly nebulization, prevented deterioration in asthma after reduction of ICS.

Interferon gamma (IFN-γ)

IFN-γ is produced by Th-1 cells and inhibits production if IL-4 and other cytokines by Th-2 cells. It also antagonizes the IgE-promoting effects of IL-4 and IL-13. INF-γ by nebulization to asthmatic patients did not significantly reduce eosinophilic inflammation induced by allergen exposure.[236] More studies are required to establish whether it has any place in asthma management. However, detection of raised IFN-γ in broncho-alveolar lavage (BAL) fluid from children and adults with asthma suggests that it is unlikely to have any value.

IL-12

Recombinant human IL-12 (rhIL-12) has severe toxic effects when administered by intravenous injections every three weeks.[239] In asthmatic patients, IL-12 administration, in a similar way to IL-5 injections, was able to reduce circulating eosinophils without inhibiting allergen responses or reducing airway hyperresponsiveness.[236] As IL-12 has its effects through promotion of IFN-γ production, it is unlikely to have a major role in asthma therapy.

Anti-IGE

IgE plays a central role in the cascade of biochemical events that result in allergic reactions.[240] The reduction in available antigen-specific IgE to bind to and sensitize mast cells would reduce IgE-mediated symptoms and improve control of allergic diseases and perhaps asthma. A recombinant humanized (IgG1) monoclonal antibody (rhuMAb-E25) is in phase III of clinical trials.[237] This antibody recognises IgE at the same site as the high-affinity receptor for IgE (FcεRI) and forms complexes with the free, unbound IgE but not with IgG or IgA. The use of rhuMAb-E25 in asthmatic patients attenuates the early- and late-phase reactions to inhaled allergens. The postulated beneficial efficacy in human asthma was investigated in 317 patients, aged 11–50 years, with moderate-to-severe perennial allergic asthma.[241] A single dose of rhuMab-E25 rapidly reduced serum-free IgE concentrations by more than 95%. The humanized antibody was well tolerated and after 20 weeks of treatment, none had antibodies against rhuMAb-E25. The primary outcome of efficacy, the daily asthma symptom score, was more improved in the active-treatment group than in the placebo group, despite the fact that all subjects received oral or inhaled corticosteroids, or both, at doses that optimized pulmonary function.[241] Although this represents an important advance in the management of asthma, repeated injections may not be feasible for the long-term treatment of moderate asthmatics and will probably be reserved for more severe forms of asthma.[236]

Phosphodiesterase inhibitors (PDE)

Increases in intracellular cyclic 3'5' adenosine monophosphate (cAMP) result in airways smooth-muscle relaxation and bronchodilation. Stimulation of β_2-receptors results in increased synthesis of cAMP by stimulating adenyl cyclase. Higher levels can also be maintained by preventing breakdown of cAMP by inhibition of cyclic nucleotide phosphodiesterases (PDE). PDE III and PDE IV inhibitors provide the greatest airway smooth-muscle relaxation in humans. Relaxation is also seen with non-selective PDE inhibitors, such as theophylline.

Owing to their bronchodilator and anti-inflammatory properties, there is considerable interest in the development of PDE4 inhibitors for the treatment of inflammatory diseases such as asthma. New PDE inhibitors are currently being developed for the treatment of asthma, although side-effects, including nausea and vomiting, have delayed the introduction of this class of drugs into clinical practice.[236] Thus, very few studies have been published concerning the efficacy of these PDE inhibitors in the treatment of asthma, especially in children. The use of these drugs is still experimental.

MUCOLYTICS AND EXPECTORANTS

The inflammatory response in the airways of asthmatic patients is frequently accompanied with mucus hypersecretion. The increased quantity of airway secretions associated to the impaired airway mucociliary clearance is an important component in airway obstruction, associated to mucosal oedema and bronchial smooth-muscle contraction.

Mucolytics are agents that break down the fibrillar molecules of mucoproteins into smaller, less viscous subunits.[242] The most effective mucolytic is acetyl cysteine. However, its use is not recommended in the treatment of asthmatics, since acetyl cysteine is highly irritating on inhalation and may provoke further bronchoconstriction.

An expectorant is an agent that is taken by mouth to produce an increased volume of sputum that can be coughed out more easily. Iodide is probably the oldest expectorant; it was in fashion for many years as a saturated solution of potassium iodide. It is no longer used owing to no proof of efficacy and to many side-effects on the skin (rash), salivary glands and thyroid gland. Guaifenasin (glyceril guaicolate) is the most popular expectorant. Despite its wide use, there is no demonstrable expectorant effect. There are no convincing studies in asthma on the expectorant action of bromhexine and its derivative, ambroxol.[242] Sputum is defined as expectorated lower respiratory secretions. An aerosol of hypertonic saline solution, generated from an ultrasonic nebulizer, permits sputum to be obtained when it is not produced spontaneously. The mechanism by which a hypertonic saline solution induces sputum is not known.[243] Induced sputum is a research tool for assessment of airway inflammation in asthma and in other pulmonary diseases.

Beta adrenergic agonists and methylxantines have beneficial but variable mucociliary effects.[244] Several products released during the inflammatory response in asthma are involved in the secretion of viscous mucus in the airways. Glucocorticoids are able to reduce mucus secretions in the airways because of inhibition of synthesis and release of inflammatory products and other mucus secretagogues. Glucocorticoids can also have a direct activity on the submucosal glands as well as the restoration of the normal epithelial/goblet cell ratio.[245]

Until appropriately controlled clinical trials have been conducted in carefully selected and homogeneous populations of asthmatic children, the benefits of mucolytic and expectorant therapy remain unknown. These drugs have been superseded by other anti-asthma drugs of proven efficacy. However, it must be remembered that the most cost-effective mucolytic preparation is water, for adequate hydration.

MUSCARINIC RECEPTOR ANTAGONISTS

The use of anticholinergics in chronic asthmatic patients has not been established. Regular treatment has not been shown to improve symptoms or diurnal variation in airway calibre.[246] Single-dose studies showed a small additional effect of either a second dose of β-agonist, terbutaline or ipratropium bromide, after a single dose of terbutaline.[247] There was a significantly greater benefit in favour of the latter two-drug combination suggesting that more trials are required to evaluate long-term use of muscarinic receptor antagonists in childhood asthma management.

Muscarinic receptor subtype antagonists

Anticholinergics, such as atropine and ipratropium bromide, block all muscarinic receptors, in a non-specific way. Blocking M_2 receptors may result in increased acetylcholine release. Tiotropium bromide is a long-acting anticholinergic drug that has some of the desirable features in the order of interaction with muscarinic receptors: $M_3 > M_1 > M_2$. Tiotropium bromide provides long-lasting bronchodilation (greater than 24 hours) and protects against methacholine-induced bronchoconstriction for 48 hours. Tiotropium has been well tolerated.[240] Clinical trials are awaited.

COMPLEMENTARY AND ALTERNATIVE MEDICINE

Complementary and alternative medicine (CAM) is a broad domain of different therapeutic procedures, not endorsed by our scientific practice of medicine, for the management of several diseases, including asthma, and mainly used in Asia.[248]

In general, in the management of asthma, these practices (acupuncture, homeopathy, herbal medicine, Ayurvedic medicine and many others) are not validated by conventional research standards, and their effectiveness is largely unproven.[249] Nevertheless, they are used by a large part of the population in the USA[250,251] and in many other countries. Owing to limited positive results and side-effects of conventional therapies in some patients; to the high costs of drugs; and to social and cultural factors, the demand from patients to use CAM for the treatment of asthma has been increasing. In this scenario, the patient must be warned that the abandonment of regular treatment is potentially dangerous, and the chosen CAM should be complementary and not an alternative to the standard treatment. Contrary to the rigorous standards required for conventional drugs, there are no requirements on efficacy and safety for homeopathic solutions and herbal remedies. There are reports of serious adverse effects associated with using CAM, and there is no support for the public perception that these treatments are 'natural' and, therefore, safe.[249]

Acupuncture, homeopathy and breathing exercises for chronic asthma were recently reviewed by the Cochrane Foundation.[252–254] The conclusion is similar: there is not enough evidence reliably to assess the possible role or to make recommendations about the value of these procedures in asthma treatment.

Herbal medicines for the treatment of asthma are especially popular in Asia. Until now, no controlled studies have been reported.[255]

The above CAM methods deserves attention in well-conducted clinical trials owing to the increase in the proportion of the population seeking CAM therapies.[256] The US National

Institutes of Health established a 'National Center for Complementary and Alternative Medicine' for the scientific evaluation of these procedures. Information and references on CAM can be obtained at http://nccam.nih.gov.

We do not endorse or recommend CAM procedures for the management of asthma in children. We believe that the therapies described throughout this chapter represent the state of art on evidence-based medicine and are able to control the disease and to improve the quality of life of millions of asthmatic children.

SUMMARY

The majority of older children with asthma can be returned to a normal existence, using a simple pharmacotherapeutic approach. For children with infrequent episodic asthma who have normal lung function between episodes, inhaled β_2-agonists can be used as necessary and may also be used for predosing to cover exercise-induced symptoms. However, there should be a low threshold for the introduction of preventive medications once the frequency of symptoms increases. If there is any evidence of abnormal spirometry between episodes, then prophylaxis is mandatory. The choice of first prophylaxis rests between four times daily sodium cromoglycate or low dose inhaled corticosteroid (200 µg/day of BDP or equivalent), twice daily.

For persistent asthma, where there is abnormal lung function between episodes, inhaled corticosteroids are necessary, and the dose should be titrated to achieve optimal control. However, before increasing the dose beyond 400 µg of BDP or equivalent per day, the use of concomitant long-acting beta-agonists or slow release theophylline or leukotriene receptor antagonists should be considered. The choice will depend on availability, cost, age of the patient and side-effect profiles.

Using evidence-based approaches, the focus of management is almost exclusively on inhaled β_2-specific agonists and inhaled corticosteroids. However, evidence also suggests that oral compounds achieve higher compliance rates, and both theophyllines and leukotriene receptor antagonists do have some anti-inflammatory properties, which suggests that they will at least have a contributory role as 'controllers' as well as having bronchodilator effects.

While there are potentially exciting new developments in asthma management under trial in adults, the only new modalities which have appeared for children with asthma in the last 30 years are leukotriene receptor antagonists.

REFERENCES

1. Maimonides M. *Treatise of Asthma*. Munter M translator. Philadelphia (PA): Lippincott, 1963.
2. Warner JO, Gotz M, Landau LI et al. Management of asthma: a consensus statement. *Arch Dis Child* 1989; **64**: 1065–79.
3. International Paediatric Asthma Consensus Group. Asthma: a follow-up statement. *Arch Dis Child* 1992; **67**: 240–8.
4. Warner JO, Naspitz CK. Third International Pediatric Consensus Statement on the management of childhood asthma. *Pediatr Pulmonol* 1998; **25**: 1–17.
5. Global Initiative for Asthma. *Global Strategy for Asthma Management and Prevention*. WHO/NHLBI Workshop Report. Bethesda (MD): National Institutes of Health Publication No. 95-3659, 1995: 1–48.
6. NIH. *Highlights of the Expert Panel Report 2: Guidelines for the diagnosis and management of asthma*. Bethesda (MD): National Institutes of Health Publication No. 97-4051A, 1997: 1–50.
7. British Asthma Guidelines Co-ordinating Committee. British Guidelines on Asthma Management: 1995 Review and Position Statement. *Thorax* 1997; **52** (Suppl): 1–21.
8. Scottish Intercollegiate Guideline Network. *An Introduction to SIGN Methodology for Development of Evidence-Based Guidelines*. Edinburgh: SIGN Publication No. 39 RCP, 1999: 1–34.
9. Agertoft LA, Pedersen S. Effects of long-term treatment with an inhaled corticosteroid on growth and pulmonary function in asthmatic children. *Respir Med* 1994; **88**: 373–81.
10. Oswald H, Phelan PD, Lannigan A et al. Childhood asthma and lung function in mid-adult life. *Pediatr Pulmonol* 1997; **23**: 14–20.
11. Gerritsen J, Koeter GH, Postma DS et al.

Airway responsiveness in childhood as a predictor of the outcome of asthma in adulthood. *Am Rev Respir Dis* 1991; **143**: 1468–9.
12. Warner JO. Review of prescribed treatment for children with asthma in 1990. *BMJ* 1995; **311**: 663–6.
13. Newhouse MT, Dolovich MB. Control of asthma by aerosols. *N Engl J Med* 1986; **315**: 870–4.
14. Page CP. Theophylline as an anti-inflammatory agent. *Eur Respir Rev* 1996; **6**: 74–8.
15. Garcia-Marcos L, Schuster A. New perspectives for asthma treatment: anti-leukotriene drugs. *Pediatr Allergy Immunol* 1999; **10**: 77–88.
16. Kavuru M, Melamed J, Gross G et al. Salmeterol and fluticasone propionate combined in a new powder inhalation device for the treatment of asthma: a randomised double-blind placebo controlled trial. *J Allergy Clin Immunol* 2000; **105**: 1108–16.
17. Nelson HS. Beta adrenergic bronchodilators. *N Engl J Med* 1995; **333**: 499–506.
18. Brittain RT, Dean M, Jack D. Sympathicominetic bronchodilator drugs. *Pharmacol Ther* 1976; **2**: 423–62.
19. Burgess CD, Windom HH, Pearce N. Lack of evidence for β$_2$ receptor selectivity: a study of metaproterranol, fenoterol, isoproterranol and ipinephrine in patients with asthma. *Am Rev Respir Dis* 1991; **143**: 444–6.
20. Wong CS, Pavord ID, Williams J et al. Bronchodilator, cardiovascular and hypocalaemic effects of fenoterol, salbutamol and terbutaline in asthma. *Lancet* 1990; **336**: 1396–9.
21. Henriksen JM, Agertoft L, Pedersen S. Bronchoprotective effect and duration of action of inhaled formoterol and salbutamol on exercise induced asthma in children. *J Allergy Clin Immunol* 1992; **89**: 1176–82.
22. Williams SJ, Winner SJ, Clark TJH. Comparison of inhaled and intravenous terbutaline in acute severe asthma. *Thorax* 1981; **36**: 629–31.
23. Pedersen S. Aerosol treatment of bronchoconstriction in children with or without a tube spacer. *N Engl J Med* 1985; **308**: 1328–30.
24. Bengtsson B, Fagerstrom PO. Extra pulmonary effects of terbutaline during prolonged administration. *Clin Pharmacol Ther* 1982; **31**: 726–32.
25. Hall IP. β$_2$-adrenoceptor polymorphisms and asthma. *Clin Exp Allergy* 1999; **29**: 1151-4.
26. Aldridge RE, Hancox RJ, Taylor DR et al. Effects of terbutaline and budesonide on sputum cells and bronchial hyperresponsiveness in asthma. *Am J Respir Crit Care Med* 2000; **161**: 1459–64.
27. Cockcroft DW, Swystun VA, Bhagat R. Interaction of inhaled β$_2$ agonist and inhaled corticosteroid on airway responsiveness to allergen and metacholine. *Am J Respir Crit Care Med* 1995; **152**: 1485–9.
28. Sears MR, Taylor DR, Print CG. Regular inhaled beta-agonist treatment in bronchial asthma. *Lancet* 1990; **336**: 1391–6.
29. Kerrebijn KF, van Essen-Zandvliet EEM, Neijens HJ. Effect of long-term treatment with inhaled corticosteroids and beta-agonists on the bronchial responsiveness of children with asthma. *J Allergy Clin Immunol* 1987; **79**: 653–9.
30. Crane J, Pearce N, Flatt A. Prescribed fenoterol and death from asthma in New Zealand. *Lancet* 1989; **1**: 917–22.
31. Spitzer WO, Suissa S, Ernst P. The use of beta-agonists and the risk of death and near death from asthma. *N Engl J Med* 1992; **326**: 501–7.
32. Mullen M, Mullen B, Carey M. The association between beta-agonist use and death from asthma. *J Am Med Assoc* 1993; **270**: 1842–5.
33. Altounyan REC. Inhibition of experimental asthma by a new compound – disodium cromoglycate (intal). *Acta Allergol* 1967; **22**: 487.
34. Norris AA. Pharmacology of sodium cromoglycate. *Clin Exp Allergy* 1996; **26**(Suppl 4): 5–7.
35. Cockcroft DW, Murdoch KY. Comparative effects of inhaled salbutamol, sodium cromoglycate and BDP on allergen induced early asthmatic responses, late asthmatic responses and increased responsiveness to histamine. *J Allergy Clin Immunol* 1987; **79**: 734–40.
36. Diaz P, Galleguillos FR, Gonzalez MC et al. Bronchoalveolar lavage in asthma: the effect of disodium cromoglycate (cromolyn) on leukocyte counts, immunoglobulins and complement. *J Allergy Clin Immunol* 1984; **74**: 41–8.
37. Walker SR, Evans ME, Richards AJ, Patterson JW. The fate of disodium cromoglycate in man. *J Pharm Pharmacol* 1972; **24**: 525–31.
38. Silverman M, Connelly NM, Balfour L et al. Long-term trial of disodium cromoglycate and isoprenaline in children with asthma. *BMJ* 1972; **3**: 378–81.
39. Eigen H, Reid JJ, Dahl R et al. Evaluation of the addition of cromolyn sodium to bronchodilator maintenance therapy in the long-term management of asthma. *J Allergy Clin Immunol* 1987; **80**: 612–21.
40. Shapiro GG, Furukawa CT, Pierson WE et al.

Double-blind evaluation of nebulised cromolyn, terbutaline and the combination for childhood asthma. *J Allergy Clin Immunol* 1988; **81:** 449–54.
41. Tasche MJA, van der Wouden JC, Eijen JHJM et al. Randomised placebo controlled trial of inhaled sodium cromoglycate in 1-4 year old children with moderate asthma. *Lancet* 1997; **350:** 1060–4.
42. Tasche MJA, Uijen JHJM, Bernsen RMD et al. Inhaled disodium cromoglycate (DSCG) as maintenance therapy in children with asthma: a systematic review. *Thorax* 2000; **55:** 913–20.
43. Price JF, Weller PH. Comparison of fluticasone propionate and sodium cromoglycate for the treatment of childhood asthma. *Respir Med* 1995; **89:** 363–8.
44. Edwards AM, Stevens MT. The clinical efficacy of inhaled nedocromil sodium (tylade) in the treatment of asthma. *Eur Respir J* 1993; **6:** 35–41.
45. Armenio L, Baldini G, Bardare M et al. Double-blind placebo controlled study of nedocromil sodium in asthma. *Arch Dis Child* 1993; **68:** 193–7.
46. The Childhood Asthma Management Program Research Group. Long-term effects of budesonide or nedocromil in children with asthma. *N Engl J Med* 2000; **343:** 1054–63.
47. Wilson JW, Djukanovic R, Howarth PH, Holgate ST. Inhaled beclomethasone dipropionate down-regulates airway lymphocyte activation in atopic asthma. *Am J Respir Crit Care Med* 1994; **149:** 86–90.
48. van Grunsven PM, Van Schayck CP, Molema J et al. Effects of inhaled corticosteroids on bronchial responsiveness in patients with 'corticosteroid naïve' mild asthma: a meta-analysis. *Thorax* 1999; **54:** 316–22.
49. Barnes PJ. Efficacy of inhaled corticosteroids in asthma. *J Allergy Clin Immunol* 1998; **102:** 531–8.
50. Lipworth BJ, Wilson AM. Dose response to inhaled corticosteroids: benefits and risks. *Sem Respir Crit Care Med* 1998; **19:** 625–46.
51. Barnes PJ, Pedersen S. Efficacy and safety of inhaled corticosteroids in asthma. *Am Rev Respir Dis* 1993; **148:** 1–26.
52. Simons FER and the Canadian Beclomethasone Dipropianate – Salmeterol Xinafoate Study Group. Comparison of beclomethasone, salmeterol and placebo in children with asthma. *N Engl J Med* 1997; **337:** 1659–65.
53. Bisgaard H, Munck SL, Neilsen JP et al. Inhaled budesonide for treatment of recurrent wheezing in early childhood. *Lancet* 1990; **336:** 649–51.
54. Mash B, Bheekie A, Jones BW. Inhaled vs. oral steroids for adults with chronic asthma. *Cochran Database Syst Review* 2000; **2:** CD002160.
55. Konig P, Shaffer J. The effect of drug therapy on long-term outcome of childhood asthma: a possible preview of the International Guidelines. *J Allergy Clin Immunol* 1996; **98:** 1103–11.
56. Williamson IJ, Matusiewicz SP, Brown PH et al. Frequency of voice problems and cough in patients using pressurized aerosol inhaled steroid preparations. *Eur Respir J* 1995; **8:** 590–2.
57. Barnes NC, Hallett C, Harris TAJ. Clinical experience with fluticasone propionate in asthma: a meta-analysis of efficacy and systemic activity compared with budesonide and beclomethasone dipropionate at half the milligram dose or less. *Respir Med* 1998; **92:** 95–104.
58. Lipworth BJ. The comparative safety/efficacy ratio of HFA-BDP. *Respir Med* 2000; **94**(Suppl D): S21–S26.
59. Lipworth BJ. Systemic adverse effects of inhaled corticosteroid therapy. A systematic review and meta-analysis. *Arch Intern Med* 1999; **159:** 941–955.
60. Brown PH, Greening AP, Crompton GK. Large volume spacer devices and the influence of high dose beclomethasone dipropionate on hypothalamic pituitary adrenal axis function. *Thorax* 1993; **48:** 233–238.
61. Crowley S, Hindmarsh PC, Honour JW, Brook CGD. Reproducibility of the cortosol response to stimulation with a low dose of ACTH: the effect of basil cortosol levels and comparison of low dose with high dose secretory dynamics. *J Endocrinol* 1993; **136:** 167–72.
62. Law CM, Marchant JL, Honour JW, Preece MA, Warner JO. Nocturnal adrenal suppression in asthmatic children taking inhaled beclomethasone diproprionate. *Lancet* 1986; **1:** 942–4.
63. Nikolaizik WH, Marchant JL, Preece MA, Warner JO. Endocrine and lung function in asthmatic children on inhaled corticosteroids. *Am J Respir Crit Care Med* 1994; **150:** 624–8.
64. Nikolaizik WH, Marchant JL, Preece MA, Warner JO. Nocturnal cortisol secretion in healthy adults before and after inhalation of Budesonide. *Am J Respir Crit Care Med* 1996; **153:** 97–101.
65. Pedersen S, Fuglsang G. Urinary cortisol excretion in children treated with high doses of inhaled corticosteroids: a comparison of budesonide and beclomethasone. *Eur Respir J* 1988; **1:** 433–5.

66. Wolthers OD, Hansen M, Juul A et al. Knemometry, urine cortisol excretion and measurements of the insulin-like growth factor axis and collagen turnover in children treated with inhaled corticosteroids. *Pediatr Res* 1997; **41:** 44–50.
67. Rao R, Gregson RK, Jones AC et al. Systemic effects of inhaled corticosteroids on growth and bone turnover in childhood asthma: a comparison of fluticasone with beclomethasone. *Eur Respir J* 1999; **13:** 87–94.
68. Hauspie R, Susanne C, Alexander F. Maturational delay and temporal growth retardation in asthmatic boys. *J Allergy Clin Immunol* 1977; **59:** 200–6.
69. Balfour-Lynn L. Growth and childhood asthma. *Arch Dis Child* 1986; **61:** 1049–55.
70. Allen DB, Mullen M, Mullen B. A meta-analysis of the effect of oral and inhaled corticosteroids on growth. *J Allergy Clin Immunol* 1994; **93:** 967–76.
71. Tinkelman DG, Reed CE, Nelson HS, Offord KP. Aerosol beclomethasone dipropionate compared with Theophylline as primary treatment for chronic, mild to moderately severe asthma in children. *Pediatrics* 1993; **92:** 64–77.
72. Silverstein MD, Younginger JW, Reed CE et al. Attained adult height after childhood asthma: effect of glucocorticoid therapy. *J Allergy Clin Immunol* 1997; **99:** 466–74.
73. Agertoft L, Pedersen S. Effect of long-term treatment with inhaled budesonide on adult height in children with asthma. *N Engl J Med* 2000; **343:** 1064–9.
74. Wolthers OD, Pedersen S. Controlled study of linear growth in asthmatic children during treatment with inhaled glucocorticoids. *Pediatrics* 1992; **89:** 839–42.
75. Wolthers OD, Pedersen S. Short term growth during treatment with inhaled fluticasone propionate and beclomethasone dipropionate. *Arch Dis Child* 1993; **68:** 673–6.
76. Agertoft L, Pedersen S. Short term knemometry and urine cortisol excretion in children treated with fluticasone propionate and budesonide: a dose response study. *Eur Respir J* 1997; **10:** 1507–12.
77. Doull IJM, Freezer NJ, Holgate ST. Growth of prepubertal children with mild asthma treated with inhaled beclomethasone dipropionate. *Am J Respir Crit Care Med* 1995; **151:** 1715–19.
78. Merkus PJFM, van Essen-Zandvliet EEN, Duiverman EJ. Long-term effect of inhaled corticosteroids on growth rate in adolescents with asthma. *Pediatrics* 1993; **91:** 1121–6.
79. Allen DB, Bronsky EA, LaForce CF et al and the Fluticasone Propionate Study Group. Growth in asthmatic children treated with fluticasone propionate. *J Pediatr* 1998; **132:** 472–477.
80. Todd G, Dunlop K, McNaboe J et al. Growth and adrenal suppression in asthmatic children treated with high dose fluticasone propionate. *Lancet* 1996; **348:** 27–29.
81. Adinoff AD, Hollister JR. Steroid induced fractures and bone loss in patients with asthma. *N Engl J Med* 1993; **309:** 265–268.
82. McEvoy CE, Ensrud KE, Bender E et al. Association between corticosteroid use and vertebral fractures in older men with chronic obstructive pulmonary disease. *Am J Respir Crit Care Med* 1998; **157:** 704–9.
83. Wong CA, Walsh LJ, Smith CJP et al. Inhaled corticosteroid use and bone mineral density in patients with asthma. *Lancet* 2000; **355:** 1399–403.
84. Baraldi E, Bollini MC, De Marchi A, Zacchello F. Effect of beclomethasone dipropionate on bone mineral content assessed by X-ray densitometry in asthmatic children: a longitudinal evaluation. *Europ Respir J* 1994; **7:** 710–14.
85. Agertoft L, Pedersen S. Bone mineral density in children with asthma receiving long-term treatment with inhaled budesonide. *Am J Respir Crit Care Med* 1998; **157:** 178–83.
86. Birkebaek NH, Esberg G, Andersen K et al. Bone and collagen turnover during treatment with inhaled dry powder budesonide and beclomethasone dipropionate. *Arch Dis Child* 1995; **73:** 524–7.
87. Simons FER, Persaud MP, Gillespie CA et al. Absence of posterior sub-capsular cataracts in young patients treated with inhaled glucocorticoids. *Lancet* 1993; **342:** 776–8.
88. Agertoft L, Larsen FE, Pedersen S. Posterior sub-capsular cataracts, bruising and hoarseness in children with asthma receiving long-term treatment with inhaled budesonide. *Eur Respir J* 1998; **12:** 130–5.
89. Mak VHF, Melchor R, Spiro S. Easy bruising as a side-effect of inhaled corticosteroids. *Eur Respir J* 1992; **5:** 1068–1074.
90. Cumming RG, Mitchell P, Leeder SR. Use of inhaled corticosteroids and the risk of cataracts. *N Engl J Med* 1997; **337:** 8–14.
91. Garbe E, Le Lorier J, Boivin J-F, Suissa S. Inhaled and nasal glucocorticoids and the risk

of ocular hypertension or open angle glaucoma. *JAMA* 1997; **27**: 722–7.
92. Pedersen S, Pedersen S, Warner JO, Price JF. Early use of inhaled steroids in children with asthma. *Clin Exp Allergy (Debate)* 1997; **27**: 995–1006.
93. Warner JO, Nikolaizik WH, Besley CR, Warner JA. A childhood asthma death in a clinical trial; potential indicators of risk. *Eur Respir J* 1998; **11**: 229–33.
94. Leung DYM, Szefler SJ. New insights into steroid resistant asthma. *Pediatr Allergy Immunol* 1998; **9**: 3–12.
95. Joad JP, Ahrens RC, Lindgren SD, Weinberger MW. Relative efficacy of maintenance therapy with theophylline, inhaled albuterol and the combination for chronic asthma. *J Allergy Clin Immunol* 1987; **79**: 78–85.
96. Kelloway JS, Wyatt RA, Adlis SA. Comparison of patient's compliance with precribed oral and inhaled asthma medications. *Arch Intern Med* 1994; **154**(12): 1349–52.
97. Aubier M, Murciano D, Viires N et al. Diaphragmatic contractility enhanced by aminophylline: role of extracellular calcium. *J Appl Physiol* 1993; **54**: 460–4.
98. Murciano D, Aubier M, Lecocquic Y et al. Effects of theophylline on diaphragmatic strengh and fatigue in patients with chronic obstructive pulmonary disease. *N Engl J Med* 1984; **311**: 349–53.
99. Linden J. Cloned adenosine A3 receptors: pharmacological properties, species differences and receptor functions. *Trends Pharmacol Sci* 1994; **15**: 298–306.
100. Barnes PJ, Pauwels RA. Theophylline in asthma: time for reappraisal? *Eur Respir J* 1994; **7**: 579–91.
101. Schudt C, Tenor H, Wendel A et al. Effect of selective phosphodiesterase (PDE) inhibitors on activation of human macrophages and lymphocytes. *Naunyn Sch Arch Pharmacol* 1992; **345**: R69 (Suppl).
102. Stephens CG, Snyderman R. Cyclic nucleotides regulate the morphologic alterations required for chemotaxis in monocytes. *J Immunol* 1982; **218**: 1192–7.
103. Spatafora M, Chiappara G, Merendino AM et al. Theophylline suppresses the release of tumor necrosis factor-α by blood monocytes and alveolar macrophages. *Eur Respir J* 1994; **7**: 223–8.
104. Kita H, Abu-Ghazaleh RI, Gleich GJ et al. Regulation of Ig-induced eosinophil degranulation by adenosine 3'5'-monophosphate. *J Immunol* 1991; **146**: 2712–18.
105. Mascali JJ, Cvietusa P, Negri J, Borish L. Anti-inflammatory effects of theophylline: modulation of cytokine production. *Ann Allergy Asthma Immunol* 1996; **77**: 34–38.
106. Minoguchi K, Kohno Y, Oda N et al. Effect of theophylline withdrawal on airway inflammation in asthma. *Clin Exp Allergy* 1998; **28**(Suppl 3): 57–63.
107. Dusdieker L, Green M, Smith GD et al. Comparison of orally administered metaproterenol and theophylline in the control of chronic asthma. *J Pediatr* 1982; **101**: 281–7.
108. Hambleton G, Weinberger M, Taylor J et al. Comparison of cromoglycate (cromolyn) and theophylline in controlling symptoms of chronic asthma: a collaborative study. *Lancet* 1977; **1**: 381–5.
109. Furukawa CT, Shapiro GG, Bierman W et al. A double-masked study comparing the effectiveness of cromolyn sodium and sustained-release theophylline in childhood asthma. *Pediatrics* 1984; **74**: 453–9.
110. Nassif EG, Wenberger M, Thompson R, Huntley W. The value of maintenance theophylline in steroid-dependent asthma. *N Engl J Med* 1981; **304**: 71–5.
111. Brenner M, Berkowitz R, Marshall N, Strunk RC. Need for theophylline in severe steroid-requiring asthmatics. *Clin Allergy* 1988; **18**: 143–50.
112. Ukena D, Harnest U, Sakalauskas R et al. Comparison of addition of theophylline to inhaled steroid with doubling the dose of inhaled steroid in asthma. *Eur Respir J* 1997; **10**: 2754–60.
113. Evans DJ, Taylor DA, Zetterstrom O et al. A comparison of low-dose inhaled budesonide plus theophylline and high-dose inhaled budesonide for moderate asthma. *N Engl J Med* 1997; **337**: 1412–18.
114. Eggleston PA, Malveaux FJ, Butz AM et al. Medications used by children with asthma living in the inner city. *Pediatrics* 1998; **101**: 349–54.
115. Hendeles L, Weinberger M, Avoidance of adverse effects during chronic therapy with theophylline. *Drug Intell Clin Pharmacol* 1980; **14**: 522–30.
116. Raj NS, Misra A, Guleria R, Pande JN. Theophylline clearance in undernourished asthma patients. *Indian J Chest Dis Allied Sci* 1998; **40(3)**: 175–8.

117. Hendeles L, Weinberger M, Szefler S. Safety and efficacy of theophylline in children with asthma. *J Pediatr* 1992; **120:** 177–83.
118. Naspitz CK, Ferguson AC, Tinkelman DG. Approaches to the treatment of chronic asthma. In: Tinkelman DG, Naspitz CK, eds. *Childhood Asthma* 2nd ed. New York: Marcel Dekker, 1993: 329–86.
119. Hui KP, Barnes NC. Lung function improvement in asthma with a cysteinyl leukotriene receptor antagonist. *Lancet* 1991; **337:** 1062–3.
120. Rouzer CA, Matsumoto T, Samuelsson B. Single protein from human leucocytes possesses 5-lipooxygenase and leukotriene A4-synthase activities. *Proc Natl Acad Sci USA* 1986; **83:** 857–61.
121. Sampson AP, Castling DP, Green CP, Price JF. Persistent increase in plasma and urinary leukotrienes after acute asthma. *Arch Dis Child* 1995; **73:** 221–5.
122. Reiss TF, Hill JB, Harman E, et al. Increased urinary excretion of LTE4 after exercise-induced bronchospasm by montelukast, a cysteinyl leukotriene receptor antagonist. *Thorax* 1997; **52:** 1030–5.
123. Taylor GW, Taylor I, Black P et al. Urinary leukotriene E4 after antigen challenge and in acute asthma and allergic rhinitis. *Lancet* 1989; **1:** 584–8.
124. Chung KF. Leukotriene receptor antagonists and biosynthesis inhibitors: potential breakthrough in asthma therapy. *Eur Respir J* 1995; **8:** 1203–13.
125. Boehner BS, Undem BJ, Lichtenstein LM. Immunological aspects of allergic asthma. *Ann Rev Immunol* 1994; **12:** 295–335.
126. Rabe KF, Munoz NM, Vita AJ et al. Contraction of human bronchial smooth muscle caused by activated human eosinophils. *Am J Physiol* 1994; **267:** 1326–34.
127. Lewis RA, Austen KF, Soberman RJ. Leukotrienes and other products of the 5-lipoxygenase pathway. Biochemistry and relation to pathobiology in human diseases. *N Engl J Med* 1990; **323:** 645–55.
128. Bisgaard H, Pedersen M. SRS – A leukotrienes decrease the activity of human respiratory cilia. *Clin Allergy* 1987; **17:** 95–103.
129. Laitinen L, Laitinen A, Haahtela T et al. Leukotriene E4 and granulocytic infiltration into asthmatic airways. *Lancet* 1993; **341:** 989–90.
130. Kohno S. Lipid mediators in bronchial asthma. *ACI International* 1998; **10**(6): 181–6.
131. Lynch KR, O'Neill GP, Liu Q et al. Characterization of the human cysteinyl leukotriene CysLT1 receptor. *Nature* 1999; **399:** 789–93.
132. Heise CE, O'Dowd BF, Figueroa DJ et al. Characterization of the human cysteinyl leukotriene 2 receptor. *J Biol Chem* 2000; **275:** 30531–6.
133. Drazen JM, Yandava CN, Dube L et al. Pharmacogenetic association between ALOX5 promoter genotype and the response to anti-asthma treatment. *Nat Genet* 1999; **22**(2): 168–70.
134. Pearlman DS, Ostrom NK, Bronsky EA et al. The leukotriene D4-receptor antagonist zafirlukast attenuates exercise-induced bronchoconstriction in children. *J Pediatr* 1999; **134**(3): 273–9.
135. Diamant Z, Grootendorst DC, Veselic-Charvat M et al. The effect of montelukast (MK-0476), a cysteinyl leukotriene receptor antagonist, on allergen-induced airway responses and sputum cell counts in asthma. *Clin Exp Allergy* 1999; **29:** 42–51.
136. Kikawa Y, Miyanomae T, Inoue Y et al. Urinary leukotriene E4 ater exercise challenge in children with asthma. *J Allergy Clin Immunol* 1992; **89:** 1111–19.
137. Kemp JP, Dockborn RJ, Shapiro GG et al. Montelukast once daily inhibits exercise-induced bronchoconstriction in 6- to 14-year-old children with asthma. *J Pediatr* 1998; **133:** 424–8.
138. Leff JA, Busse WW, Pearlman D, et al. Montelukast, a leukotriene receptor antagonist, for the treatment of mild asthma and exercise-induced bronchoconstriction. *N Engl J Med* 1998; **339:** 147–52.
139. Bronsky EA, Kemp JP, Zhang J et al. Dose-related protection of exercise-induced bronchoconstriction by montelukast, a cysteinyl leukotriene-receptor antagonist, at the end of a once-daily dosing interval. *Clin Pharmacol Ther* 1997; **62:** 556–61.
140. Villaran C, O'Neill SJ, Helbling A et al. Montelukast versus salmeterol in patients with asthma and exercise-induced bronchoconstriction. *J Allergy Clin Immunol* 1999; **104**(3 Pt 1): 547–53.
141. Busse W, Nelson H, Wolfe et al. Comparison of inhaled salmeterol and oral zafirlukast in patients with asthma. *J Allergy Clin Immunol* 1999; **103:** 1075–80.
142. Knorr B, Larson P, Nguyen HAH et al.

Montelukast dose selection in 6- to 14-year-olds: comparison of single-dose pharmacokinetics in children and adults. *J Clin Pharmacol* 1999; **39**: 1–8.
143. Malmstrom K, Rodriguez-Gomez G, Guerra J et al. Oral montelukast, inhaled beclomethasone, and placebo for chronic asthma. *Ann Intern Med* 1999; **130**: 487–95.
144. Laviolette M, Malmstrom K, Lu S et al. Montelukast added to inhaled beclometasone in treatment of asthma. *Am J Respir Crit Care Med* 1999; **160**(6): 1862–8.
145. Bisgaard H, Loland L. NO in exhaled air of asthmatic children is reduced by the leukotriene receptor antagonist montelukast. *Am J Respir Crit Care Med* 1999; **160**(4): 1227–31.
146. Bratton DL, Lanz MJ, Miyazawa N et al. Exhaled nitric oxide before and after montelukast sodium therapy in school-age children with chronic asthma: a preliminary study. *Pediatr Pulmonol* 1999; **28**: 401–7.
147. Bisgaard H, Nielsen KG. Bronchoprotection with a leukotriene receptor antagonist in asthmatic pre-school children. *Am J Respir Crit Care Med* 2000; **162**(1): 187–90.
148. Roquet A, Dahlen B, Kumlim M et al. Combined antagonism of leukotrienes and histamine produces predominant inhibition of allergen-induced early and late phase airway obstruction in asthmatics. *Am J Respir Crit Care Med* 1997; **1155**: 1856–63.
149. Reicin A, White R, Weinstein SF et al. Montelukast, a leukotriene receptor antagonist, in combination with loratadine, a histamine receptor antagonist, in the treatment of chronic asthma. *Arch Intern Med* 2000; **160**: 2481–8.
150. Reiss TF, Chervinsky P, Dockhorn RJ et al. Montelukast, a once-daily leukotriene receptor antagonist, in the treatment of chronic asthma: a multicenter randomized double-blind trial. *Arch Intern Med* 1998; **158**: 1213–20.
151. Knorr B, Matz J, Bernstein JA et al. Montelukast for chronic asthma in 6- to 14-year-old children. *JAMA* 1998; **279**: 1181–6.
152. Pearlman DS, Lampl KL, Dowling PJ et al. Effectiveness and tolerability of zafirlukast for the treatment of asthma in children. *Clin Ther* 2000; **22**: 732–47.
153. Bisgaard H, Franchi LM, Maspero JF et al. Long-term safety of montelukast in 2- to 5-year old children with asthma. *Eur Resp J* 2000; **16** (Suppl 31): 307(s).
154. Knorr B, Franchi L, Maspero J et al. Montelukast improves daytime and overnight astha symptoms over a 12-week tretament period in 2- to 5-year olds. *Eur Resp J* 2000; **16** (Suppl 31): 307(s).
155. Chanarin N, Johnston SL, Leukotrienes as a target in asthma therapy. *Drugs* 1994; **47**(1): 12–24.
156. Smith LJ. Pharmacology and safety of the leukotriene antagonists. *Clin Rev Allergy Immunol* 1999; **17**: 195–212.
157. Kiroshita M, Shiraishi T, Koga T et al. Churg–Strauss syndrome after corticosteroid withdrawal in an asthmatic patient treated with pranlukast. *J Allergy Clin Immunol* 1999; **103**: 534–5.
158. Merck Sharp & Dohme. *Montelukast Product Monograph*. New Jersey: Merck Sharpe & Dohme, March 1998.
159. Granneman GR, Braeckman RA, Locke CS et al. Effect of zileuton on theophylline pharmacokinetics. *Clin Pharmacokinet* 1995; **29**(Suppl 2): 77–83.
160. Adkins JC, Brogden RN. Zafirlukast. A review of its pharmacology and therapeutic potential in the management of asthma. *Drugs* 1998; **55**: 121–44.
161. Drazen JM, Israel E, O'Byrne PM. Treatment of asthma with drugs modifying the leukotriene pathway. *N Engl J Med* 1999; **340**: 197–206.
162. Smith LJ. Newer asthma therapies. *Ann Int Med* 1999; **130**: 531–2.
163. Bigby TD. Regulation of expression of the 5-lipooxygenase pathway. *Clin Rev Allergy Immunol* 1999; **17**: 43–58.
164. Azevedo I, de Blic J, Scheimann P et al. Enhanced arachidonics acid metabolism in alveolar macrophages from wheeze infants. Modulation by dexamethasone. *Am J Respir Crit Care Med* 1995; **152**: 1208–14.
165. Uz T, Dwivedi Y, Savani PD et al. Glucocorticoids stimulate inflammatory 5-lipooxygenase gene expression and protein translocation in the brain. *J Neurochem* 1999; **73**: 693–9.
166. Dahlen SE. Leukotrienes. In: *Inflammatory Mechanisms in Asthma*. Holgate ST, Busse, WW, eds. New York: Marcel Dekker, Inc., 1998: 679–733.
167. Lofdahl CG, Reis TF, Leff JA et al. Randomized placebo controlled trial of effect of a leukotriene receptor antagonist, montelukast, on tapering inhaled corticosteroids in asthmatic patients. *BMJ* 1999; **319**: 87–90.
168. Verberne AAPH, Hop WCJ, Bos AB, Kerrebijn

KF. Effect of a single dose of inhaled salmeterol on baseline airway calibre and metacholine induced airway obstruction in asthmatic children. *J Allergy Clin Immunol* 1993; **91**: 127–34.
169. Roberts JA, Bradding P, Britten KM et al. The long acting β₂ agonist salmeterol xinafoate: effects on airway inflammation in asthma. *Eur Respir J* 1999; **14**: 275–82.
170. Verbene AAPH, Frost C, Roorda RJ et al. One-year treatment with salmeterol compared with beclomethasone in children with asthma. *Am J Respir Crit Care Med* 1997; **156**: 688–95.
171. Yates DH, Kharitonov SE, Barnes PJ. An inhaled glucocorticoid does not prevent tolerance to the broncho protective effect of a long acting inhaled β₂ agonist. *Am J Respir Crit Care Med* 1996; **154**: 1603–7.
172. Greening AP, Ind PW, Northfield M et al. Added salmeterol vs. higher dose corticosteroid in asthma patients with symptoms on existing inhaled corticosteroid. *Lancet* 1994; **344**: 219–24.
173. Woolcock A, Lundback B, Ringdal N et al. Comparison of addition of salmeterol to inhaled steroids with doubling of the dose of inhaled steroid. *Am J Respir Crit Care Med* 1996; **153**: 1481–8.
174. Davies B, Brooks G, Devoy M. The efficacy and safety of salmeterol compared to theophylline: meta-analysis of 9 controlled studies. *Respir Med* 1998; **92**: 256–63.
175. Pauwels RA, Lofdahl CG, Postma DS et al. Effect of inhaled formoterol and budesonide on exacerbations of asthma. *N Engl J Med* 1997; **337**: 1412–18.
176. Palmqvist M, Persson D, Lazer L et al. Inhaled dry powder formoterol and salmeterol in asthmatic patients: onset of action, duration of effect and potency. *Eur Respir J* 1997; **10**: 2484–9.
177. Shrewsbury S, Pyke S, Britton M. Meta-analysis of increased dose of inhaled steroid or addition of salmeterol in symptomatic asthma. *BMJ* 2000; **320**: 1368–73.
178. Kavuru M, Melamed J, Gross G et al. Salmeterol and fluticasone propionate combined in a new powder inhalation device for the treatment of asthma: a randomised double-blind placebo controlled trial. *J Allergy Clin Immunol* 2000; **105**: 1108–16.
179. Van den Berg NJ, Ossip MS, Hederos CA et al. Salmeterol/fluticasone propionate (50/100 μgm) in combination in a discus inhaler (seratide) is effective and safe in children with asthma. *Pediatr Pulmonol* 2000; **30**: 97–105.
180. Edelman JM, Turpin JA, Bronsky EA et al. Oral montelukast compared with inhaled salmeterol to prevent exercise induced bronchoconstriction. *Ann Intern Med* 2000; **132**: 97–104.
181. Gordon DS. Intravenous immunoglobulin: historical perspectives. *Am J Med* 1987; **83**(Suppl 4A): 1–3.
182. Gelfand EW, Landwehr LP, Mazer B. Intravenous immune globulin: an alternative therapy in steroid dependent allergic diseases. *Clin Exp Immunol* 1996; **104**(Suppl 1): 61–6.
183. Amran D, Renz H, Lack G et al. Supression of cytokine dependent human T-cell proliferation by intravenous immunoglobulin. *Clin Immunol Immunopathol* 1994; **73**: 180–6.
184. Spahn JD, Leung DYM, Chan MTSC et al. Mechanisms of glucocorticoid reduction in asthmatic subjects treated with intravenous immunoglobulin. *J Allergy Clin Immunol* 1999; **103**: 421–6.
185. Hashimoto F, Sakiyama Y, Matsumoto S. The supressive effect of gammaglobulin preparations on in vivo pokeweed mitogen-induced immunoglobulin production. *Clin Exp Immunol* 1986; **65**: 409–15.
186. Kazatchkine MD, Dietrich G, Hurez V et al. V region-mediated selection of autoreactive repertories by intravenous immunoglobulin (IvIg). *Immunol Rev* 1994; **139**: 79–107.
187. Vrugt B, Wilson S, van Venzel E et al. Effects of high dose intravenous immunoglobulin in two severe corticosteroid insensitive patients. *Thorax* 1997; **52**: 662–4.
188. Page R, Friday G, Stillwagon P et al. Asthma and selective immunoglobulin subclass deficiency: improvement of asthma after immunoglobulin replacement therapy. *J Pediatr* 1988; **112**: 127–31.
189. Mazer BD, Gelfand EW. An open-label study of high-dose intravenous immunoglobulin in severe childhood asthma. *J Allergy Clin Immunol* 1991; **87**: 976–83.
190. Landwehr LP, Jeppson JD, Katlan MG et al. Benefits of high-dose IV immunoglobulin in patients with severe steroid-dependent asthma. *Chest* 1998; **114**: 1349–56.
191. Salmun LM, Barlan I, Wolf HM et al. Effect of intravenous immunoglobulin on steroid consumption in patients with severe asthma: A double-blind, placebo-controlled, randomized trial. *J Allergy Clin Immunol* 1999; **103**: 810–15.
192. Niggemann B, Leupold W, Shuster A et al. Prospective, double-blind, placebo-controlled,

multicentre study on the effect of high-dose, intravenous immunoglobulin in children and adolescents with severe bronchial asthma. *Clin Exp Allergy* 1998; **28:** 205–10.
193. Kishiyama JL, Valacer D, Cunningham-Rundles C et al. A multicenter, randomised, double-blind, placebo-controlled trial of high-dose intravenous immunoglobulin for oral corticosteroid-dependent asthma. *Clin Immunol* 1999; **91:** 126–33.
194. Gelfand EW. Use of intravenous immunoglobulin in severe steroid-dependent asthma. In: Barnes PJ, Grunstein MM, Leff AR, Woolcock AJ, eds. *Asthma*, 1st ed, Philadelphia: Lippincott-Raven, 1997: 1683–8.
195. Schiff RI. Intravenous gammaglobulin, 2: pharmacology, clinical uses and mechanisms of action. *Pediatr Allergy Immunol* 1994; **5:** 127–56.
196. Yap PL. The viral safety of intravenous immune globulin. *Clin Exp Immunol* 1996; **104:** 35–42.
197. Renal insufficiency and failure associated with IVIG therapy. *MMWR* 1999; **48:** 518–21.
198. Suárez CR, Pickett WC, Bell DH, Effect of low dose of methotrexate on neutrophil chemotaxis induced by leukotriene B4 and Complement C5a. *J Rheumatol* 1987; **14:** 9–13.
199. Segal R, Mozes E, Yaron M. The effects of methotrexate on the production and activity of interleukin-1. *Arthritis Rheum* 1989; **32:** 370–6.
200. Aaron SD, Dales RE, Pham B. Management of steroid-dependent asthma with methotrexate: a meta-analysis of randomized clinical trials. *Respir Med* 1998; **92**(8): 1059–65.
201. Marin MG. Low-dose methotrexate spares steroid usage in steroid-dependent asthmatic patients: a meta-analysis. *Chest* 1997; **112:** 29–33.
202. Vrugt B, Wilson S, Bron A et al. Low-dose methotrexate treatment in severe glucorticoid-dependent asthma: effect on mucosal inflammation and in vitro sensitivity to glucorticoids of mitogen-enduced T cell proliferation. *Eur Respir J* 2000; **15:** 478–85.
203. Stempel DA, Lammert J, Mullarkey MF. Use of methotrexate in the treatment of steroid-dependent adolescent asthmatics. *Ann Allergy* 1991; **67**(3): 346–8.
204. Guss S, Portnoy J. Methotrexate treatment of severe asthma in children. *Pediatrics* 1992; **89:** 635–9.
205. Solé D, Costa-Carvalho BT, Soares FJP et al. Methotrexate in the treatment of corticodependent asthmatic children. *J Invest Allergol Clin Immunol* 1996; **6**(2): 126–30.
206. Moss RB. Alternative pharmacotherapies for steroid-dependent asthma. *Chest* 1995; **107:** 817–25.
207. Bleyer WA. Clinical pharmacology and therapeutic drug monitoring of methotrexate. *Am Assoc Clin Chemistry* 1985; **6:** 1–5.
208. Lammert JK, Mullarkey MF. Promises and problems with the use of methotrexate in the asthmatic patient. *Immunol Allergy Clin N Am* 1991; **11:** 65–79.
209. Honma M, Tamura G, Shirato K et al. Effect of an oral gold compound, auranofin, on non-specific bronchial hyperresponsiveness in mild asthma. *Thorax* 1994; **49:** 649–51.
210. Bernstein IL, Bernstein DI, Dubb JW et al. A placebo-controlled multicenter study of auranofin in the treatment of patients with corticosteroid-dependent asthma. Auranofin Multicenter Drug Trial. *J Allergy Clin Immunol* 1996; **98:** 317–24.
211. Loh LC, Barnes NC. Immunotherapeutic approaches to the drug therapy in severe asthma, including immunosuppressants and intravenous immunglobulin. In: Holgate ST, Boushey HA, Fabbri LM, eds. *Difficult Asthma*. London: Martin Dunitz, 1999: 477–92.
212. Giannini EH, Brewer EJ, Pearson DA. Auranofin in the treatment of juvenile rheumathoid arthritis. *J Pediatr* 1983; **102:** 1138–41.
213. Nizankowska E, Soja J, Pinis G et al. Treatment of steroid-dependent bronchial asthma with cyclosporin. *Eur Respir J* 1995; **8:** 1091–9.
214. Lock SH, Kay Ab, Barnes NC. Double-blind, placebo-controlled study of cyclosporin A as a corticosteroid-aoaring agent in corticosteroid-dependent asthma. *Am J Resp Crit Care Med* 1996; **153:** 509–14.
215. Sihra BS, Kon OM, Durham SR et al. Effect of cyclosporin A on the allergen-induced late asthmatic reaction. *Thorax* 1997; **52:** 447–52.
216. Mori A, Kaninuma O, Ogawa K et al. Control of Il-5 production by human helper T cells as a treatment for eosinophilic inflammation: Comparison of in vitro and in vivo effects between selective and nonselective cytokine synthesis inhibitors. *J Allergy Clin Immunol* 2000; **106:** S58–64.
217. Balfour-Lynn I. Difficult asthma; beyond the guidelines. *Arch Dis Child* 1999; **80:** 201–6.
218. Coren ME, Rosenthal M, Bush A. The use of cyclosporin in corticosteroid dependent asthma. *Arch Dis Child* 1997; **77:** 522–6.

219. Szefler SJ, Rose JQ, Ellis EF et al. The effect of troleandomycin on methylprednisolone elimination. *J Allergy Clin Immunol* 1980; **66:** 447–51.
220. LaForce CF, Szefler SJ, Miller MF et al, Inhibition of methylprednisolone elimination in the presence of erythromycin therapy. *J Allergy Clin Immunol* 1983; **72:** 34–9.
221. Fost DA, Leung DY, Martin RJ et al. Inhibition of methylprednisolone elimination in the presence of clarithromycin therapy. *J Allergy Clin Immunol* 1999; **103**(6): 1031–5.
222. Amayasu H, Yoshida S, Ebana S et al. Clarythromycin supresses bronchial hyperresponsiveness associated with eosinophilic inflammation in patients with asthma. *Ann Allergy Asthma Immunol* 2000; **84:** 594–8.
223. Shoji T. Yoshida S, Sakamoto H et al. Antiinflammatory effect of roxitromycin in patients with aspirin-intolerant asthma. *Clin Exp Allergy* 1999; **29:** 950–6.
224. Eitches RW, Rachelefsky GS, Katz RM et al. Methylprednisolone and troleandromycin in treatment of steroid-dependent asthmatic children. *AJDC* 1985; **139:** 264–8.
225. Ball BD, Hill MR, Brenner M et al. Effect of low dose troleandomycin on glucocorticoid pharmacokinetics and airway hyperresponsiveness in severely asthmatic children. *Ann Allergy* 1990; **65:** 37–45.
226. Flotte TR, Loughlin GM. Benefits and complications of troleandromycin (TAO) in young children with steroid-dependent asthma. *Pediatr Pulmonol* 1991; **10**(3): 178–82.
227. Kamada AK, Hill MR, Ikle DN et al. Efficacy and safety of low-dose troleandomycin therapy in children with severe, steroid-requiring asthma. *J Allergy Clin Immunol* 1993; **91:** 873–82.
228. Koh YY, Lee Mh, Sun YH et al. Effect of roxithromycin on airway responsiveness in children with bronchiectasis: a double-blind, placebo-controlled study. *Eur Respir J* 1997; **10:** 994–9.
229. Avila PC, Boushey A. Macrolides. Asthma, inflammation and infection. *Ann Allergy Asthma Immunol* 2000; **84:** 565–8.
230. Koyama T, Takizawa H, Kawasaki S et al. Fourteen-member macrolides inhibit interleukin-8 release by human eosinophils from atopic donors. *Antimicrob Agents Chemother* 1999; **43:** 907–11.
231. Abe S, Nakamura H, Inoue S et al. Interleukin-8 gene repression by clarithromycin is mediated by the activator protein 1-binding site in human bronchial epithelial cells. *Am J Resp Cell Mol Biol* 2000; **22:** 51–60.
232. Suez D, Szefler SJ. Excessive accumulation of mucus in children with asthma: a potential role for erythromycin. *J Allergy Clin Immunol* 1986; **77:** 330–4.
233. Zeiger RS, Schatz M, Sperling W et al. Efficacy of trolendromycin in outpatients with severe corticosteroid dependent asthma. *J Allergy Clin Immunol* 1980; **66:** 438–46.
234. Szefler SJ, Ellis EF, Brenner M et al. Steroid-specific and anticonvulsivant interaction aspects of troleandromycin-steroid therapy. *J Allergy Clin Immunol* 1982; **69**(5): 455–60.
235. Barnes PJ. Therapeutic strategies for allergic diseases. *Nature* 1999; **402:** B31–B38.
236. Barnes PJ. New directions in allergic diseases: mechanism-based anti-inflammatory therapies. *J Allergy Clin Immunol* 2000; **106:** 5–16.
237. Glennie MJ, Johnson PWM. Clinical trials of antibody therapy. *Immunol Today* 2000; **21:** 403–10.
238. Leckie MJ, Brincke A, Jordan J et al. SB 240563, a humanized anti-IL-5 monoclonal antibody. Initial single dose safety and activity in patients with asthma. *Am J Respir Crit Care Med* 1999; **159:** A624.
239. Leonard JP. Sherman ML, Fisher GL et al. Effects of single-dose interleukin-12 exposure on interleukin-12 associated toxicity and interferon-gamma production. *Blood* 1997; **90:** 2541–8.
240. Casale TB. Future perspectives on asthma treatment. In: Neffen HE, Baenaa-Cagnani CE, Fabbri L et al. *Asthma – A Link Between Environment, Immunology and the Airways*. Hogrefe & Huber Publishers, USA. 1999: 190–9.
241. Millgrom H, Fick RB, Su JQ et al. Treatment of allergic asthma with monoclonal anti-IgE antibody. *N Engl J Med* 1999; **341:** 1966–73.
242. Ziment I. Hydration, humidification and therapy. In: Weiss EB, Segal MS, Stein M. eds. *Bronchial Asthma*. Boston: Little, Brown & Company, 1985: 756–75.
243. Gibson PG, Hargreave FE. Evidence from induced sputum. In: Holgate ST, Busse WW. *Inflammatory Mechanisms in Asthma*. Marcel Dekker, Inc., New York. 1998: 75–88.
244. Nelson HS. β-adrenergic agonists. In: Barnes PJ et al, eds. *Asthma*. Lippincott-Raven, New York. 1997: 1507–21.
245. Stellato C, Schwiebert LM, Schleimer RP. Mechanisms of glucocorticosteroid action. In:

Barnes PJ et al, eds. *Asthma*. Lippincott-Raven, New York. 1997: 1569–96.
246. Sly PD, Landau LI, Olinsky A. Failure of ipratropium bromide to modify the diurnal variation of asthma in asthmatic children. *Thorax* 1987; **42:** 357–60.
247. Greenough A, Yuksel B, Everett L, Price JF. Inhaled ipratropium bromide and terbutaline in asthmatic children. *Respir Med* 1993; **87:** 111–14.
248. Zollman C, Vickers A. What is complementary medicine? *BMJ* 1999; **319:** 693–696.
249. Global Strategy for Asthma Management and Prevention. NHLBI/WHO Workshop Report. National Institutes of Health, Publication No. 95–36559, 1995.
250. Eisenberg DM, Kessler RC, Foster C et al. Unconventional medicine in the United States. Prevalence, costs, and patterns of use. *N Engl J Med* 1993; **328:** 246–52.
251. Eisenberg DM, Davis RB, Ettner SL. Trends in alternative medicine use in the United States, 1990–1997: results of a follow-up national survey. *JAMA* 1998; **280:** 1569–75.
252. Linde K, Jobst K, Panton J. Acupuncture for chronic asthma. *Cochrane Database Syst Rev* 2000; (2): CD000008.
253. Linde K, Jobst KA. Homeopathy for chronic asthma. *Cochrane Database Syst Rev* 2000; (2): CD000353.
254. Holloway E, Ram FS. Breathing exercises for asthma. *Cochrane Database Syst Rev* 2000; (3): CD001277.
255. Chanez P, Bousquet J, Godard P, Michel JF. Controversial forms of treatment for asthma. *Clin Rev Allergy Immunol* 1996; **14:** 247–52.
256. Ziment I, Tashkin DP. Alternative medicine for allergy and asthma. *J Allergy Clin Immunol* 2000; **106:** 603–14.

9

Assessment and treatment of acute asthma in children and adolescents

Gary L Larsen, Giuseppe N Colasurdo

Introduction • Pathology of acute asthma • Physiological characteristics of acute asthma • Approach to children/adolescents with acute asthma • Summary

INTRODUCTION

Acute asthma may be defined as airway obstruction that becomes clinically manifest over a relatively short period of time. The clinical manifestations include some combination of shortness of breath, cough, wheezing, and chest tightness. The obstruction may be mild and self-limited (exercise-induced asthma that resolves without therapy), or may be life threatening if not immediately addressed.[1] Between these extremes one finds all gradations of obstruction that must be appropriately assessed and effectively managed to minimize morbidity and prevent mortality. This chapter deals with these episodes when control of this disease is lost.

The effective management of acute asthma in children is based in part on an understanding of the pathology and physiology of this disease. The former is important because it reminds the clinician of the components of obstruction that are not readily amenable to treatment and take time to resolve. The physiology is critical in that measures of pulmonary physiology are utilized to quantify the severity of an episode and to guide therapy. This chapter will focus on a brief review of pathology and physiology before discussing assessment and therapy of acute episodes. Whenever possible, studies involving children and adolescents are cited. Investigations into the disease in infants and adults are also cited when they give insight into pathogenesis.

PATHOLOGY OF ACUTE ASTHMA

It has been known for decades that fatal asthma is associated with marked inflammation within airways.[2-4] When asthma is the terminal event, one finds a combination of obstruction of airways with mucus and cellular debris, loss of airway epithelium, subepithelial collagen deposition, and airway wall thickening (smooth muscle hypertrophy, edema, goblet cell hyperplasia, infiltration of inflammatory cells). This has been noted in autopsy material from not only adults but also pediatric patients of various ages.[5] Furthermore, with the more recent use of bronchoalveolar lavage and biopsy to address disease pathogenesis, it is now apparent that asthma that is clinically mild is also characterized by airway inflammation.[6,7] The most frequently identified features of this inflammation include infiltration of airways by eosinophils, activation of T-cells within airways, an increase in mast cell numbers, and desquamation of airway epithelium.[8] These invasive clinical studies have been performed primarily in adults. Although information on pediatric patients is limited, work employing lavage in older children and adolescents suggests that findings within their lungs are similar to the abnormalities described in adults.[9] In addition, Cutz and coworkers[10] found that biopsies obtained from children with severe but stable asthma had features that were also found when the disease led to death. This observation is especially important to keep in mind when considering the length of time it may take lung function to return to an acceptable level following an acute episode of the disease (see below).

PHYSIOLOGICAL CHARACTERISTICS OF ACUTE ASTHMA

Asthma is characterized by several physiological abnormalities: hyperresponsiveness of airways, variable airflow limitation, and reversible airway obstruction. Given these features, asthma is a disease that is best characterized in a quantitative manner by tests of lung function. Several measures of lung mechanics have been used to characterize asthma during both symptomatic and asymptomatic phases of the disease.[11] These measures include: lung volumes, the pressure–volume characteristics of the lung, resistance to airflow, and flow rates. A discussion of each of these measures has been recently presented.[12] The present discussion will focus on measures most likely to be used by practicing physicians to assess acute asthma: flow rates and lung volumes. These considerations follow a general discussion of airway hyperresponsiveness, a fundamental feature of this disease.[13,14] This section also includes a review of the changes that occur in arterial blood gases as the severity of obstruction increases.

Increased airway responsiveness

Airway responsiveness is commonly defined as the ease with which airways narrow in response to various nonallergic and non-sensitizing stimuli including inhaled pharmacologic agents (histamine, methacholine) as well as natural physical stimuli (exercise, exposure to cold air). Heightened airway responsiveness to several stimuli is a hallmark of asthma.[13,14] Even when conventional assessments of lung function are normal in children with chronic asthma, the airways commonly exhibit a heightened responsiveness or 'twitchiness.' The most common method of quantifying airway responsiveness is to assess lung function before and after inhaling increasing concentrations of methacholine. The more responsive the airways, the less the amount of methacholine needed to decrease lung function.

The level of airway responsiveness has been noted to correlate roughly with the severity of disease in adults[13] as well as children.[15,16] Thus, asthmatics who are most responsive are generally the most symptomatic (wheeze, cough, chest tightness) and require the most medications. Although there can be great variability in responsiveness within groups of patients classified by disease severity,[17] the concept that the level of responsiveness correlates with disease severity is important when considering acute asthma. In this respect, the level of airway responsiveness is not static in either normal individuals or those with asthma, but may increase or decrease in response to various stimuli. When airway responsiveness increases, control of the disease is often lost. In other words, this is the time when asthmatics develop signs and symptoms of their disease. In general, stimuli that increase responsiveness are found in our environment and induce or exacerbate airway inflammation. For children, these stimuli commonly include viral respiratory infections, air pollutants (including cigarette smoke), and allergens.

A viral infection of the respiratory tract is a common antecedent to an acute episode of asthma in children.[18] The fact that these infections can increase airway responsiveness has been recognized for over two decades.[19] This has been documented for several respiratory viruses including the respiratory syncytial virus,[20] influenza A,[21] and rhinovirus.[22] In terms of air pollutants, both nitrogen dioxide[23] and ozone[24,25] have been shown to enhance airway responsiveness. Cigarette smoke is arguably the most serious environmental air pollutant in terms of the respiratory health of children and has been implicated in the onset and perpetuation of asthma.[26–28] Finally, exposure of atopic individuals to allergens can lead to significant increases in airway responsiveness that persist for days to months.[29–31] Although these three classes of precipitants are usually considered separately, they likely interact in an asthmatic's environment in ways that lead to instability of the disease.[22]

Flow rates

The usual method of assessing the degree of airflow limitation is to measure lung function during a maximal forced exhalation.[32] For this maneuver, the subject exhales forcibly from total lung capacity (TLC) to residual volume (RV) either into a spirometer or through a flowmeter, where flow is integrated to give volume. The results are usually expressed in one of two ways: as a time-based recording of expired volume (spirogram) or as a plot of instantaneous airflow against lung volume (maximal expiratory flow–volume (MEFV) curve). The tests of lung function derived from a spirogram are the forced vital capacity (FVC), the 1 second forced expiratory volume (FEV_1), and the forced expiratory flow from 25% to 75% of the FVC (FEF_{25-75}). From the flow–volume curve, the maximal expiratory flow rate (MEFR) achieved approximates the peak expiratory flow rate (PEFR) obtained from a flow meter. Flow at 50% of the vital capacity as well as flows at lower lung volumes are also generated as part of this maneuver. Since airflow is related to lung volume, plethysmography combined with the MEFV maneuver plotted as a flow–volume curve or loop allows assessment of the relationship between airflow and an absolute lung volume (Figure 9.1). Measuring flow rates in this manner may be especially informative when an isovolume shift occurs (discussed below).

In asthmatic patients, the expected pattern of altered flow rates during acute exacerbations has been described. On spirometry, both the FEV_1 and FEF_{25-75} are diminished, although the FEV_1 is more preserved as a percentage of predicted than the FEF_{25-75}. On the MEFV curve, the overall shape of the flow–volume loop usually changes and there is a scooping out of the distal portion of the loop as one of the first abnormalities (Figure 9.1). Flows at low lung volumes are also the last to return to normal. The MEFR, like its counterpart FEV_1, is preserved more during the acute attacks and, likewise, is quicker to normalize.

In a minority of episodes of acute asthma, the spirogram or MEFV curve alone will not reflect significant airway obstruction. However, if these subjects are studied with both an MEFV maneuver plus plethysmography to assess lung volumes, they will be noted to have a parallel displacement to a higher lung volume of the flow–volume curve without a change in the configuration of the curve itself.[33] Thus, if flow is measured as a percentage of the vital capacity, no change in flow is appreciated. However, when the same curve is plotted as a function of the absolute lung volumes present before and after onset of symptoms, substantial changes in flow become apparent at isovolumes. This represents an isovolume shift to a higher lung volume. The factors responsible for isovolume shifts are undefined, but may include complete closure of some airways with subsequent loss of the contribution of these units to the flow–volume pattern.

In acute severe asthma, loss of symptoms and signs of asthma does not mean that lung function has returned to normal. Classical studies by McFadden and coworkers[34] demonstrated that when patients with acute severe asthma became asymptomatic, the overall mechanical function of their lungs in terms of the FEV_1 was still only 40–50% of predicted normal values. Thus, loss of clinical signs of airway obstruction does not mean there has been physiologic recovery.

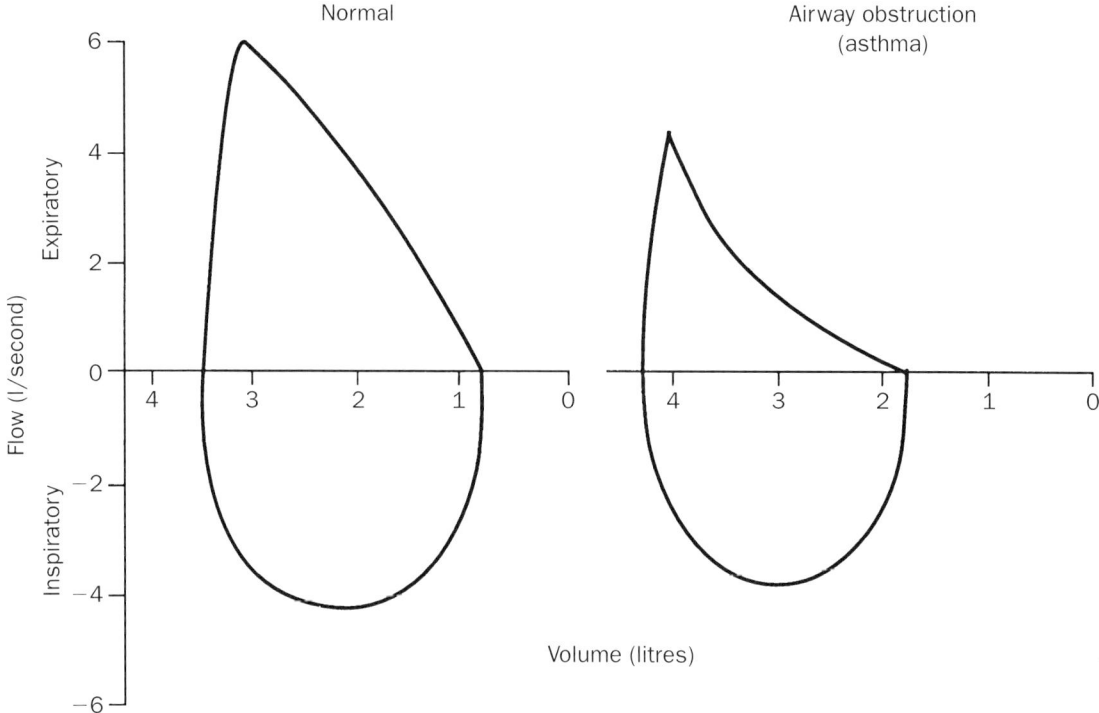

Figure 9.1 Maximal inspiratory and expiratory curves that together constitute a flow–volume loop are shown in a patient with asthma when the disease is under control (left loop) and during acute asthma (right loop). Flow is shown on the y-axis and absolute lung volume is displayed on the x-axis. The point of maximal inspiration (total lung capacity) is the point of zero flow on the left side of the loops, and the point of maximal expiration (residual volume) is at the point of zero flow on the right side of the loops. During an acute episode of wheezing, hyperinflation is noted with an increase in residual volume. In addition, expiratory flow rates decrease as demonstrated in the maximal expiratory portion of the curve, which becomes concave in shape. With milder episodes as shown in this example, the inspiratory portion of the loop is fairly well preserved. With more severe obstruction, inspiratory flows will be more compromised. (From Wenzel and Larsen.[32])

The use of peak flow meters within the home is an inexpensive method of monitoring a flow rate to assess asthma stability.[35] Significant changes in PEFR may be manifest before symptoms are evident. These devices may be especially helpful in defining the presence and severity of nocturnal asthma in individual patients.[36] Given that excessive diurnal variations in lung function during recovery from status asthmaticus have been associated with an increased risk of sudden death,[37] this vulnerable period of time should be monitored very closely within both the hospital and home environment. In more severely affected patients, monitoring the PEFR as part of their daily routine allows for earlier recognition of loss of control with more timely intervention. The normal diurnal variation of PEFR (i.e. the difference between morning and evening measurements) is less than 10%. A PEFR variability of greater than 15–20% has been used as one defining feature of nocturnal asthma, a common clinical manifestation of more severe asthma in both children and adults. Patients with nocturnal asthma should be regarded as having more severe disease as well as loss of asthma control, and should be appropriately treated.

Lung volumes

During acute exacerbations of asthma, all the various capacities and volumes of gas contained in the lung may be altered to some extent. The residual volume, functional residual capacity (FRC), and total lung capacity are usually increased (RV $\geqslant$ FRC > TLC) whereas the vital capacity (VC) and its subdivisions are decreased (Figure 9.1). These alterations have been described during natural exacerbations of asthma in both adults[38] and children.[39] Although laboratory-induced changes in lung volumes (exercise, histamine challenge) may be immediately normalized with inhalation of a bronchodilator, it may take weeks after an episode of severe acute asthma for the RV to return to a normal range.[11] The mechanisms responsible for the increases in RV, FRC (hyperinflation) and TLC (overdistension) are not completely understood. However, several factors have been identified that may contribute, including a generalized decrease in the elastic properties of the lung, a ball-valve phenomenon caused by swollen and mucus-plugged airways, and tonic activity in the intercostal muscles and diaphragm during episodes of obstruction.[11]

Arterial blood gases and the severity of airway obstruction

Several studies of acute asthma have attempted to correlate arterial blood gases with the level of airway obstruction. One of the classic descriptions is the study of McFadden and Lyons.[40] These authors chose a large study population (101 subjects) who, because of age (14 to 45 years old) and medical history, were unlikely to have asthma complicated by bronchitis and emphysema. This study and others cited below provide an important description of the expected abnormalities in gas exchange as a function of the degree of airway obstruction.

Oxygen tension
McFadden and Lyons[40] reported that the characteristic blood gas pattern in patients who were experiencing acute asthma was hypoxemia associated with respiratory alkalosis. The hypoxemia was the most consistent abnormality, found in 91 of the 101 subjects in the study. An approximately linear correlation was found between values of FEV_1 and arterial oxygen tension (Figure 9.2 (top)). Patients with an FEV_1 of 50–85% of their predicted normal value were classified as having mild airway obstruction, those with values of 26–50% as having moderate obstruction, and those with values of less than 25% predicted as having severe obstruction. The mean values of arterial oxygen tension (in mm Hg as measured at sea level) ranked by disease severity were: 82.8, 71.3, and 63.1, respectively. Thus, there was almost a 20 mm Hg difference in arterial oxygen tensions between the mild and severe groups. Just as important, it was also noted that some degree of hypoxemia was encountered at all levels of airway obstruction. Weng et al.[41] noted similar findings in children 14 months to 14 years of age, reporting that all symptomatic asthma patients were hypoxemic with the level of hypoxemia correlating with the degree of airflow obstruction.

Several mechanisms may contribute to the hypoxemia described above. The primary mechanism for the depressed oxygen tension in asthma is felt to be an alteration in ventilation–perfusion ratios.[40,41] In severely obstructed subjects in whom atelectatic alveoli are still being perfused, transitory anatomic shunts might also contribute to the hypoxemia. In the most severely obstructed subjects, alveolar hypoventilation with hypercapnia may also be important.

The normal response of the body to a decrease in arterial oxygen tension is to increase ventilation. A reduced chemosensitivity to hypoxia coupled with a blunted perception of dyspnea could predispose patients to fatal asthma attacks. Kikuchi and colleagues[42] found that patients with a history of near-fatal asthma had respiratory responses to hypoxia that were significantly lower than responses found in normal subjects and in asthmatics without near-fatal attacks. The lower hypoxic response was seen in conjunction with a blunted perception

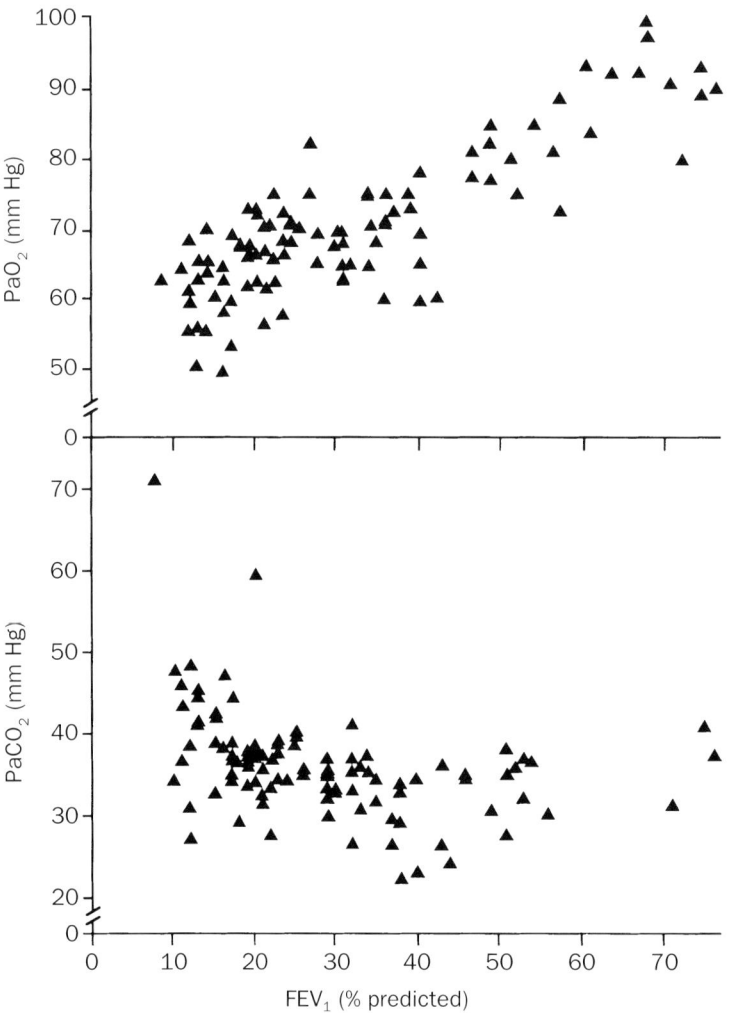

Figure 9.2 The relationship between arterial oxygen (mm Hg) and degree of airway obstruction (FEV$_1$ as a percentage of predicted) is shown in the top panel, and the relationship between arterial carbon dioxide (mm Hg) and FEV$_1$ is shown in the bottom panel. Although the level of hypoxemia correlates with the level of airway obstruction, an elevation in carbon dioxide levels is seen only when FEV$_1$ is markedly compromised. (From McFadden and Lyons.[40])

of dyspnea. These abnormalities could occur because of pre-existing genetic factors and/or adaptation of the body to recurrent hypoxia. The relative contribution of these factors is undefined.

Carbon dioxide tension
McFadden and Lyons[40] demonstrated that the characteristic blood gas pattern found in asthmatics experiencing acute attacks was hypoxemia associated with respiratory alkalosis. In terms of carbon dioxide tensions, their study suggested that most attacks were associated with alveolar hyperventilation, and that hypercapnia was not likely to occur until extreme degrees of obstruction were reached. Plotting airways obstruction (percent predicted FEV$_1$) against the carbon dioxide tension graphically indicated that hypercapnia was not seen until the FEV$_1$ fell to less than 20% of its predicted value (Figure 9.2 (bottom)). Thus, the conventional admonition that a 'normal' PaCO$_2$ in a patient with acute asthma is cause for concern.

Arterial values of pH
Values of arterial pH in acute asthma have generally reflected the respiratory alkalosis noted above. In the study of McFadden and

Lyons,[40] 73 of the 101 subjects had a respiratory alkalosis (mean pH, 7.46), 21 a normal pH, and seven had a respiratory acidosis (mean pH 7.32). Weng et al.[41] reported similar results in children. A metabolic acidosis may also be seen in acute asthma. Although this is rarely seen in adults, it has been noted in combination with a respiratory acidosis in children with severe asthma.[41,43] When this disturbance of acid/base balance is present, it is usually associated with very severe airway obstruction.[44] Although the mechanisms responsible for the development of the metabolic acidosis remain to be clarified, subjects with a metabolic acidosis are in imminent danger of development of respiratory failure.[41]

Table 9.1 Diseases that may masquerade as acute asthma in children and adolescents

Vocal cord dysfunction
Gastroesophageal reflux ± aspiration
Bronchiolitis obliterans
Tracheomalacia and/or bronchomalacia
Interstitial lung disease
Hypersensitivity pneumonia
Mediastinal mass
Anaphylaxis

APPROACH TO CHILDREN/ADOLESCENTS WITH ACUTE ASTHMA

The approach to acute asthma in pediatric patients is first discussed in terms of diseases that may mimic this problem. Factors that can cause the child with established asthma to have more severe disease and thus more episodes of acute deterioration are then presented. This is followed by a discussion of the assessment of acute asthma and a review of therapy in various settings from the home to the intensive care unit.

Diseases that masquerade as acute asthma

Shortness of breath, cough, wheezing, and chest tightness are not specific to asthma. Thus, children that present in this manner may have medical problems other than asthma. The differential diagnosis of wheezing and dyspnea in pediatric subjects is influenced by the age of the patient. The younger the child, the more one has to consider congenital problems involving the airways. This is especially true for infants and toddlers, as discussed in other chapters within this text. In older children and adolescents, the confounding conditions will be more similar to the problems seen in adults. Diseases that can masquerade as acute asthma in children and adolescents are listed in Table 9.1. This list is not totally inclusive, but rather is based in large part on the experience of the authors. Although many diagnoses in this table are familiar to practitioners who deal with children, specific information on vocal cord dysfunction plus more general comments about several other problems on the list are presented.

Vocal cord dysfunction (VCD), a functional disorder of vocal cords which mimics attacks of asthma and/or upper airway obstruction, has recently received widespread attention.[45,46] Paroxysms of wheezing and dyspnea seen with VCD are refractory to standard therapy for asthma. During symptomatic episodes, the maximal expiratory and inspiratory flow–volume loop resembles a variable extrathoracic obstruction (Figure 9.3). The diagnosis is confirmed by laryngoscopy, which demonstrates that the wheezing and/or stridor are associated with paradoxic adduction of the vocal cords during inspiration and sometimes during the entire respiratory cycle. Both the flow–volume loops and the laryngoscopy findings are completely normal when the subjects are asymptomatic. In the vast majority of patients, VCD is subconscious and may be associated with stress. In pediatric patients as young as 4 years of age, underlying factors such as stress related to athletic or academic performance may be found.[47] It must be noted that VCD and asthma frequently coexist in children.[47] Truncation of the inspiratory portion of the flow–volume loop

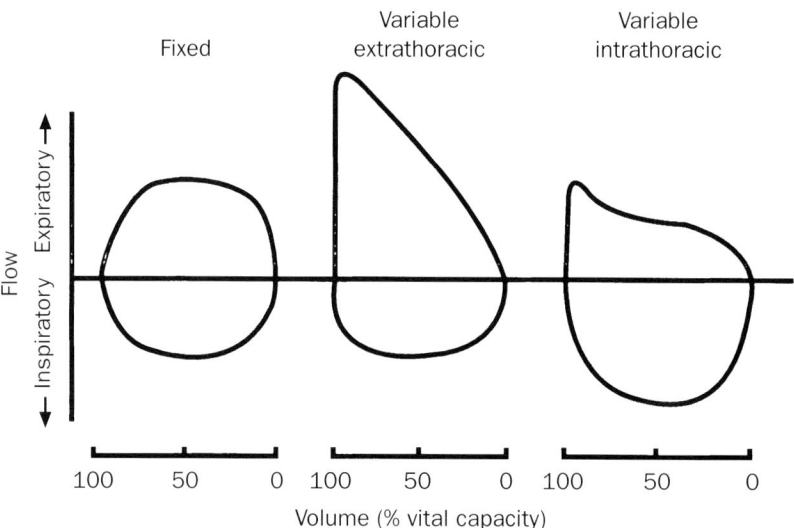

Figure 9.3 Flow–volume loops are displayed for various types of obstructive lesions in the proximal airways (larynx and trachea) which may present with wheezing. For comparison, the normal contour of a flow–volume loop is shown on the left side of Figure 9.1. With a lesion that is circumferential, preventing either compression or dilation of the airway with respiratory efforts, a fixed pattern is seen with truncation of both the inspiratory and expiratory curves. Subglottic stenosis and vascular rings that surround an airway might present with such a pattern. If a lesion permits compression or dilation with respiration, the pattern will depend on whether the lesion is intrathoracic or extrathoracic. With extrathoracic lesions (vocal cord dysfunction), the inspiratory curve is more affected. An intrathoracic lesion (mass that compresses only part of the airway) will have more of an effect on expiratory flow rates. (From Wenzel and Larsen.[32])

together with a concave shape of the expiratory curve may then be found. Treatment of VCD is primarily accomplished through speech therapy as well as psychotherapy.[46] Although rarely needed, breathing a mixture of 70% helium and 30% oxygen can relieve dyspnea and abort acute attacks.

Gastroesophageal reflux (GER) with possible aspiration has been associated with persistent wheezing in infants.[48] In older children and adolescents, GER without apparent aspiration has been associated with acute wheezing when this occurs during sleep.[49,50] The mechanism for this association appears to be the development of esophagitis with reflex airway obstruction occurring via vagal pathways.

Children with bronchiolitis obliterans have experienced insults to their lungs (adenovirus infection, Stevens–Johnson syndrome with pulmonary involvement, etc.) which have led to scarring within small airways and severe airway obstruction.[51] They may present with dyspnea/wheezing leading to the impression that they have acute asthma. The correct diagnosis may be suggested by a chest X-ray or by the lack of significant reversal of the airway obstruction with therapy including corticosteroids. Pediatric patients with interstitial lung disease may also present with dyspnea and poor air exchange on physical examination.[52,53] Although these patients have a diminished FEV_1, the FEV_1/FVC ratio is normal.

Factors that increase the frequency of acute asthma

The primary objective in the therapy of acute asthma is to quickly treat hypoxemia and to reverse airway obstruction (see below).

However, those who treat acute deterioration should be aware of various factors that may lead to repeated loss of control of this disease. When a child with asthma develops more severe disease and frequent episodes of acute asthma, several complicating conditions should be considered. For example, in an atopic asthmatic child, introduction of allergens into the environment might lead to increased nocturnal awakenings and other clinical features of acute asthma. Other environmental factors may also be contributing to compromised asthma control, such as cigarette smoke, indoor and outdoor pollutants, and irritants. In addition, sinusitis has long been recognized to be associated with asthma.[54] The suggestion that upper airway inflammation (sinusitis) contributes to the pathogenesis of asthma has been derived from observations that asthma sometimes improves dramatically after medical and/or surgical treatment of sinusitis. A recent study in humans with sinusitis demonstrated that airway hyperresponsiveness may be sustained by reflexes originating in pharyngeal receptors made hypersensitive by seeding of the inflammatory process from above.[55] After therapy with antibiotics and nasal steroids, lower airway responsiveness significantly improved in this latter study. The potential importance of gastroesophageal reflux in producing acute episodes of nocturnal wheezing has been noted above.[49,50] An allergic bronchopulmonary syndrome may also complicate asthma in children.[56] Although allergic bronchopulmonary aspergillosis is the most commonly recognized syndrome, it is now apparent that a variety of molds will cause a similar clinical picture.[57] In the asthma patient with frequent instability associated with an elevated serum IgE, peripheral blood eosinophilia, and transient or fixed radiographic infiltrates, an evaluation should be performed after the acute episode has been treated. The evaluation should include immediate hypersensitivity skin tests to molds as well as tests for precipitating antibodies and mold-specific IgE. If not recognized and treated early, the sequelae of the syndrome include central bronchiectasis, irreversible abnormalities of lung function, pulmonary fibrosis, and respiratory failure.[58] Psychosocial factors must also be considered when asthma recurs frequently and/or leads to prolonged hospitalizations.[59] Lack of compliance with a medical regimen may not only lead to instability, but is also a risk factor for death caused by this disease.[35]

Assessment of the child/adolescent with acute asthma

Children and adolescents with asthma together with their families should be educated about the precipitants of disease and the signs and symptoms that signify loss of control. They must be able to recognize acute symptoms promptly so that an appropriate response can be initiated. To facilitate this process, those who provide care (parents, guardians, school officials, etc.) should be given an action plan that provides specific, practical instructions in the event of an acute episode. Examples of such a plan can be found in the most recent Expert Panel Report.[35] Families must be encouraged to seek assistance when a beneficial response to medical therapy is not obvious or anytime questions arise.

In assessing a child with acute asthma, several historical facts should be considered by the treating physician, including the precipitant of the episode, time of onset, and duration of symptoms. Delay in seeking medical attention, and denial on the part of subjects and their families are characteristics of near-fatal asthma in childhood.[60] Thus, when an acute episode occurs it is important to have an appreciation of the severity of disease in a child as well as the family dynamics. Knowledge of these factors and the assessment skills of those providing care is essential when giving advice via the telephone. Information on current medication use with time of last administration is also important. A history of previous hospitalizations (especially in the recent past and to an intensive care unit) will also influence the decision-making process. A past history of possible life-threatening events (respiratory arrest, hypoxic seizures, need for mechanical ventilation, etc.)

should also be sought. Although several factors have been noted to identify the fatality-prone asthmatic,[35,42] the treating physician should also recall that children with 'mild' disease may suffer fatal asthma.[61]

The severity of acute asthma may be gauged by findings on physical examination as well as through tests of lung function and the adequacy of oxygenation and ventilation (oximetry, arterial blood gases). In the examination, use of accessory muscles of respiration, particularly the sternocleidomastoid muscle, is an indication of significant airflow obstruction.[62] The presence of a pulsus paradoxus of >20 mm Hg[63,64] is also a useful indicator of severe airflow limitation in children with acute asthma. The presence of a 'quiet chest' in an anxious patient struggling to breathe is an ominous finding.

Although it is critical to recognize and appreciate the importance of these physical findings, quantitative assessments are also of great value in the patient with acute asthma. In asthmatics who are extremely breathless, tests of lung mechanics, though highly desirable, may be difficult or impossible to obtain. When tests can be performed, assessments commonly include PEFR and FEV_1. Although flow rates upon presentation are important to record, lack of improvement in lung function after initial treatment may be a better predictor of the need for hospitalization than the pretreatment value.[65]

In critically ill children, arterial blood gases may need to be performed at presentation and then serially as dictated by abnormalities in gas exchange and clinical status. The expected abnormalities in terms of arterial oxygen and carbon dioxide levels as a function of the level of obstruction (FEV_1) were discussed above and are displayed in Figure 9.2. In most clinical settings, advances made in non-invasive monitoring allow for relatively quick assessments in patients with acute asthma regardless of age or degree of obstruction. These methods include oximetry and transcutaneous measurements of oxygen and/or carbon dioxide. The latter has been applied primarily to infants and children, but has also been utilized in older pediatric patients.[66] Oximetry has become the most widely applied and clinically useful tool for assessing oxygenation in emergent situations. Oximeters offer a rapid and reliable non-invasive method of assessing the most vital physiologic consequence of obstructed breathing. Physical signs of hypoxemia such as irritability, pallor and cyanosis are variable and may not be present at mild to moderate levels of oxygen desaturation. In children, oximetry provides a gauge of the acuity of their asthma and may be helpful in decision making about the need for hospitalization. In a study from Australia, Geelhoed and associates[67] found that the initial arterial oxygen saturation was highly predictive of outcome in pediatric asthma patients in an emergency department. A saturation of 91% was found to discriminate between favorable and unfavorable outcomes as defined in part by the need for subsequent care after the initial visit. In addition, continuous measurements of oxygen saturation during therapy helps minimize fluctuations in oxygenation which may be the consequence of both the disease and the therapy provided to the patient. In regard to the latter, lung mechanics may improve after inhalation of a β_2-adrenergic agonist while oxygenation deteriorates.[68] This phenomenon has been attributed in part to the vasodilatory effect of the drugs on the pulmonary vessels, counteracting local vasoconstrictive factors in the lung. Both oximetry and electrodes that assess transcutaneous oxygen provide a non-invasive approach that allow quick responses to fluctuating oxygen needs.

In children with mild episodes of acute asthma, chest radiographs will likely show hyperinflation and peribronchial thickening. For most children that respond to outpatient therapy for the acute episode, radiographs of the chest are not necessary unless there is suspicion of complicating processes (localized rales or decreased breath sounds, localized wheezing, increased temperature). On the other hand, children requiring hospitalization will often have this study performed to assess for atelectasis, pneumomediastinum, and/or pneumonic consolidation.[69,70]

Therapy of acute asthma in children and adolescents

The therapeutic approach to the pediatric patient with an acute exacerbation of asthma that does not easily respond to inhaled β_2-adrenergic agonists in the home setting can be organized in several ways. This section will review the therapeutic agents most commonly used to treat acute asthma (inhaled β_2-agonists, corticosteroids, inhaled anticholinergic agents, intravenous aminophylline or theophylline). Doses of conventional medications as well as routes of administration are listed in Table 9.2. This will be followed by a discussion of mechanical ventilation. Finally, other forms of therapy that are sometimes employed but are not as well studied or are more controversial in terms of benefit will be listed.

The point must again be made that delay in seeking medical attention as well as underuse or delay in initiation of oral corticosteroids may contribute to the subsequent need for admission to an intensive care unit.[71] A physician must balance the advantages of early therapy by the family within the home when the episode appears mild versus the advantages of personally assessing the patient within an outpatient setting. The education of patient and care givers regarding what can safely be done in the home and when help must be sought have to be continually reviewed and discussed. This will vary from patient to patient because of several factors including the ability of care givers to assess and provide effective management early in the course of the episode.

Table 9.2 Medications for treating acute asthma in children and adolescents

Medication	Route	Dose*	Frequency of administration
Oxygen	Inhalation	1–3 LPM	Continuously until PaO_2 > 92% on room air
Albuterol (salbutamol)	Inhalation – nebulization	0.15 mg/kg	q20 minutes × 3, then prn
		0.30–0.50 mg/kg per hour	Continuous nebulization
	– MDI	4–8 puffs	q20 minutes × 3, then q1–4 hours
Terbutaline	Intravenous	10 µg/kg	Initial infusion over 10 minutes
		0.10–4.0 µg/kg per hour	Continuous infusion
Prednisone	Oral	1 mg/kg	Two times a day
Prednisolone	Oral	1 mg/kg	Two times a day
Methylprednisolone	Intravenous	1 mg/kg	q6 hours
Ipratropium bromide	Inhalation – nebulization	250 µg	q20 minutes × 3, then q3–6 hours

* Doses of most medications are based on recommendations found in the second Expert Panel Report of the National Heart, Lung, and Blood Institute National Asthma Education Program.[35] Use of intravenous terbutaline is discussed in the first Expert Panel Report.[110]

Whenever there are concerns expressed by those responsible for delivering care, children should be seen and evaluated by medical personnel.

Pharmacotherapy

A selective β_2-adrenergic agonist (usually albuterol (salbutamol)) is administered by inhalation to accomplish the primary goal of rapidly reversing airway obstruction. Inhaled adrenergic agonists have replaced subcutaneous administration of this class of drugs as the treatment of choice owing to equal efficacy as well as the fact that injections can be avoided in children who are already anxious.[72] In instances when the episode is mild and the therapy is initiated early, administration of one respiratory treatment via metered dose inhaler (two actuations) or by nebulization (0.5 ml of a 5 mg/ml solution in 3 ml normal saline) may lead to substantial and prolonged bronchodilation. A good response is commonly defined as a return of the PEFR to greater than 80% predicted or personal best with the response sustained for 4 hours.[35] Children who improve with home bronchodilator therapy may then safely repeat this treatment as frequently as every 4 hours. Serial measurement of peak flow before and after therapy is a useful way not only to assess the severity of acute asthma but also to monitor the response to treatment.

A lack of response or an incomplete response to inhalation of a β_2-adrenergic agonist in a patient with asthma should always be a concern, and is reason for evaluation and treatment by a physician. Despite a poor response, this class of drugs is still central to the therapy of the disease when it reaches a more critical state. In the appropriately monitored patient, albuterol (salbutamol) may be administered by small volume nebulization either continuously (0.3–0.5 mg/kg per hour; maximum = 15 mg/hour) or intermittently (0.15 mg/kg per dose every 20 minutes for 1–2 hours; minimum = 1.25 mg/dose; maximum = 5 mg/dose) as dictated by the clinical picture. These doses are based in part on studies that addressed the effects of drug dose and frequency of administration in children,[73–75] and are similar to doses recommended in the Expert Panel Report of the National Heart, Lung, and Blood Institute National Asthma Education Program.[35] Because of the hypoxia commonly seen when asthmatics present for care and the fact that hypoxia may also develop with administration of β_2-agonists (reviewed above), this drug should be administered with oxygen.

Recent reports have demonstrated the utility of using a metered-dose inhaler with a spacer device to deliver adrenergic agonists in the face of acute asthma.[76–78] In one study, an average of eight puffs (range 4–14 puffs) was required to achieve an acceptable improvement in airflow rate with minimal side-effects.[76] Although this number of actuations is large compared with the number commonly used to treat mild asthma,[79] the actual dose of β_2-agonist (μg/kg) was only 20% of that delivered to a control group by conventional small volume nebulization.[76] The cost and time savings of this delivery method must be balanced against various concerns with this form of treatment, including the message transmitted to patients and families that this approach might be employed at home without the need to seek medical attention. The consequences of the latter are currently undefined.

In the patient who is not responding to continuous nebulized administration of albuterol (salbutamol) (combined with intravenous steroids and theophylline ± inhaled ipratropium bromide as discussed below), intravenous infusion of a selective β_2-agonist may be added in an attempt to avoid mechanical ventilation.[80–82] An arterial line is necessary in this situation to monitor closely the effect of this therapy on the $PaCO_2$. When using these agents in this or other manners that lead to administration of high doses of drugs, the potential for cardiac toxicity must be kept in mind. Thus, monitoring of CPK-MB levels as well as electrocardiograms is recommended.[83] Serum potassium should also be monitored closely in this situation because of the combined effects of sympathomimetics and corticosteroids in decreasing serum potassium.[84] Hypokalemia should be corrected to minimize risks of cardiac toxicity.

The early administration of corticosteroids is

important in the treatment of acute asthma that is either poorly or only partially responsive to β_2-agonists. For ambulatory patients, the benefits of prompt intervention with short courses of oral corticosteroid to prevent progression of asthma have been demonstrated.[85–89] Collectively, these studies suggest that oral corticosteroids given to outpatients prevent hospitalization, reduce symptoms, and improve pulmonary function. In general, a dose of 1–2 mg/kg per day of either prednisone or prednisolone is given in two divided doses for a minimum of 3–5 days.

The utility of intravenous administration of corticosteroids to hospitalized asthmatic children has also been shown.[90,91] Methylprednisolone may be the preferred glucocorticoid, in part because of its preferential penetration into the lung.[92,93] The starting dose for children with acute asthma who require hospitalization is commonly 1 mg/kg given every 6 hours. It should be noted that hospitalized children have also shown significant benefit from oral corticosteroids.[94,95] The decision regarding use of an oral versus intravenous route within an inpatient setting must be made on the basis of clinical criteria that include the severity of the episode as well as the ability of the patient to tolerate medications/fluids orally.

Short courses of high dose corticosteroids as used to treat acute asthma are usually well tolerated. Although hypokalemia and hyperglycemia may be seen, the more serious complication of prolonged muscle weakness may evolve when this class of medication is used with non-depolarizing muscle relaxants during mechanical ventilation (see below). Long-term suppression of the hypothalamic–pituitary–adrenal axis is usually not seen when corticosteroids are used for 5 or fewer days[96] but is a concern when this pattern of administration is repeated several times a year.[97]

Inhaled anticholinergic agents may be beneficial in the treatment of acute asthma in pediatric patients. Several studies have shown additional bronchodilation when ipratropium bromide is combined with an inhaled adrenergic agent in older children and adolescents with acute asthma.[98–101] This additive effect is shown in Figure 9.4.[101] A study of the dose–response relationship of this drug in 9–17-year-old asthmatics demonstrated dose-dependent bronchodilation that became significant at a dose of 75 µg.[102] A plateau was reached at a dose of 250 µg, leading to the commonly recommended dose of 250 µg. This dose may be given every 20 minutes for 3 doses and then every 2–4 hours thereafter.[35,101]

Intravenous administration of aminophylline used to be commonly employed in the therapy of acute asthma. However, recent studies suggest this therapy adds little except toxicity when added to more conventional therapy in children with mild to moderate illness.[103–107] However, current data are inadequate to judge whether this drug is beneficial in the severely ill child who is not responding to therapy and who may be progressing toward respiratory failure.[108] In this instance, many physicians will also treat with intravenous aminophylline or theophylline. A parenteral form of theophylline without ethylenediamine is available and is recommended when used for the therapy of severe status asthmaticus.[109] Loading doses and constant infusion rates are based on the age of the patient and are calculated to obtain a mean steady state concentration of approximately 15 µg/ml. These doses and rates are included in the first Expert Panel Report.[110] Serum concentrations must be serially monitored when aminophylline or theophylline is administered.

Mechanical ventilation

When therapeutic efforts at reversing airway obstruction are unsuccessful as judged by various criteria (Table 9.3), mechanical ventilation must be added to the pharmacologic regimen. As reviewed previously, an increase in $PaCO_2$ is seen when airflow is markedly compromised (Figure 9.2). Although retention of carbon dioxide is a critical finding in an asthmatic, it no longer constitutes an absolute indication for intubation and mechanical ventilation.[111] The morbidity and mortality associated with mechanical ventilation have prompted new approaches to this form of intervention which may decrease adverse outcomes.[112–116] Ventilator

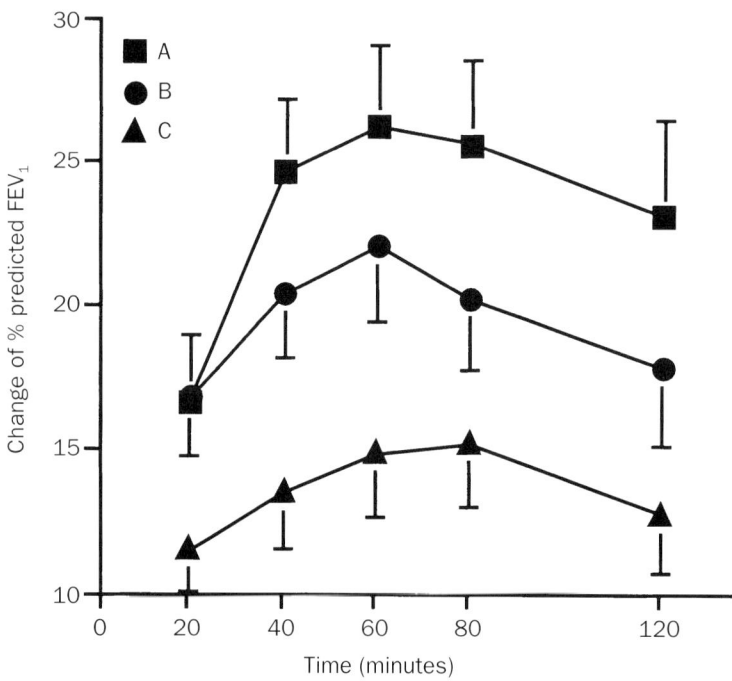

Figure 9.4 The mean change of percent predicted FEV_1 with time in three groups of pediatric patients with acute asthma where the FEV_1 was less than 50% of that predicted at presentation. All three groups received three treatments of albuterol (salbutamol) in the first hour (0.15 mg/kg per dose). Group A ($n = 40$) also received three doses of ipratropium (250 μg/dose) over the first hour, whereas Group B ($n = 39$) received only one dose of ipratropium during this same period of time. Group C ($n = 41$) received only albuterol (salbutamol) and no ipratropium. The children receiving albuterol (salbutamol) plus ipratropium (Groups A and B) had significantly greater improvement in lung function compared with the group that received albuterol (salbutamol) only. Patients receiving three doses in the first hour of therapy (Group A) had the greatest response. (From Schuh et al.[101])

strategies that decrease mean airway pressure (through pressure or volume limitation) with a resultant 'permissive hypercapnia' have been associated with improved clinical outcomes.[112] Employing this approach, elevated $PaCO_2$ levels are tolerated, provided adequate oxygenation and a pH $\geqslant 7.20$ can be maintained. This method of ventilation significantly decreases the risk of barotrauma because high peak pressures are avoided.[117]

Several important complications in addition to barotrauma may result from mechanical ventilation. Prolonged therapeutic paralysis during mechanical ventilation when used with corticosteroids has been associated with a myopathy that may be severe.[118,119] This risk is decreased if short-term paralysis (<48 hours) can be used to provide satisfactory hypoventilation during the initial period of ventilation. Other significant complications include the development of intrinsic positive end-expiratory pressure (PEEP). This occurs because severe airway obstruction is associated with long time constants in the lung and the need for prolonged expiratory times to empty respiratory units. If expiratory times on the ventilator are not long enough to allow the lungs to deflate, auto-PEEP develops. This may interfere with venous return and cause hypotension. To prevent this problem, low levels of PEEP (up to 3 cm H_2O) and low ventilatory rates with high inspiratory flows are employed to provide low inspiratory/expiratory ratios and prolonged expiratory times. Another complication is atelectasis. Although this usually responds to conservative management (frequent suctioning and use of chest physiotherapy as tolerated), flexible bronchoscopy has been employed to remove mucus plugs. However, this may lead to increased airway obstruction in response to manipulation of the airway.[111]

Pressure-support ventilation has also been employed in a small series to treat four asthmatic children with respiratory failure.[120] This approach allowed each patient to determine their own respiratory pattern and to maintain

Table 9.3 Indications for mechanical ventilation of children and adolescents with acute asthma

Rapidly increasing pulsus paradoxus
Decreasing pulsus paradoxus in an exhausted patient
Deteriorating mental status (lethargy or agitation)
Cardiac arrhythmia or arrest
Respiratory arrest
Inability to speak
Unresolving lactic acidosis
Diaphoresis in the recumbent position
Silent chest in spite of vigorous respiratory effort
Hypoxemia (PaO_2 < 60 mm Hg) unrelieved by 100% oxygen*
$PaCO_2$ > 60 mm Hg and rising more than 5 mm Hg/hour*

* Relative indication.

forced exhalation. Thus, patient–ventilator asynchrony was eliminated and the chances of airleak syndromes were reduced.

Other forms of therapy
Other forms of therapy have been employed in pediatric outpatient as well as in inpatient settings including intensive care units. Although almost all patients respond to the more conventional therapies outlined above, the treatments discussed in this section offer additional approaches that with time may become more generally accepted and utilized. In addition, certain approaches have been used when traditional forms of therapy have been unsuccessful (use of anesthetic agents). Physicians caring for patients with asthma should know that these extraordinary treatments have been employed with some success. These therapies are briefly noted with citations provided for readers desiring additional information.

In patients with asthma, the inhalation of the low density gas helium may reduce the work of breathing by changing turbulent to laminar flow in obstructed portions of central airways. In a recent double-blind study involving 18 children in an emergency department or intensive care unit, inhalation of heliox (80% helium, 20% oxygen mixture) for 15 minutes in addition to administration of oxygen (nasal cannula) together with continuous albuterol (salbutamol) nebulizations and intravenous methylprednisolone significantly lowered the pulsus paradoxus, increased the peak flow, and decreased the dyspnea index.[121] In addition, the authors felt that this therapy prevented the need for mechanical ventilation in three patients. Unfortunately, experience with heliox in pediatric patients with acute severe asthma has not always demonstrated a benefit.[122] The reason for the differences in outcome between these studies is not readily apparent, suggesting that additional investigations are needed to define factors that determine response to this therapy.

Intravenous infusions of magnesium sulfate have been noted to significantly improve short-term pulmonary function in children with moderate to severe asthma via mechanisms that are poorly understood. This clinical effect was recently demonstrated in a randomized, placebo-controlled, double-blind study in 6–18-year-old children in an emergency department who had a peak expiratory flow rate of less than 60% predicted after three nebulizer treatments with a β_2-agonist.[123] In this study, an intravenous infusion of 25 mg/kg (up to a maximum dose of 2 g) was added to the subsequent conventional therapy, and this led to a lower hospitalization rate as well as more rapid improvement in lung function. Slow infusions are utilized to prevent alterations in blood pressure and heart rate. Additional side-effects can include flushing, nausea, vomiting, dry mouth and malaise. Muscle weakness and respiratory depression as well as loss of deep tendon reflexes occur when serum magnesium levels exceed 12 mmol/l.[124]

Respiratory failure that remains refractory to pharmacotherapy plus mechanical ventilation has been successfully treated with anesthetic agents. These medications have included inhalation agents such as halothane[125] and isoflurane[126] as well as ketamine delivered by intravenous infusion.[127] Since only a few hospitalized patients require mechanical ventilation and most do well with conventional treatment, future large controlled trials of general anesthesia in the treatment of refractory severe asthma are unlikely. Thus, we will continue to rely on case reports or manuscripts in which a small number of patient experiences are chronicled. Yet, examination of the literature suggests use of anesthetic agents represents a reasonable intervention in selected patients.[128]

SUMMARY

During acute episodes of asthma, marked decreases in flow rates together with hyperinflation of the lungs are seen in tests of lung mechanics. In addition, hypoxemia is a common finding in subjects with wheezing, and hypercapnia develops as a late consequence of severe airflow obstruction. Clinical signs and symptoms of obstruction resolve before tests of lung function which may not normalize for some time. In a subgroup of asthmatic patients, lung function will never completely normalize. With the development of acute asthma, control is regained through inhalations of a β_2-agonist, which may be given continuously if necessary. In addition, for episodes that do not quickly respond to inhaled β_2-agonist, oral or intravenous corticosteroids are used. Intravenous theophylline as well as inhaled ipratropium bromide and intravenous administration of a β_2-agonist may help prevent the need for mechanical ventilation in the most severe patients. A fundamental knowledge of the pathophysiology of acute severe asthma is necessary to provide effective treatment for patients with this potentially life-threatening condition.

ACKNOWLEDGEMENTS

This work was supported in part by Grant No. HL 36577 from the National Institutes of Health. The authors thank Ms Stephanie Park for her assistance in the preparation of this manuscript.

REFERENCES

1. O'Hollaren MT, Yuninger JW, Offord KP et al. Exposure to an aeroallergen as a possible precipitating factor in respiratory arrest in young patients with asthma. *N Engl J Med* 1991; **324:** 359–63.
2. Persson CGA. Centennial notions of asthma as an eosinophilic, desquamative, exudative, and steroid-sensitive disease. *Lancet* 1997; **350:** 1021–4.
3. Dunnill MS. The pathology of asthma, with special reference to changes in the bronchial mucosa. *J Clin Pathol* 1960; **13:** 27–33.
4. Dunnill MS, Massarella GR, Anderson JA. A comparison of the quantitative anatomy of the bronchi in normal subjects, in status asthmaticus, in chronic bronchitis, and in emphysema. *Thorax* 1969; **24:** 176–9.
5. Richards W, Patrick JR. Death from asthma in children. *Am J Dis Child* 1965; **110:** 4–23.
6. Beasley R, Roche WR, Roberts JA, Holgate ST. Cellular events in the bronchi in mild asthma and after bronchial provocation. *Am Rev Respir Dis* 1989; **139:** 806–17.
7. Vignola AM, Chanez P, Campbell AM et al. Airway inflammation in mild intermittent and in persistent asthma. *Am J Respir Crit Care Med* 1998; **157:** 403–9.
8. Djukanović R, Roche WR, Wilson JW et al. Mucosal inflammation in asthma. *Am Rev Respir Dis* 1990; **142:** 434–57.
9. Ferguson AC, Whitelaw M, Brown H. Correlation of bronchial eosinophil and mast cell activation with bronchial hyperresponsiveness in children with asthma. *J Allergy Clin Immunol* 1992; **90:** 609–13.
10. Cutz E, Levison H, Cooper DM. Ultrastructure of airways in children with asthma. *Histopathology* 1978; **2:** 407–21.
11. McFadden ER Jr. Development, structure, and physiology in the normal lung and in asthma. In: Middleton E Jr, Reed CE, Ellis EF, Adkinson NF Jr, Yuninger JW, Busse WW, eds. *Allergy: Principles and Practice*, 5th edn. St Louis: Mosby, 1998, 508–19.
12. Larsen GL, Brugman SM. Severe asthma in children. In: Barnes PJ, Grunstein MM, Leff A,

13. Woolcock AJ, eds. *Asthma*. Philadelphia: Lippincott-Raven, 1997, 1955–75.
13. Hargreave FE, Dolovich J, O'Byrne PM et al. The origin of airway hyperresponsiveness. *J Allergy Clin Immunol* 1986; **78:** 825–32.
14. Colasurdo GN, Larsen GL. Airway hyperresponsiveness. In: Busse W, Holgate S, eds. *Asthma and Rhinitis*. Boston: Blackwell Scientific Publications, 1994, 1044–56.
15. Murray AB, Ferguson AC, Morrison B et al. Airway responsiveness to histamine as a test for overall severity of asthma in children. *J Allergy Clin Immunol* 1981; **68:** 119–24.
16. Avital A, Noviski N, Bar-Yishay E et al. Nonspecific bronchial reactivity in asthmatic children depends on severity but not on age. *Am Rev Respir Dis* 1991; **144:** 36–8.
17. Amaro-Galvez R, McLaughlin FJ, Levison H et al. Grading severity and treatment requirements to control symptoms in asthmatic children and their relationship with airway hyperreactivity to methacholine. *Ann Allergy* 1987; **59:** 298–302.
18. Rakes GP, Arruda E, Ingram JM et al. Rhinovirus and respiratory syncytial virus in wheezing children requiring emergency care. *Am J Respir Crit Care Med* 1999; **159:** 785–90.
19. Empey DW, Laitenen LA, Jacobs L et al. Mechanisms of bronchial hyperreactivity in normal subjects after upper respiratory tract infection. *Ann Rev Respir Dis* 1976; **113:** 131–9.
20. Hall WJ, Hall CB, Speers DM. Respiratory syncytial virus infection in adults. Clinical, virologic, and serial pulmonary function studies. *Ann Intern Med* 1978; **88:** 203–5.
21. Little JW, Hall WJ, Douglas RG et al. Airway hyperreactivity and peripheral airway dysfunction in influenza A infection. *Am Rev Respir Dis* 1978; **118:** 295–303.
22. Lemanske RF Jr, Dick EC, Swenson CA et al. Rhinovirus upper respiratory infection increases airway hyperreactivity and late asthmatic reactions. *J Clin Invest* 1989; **83:** 1–10.
23. Bauer MA, Utell MJ, Morrow PE et al. Inhalation of 0.3 ppm nitrogen dioxide potentiates exercise-induced bronchospasm in asthmatics. *Am Rev Respir Dis* 1986; **134:** 1203–8.
24. Seltzer J, Bigby BG, Stulbarg M et al. O_3-induced change in bronchial reactivity to methacholine and airway inflammation in humans. *J Appl Physiol* 1986; **60:** 1321–6.
25. Zwick H, Popp W, Wagner C et al. Effects of ozone on the respiratory health, allergic sensitization, and cellular immune system in children. *Am Rev Respir Dis* 1991; **144:** 1075–9.
26. Martinez FD, Antognoni G, Macri F et al. Parental smoking enhances bronchial responsiveness in nine-year-old children. *Am Rev Respir Dis* 1988; **138:** 518–23.
27. Fielder HMP, Lyons RA, Heaven M et al. Effect of environmental tobacco smoke on peak flow variability. *Arch Dis Child* 1999; **80:** 253–6.
28. Burr ML, Anderson HR, Austin JB et al. Respiratory symptoms and home environment in children: a national survey. *Thorax* 1999; **54:** 27–32.
29. Cartier A, Thomson NC, Frith PA et al. Allergen-induced increase in bronchial responsiveness to histamine: relationship to the late asthmatic response and change in airway caliber. *J Allergy Clin Immunol* 1982; **70:** 170–7.
30. Boulet LP, Cartier A, Thomson NC et al. Asthma and increases in nonallergic bronchial responsiveness from seasonal pollen exposure. *J Allergy Clin Immunol* 1983; **71:** 399–406.
31. Mussaffi H, Springer C, Godfrey S. Increased bronchial responsiveness to exercise and histamine after allergen challenge in children with asthma. *J Allergy Clin Immunol* 1986; **77:** 48–52.
32. Wenzel SE, Larsen GL. Assessment of lung function: pulmonary function testing. In: Bierman CW, Pearlman DS, Shapiro GS, Busse WW, eds. *Allergy, Asthma, and Immunology from Infancy to Adulthood*, 3rd edn. Philadelphia: WB Saunders, 1996, 157–72.
33. Olive JT Jr, Hyatt RE. Maximal expiratory flow and total respiratory resistance during induced bronchoconstriction in asthmatic subjects. *Am Rev Respir Dis* 1972; **106:** 366–76.
34. McFadden ER Jr, Kiser R, deGroot WJ. Acute bronchial asthma. Relations between clinical and physiologic manifestations. *N Engl J Med* 1973; **288:** 221–5.
35. National Asthma Education and Prevention Program. *Expert Panel Report II, Guidelines for the Diagnosis and Management of Asthma*. Bethesda, MD: National Heart, Lung and Blood Institute, 1997.
36. Martin RJ. Nocturnal asthma. *Clinics Chest Med* 1992; **13:** 533–50.
37. Hetzel MR, Clark TJH, Branthwaite MA. Asthma: analysis of sudden deaths and ventilatory arrests in hospitals. *Br Med J* 1977; **1:** 808–11.
38. Woolcock AJ, Read J. Lung volumes in exacerbations of asthma. *Am J Med* 1966; **41:** 259–73.

39. Weng TR, Levison H. Pulmonary function in children with asthma at acute attack and symptom-free status. *Am Rev Respir Dis* 1969; **99**: 719–28.
40. McFadden ER Jr, Lyons HA. Arterial-blood gas tension in asthma. *N Engl J Med* 1968; **278**: 1027–32.
41. Weng TR, Langer HM, Featherby EA, Levison H. Arterial blood gas tensions and acid–base balance in symptomatic and asymptomatic asthma in childhood. *Am Rev Respir Dis* 1970; **101**: 274–82.
42. Kikuchi Y, Okabe S, Tamura G et al. Chemosensitivity and perception of dyspnea in patients with a history of near-fatal asthma. *N Engl J Med* 1994; **330**: 1329–34.
43. Downes JJ, Wood DW, Striker TW, Pittman JC. Arterial blood gas and acid–base disorders in infants and children with status asthmaticus. *Pediatrics* 1968; **42**: 238–49.
44. Appel D, Rubenstein R, Schrager K, Williams MH Jr. Lactic acidosis in severe asthma. *Am J Med* 1983; **75**: 580–4.
45. Christopher KL, Wood RP, Eckert C et al. Vocal-cord dysfunction presenting as asthma. *N Engl J Med* 1983; **308**: 566–70.
46. Martin RJ, Blager FB, Gay ML, Wood RP. Paradoxic vocal cord motion in presumed asthmatics. *Semin Respir Med* 1987; **8**: 332–7.
47. Brugman SM, Howell JH, Rosenberg DM et al. The spectrum of pediatric vocal cord dysfunction. *Am J Respir Crit Care Med* 1994; **149**(2): A353.
48. Eid NS, Shepherd RW, Thomson MA. Persistent wheezing and gastroesophageal reflux in infants. *Pediatr Pulmonol* 1994; **18**: 39–44.
49. Martin ME, Grunstein MM, Larsen GL. The relationship of gastroesophageal reflux to nocturnal wheezing in childhood asthma. *Ann Allergy* 1982; **49**: 318–22.
50. Davis RS, Larsen GL, Grunstein MM. Respiratory response to intraesophageal acid infusion in asthmatic children during sleep. *J Allergy Clin Immunol* 1983; **72**: 393–8.
51. Hardy KA, Schidlow DV, Zaeri N. Obliterative bronchiolitis in children. *Chest* 1988; **93**: 460–6.
52. Fan LL, Mullen ALW, Brugman SM et al. Clinical spectrum of chronic interstitial lung disease in children. *J Pediatr* 1992; **121**: 867–72.
53. Fan LL, Langston C. Chronic interstitial lung disease in children. *Pediatr Pulmonol* 1993; **16**: 184–96.
54. Rachelefsky GS, Katz RM, Siegel SC. Chronic sinus disease with associated reactive airways disease in children. *Pediatrics* 1984; **73**: 526–9.
55. Bucca C, Rolla G, Scappaticci E et al. Extrathoracic and intrathoracic airway responsiveness in sinusitis. *J Allergy Clin Immunol* 1995; **95**: 52–9.
56. Wang JLF, Patterson R, Mintzer R et al. Allergic bronchopulmonary aspergillosis in pediatric practice. *J Pediatr* 1979; **94**: 376–81.
57. Lee TM, Greenberger PA, Oh S et al. Allergic bronchopulmonary candidiasis: case report and suggested diagnostic criteria. *J Allergy Clin Immunol* 1987; **80**: 816–20.
58. Greenberger PA, Miller TP, Roberts M, Smith LL. Allergic bronchopulmonary aspergillosis in patients with and without evidence of bronchiectasis. *Ann Allergy* 1993; **70**: 333–8.
59. Morray B, Redding G. Factors associated with prolonged hospitalization of children with asthma. *Arch Pediatr Adolesc Med* 1995; **149**: 276–9.
60. Martin AJ, Campbell DA, Gluyas PA et al. Characteristics of near-fatal asthma in childhood. *Pediatr Pulmonol* 1995; **20**: 1–8.
61. Robertson CF, Rubinfeld AR, Bowes G. Pediatric asthma deaths in Victoria: the mild are at risk. *Pediatr Pulmonol* 1992; **13**: 95–100.
62. Commey JOO, Levison H. Physical signs in childhood asthma. *Pediatrics* 1976; **58**: 537–41.
63. Galant SP, Groncy CE, Shaw KC. The value of pulsus paradoxus in assessing the child with status asthmaticus. *Pediatrics* 1978; **61**: 46–51.
64. Martell JAO, Lopez JGH, Harker JEG. Pulsus paradoxus in acute asthma in children. *J Asthma* 1992; **29**: 349–52.
65. Schuh S, Johnson D, Stephens D et al. Hospitalization patterns in severe acute asthma in children. *Pediatr Pulmonol* 1997; **23**: 184–92.
66. Holmgren D, Sixt R. Transcutaneous and arterial blood gas monitoring during acute asthmatic symptoms in older children. *Pediatr Pulmonol* 1992; **14**: 80–4.
67. Geelhoed GC, Landau LI, LeSouëf PN. Predictive value of oxygen saturation in emergency evaluation of asthmatic children. *Br Med J* 1988; **297**: 395–6.
68. Holmgren D, Sixt R. Effects of salbutamol inhalations on transcutaneous blood gases in children during the acute asthmatic attack: from acute deterioration to recovery. *Acta Paediatr* 1994; **83**: 515–19.
69. Eggleston PA, Ward BH, Pierson WE et al. Radiographic abnormalities in acute asthma in

children. *Pediatrics* 1974; **54:** 442–9.
70. Gershel JC, Goldman HS, Stein REK et al. The usefulness of chest radiographs in first asthma attacks. *N Engl J Med* 1983; **309:** 336–9.
71. Stein R, Canny GJ, Bohn DJ et al. Severe acute asthma in a pediatric intensive care unit: six years' experience. *Pediatrics* 1989; **83:** 1023–8.
72. Becker AB, Nelson NA, Simons FER. Inhaled salbutamol (albuterol) vs injected epinephrine in the treatment of acute asthma in children. *J Pediatr* 1981; **102:** 465–9.
73. Robertson CF, Smith F, Beck R, Levison H. Response to frequent low doses of nebulized salbutamol in acute asthma. *J Pediatr* 1985; **106:** 672–4.
74. Schuh S, Parkin P, Rajan A et al. High- versus low-dose, frequently administered, nebulized albuterol in children with severe, acute asthma. *Pediatrics* 1989; **83:** 513–18.
75. Schuh S, Reider MJ, Canny G et al. Nebulized albuterol in acute childhood asthma: comparison of two doses. *Pediatrics* 1990; **86:** 509–13.
76. Benton G, Thomas RC, Nickerson BG et al. Experience with a metered-dose inhaler with a spacer in the pediatric emergency department. *Am J Dis Child* 1989; **143:** 678–81.
77. Kerem E, Levison H, Schuh S et al. Efficacy of albuterol administered by nebulizer versus spacer device in children with acute asthma. *J Pediatr* 1993; **123:** 313–17.
78. Lin Y-Z, Hsieh K-H. Metered dose inhaler and nebulizer in acute asthma. *Arch Dis Child* 1995; **72:** 214–18.
79. Schuh S, Johnson D, Stephens D et al. Comparison of albuterol delivered by a metered dose inhaler with a spacer versus a nebulizer in children with mild acute asthma. *J Pediatr* 1999; **135:** 22–7.
80. Pierce RJ, Payne CR, Williams SJ et al. Comparison of intravenous and inhaled terbutaline in the treatment of asthma. *Chest* 1981; **79:** 506–11.
81. Bohn D, Kalloghlian A, Jenkins J et al. Intravenous salbutomol in the treatment of status asthmaticus in children. *Crit Care Med* 1984; **12:** 892–6.
82. Van Renterghem D, Lamont H, Elinck W et al. Intravenous versus nebulized terbutaline in patients with acute severe asthma: a double-blind randomized study. *Ann Allergy* 1987; **59:** 313–16.
83. Maguire JF, O'Rourke PP, Colan SD et al. Cardiotoxicity during treatment of severe childhood asthma. *Pediatrics* 1991; **88:** 1180–6.
84. Spangler DL. Review of side effects associated with beta agonists. *Ann Allergy* 1989; **62:** 59–62.
85. Shapiro GG, Furukawa CT, Pierson WE et al. Double-blind evaluation of methylprednisolone versus placebo for acute asthma episodes. *Pediatrics* 1983; **71:** 510–14.
86. Deshpande A, McKenzie SA. Short course of steroids in home treatment of children with acute asthma. *Br Med J* 1986; **293:** 169–71.
87. Harris JB, Weinberger MM, Nassif E et al. Early intervention with short courses of prednisone to prevent progression of asthma in ambulatory patients incompletely responsive to bronchodilators. *J Pediatr* 1987; **110:** 627–33.
88. Scarfone RJ, Fuchs SM, Nager AL, Shane SA. Controlled trial of oral prednisone in the emergency department treatment of children with acute asthma. *Pediatrics* 1993; **92:** 513–18.
89. Horowitz L, Zafrir O, Gilboa S et al. Acute asthma. Single dose oral steroids in paediatric community clinics. *Eur J Pediatr* 1994; **153:** 526–30.
90. Pierson WE, Bierman CW, Kelley VC. A double-blind trial of corticosteroid therapy in status asthmaticus. *Pediatrics* 1974; **54:** 282–8.
91. Younger RE, Gerber PS, Herrod HG et al. Intravenous methylprednisolone efficacy in status asthmaticus of childhood. *Pediatrics* 1987; **80:** 225–30.
92. Braude AC, Rebuck AS. Prednisone and methylprednisolone disposition in the lung. *Lancet* 1983; **2:** 995–7.
93. Greos LS, Vichyanond P, Bloedow DC et al. Methylprednisolone achieves greater concentrations in the lung than prednisolone. A pharmacokinetic analysis. *Am Rev Respir Dis* 1991; **144:** 586–92.
94. Loren ML, Chai H, Leung P et al. Corticosteroids in the treatment of acute exacerbations of asthma. *Ann Allergy* 1980; **45:** 67–71.
95. Becker JM, Arora A, Scarfone RJ et al. Oral versus intravenous corticosteroids in children hospitalized with asthma. *J Allergy Clin Immunol* 1999; **103:** 586–90.
96. Zora JA, Zimmerman D, Carey TL et al. Hypothalamic–pituitary–adrenal axis suppression after short-term, high-dose glucocorticoid therapy in children with asthma. *J Allergy Clin Immunol* 1986; **77:** 9–13.
97. Dolan LM, Kesarwala HH, Holroyde JC, Fischer TJ. Short-term, high-dose systemic steroids in children with asthma: the effect on the hypo-

thalamic–pituitary–adrenal axis. *J Allergy Clin Immunol* 1987; **81**: 80–7.
98. Beck R, Robertson C, Galdès-Sebaldt M, Levison H. Combined salbutamol and ipratropium bromide by inhalation in the treatment of severe acute asthma. *J Pediatr* 1985; **107**: 605–8.
99. Watson WTA, Becker AB, Simons FER. Comparison of ipratropium solution, fenoterol solution, and their combination administered by nebulizer and face mask to children with acute asthma. *J Allergy Clin Immunol* 1988; **82**: 1012–18.
100. Reisman J, Galdes-Sebalt M, Kazin F et al. Frequent administration by inhalation of salbutamol and ipratropium bromide in the initial management of severe acute asthma in children. *J Allergy Clin Immunol* 1988; **81**: 16–20.
101. Schuh S, Johnson DW, Callahan S et al. Efficacy of frequent nebulized ipratropium bromide added to frequent high-dose albuterol therapy in severe childhood asthma. *J Pediatr* 1995; **126**: 639–45.
102. Davis A, Vickerson F, Worsley G et al. Determination of dose–response relationship for nebulized ipratropium in asthmatic children. *J Pediatr* 1984; **105**: 1002–5.
103. Carter E, Cruz M, Chesrown S et al. Efficacy of intravenously administered theophylline in children hospitalized with severe asthma. *J Pediatr* 1993; **122**: 470–6.
104. DiGiulio GA, Kercsmar CM, Krug SE et al. Hospital treatment of asthma: lack of benefit from theophylline given in addition to nebulized albuterol and intravenously administered corticosteroid. *J Pediatr* 1993; **122**: 464–9.
105. Strauss RE, Wertheim DL, Bonagura VR, Valacer DJ. Aminophylline therapy does not improve outcome and increases adverse effects in children hospitalized with acute asthmatic exacerbations. *Pediatrics* 1994; **93**: 205–10.
106. Bien JP, Bloom MD, Evans RL et al. Intravenous theophylline in pediatric status asthmaticus. A prospective, randomized, double-blind, placebo-controlled trial. *Clin Pediatr* 1995; **34**: 475–81.
107. Needleman JP, Kaifer MC, Nold JT et al. Theophylline does not shorten hospital stay for children admitted for asthma. *Arch Pediatr Adolesc Med* 1995; **149**: 206–9.
108. Weinberger MM, Theophylline: when should it be used? *J Pediatr* 1993; **122**: 403–5.
109. Weinberger MM. Why adulterate theophylline? *Ann Allergy* 1993; **71**: 419.
110. National Heart, Lung, and Blood Institute National Asthma Education Program. Expert Panel Report, guidelines for the diagnosis and management of asthma. *J Allergy Clin Immunol* 1991; **88**(2): 425–534.
111. DeNicola LK, Monem GF, Gayle MO, Kissoon N. Treatment of critical status asthmaticus in children. *Ped Clin N America* 1994; **41**: 1293–324.
112. Darioli R, Perret C. Mechanical controlled hypoventilation in status asthmaticus. *Am Rev Respir Dis* 1984; **129**: 385–7.
113. Dworkin G, Kattan M. Mechanical ventilation for status asthmaticus in children. *J Pediatr* 1989; **114**: 545–9.
114. Williams TJ, Tuxen DV, Scheinkestel CD et al. Risk factors for morbidity in mechanically ventilated patients with acute severe asthma. *Am Rev Respir Dis* 1992; **146**: 607–15.
115. Bidani A, Tzouanakis AE, Cardenas VJ, Zwischenberger JB. Permissive hypercapnia in acute respiratory failure. *JAMA* 1994; **272**: 957–62.
116. Tuxen DV. Permissive hypercapnic ventilation. *Am J Respir Crit Care Med* 1994; **150**: 870–4.
117. Cox RG, Barker GA, Bohn DJ et al. Efficacy, results, and complications of mechanical ventilation in children with status asthmaticus. *Pediatr Pulmonol* 1991; **11**: 120–6.
118. Douglass JA, Tuxen DV, Horne M et al. Myopathy in severe asthma. *Am Rev Respir Dis* 1992; **146**: 517–19.
119. Hansen-Flaschen J, Cowen J, Raps EC. Neuromuscular blockade in the intensive care unit: more than we bargained for. *Am Rev Respir Dis* 1993; **147**: 234–6.
120. Wetzel RC. Pressure-support ventilation in children with severe asthma. *Crit Care Med* 1996; **24**: 1603–5.
121. Kudukis TM, Manthous CA, Schmidt GA et al. Inhaled helium–oxygen revisited: effect of inhaled helium–oxygen during the treatment of status asthmaticus in children. *J Pediatr* 1997; **130**: 217–24.
122. Carter ER, Webb CR, Moffitt DR. Evaluation of heliox in children hospitalized with acute severe asthma. *Chest* 1996; **109**: 1256–61.
123. Ciarallo L, Sauer AH, Shannon MW et al. Intravenous magnesium therapy for moderate to severe pediatric asthma: results of a randomized, placebo-controlled trial. *J Pediatr* 1996; **129**: 809–14.
124. Noppen M, Vanmaele L, Impens N, Schandevyl

W. Bronchodilating effect of intravenous magnesium sulfate in acute severe bronchial asthma. *Chest* 1990; **97**: 373–6.
125. Schwartz SH. Treatment of status asthmaticus with halothane. *JAMA* 1984; **251**: 2688–9.
126. Otte RW, Fireman P. Isoflurane anesthesia for the treatment of refractory status asthmaticus. *Ann Allergy* 1991; **66**: 305–9.
127. Rock MJ, Reyes de la Rocha S, L'Hommedieu CS, Truemper E. Use of ketamine in asthmatic children to treat respiratory failure refractory to conventional therapy. *Crit Care Med* 1986; **14**: 514–16.
128. Roy TM, Pruitt VL, Garner PA, Heine MF et al. The potential role of anesthesia in status asthmaticus. *J Asthma* 1992; **29**: 73–7.

10

Exercise-induced asthma in children and adolescents and its relationship to sports

Kai-Håkon Carlsen

Pathogenesis of EIA • **Diagnosis of EIA** • **EIA, physical training athletes and sport** • **Management of EIA** • **Conclusions**

Exercise-induced asthma (EIA) has long been recognized as a specific entity and characteristic of asthma and was described as early as 2000 years ago in Cappadocia.[1] Exercise-induced asthma is one major distinctive feature of childhood asthma especially in patients without anti-inflammatory treatment. It has been maintained that 70–80% of untreated asthmatics suffer from EIA.[2] Backer and Ulrik reported that 16% of a random sample of 494 Danish children and adolescents experienced more than 10% reduction in FEV_1 after a standardized exercise test.[3] Exercise-induced asthma may cause limitations in their daily life for asthmatic children, and it has been documented that many asthmatic children suffer such limitations.[4,5] It is important for children's self-esteem that they participate in play and sports, and mastering EIA is considered an essential part of successful management of asthma.[6] Furthermore, EIA may be regarded as a measure of bronchial hyperresponsiveness,[7,8] and quantifying EIA in a standardized way may help in monitoring asthma. In relationship to sports there is another link between physical training and asthma. Several reports indicate that heavy endurance training in itself may be a causative factor for bronchial hyperresponsiveness and asthma.[9,10]

PATHOGENESIS OF EIA

Presently, there are two main theories to explain the relationship between physical activity and EIA. Firstly, the theory of airway cooling due to respiratory heat loss with rewarming by secondary hyperaemia and pulmonary vasodilatation will be considered.[11] As the inspiratory air is rapidly saturated with water vapour during breathing, the temperature of the inspiratory air also increases. Through thermal mapping McFadden and coworkers demonstrated that the temperature increased from $32.0 \pm 0.05°C$ in the upper trachea to $35.5 \pm 0.3°C$ in the subsegmental bronchi during quiet breathing (ventilation 15 l/min) of room air ($26.7 \pm 0.5°C$).[12] During increasing ventilation the temperature fell, and with a maximum ventilation of 100–120 l/min the temperature in the upper trachea was $29.2 \pm 0.5°C$, and $33.9 \pm 0.8°C$ in the subsegmental bronchi. During maximum ventilation with frigid air ($-18.6 \pm 1.2°C$) the upper tracheal temperature was $20.5 \pm 0.6°C$ and the subsegmental bronchial temperature was $31.6 \pm 1.2°C$.[12] Airway cooling may stimulate receptors in the airways, causing bronchial constriction through a reflex pathway. Furthermore, owing to pulmonary vasoconstriction induced by the cold air, a secondary reactive hyperaemia may occur, with resulting oedema and airways narrowing.[11]

Secondly, there is substantial evidence to indicate that EIA is effected through the release of mediators from mast cells and other inflammatory cells of the airways.[13] Recently increased levels of the mast cell mediator 9α, 11β prostaglandin F_2 were found in urine after exercise challenge in patients with EIA compared with patients without EIA, but this was not found for leukotriene E_4 (LTE_4) and N-methylhistamine.[14] However, in a study including more patients, Reiss et al. also found increased levels of LTE_4 after exercise challenge.[15] We have described signs of eosinophil and neutrophil activation (increased s-ECP and s-MPO) in top athletes after heavy training exercises, but not after moderate training exercises.[16] The mediator release provoked by exercise is the main reason for considering EIA an indirect measure of bronchial reactivity.[17]

The lower respiratory tract is lined with ciliary epithelium coated with periciliary fluid. As the airways are divided into an increasing number of bronchial generations, the amount of periciliary fluid increases exponentially.[18] During breathing, respiratory vapour loss increases rapidly with increasing ventilatory rate.[19] It is debated whether the main stimulus behind the exercise-induced bronchoconstriction is water loss occurring during hyperventilation caused by exercise,[20] or a temperature gradient over the airways caused by respiratory heat loss.[21,22] The main factor causing the mediator release is now thought to be the change in osmolarity of the periciliary fluid lining the surface of the respiratory mucosal membranes, whether it is caused by respiratory heat loss or respiratory water loss. The increase in chloride ions on the luminal side of the bronchial epithelium is thought to be the stimulus for mediator release. This is supported by the finding that inhaled furosemide, which inhibits the secretion of chloride ions into the bronchial lumen in vitro,[23] protects against exercise-induced asthma.[24] The increased extracellular osmolarity thus leads to influx into the cell, particularly of Na^+ and Cl^-. Ca^{2+} follows Cl^- passively into the cell and this activates phospholipase in the cellular membranes, leading to activation of phospholipase II, thus increasing the output of leukotrienes and causing mediator release.

The mechanisms may be better understood by learning from findings in athletes. Mediator release from eosinophils and neutrophils increased both in healthy and asthmatic athletes after heavy exercise. s-ECP and s-MPO increased significantly 2–4 hours after heavy exercise, but not after moderate exercise in Norwegian Olympic cross-country skiers.[16] Heavy exercise may increase airway inflammation, and thus bronchial responsiveness. This increase in bronchial responsiveness has previously been demonstrated in Norwegian competitive swimmers after heavy swimming exercise.[25] Inflammatory changes with lymphoid aggregates in bronchial biopsies have also been demonstrated much more frequently in heavily trained young skiers without asthma, but with increased airways responsiveness to cold air compared with control subjects.[26]

EIA and late asthmatic reactions

Late allergic reactions are thought to increase airway inflammation and bronchial hyperresponsiveness.[27] In a similar way, late bronchoconstrictive reactions after exercise have been described in a limited group of children with an early bronchial reaction to exercise.[28–31] A relationship between late asthmatic reactions to exercise and increase in inflammatory mediators during exercise has also been described.[29]

However, difficulties in reproducing the late reaction to exercise have cast doubt on the existence of a true late asthmatic reaction to exercise.[32–34] It has been recommended that studies of late asthmatic reactions should be compared with control days without exercise, since late asthmatic reactions after exercise might be confused with spontaneous variation in lung function.[34] Sano et al. reported that 28.1% of a group of 32 children with EIA also had a late response to exercise (within 8 hours of the exercise test).[31] They compared the lung function after exercise with the spontaneous variation in lung function in the same group of children. There was a significant difference between lung function after exercise and the spontaneous variation in lung function in the same children.[31] Their findings are confirmed by the recent report of Chhabra and Ojha, who demonstrated a late response to exercise in eight out of 16 patients with EIA comparing the findings after exercise with the spontaneous variation in lung function on a control day.[35]

The magnitude of EIA is determined in part by the exercise load and climatic conditions during exercise.[36] From combining the exercise with cold dry air inhalation during exercise, there may be a significantly greater reduction in lung function.[37] This may also influence the occurrence of late asthmatic reactions after exercise. In the study of Sano et al. exercise was combined with inhalation of dry and moderately cold air (+5°C).[31] Furthermore, the use of anti-inflammatory medication (e.g. inhaled steroids) reduces the occurrence of EIA, and may also influence the occurrence of late asthmatic reactions after exercise. In the study of Sano et al. the patients had not taken anti-inflammatory drugs in the last month before the study. Thus, the effects of exercise load, environmental factors and use of asthma medication should also be taken into consideration in later studies of this phenomenon.

DIAGNOSIS OF EIA

There are several differential diagnoses to EIA, such as exercise-induced laryngeal stridor[38,39] or hyperventilation. A diagnosis of EIA ought to be made before starting treatment. An exact clinical history, examination with lung function measurements before and after inhalation of a β_2-agonist, before and after a standardized exercise test such as treadmill running and/or a cold-air inhalation test, and measurement of BHR by metacholine inhalation are parts of the diagnostic process. The extent of diagnostic procedures to be employed will vary from case to case. One important part of the diagnostic process is to follow the patient to evaluate the treatment effect.

Exercise-induced bronchoconstriction may be diagnosed in different ways, and by employing different sorts of exercise. To be able to compare the results of testing between different individuals, and to compare results from the same individual at different times, it is important to standardize the test. Tests with free running, step tests, cycling, and running on a motor-driven treadmill have all been standardized and used in the diagnosis of exercise-induced bronchoconstriction. Running provokes exercise-induced bronchoconstriction in children more easily than cycling, probably because the muscles used during running are usually better trained than the muscles used during cycling in most children. As early as the 1970s a series of experiments were performed to standardize tests to diagnose EIA. It was found that running was better suited for provoking EIA than was cycling.[40] Furthermore, it was found that running for 6–8 minutes provoked greater decrease in post-exercise FEV_1 than running for shorter or longer time periods. The exercise load should be submaximal, that is about 70–80% of maximum exercise.[41] Experience has shown that running on a motor-driven treadmill is particularly useful and easy to standardize. In our laboratory, running on a motor-driven treadmill with submaximal load is used. The treadmill has an inclination of 5.5%, and during running the speed of the treadmill is previously gradually increased until a steady-state heart rate of at least 170 beats per minute is reached. However, the widespread use of inhaled steroids reduces the amount of EIA, and it has been found that a heavier exercise load should now be employed in testing for EIA. Increased sensitivity of the exercise test has been demonstrated by increasing the exercise load to a heart rate of at least 95% of the calculated maximum.[42] Maximum heart rate is approximately calculated from 220 minus the age of the patient. The heart rate has to be measured, and can be done so electronically with devices such as the Sport-Tester PE 3000®. The child then runs for 6 minutes at this steady state. The running is performed with a room temperature of approximately 20°C and a relative humidity of approximately 40%. Lung function is measured before running, immediately after cessation of running and after 3, 6, 10, 15 and 20 minutes after running. FEV_1 is usually the lung function parameter employed, and a fall of 15% is most often used as a sign of exercise-induced bronchoconstriction. Some authors also use 10% reduction in FEV_1 from before to after exercise as a criterion of exercise-induced bronchoconstriction.[3,43] Instead of expressing EIA as percent reduction in FEV_1 from the baseline value, results can be expressed as percentages of predicted values, thus taking into account the baseline lung function. Figure 10.1 demonstrates the course of an exercise test. In addition to diagnosing EIA, the reduction in FEV_1 after standardized exercise may be considered a measure of nonspecific bronchial reactivity and used to evaluate the severity of asthma, as well as the effects of therapy. This measure of nonspecific bronchial reactivity is an indirect measure,[17] since it is thought to work though the release of mediators.[2] It has been shown to correlate well to direct measures of bronchial reactivity, such as histamine or metacholine bronchial provocation.[8] Furthermore it is a useful physiologic measure, since it reflects the effect of everyday activities upon the asthmatic child.

Studies have shown that this test has a very high specificity for the diagnosis of asthma, but a rather low sensitivity when compared with histamine or metacholine bronchial provocation.[7,44] When an extra stimulus is added to the exercise test, by combining running on a treadmill with the inhalation of dry cold air of −20°C (Figure 10.1), the high specificity is maintained, but the sensitivity is markedly increased.[37]

In young preschool children the objective diagnosis of EIA may be difficult. It is important to be aware of exercise-induced wheeze or cough in the kindergarten. Objective diagnosis may be obtained by letting the young children exercise during playing, while recording heart rate electronically to obtain data about exercise load. After attaining a heart rate of 180–190 per minute over several minutes, the child may start wheezing with audible rhonchi and sibilating rhonchi. Thus, a useful diagnosis of exercise-induced wheeze may be obtained.

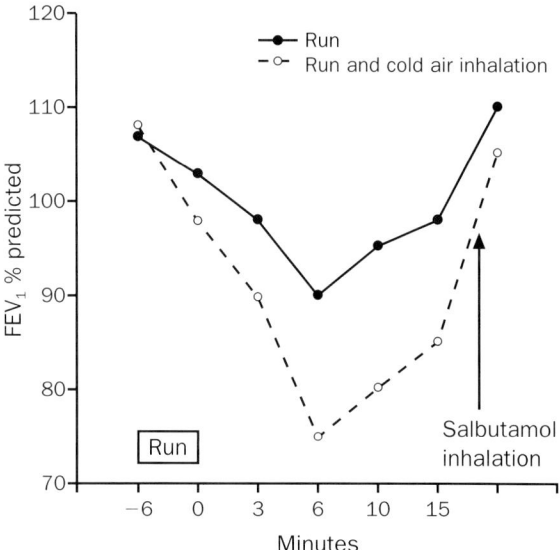

Figure 10.1 Lung function before and after running on a motor-driven treadmill with and without simultaneous inhalation of cold dry air at −15°C.

EIA, PHYSICAL TRAINING ATHLETES AND SPORT

Different types of exercise tend to provoke EIA to a different degree. Running is the type of exercise best suited to provoke EIA. Cycling and especially swimming, perhaps due to the humid conditions during swimming, will not provoke EIA to the same extent as running.[45] Several studies indicate that frequent heavy physical exercise may contribute to increased bronchial responsiveness. Highly-trained elite athletes have been reported to have an increased incidence of asthma and EIA. This has been reported from a number of different types of sports, the common denominator being that they are endurance sports. It was reported that elite American football players had a very high incidence of bronchial hyperreactivity (PC_{20} metacholine) compared to volleyball players,[46] and during the XXIII Summer Olympic Games 41 Olympic medals, including 15 gold medals and 21 silver medals, were won by American athletes suffering from exercise-induced bronchoconstriction.[47] Increased prevalence of EIA has been reported among elite cross-country skiers,[9,48] swimmers,[25] long-distance runners[49] and figure skaters.[46,50]

This high prevalence of exercise-induced bronchoconstriction among elite athletes raises the question of whether physical training with a high intensity level may in itself enhance bronchial reactivity. Several studies with different types of physical exercise suggest that short-term exercise with a high intensity level increases bronchial reactivity.[25,51,52] Suzuki et al. found an increase in bronchial reactivity in asthmatics from before to after cycling,[52] but Zawadski et al. could not confirm this. However, the latter study was performed with a moderate exercise load.[53] In a previous study of elite competition swimmers in Norway, bronchial reactivity from histamine provocation (PC_{20}) was measured before and after a heavy swimming session, with three main intervals of 1000 m swimming: the first interval was 5% below the calculated anaerobic threshold; the second interval was at the calculated anaerobic threshold; and the third session was 5% above the calculated anaerobic threshold. $PC_{20\text{-histamine}}$ was found to decrease from before to after the swimming procedure in both asthmatic swimmers and non-asthmatic swimmers. The decrease in $PC_{20\text{-histamine}}$ (the increase in bronchial reactivity) was significantly correlated to the exercise load, as measured by the change in serum-lactate and base excess.[8]

Exercise testing in the laboratory at a sub-maximal level is not comparable to the exercise intensity that elite athletes in endurance sports employ during their training. In the predisposed individual, high intensity training for 2–4 hours daily for several years may provoke airways inflammation, especially when combined with unfavourable environmental conditions such as cold air temperature or air pollution.[54,55] Norwegian studies suggest that bronchial reactivity in elite cross-country skiers increases during the most active training and competitive season (January and February), and improves when the training intensity decreases.[56] Furthermore, after having trained for many years the prevalence of asthma among the elite skiers increased markedly from approximately 6% when the skiers were 20 years old up to over 20% when the skiers had reached the age of 30 years. This was not found in the control group.[9] This suggests that heavy long-lasting exercise may induce bronchial hyperresponsiveness in susceptible individuals. Moreover a Swedish study reported high prevalence of asthma among top cross-country skiers.[48]

It should be remembered that the physically active child and the training athlete are more exposed to pollutants and allergens in ambient air owing to hyperventilation and inhalation of larger amounts of air. It has been demonstrated that in indoor pools swimmers may be exposed to levels of chlorine at the limit of maximum allowed levels in industry.[57] In summer sports increased prevalence of asthma was found among long-distance runners. They also had more frequent allergy to seasonal allergens such as birch and grass pollen.[58] Thus, a combination of endurance training and an environmental hazard such as cold air, seasonal allergens, pollutants or respiratory virus infections tends to increase the occurrence of asthma among athletes. During physical exercise the minute ventilation and the volume of inhaled air increase, and the magnitude of possible environmental agents inhaled will increase to a great extent. For the different types of endurance sports, different types of environmental hazard may influence the development of bronchial hyperresponsiveness and asthma. In skiing and other outdoor winter sports it may be the cold air inhaled in great amounts during exercise; for swimmers it may be increased chlorine levels inhaled during swimming in indoor pools; and for endurance summer sports it may be inhalation of pollen or mould spores. For all sorts of training and sports, respiratory tract infections represent a hazard and endurance training should not be performed during a respiratory infection.[59]

MANAGEMENT OF EIA

General therapeutic measures

Treatment strategies involve environmental measures, practices related to training, and drug treatment. Physical warming-up is one of the general practices related to training procedures. This is an important way of preventing EIA. Protection against cold air inhalation is also important. Various equipment may be used which employs the principle of warm air exchange. Expired air at 37°C warms up the inspired air. In common use in Scandinavia are Jonaset®, Jonaset Sport® (made in Finland) and Lungplus® (made in Sweden). In this equipment expired warm humid air moves through a metal grid during breathing, warming up the incoming air. To avoid developing BHR, athletes should not perform endurance training or participate in competition during ongoing viral respiratory infections or during cold air temperatures. Furthermore intense physical activity in polluted air should be avoided.

Drug treatment of exercise-induced asthma

The medical drug treatment of EIA consists of premedication shortly before physical activity or training and prophylactic treatment. The prophylactic treatment mainly consists of anti-inflammatory treatment. Furthermore, symptoms occurring through exercise must be treated.

Prophylactic anti-inflammatory treatment
In order to master physical activity, the asthmatic disorder should be treated optimally to improve bronchial hyperresponsiveness and to maintain good control of disease activity. The usual guidelines for treating asthma should be followed. Anti-inflammatory treatment is presently the cornerstone in treating asthma, and is also crucial for controlling EIA. Inhaled steroids are the most important treatment. After only 1 week's treatment with inhaled steroids (budesonide) in asthmatic well-trained athletes a marked reduction in EIA was observed, as measured by the fall in FEV_1 after a standardized treadmill run.[60] A similar result was observed 15 years ago in asthmatic children, but in order to obtain a significant reduction of the fall in MEF_{25-75}, a measure of peripheral bronchial obstruction, further treatment of 3–4 weeks was necessary.[61] It is also demonstrated that a more rapidly occurring effect on EIA is obtained with inhaled steroids than upon BHR as measured by metacholine bronchial provocation. After 2–3 months' treatment with inhaled steroids, the anticipated improvement of EIA is obtained.[43] On the other hand, ongoing improvement of BHR, measured by metacholine provocation, has been observed for up to 22 months.[62]

Another treatment principle that has recently been introduced is the use of leukotriene antagonists, taken orally. There are two main groups of leukotriene antagonists: leukotriene synthesis inhibitors and leukotriene receptor antagonists. These drugs reduce EIA. After one single dose leukotriene antagonists are significantly better than placebo against EIA,[63] and 2 days' treatment with a leukotriene synthesis inhibitor (zileuton) caused a protection of 40% against EIA.[64] Moreover in children the use of montelukast, a leukotriene receptor antagonist, led to a significant reduction in EIA after only 2 days' treatment in both children and adults.[65,66] It remains to be demonstrated whether continuous use of leukotriene receptor antagonists provides an additional anti-inflammatory effect and increased improvement of EIA over time.

The other anti-inflammatory asthma drugs, which have been used for many years, are disodium cromoglycate (DSCG) and the related, more recently introduced nedocromile sodium. Some studies report an improvement of BHR after the use of DSCG, but other studies cannot confirm this finding.[67,68] The most often reported effect of DSCG and nedocromile sodium upon EIA is when taking the drugs before exercise.[69]

Treatment before exercise
A number of different drugs may be taken before exercise to protect against EIA. The effect of using any of these drugs should be evaluated

by performing an exercise test or by a follow-up consultation. When no effect is observed, the treatment should be adjusted, or, especially if the diagnosis of EIA is based upon history alone, the diagnosis should be reconsidered. The most usual therapeutic drugs employed before exercise are inhaled β_2-agonists, DSCG or nedocromile sodium and, more rarely, inhaled ipratropium bromide.[70] Both DSCG and nedocromile sodium have been demonstrated to be useful in the pretreatment of EIA.[69,71,72] Taken within 15 minutes before physical activity, they reduce the fall in lung function provoked by the activity. It has been demonstrated that DSCG, in addition to protecting against EIA, also reduces ventilation and energy consumption during running.

Maximum oxygen uptake was significantly lower when the children inhaled DSCG or the β_2-agonist salbutamol before running when compared with placebo.[73] It has later been shown that DSCG reduces the ventilatory work in children suffering from EIA, but not in healthy children.[74] This suggests that the energy consumption during exercise is higher in untreated than in treated asthmatic children, adolescents and athletes to participate in sports and physical activity on an equal level with healthy children, adolescents and athletes.

Both DSCG and the inhaled β_2-agonist terbutaline have been found to protect against EIA for up to 2 hours after inhalation, whereas the combination DSCG and terbutaline protected for 4 hours. Thus, combining the two drugs prolonged the protection.[75] It has been maintained that an inhaled β_2-agonist is preferable when there is baseline bronchial constriction, whereas DSCG should be used when the subject does not demonstrate signs of bronchial constriction before the physical activity.[70] It is important that DSCG is taken in adequately high doses; 20 mg is to be preferred. This makes treatment impractical, and inhaled β_2-agonists are often preferred.

Inhaled β_2-agonists are often preferred as protective treatment before physical activity. The protective effect against EIA is usually very good, both when bronchial constriction is present before exercise and when it is not.[70] The short-acting inhaled β_2-agonists salbutamol and terbutaline are usually preferred. Inhaled β_2-agonists have better effect than when the drugs are taken orally. The recommended dose of inhaled salbutamol is 0.2–0.4 mg, corresponding to an inhaled dose of 0.25–0.5 mg terbutaline.

Long-acting β_2-agonists for inhalation have recently been introduced: salmeterol and formoterol. Both have been demonstrated to have good protective effect against EIA.[76–78] Children with EIA will benefit from a long-acting protective drug, since they do not plan their activity beforehand. In athletes performing endurance sports, a long-acting β_2-agonist may be of benefit, since the usual β_2-agonists may last too short a time. In addition the use of a long-acting β_2-agonist may improve symptom control and quality of life both in the asthmatic athlete and in asthmatic children and adolescents.[79,80] However, the development of tolerance against the protective effect for exercise-induced bronchoconstriction has been described after 4 weeks' regular daily treatment with long-acting β_2-agonists.[81]

Ipratropium bromide may be effective in protecting against EIA in singular patients, but is less useful than inhaled β_2-agonists.[70,82] However, in certain subjects ipratropium bromide should be tried. Sometimes an additional protective effect may be obtained when ipratropium bromide is added to an inhaled β_2-agonist.[83] This underlines the importance of trying out the effects of prescribed drugs.

Lately a protective effect of inhaled furosemide[24] and inhaled heparin[84] upon EIA has been described. This is of considerable theoretical interest, but these drugs do not represent a therapeutic alternative to the other treatments.

The latest group of drugs reported to have an effect upon EIA are the leukotriene antagonists (consisting of leukotriene synthesis inhibitors and leukotriene receptor antagonists).[15,64] The magnitude of EIA is reduced, but EIA is not completely eliminated.[65,66,85] However, in a recent randomized, double-blind, placebo-controlled study the protective effect against EIA was approximately equal to the protection from inhaled salmeterol 3 days after starting regular treatment, but better than salmeterol after 4 and 8 weeks without the development of tolerance seen with salmeterol.[86]

As exercise-induced wheeze in young preschool children may inhibit normal play and physical activity, this should generally be treated according to the same principle as EIA in older children.

The relationship to doping

> But also the danger of 'manufacturing' a programmed athlete, medically prepared to attain the highest performance at the very risk of endangering health, and sometimes even his or her life.[87]

Systematic use of medical drugs has been employed to improve performance in healthy top athletes in most types of sport. Frequent use of any type of drug may cause suspicion that the drugs are used for this purpose, and not to treat medical illness. The frequent occurrence of EIA in participants in endurance sports has led to a high consumption of asthma drugs in these branches of athletics.[9] Thus, it has been discussed whether inhaled β_2-agonists in particular could improve performance, especially endurance performance. In animals it has been demonstrated that oral β_2-agonists (clenbuterol) in high doses may cause an increase in muscle mass. This has entailed restrictions in the international doping regulations. Both inhaled steroids and inhaled β_2-agonists are allowed for use in sports in asthmatic athletes. Systemic β_2-agonists and systemic steroids are not allowed. Since 1993 the inhaled β_2-agonists salbutamol and terbutaline were allowed for use by asthmatics in sports, and, after studies demonstrating that neither salbutamol, terbutaline nor salmeterol improves performance in sports,[88–91] salmeterol too has been allowed for use in sports since 1 February 1996. As regards formoterol, a recent study could not demonstrate any effect upon endurance performance in healthy well-trained athletes,[92] but use of this drug in sports is presently not allowed by the International Olympic Committee, Medical Commission.

CONCLUSIONS

The asthmatic condition should be treated optimally in athletes and children suffering from EIA. This usually includes the use of inhaled steroids, which reduce BHR and EIA considerably. However, additional protective medication before exercise is often needed. Inhaled β_2-agonists, usually short acting, are most often used. Exercise-induced asthma is usually well controlled combining inhaled steroids and inhaled β_2-agonists. Long-acting inhaled β_2-agonists may be necessary, especially in severe asthma, but also in children, who do not plan their physical activity in the same way as athletes do. In sport the use of asthma drugs is restricted, and athletes have the responsibility to know the doping rules. However, the physician also should know these rules, to avoid prescribing drugs not permitted for use in sports. For individual patients and athletes it is important that the effectiveness of the prescribed treatment be reassessed.

In addition to medical treatment, certain preventive measures should be implemented to help the athlete avoid the dangers of heavy endurance training and competition. Endurance training and competition should not be performed during a respiratory tract infection, nor in cold temperatures (below $-10°C$) without cold-protection equipment; and in indoor swimming pools, adequate ventilation should be ensured in order not to expose swimmers to high levels of chlorine in inhaled air.

Asthmatic children and participation in sports

When can be concluded for asthmatic children? On one hand, participation in physical activity, play and sport is important for the asthmatic child, but the asthmatic child should learn to take certain precautions, such as avoiding physical activity in ambient cold air and ambient pollution. Rather than avoiding physical activity and sport, the asthmatic child should be helped to participate with others in sport, since the mastering of sports and physical activity is a good measure of mastering asthma. The physician treating children and adolescents with EIA should have good knowledge about the doping rules and prescribe only drugs whose use is permitted in sport.

REFERENCES

1. Adams F. *The Extant Works of Aretaeus, the Cappadocian.* London: Sydenham Society, 1856.
2. Lee TH, Anderson SD. Heterogeneity of mechanisms in exercise-induced asthma. *Thorax* 1985; **40**: 481–7.
3. Backer V, Ulrik CS. Bronchial responsiveness to exercise in a random sample of 494 children and adolescents from Copenhagen. *Clin Exp Allergy* 1992; **22**: 741–7.
4. Taylor WR, Newacheck PW. Impact of childhood asthma upon health. *Pediatrics* 1992; **90**: 657–62.
5. Lenney W, Well NEJ, O'Neill BA. The burden of paediatric asthma. *Eur Respir Rev* 1994; **4**: 49–62.
6. International Paediatric Consensus Group on Asthma. Asthma: a follow up statement from an international paediatric asthma consensus group. *Arch Dis Child* 1992; **67**(2): 240–8.
7. Godfrey S, Springer C, Noviski N, Maayan Ch, Avital A. Exercise but not metacholine differentiates asthma from chronic lung disease in children. *Thorax* 1991; **46**: 488–92.
8. Carlsen KH, Bech R, Oseid S, Schrøder E. Bronchial reactivity measured by exercise-induced asthma test and PC-20-histamine: a comparison of two methods. In: Morehouse CA, ed. *Children and Exercise XII.* Champaign, IL: Human Kinetics Publishers, 1986, 295–300.
9. Heir T, Oseid S. Self-reported asthma and exercise-induced asthma symptoms in high-level competitive cross-country skiers. *Scand J Med Sci Sports* 1994; **4**: 128–33.
10. Helenius IJ, Tikkanen HO, Haahtela T. Association between type of training and risk of asthma in elite athletes. *Thorax* 1997; **52**: 157–60.
11. Gilbert IA, McFadden ER Jr. Airway cooling and rewarming. The second reaction sequence in exercise-induced asthma. *J Clin Investigation* 1992; **90**: 699–704.
12. McFadden ER Jr, Pichurko BM, Bowman HF, Ingenito E, Burns S, Dowling N et al. Thermal mapping of the airways in humans. *J Appl Physiol* 1985; **58**: 564–70.
13. Lee TH, Nagakura T, Papageorgiou N, Cromwell O, Ikura Y, Kay AB. Mediators in exercise-induced asthma. *J Allergy Clin Immunol* 1994; **73**: 634–9.
14. O'Sullivan S, Rooquet A, Dahlén B, Larsen F, Eklund A, Kumlin M et al. Evidence for mast cell activation during exercise-induced bronchoconstriction. *Eur Respir J* 1998; **12**: 345–50.
15. Reiss TF, Hill JB, Harman E, Zhang J, Tanaka WK, Bronsky E et al. Increased urinary excretion of LTE4 after exercise and attenuation of exercise-induced bronchospasm by montelukast, a cysteinyl leukotriene receptor antagonist. *Thorax* 1997; **52**: 1030–5.
16. Rønsen O, Hem E, Edvardsen E, Halvorsen R, Carlsen KH. Changes in airways inflammatory markers during high intensity training in elite cross country skiers. *Eur Respir J* 1995; **8**: 473S.
17. Pauwels R, Joos G, Van der Straten M. Bronchial responsiveness is not bronchial responsiveness is not asthma. *Clin Allergy* 1988; **18**: 317–21.
18. Anderson SD. Exercise-induced asthma: stimulus, mechanism and management. In: Barnes PJ, Roger IW, Thomson NC, eds. *Asthma. Basic Mechanisms and Clinical Management.* London: Academic Press, 1988, 503–22.
19. Anderson SD, Schoeffel RE, Black JL, Daviskas E. Airway cooling as the stimulus to exercise-induced asthma. A re-evaluation. *Eur Respir J* 1985; **67**: 20–30.
20. Sheppard D, Eschenbacher WL. Respiratory water loss as a stimulus to exercise-induced bronchoconstriction. *J Allergy Clin Immunol* 1984; **73**: 640–2.
21. Anderson SD, Daviskas E. The airway microvasculature and exercise induced asthma. *Thorax* 1992; **47**: 748–52.
22. Lee TH, Assoufi BK, Kay AB. The link between exercise, respiratory heat exchange, and the mast cell in bronchial asthma. *Lancet* 1983; **1**: 520–2.
23. Widdicombe JH, Nathanson IT, Highland E. Effects of 'loop' diuretics on ion transport by dog tracheal epithelium. *Am J Physiol* 1983; **245**: C388–96.
24. Bianco S, Vaghi A, Robuschi M, Pasargiklian M. Prevention of exercise-induced bronchoconstriction by inhaled frusemide. *Lancet* 1988; **2**: 252–5.
25. Carlsen KH, Oseid S, Odden H, Mellbye E. The response to heavy swimming exercise in children with and without bronchial asthma. In: Oseid S, Carlsen KH, eds. *Children and Exercise XIII.* Champaign, IL: Human Kinetics Publishers, 1989, 351–60.

26. Sue-Chue M, Karjalainen EM, Altraja A, Laitinen A, Laitinen LA, Naess AB et al. Lymphoid aggregates in endobronchial biopsies from young elite cross-country skiers. *Am J Respir Crit Care Med* 1998; **158:** 597–601.
27. Cockcroft DW, Ruffin RE, Dolovich J, Hargreave FE. Allergen-induced increase in non-allergic bronchial reactivity. *Clin Allergy* 1977; **7:** 503–13.
28. Bierman CW, Spiro SG, Petheran DJ. Late response in exercise-induced asthma. *J Allergy Clin Immunol* 1980; **65:** 206.
29. Lee TH, Nagakura T, Papageorgiou N, Iikura Y, Kay AB. Exercise-induced late asthmatic reactions with neutrophil chemotactic activity. *New Engl J Med* 1983; **308:** 1502–5.
30. Boner AL, Niero E, Antolini I, Warner JO. Biphasic (early and late) asthmatic responses to exercise in children with severe asthma, resident at high altitude. *Eur J Pediatr* 1985; **144:** 164–6.
31. Sano F, Sole D, Naspitz CK. Prevalence and characteristics of exercise-induced asthma. *Pediatr Allergy Immunol* 1998; **9:** 181–5.
32. Boner AL, Vallon G, Chiesa M, Spezia E, Fambri L, Sette L. Reproducibility of late phase pulmonary response to exercise and its relationship to bronchial hyperreactivity in children with chronic asthma. *Pediatr Pulmonol* 1992; **14:** 156–9.
33. Hofstra WB, Sterk PJ, Neijens HJ, Kouwenberg JM, Mulder PG, Duiverman E. Occurrence of a late response to exercise in asthmatic children: multiple regression approach using time-matched baseline and histamine control days. *Eur Respir J* 1996; **9:** 1348–55.
34. Peroni DG, Boner AL. Exercise-induced asthma: is there space for late-phase reactions? *Eur Respir J* 1996; **9:** 1335–8.
35. Chhabra SK, Ojha UC. Late asthmatic response in exercise-induced asthma. *Ann Allergy Asthma Immunol* 1998; **80:** 323–7.
36. Noviski N, Bar-Yishay E, Godfrey S. Exercise intensity determines and climatic conditions modify the severity of exercise-induced asthma. *Am Rev Respir Dis* 1987; **136:** 592–4.
37. Carlsen KH, Engh G, Mørk M, Schrøder E. Cold air inhalation and exercise-induced bronchoconstriction in relationship to metacholine bronchial responsiveness. Different patterns in asthmatic children and children with other chronic lung diseases. *Respir Med* 1998; **92:** 308–15.
38. Landwehr LP, Wood RP, Blager FB, Milgrom H. Vocal cord dysfunction mimicking exercise-induced bronchospasm in adolescents. *Pediatrics* 1996; **98:** 971–4.
39. McFadden ER Jr, Zawadski DK. Vocal cord dysfunction masquerading as exercise-induced asthma. A physiologic cause for 'choking' during athletic activities. *Am J Respir Crit Care Med* 1996; **153:** 942–7.
40. Anderson SD, Silverman M, Tai E, Godfrey S. Specificity of exercise in exercise-induced asthma. *Br Med J* 1971; **4:** 814–15.
41. Godfrey S, Silverman M, Anderson SD. The use of the treadmill for assessing exercise-induced asthma and the effect of varying the severity and duration of exercise. *Pediatrics* 1975; **56**(5 pt-2 suppl): 893–8.
42. Engh G, Mørk M, Carlsen KH. Exercise induced bronchoconstriction depends on exercise load. *Am J Respir Crit Care Med* 1998; **157:** A621.
43. Waalkens HJ, van Essen-Zandvliet EE, Gerritsen J, Duiverman EJKK, Knol K. The effect of an inhaled corticosteroid (budesonide) on exercise-induced asthma in children. Dutch CNSLD Study Group. *Eur Respir J* 1993; **6:** 652–6.
44. Avital A, Springer C, Bar Yishay E, Godfrey S. Adenosine, methacholine, and exercise challenges in children with asthma or paediatric chronic obstructive pulmonary disease. *Thorax* 1995; **50:** 511–16.
45. Bar-Or O, Inbar O. Swimming and asthma. Benefits and deleterious effects. *Sport Med* 1992; **14:** 397–405.
46. Weiler JM, Metzger J, Donnelly AL, Crowley ET, Sharath MD. Prevalence of bronchial responsiveness in highly trained athletes. *Chest* 1986; **90:** 23–8.
47. Pierson WE. Exercise-induced bronchospasm in the XXIII Summer Olympic Games. *N Engl Reg Allergy Proc* 1988; **9:** 209–13.
48. Larsson K, Ohlsen P, Larsson L, Malmberg P, Rydstrom PO, Ulriksen H. High prevalence of asthma in cross country skiers. *Br Med J* 1993; **307:** 1326–9.
49. Helenius IJ, Tikkanen HO, Haahtela T. Occurrence of exercise induced bronchospasm in elite runners: dependence on atopy and exposure to cold air and pollen. *Br J Sports Med* 1998; **32:** 125–9.
50. Mannix ET, Farber MO, Palange P, Galassetti P, Manfredi F. Exercise-induced asthma in figure skaters. *Chest* 1996; **109:** 312–15.
51. Magnussen H, Reuss G, Jörres R. Airway response to metacholine during exercise induced refractoriness in asthma. *Thorax* 1986; **41:** 667–70.
52. Suzuki S, Chonan T, Sasaki H, Takishima T. Bronchial hyperresponsiveness to metacholine

after exercise in asthmatics. *Ann Allergy* 1985; **54:** 136–41.
53. Zawadski DK, Lenner KA, McFadden ER Jr. Effect of exercise on nonspecific airway reactivity in asthmatics. *J Appl Physiol* 1988; **64:** 812–16.
54. Mahler DA, Loke J. Lung function after marathon running at warm and cold ambient temperatures. *Am Rev Respir Dis* 1981; **124:** 154–7.
55. Adams WC. Effects of ozone exposure at ambient air pollution episode levels on exercise performance. *Sport Med* 1987; **4:** 395–424.
56. Heir T, Larsen S. The influence of training intensity, airway infections and environmental conditions on seasonal variations in bronchial responsiveness in cross-country skiers. *Scand J Med Sci Sports* 1995; **5:** 152–9.
57. Drobnic F, Freixa A, Casan P, Sanchis J, Guardino X. Assessment of chlorine exposure in swimmers during training. *Med Sci Sports Exerc* 1996; **28:** 271–4.
58. Helenius IJ, Tikkanen HO, Haahtela T. Association between type of training and risk of asthma in elite athletes. *Thorax* 1997; **52:** 157–60.
59. Heir T, Aanestad G, Carlsen KH, Larsen S. Respiratory tract infection and bronchial responsiveness in elite athletes and sedentary control subjects. *Scand J Med Sci Sports* 1995; **5:** 94–9.
60. Papalia SM. Aspects of inhaled budesonide use in asthma and exercise. (Doctoral thesis.) Perth: Department of Human Movement, University of Western Australia, 1996.
61. Henriksen JM, Dahl R. Effects of inhaled budesonide alone and in combination with low-dose terbutaline in children with exercise-induced asthma. *Am Rev Respir Dis* 1983; **128:** 993–7.
62. van Essen-Zandvliet EE, Hughes MD, Waalkens HJ, Duiverman EJ, Pocock SJ, Kerrebijn KF et al. Effects of 22 months of treatment with inhaled corticosteroids and/or beta-2 agonists on lung function, airway responsiveness, and symptoms in children with asthma. *Am Rev Respir Dis* 1992; **146:** 547–54.
63. Robuschi M, Riva E, Fuccella LM, Vida E, Barnabe R, Rossi M et al. Prevention of exercise-induced bronchoconstriction by a new leukotriene antagonist (SK&F 104353). A double-blind study versus disodium cromoglycate and placebo. *Am Rev Respir Dis* 1992; **145:** 1285–8.
64. Meltzer SS, Hasday JD, Cohn J, Bleecker ER. Inhibition of exercise-induced bronchospasm by zileuton: a 5-lipoxygenase inhibitor. *Am J Respir Crit Care Med* 1996; **153:** 931–5.
65. Kemp JP, Dockhorn RJ, Shapiro GG, Nguygen HH, Reiss TF, Seidenberg BC et al. Montelukast once daily inhibits exercise-induced bronchoconstriction in 6- to 14-year-old children with asthma. *J Pediatr* 1998; **133:** 424–8.
66. Leff JA, Busse WW, Pearlman D, Bronsky E, Kemp J, Hendeles L et al. Montelukast, a leukotriene-receptor antagonist, for the treatment of mild asthma and exercise-induced bronchoconstriction. *N Engl J Med* 1998; **339:** 147–52.
67. Hoag JE, McFadden ER Jr. Long-term effect of cromolyn sodium on nonspecific bronchial hyperresponsiveness: a review. *Ann Allergy* 1991; **66:** 53–63.
68. Carlsen KH, Larsson K. The efficacy of inhaled disodium cromoglycate and glucocorticoids. *Clin Exp Allergy* 1996; **26**(suppl 4): 8–17.
69. Benedictis FM, Tuteri G, Bertotti A, Bruni L, Vaccaro R. Comparison of the protective effects of cromolyn sodium and nedocromil sodium in the treatment of exercise-induced asthma in children. *J Allergy Clin Immunol* 1994; **94:** 684–8.
70. Anderson SD. Drugs and the control of exercise-induced asthma. *Eur Respir J* 1993; **6:** 1090–2.
71. Comis A, Valletta EA, Sette L, Andreoli A, Boner AL. Comparison of nedocromil sodium and sodium cromoglycate administered by pressurized aerosol, with and without a spacer device in exercise-induced asthma in children. *Eur Respir J* 1993; **6:** 523–6.
72. Oseid S, Mellbye E, Hem E. Effect of nedocromil sodium on exercise-induced bronchoconstriction exacerbated by inhalation of cold air. *Scand J Med Sci Sports* 1995; **5:** 88–93.
73. Zanconato S, Baraldi E, Santuz P, Magagnin G, Zacchello F. Effect of inhaled disodium cromoglycate and albuterol on energy cost of running in asthmatic children. *Pediatr Pulmonol* 1990; **8:** 40–4.
74. Baraldi E, Santuz P, Magagnin G, Filippone M, Zacchello F. Effect of disodium cromoglycate on ventilation and gas exchange during exercise in asthmatic children with a postexertion FEV1 fall less than 15 percent. *Chest* 1994; **106:** 1083–8.
75. Woolley M, Anderson SD, Quigley BM. Duration of protective effect of terbutaline sulfate and cromolyn sodium alone and in combination on exercise-induced asthma. *Chest* 1990; **97:** 39–45.
76. Green CP, Price JF. Prevention of exercise induced asthma by inhaled salmeterol xinafoate. *Arch Dis Child* 1992; **67:** 1014–17.

77. Carlsen KH, Røksund O, Olsholt K, Njå F, Leegaard J, Bratten G. Overnight protection by inhaled salmeterol on exercise-induced asthma in children. *Eur Respir J* 1995; **8:** 1852–5.
78. Boner AL, Spezia E, Piovesan P, Chiocca E, Maiocchi G. Inhaled formoterol in the prevention of exercise-induced bronchoconstriction in asthmatic children. *Am J Respir Crit Care Med* 1994; **149:** 935–9.
79. Steffensen I, Faurschou P, Riska H, Rostrup J, Wegener T. Inhaled formoterol dry powder in the treatment of patients with reversible obstructive airway disease. A 3-month, placebo-controlled comparison of the efficacy and safety of formoterol and salbutamol, followed by a 12-month trial with formoterol. *Allergy* 1995; **50:** 657–63.
80. Juniper EF, Johnston PR, Borkhoff CM, Guyatt GH, Boulet LP, Haukioja A. Quality of life in asthma clinical trials: comparison of salmeterol and salbutamol. *Am J Respir Crit Care Med* 1995; **151:** 66–70.
81. Ramage L, Lipworth BJ, Ingram CG, Cree IA, Dhillon DP. Reduced protection against exercise induced bronchoconstriction after chronic dosing with salmeterol. *Respir Med* 1994; **88:** 363–8.
82. Finnerty JP, Holgate ST. The contribution of histamine release and vagal reflexes, alone and in combination, to exercise-induced asthma. *Eur Respir J* 1993; **6:** 1132–7.
83. Greenough A, Yuksel B, Everett L, Price JF. Inhaled ipratropium bromide and terbutaline in asthmatic children. *Respir Med* 1993; **87:** 111–14.
84. Garrigo J, Danta I, Ahmed T. Time course of the protective effect of inhaled heparin on exercise-induced asthma. *Am J Respir Crit Care Med* 1996; **153:** 1702–7.
85. Pearlman DS, Ostrom NK, Bronsky EA, Bonuccelli CM, Hanby LA. The leukotriene D4-receptor antagonist zafirlukast attenuates exercise-induced bronchoconstriction in children. *J Pediatr* 1999; **134:** 273–9.
86. Villaran C, O'Neill SJ, Helbling A, Van Noord JA, Lee TH, Chuchalin AG et al. Montelukast versus salmeterol in patients with asthma and exercise-induced bronchoconstriction. *J Allergy Clin Immunol* 1999; **104:** 547–53.
87. Samaranch JA. *The Olympic Book of Sports Medicine.* London: Blackwell Scientific Publications, 1988.
88. Meeuwisse WH, McKenzie DC, Hopkins S, Road JD, Hopkins SR. The effect of salbutamol on performance in nonasthmatic athletes. *Med Sci Sports Exercise* 1992; **24:** 1161–6.
89. Morton AR, Papalia SM, Fitch KD. Is salbutamol ergogenic? The effects of salbutamol on physical performance in the high-performance nonasthmatic athletes. *Clin J Sport Med* 1992; **2:** 93–7.
90. Carlsen KH, Ingjer F, Thyness B, Kirkegaard H. The effect of inhaled salbutamol and salmeterol on lung function and endurance performance in healthy well-trained athletes. *Scand J Med Sci Sports* 1997; **7:** 160–5.
91. Heir T, Stemshaug H. Saltbutamol and high-intensity treadmill running in nonasthmatic highly conditioned athletes. *Scand J Med Sci Sports* 1995; **5:** 231–6.
92. Carlsen KH, Hem E, Stensrud T, Held T, Herland K, Mowinckel P. Formoterol turbuhaler does not improve endurance performance in healthy well-trained athletes. *Am J Respir Crit Care Med* 1999; **159:** A412.

11

Upper airways disease and asthma

Jonathan Corren, Gary Rachelefsky

Introduction • Historical considerations • Population studies linking upper airway disease and asthma • Inflammation in rhinitis, sinusitis, and asthma • Pathophysiologic mechanisms connecting the upper and lower airways • Effects of nasal and sinus therapies upon the lower airways • Conclusions

INTRODUCTION

The coexistence of rhinitis and sinusitis with asthma became widely appreciated by physicians during the past century. Only recently, however, have researchers begun to realize that the upper airway actively modulates lung function in a number of important ways. This dynamic relationship between the upper and lower airways has important therapeutic implications for all clinicians who treat asthma. In fact, there is an emerging body of data suggesting that aggressive treatment of allergic rhinitis and chronic sinusitis may improve asthma outcomes.

In this chapter, we will focus upon the interrelationship between allergic rhinitis and sinusitis and asthma in children and adolescents. After considering the historical background, we will review data from epidemiologic, experimental, and clinical studies, and discuss potential areas of future research.

HISTORICAL CONSIDERATIONS

Galen, one of the fathers of Western medicine and a respected authority on disease during the second century AD, has been credited as the first physician to note an association between upper airway disorders and bronchial asthma.[1] He believed that secretions dripped from the skull into the lower airways and thereby aggravated both chronic cough and asthma. To help alleviate symptoms of asthma, he recommended purging of the nasal passages with water to prevent these secretions from reaching the chest cavity. This treatment was widely practiced by physicians throughout southern Europe and Egypt until the mid 17th century, when anatomists failed to demonstrate a direct connection between the interior of the skull and the lungs.

The concept of a link between upper airway disorders and asthma lay dormant until early in the 20th century, when otolaryngologists began to observe that severe asthma improved after the treatment of sinusitis. In a seminal paper written in 1919, Sluder hypothesized that asthma was largely caused by a neural reflex originating in the nose.[2] In 1925, Gottlieb expanded the possible mechanisms by which nasal and sinus diseases might aggravate asthma, including postnasal drip of secretions into the lungs and a tendency to breathe cold air directly into the mouth.[3] These postulated mechanisms remain essentially unchanged today.

POPULATION STUDIES LINKING UPPER AIRWAY DISEASE AND ASTHMA

Allergic rhinitis

A large number of cross-sectional studies have demonstrated that rhinitis and asthma commonly occur together in children and adolescents. Many studies have reported that nasal symptoms occur in 28–78% of adolescent and young adult patients with asthma,[4–6] compared with approximately 5–20% of the general population.[7] A more recent study which utilized a standardized questionnaire demonstrated that rhinitis is present in 93% of asthmatic adolescents.[8] Conversely, asthma has also been shown to afflict up to 38% of patients with allergic rhinitis,[4,6] which is significantly higher than the 3–5% prevalence noted in the general population.[9]

Both investigators and patients are interested in whether nasal allergy predisposes patients to the development of asthma. In children and adolescents who have both rhinitis and asthma, upper airway symptoms either precede or start at the same time as asthma in 59–85% of cases.[6,8,10,11] Data from two prospective studies suggest that the risk of developing asthma in patients with pre-existing allergic rhinitis is substantial. Johnstone followed a group of children with ragweed-allergic rhinitis over a period of 5 years and found that approximately 50% of the subjects developed asthma.[12] In a later study, Settipane et al prospectively followed a large group of college freshmen for 23 years to determine the natural history of their atopic disease.[13] Students who reported nasal symptoms at the beginning of the observation period developed asthma three times more often (10.5%) than individuals without rhinitis (3.6%).

Although patients with rhinitis appear to be more likely to develop asthma, it has not been possible to predict which patients are at greatest risk for manifesting lower airway symptoms. Children and adolescents with allergic rhinitis and no clinical evidence of asthma frequently exhibit bronchial hyperresponsiveness to bronchoconstrictor agents such as methacholine or histamine.[14–17] The mechanisms underlying this hyperresponsiveness are unclear, but recent evidence suggests that it is associated with a familial predisposition that may have a genetic basis.[18] This high incidence of hyperresponsiveness in rhinitic patients has caused some investigators to postulate that bronchial hyperreactivity may represent an intermediate phase between nasal allergy and symptomatic asthma. Though at least two small investigations have suggested that lower airway hyperresponsiveness confers a higher risk for developing symptoms and signs of asthma,[16,17] future well-powered, prospective studies will be needed to confirm these findings.

Recent large-scale population-based surveys have attempted to correlate the presence of rhinitis with asthma severity and health care costs attributable to asthma. In an analysis of 1261 adolescent and young adult asthmatics, Huse et al compared patients with significant nasal allergy with those that had mild or no symptoms of nasal disease.[19] These investigators noted that patients with more severe rhinitis were much more likely to have nocturnal awakening caused by asthma (19.6% versus 11.8%), 'moderate to severe asthma' as defined by the National Asthma Education Program (60.2% versus 51.2%), or work loss related to asthma (24.1% versus 21.1%). Similarly, Halpern and co-workers observed that patients with symptomatic rhinitis used more asthma medications, particularly more inhaled and supplemental oral corticosteroids.[20]

Although asthma appears to be more severe in patients with rhinitis, there is evidence that nasal disease is also worse in patients with asthma. Researchers at Johns Hopkins University reported that asthmatic subjects report a higher degree of nasal sensitivity to a variety of allergens and non-specific irritants than patients without asthma.[21] These recent investigations imply that both allergic rhinitis and asthma are more severe in the presence of the other disease. Taken in total, these data suggest two possibilities: (1) patients with both rhinitis and asthma may have a more severe, global form of airway disease with greater degrees of dysfunction than patients with isolated upper or lower airway disease; and (2) rhinitis may be contributing to lower airway dysfunction and increased asthma severity. Whereas the first possibility is speculative, the second hypothesis may be tested via both provocational studies and therapeutic trials.

Sinusitis

During the early part of the 20th century, physicians began to document the high incidence of sinusitis in both pediatric and adult patients with asthma. In the 1930s, Chobot found that the incidence of sinusitis (based on clinical symptoms) was as high as 70% in asthmatic children.[22] Conversely, a large retrospective study of children and adults with chronic sinusitis noted a 12% incidence of asthma.[23] In this study, only one-third of patients with both diseases reported that sinusitis preceded their lower airway symptoms.

A number of studies have investigated the incidence of sinus radiograph abnormalities in children with persistent wheezing. Between 31% and 53% of chronic asthma patients have abnormal plain sinus radiographs, and 21–31% have markedly abnormal findings (defined as opacification of one or both maxillary sinuses, air-fluid levels, or mucosal thickening greater than 5 mm)[24–27] (Table 11.1). These radiographic findings appear to represent more than radiologic artifact, since only 6% of healthy children older than 1 year demonstrate similar radiographic changes. Further, studies utilizing more specific imaging methods, such as computed tomography, have also demonstrated a high (approximately 40%) incidence of significant sinus abnormalities.[28]

The incidence of sinus abnormalities in patients presenting to the hospital with acute asthma was examined recently in a prospective study.[29] The authors determined that 19 of 65 patients had CT evidence of extensive sinus disease, and that mucosal thickening of the nasal passages and ethmoid and sphenoid sinuses was significantly more common in the asthmatics than in a group of controls. Five months later, 13 of the 19 patients underwent repeat CT scans; 11 demonstrated resolution of mucosal changes without any specific treatment for sinusitis. These results suggest that acute sinus inflammation is common in patients with acute exacerbations of asthma and that it often improves spontaneously over time without antimicrobial therapy.

Table 11.1 Incidence of chronic sinusitis in asthma: X-ray studies

Study	N	Age	Total abnormalities	Significant abnormalities
Ref. 24	52	19–60	62	NA
Ref. 25	70	3–16	52	27
Ref. 26	217	9–70	47	21
Ref. 27	138	6–19	31	31

INFLAMMATION IN RHINITIS, SINUSITIS, AND ASTHMA

The histopathology of asthma is noteworthy for several key features, including: cellular inflammation with increased numbers of eosinophils, lymphocytes, and mast cells; mucosal edema; increased goblet cell numbers and mucus production; epithelial desquamation; and smooth muscle hyperplasia and constriction. Most of these features, with the exception of smooth muscle changes and epithelial desquamation, are shared by both allergic rhinitis and chronic sinusitis. The immunologic basis of these three disorders is also similar, with CD4/TH2 lymphocytes predominating in the tissue and releasing a number of instrumental cytokines and chemokines, including interleukins 4, 5, and 13, GM-CSF, TNF-α, RANTES, and eotaxin.[30]

PATHOPHYSIOLOGIC MECHANISMS CONNECTING THE UPPER AND LOWER AIRWAYS

Although rhinitis, sinusitis, and asthma may reflect the same pathogenetic process occurring in different parts of the airway, the nose also has the capacity to actively modulate lung function. A large number of animal experiments were performed, starting in the 1960s, which demonstrated that the nose played an active role in regulating lower airway patency. As a result of these animal studies and subsequent studies in both healthy and asthmatic adults, several potential theories have been invoked to explain the functional relationship between upper and lower airway disease (Table 11.2).

Nasal-bronchial reflex

Increasingly sophisticated studies began to emerge in the late 1960s and focused upon the effects of mucosal irritants on lower airway function. In 1969, Kaufman et al applied silica particles onto the nasal mucosa of healthy, non-asthmatic individuals and noted significant, immediate increases in lower airway resistance.[31] Bronchospasm induced by nasal silica was blocked by both resection of the trigeminal nerve[32] and systemic administration of atropine. Fontanari and co-workers recently re-evaluated the possibility of a neural connection between the upper and lower airway, using cold, dry air as the nasal stiumulus.[33] These investigators demonstrated that isolated nasal inhalation of very cold air caused an immediate and clinically relevant increase in lower airway resistance They also demonstrated that this change in pulmonary function was prevented by both topical nasal anesthesia and cholinergic blockade induced by inhaled

---

Table 11.2 Putative mechanisms connecting upper and lower airways

Direct mechanisms

- Nasal-bronchial reflex
- Postnasal drip of inflammatory material
- Systemic absorption of inflammatory cells/mediators from nasal into pulmonary circulation
- Reduction in β-adrenergic responsiveness

Indirect mechanisms

- Nasal obstruction causes increased mouth breathing of cold, dry air or particulate matter

ipratroprium bromide. The studies by Kaufman and Fontanari strongly suggest the presence of a reflex arc connecting irritant afferent receptors in the upper airway to cholinergic efferent nerves in the lower airway.

Subsequent studies performed during the 1970s through the early 1990s utilized challenge materials considered to be more biologically relevant to human disease, including histamine, whole pollen particles, and allergenic extracts. Yan and Salome performed nasal histamine challenges in subjects with perennial rhinitis and stable asthma and observed that FEV_1 was reduced by 10% or more immediately following provocation in 8 of 12 subjects.[34] Importantly, radiolabeling studies were performed as part of this study which demonstrated that histamine was not deposited into the lower airways. However, a large number of other studies that employed histamine[35–37] and/or allergen[35–39] failed to invoke bronchoconstriction following nasal provocation. This discrepancy in results may be partly explained by the type of patients who participated in these studies. Yan investigated subjects who had perennial, symptomatic rhinitis and asthma and therefore had chronic, ongoing inflammatory disease in both the upper and lower respiratory tracts. The majority of other studies, however, studied patients who were outside of their pollen season and were without active rhinitis or asthma. The absence of priming in these studies may have had a significant effect upon the results.

In addition to neurally mediated bronchospasm, it has also been postulated that a nasal allergic reaction might alter lower airway responsiveness. Corren et al investigated the effects of nasal allergen provocation on non-specific bronchial responsiveness to methacholine.[39] Ten subjects with seasonal allergic rhinitis and asthma were selected for study; all patients related worsening of their asthma to the onset of hay fever symptoms. Non-specific bronchial responsiveness was significantly increased 30 minutes after nasal challenge and persisted for 4 hours (Figure 11.1). As radionuclide studies demonstrated no evidence of allergen deposition into the lungs, it seems unlikely that these increases in airway reactivity can be attributed to direct effects of allergen. In addition, the rapidity with which these changes occurred strongly suggests the possibility of a reflex mechanism.

Other investigators have postulated that chronic sinusitis may induce bronchial hyperresponsiveness via pharyngeal-bronchial reflexes. In a study of 24 patients with chronic sinusitis but without asthma, Rolla et al determined that 19 had lower airway hyperresponsiveness to inhaled histamine.[40] Airway reactivity was significantly associated with duration of sinusitis, increased nasal lavage fluid eosinophils, and increased pharyngeal submucosal nerve density (from biopsy specimens). The authors speculated that chronic sinusitis may result in secondary pharyngeal inflammation characterized by an increase in pharyngeal nerve density. Upper airway irritants are then able to activate reflexes originating in the pharynx that mediate bronchospasm.

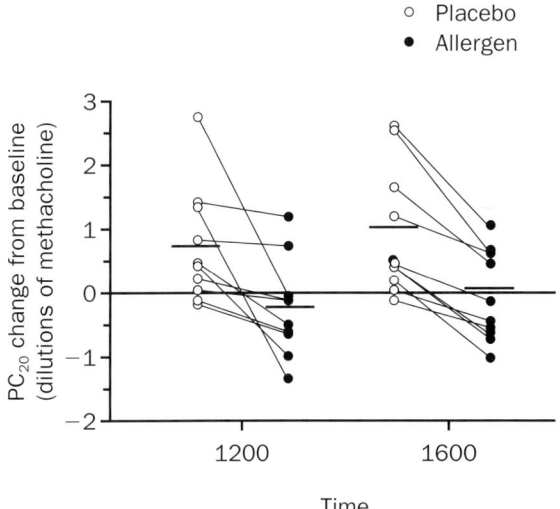

Figure 11.1 Changes in PC_{20} from baseline 0800 (8 am) at 1200 (12 pm) and 1600 (4 pm) in individual subjects after nasal challenge. Data are expressed in doubling dilutions of methacoline, and means are indicated with horizontal bars. $N = 10$ for both treatments. (Reprinted with permission from ref. 39.)

Postnasal drip of inflammatory material

Asthmatic patients frequently complain that postnasal drip triggers episodes of coughing and wheezing. Early studies investigating the possibility of aspiration of nasal secretions demonstrated that substances placed in the upper respiratory tract could later be recovered from the tracheobronchial tree.[41,42] More recently, Huxley et al investigated pharyngeal aspiration during sleep in both healthy subjects and in patients with depressed sensorium.[43] With the use of a radiolabeled marker that was intermittently released into the nose, pulmonary aspiration was detected in a significant number of both the normal and ill subjects. Bardin et al, however, were unable to document significant aspiration of radionuclide in a study of 13 patients with chronic rhinosinusitis and asthma.[44] Although postnasal drip seems like a plausible explanation connecting nasal disease to asthma, more definitive studies in humans are required to confirm this theory.

Mouth breathing caused by nasal obstruction

Nasal blockage resulting from tissue swelling and secretions may cause a shift from the normal pattern of nasal breathing to predominantly mouth breathing. Previous work has shown that mouth breathing associated with nasal obstruction results in worsening of exercise-induced bronchospasm, whereas exclusive nasal breathing significantly reduced asthma following exercise[45] (Figure 11.2). Improvements in asthma associated with nasal breathing may be the result of superior humidification and warming of inspired air before it reaches the lower airways.[46] Similarly, it would be expected that airborne allergens and pollutants would also be less likely to enter the lungs during periods of normal nasal function.

It is difficult to determine which of these experimental mechanisms is most important in linking the nose to the lower airways. In all likelihood, however, several of these phenomena may contribute in some way to alterations in lung physiology in patients with allergic rhinitis and asthma.

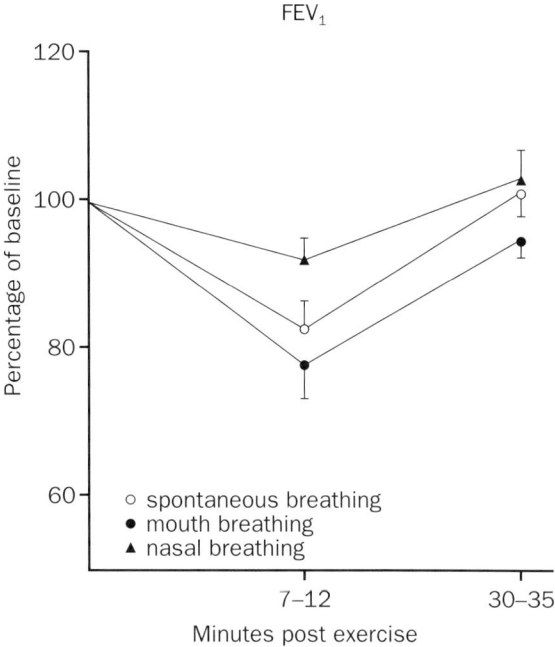

Figure 11.2 Changes of the forced expiratory volume in 1 second (FEV_1) after exercise. Exercise was performed with mouth breathing (●), nasal breathing (▲), and spontaneous breathing (○). Mean ± SE values are shown. (Reprinted with permission from ref. 45.)

Systemic absorption of inflammatory factors

Investigators have postulated that inflammation may spread from the nose and sinuses to the lower airways via the systemic circulation. Recently, Braunstahl and colleagues performed segmental bronchial provocation in patients with allergic rhinitis and no asthma.[47] Interestingly, they demonstrated increases in eosinophils in both blood and airway tissue (nasal and bronchial lamina propria) as well as late reductions in both pulmonary and nasal function. These results suggest that an inflammatory reaction localized to a small segment of the airway does spread to the systemic circulation and then to non-contiguous areas of the respiratory tract. These findings make a strong case for the possibility that inflammation may also spread from the upper airways to the lungs.

EFFECTS OF NASAL AND SINUS THERAPIES UPON THE LOWER AIRWAYS

Allergic rhinitis

Physicians often note anecdotally that treatment of allergic rhinitis results in improvements in asthma symptoms and pulmonary function. However, there have been relatively few well-controlled, large-scale clinical trials that have attempted to quantify this effect.

Intranasal corticosteroids
Several small studies have examined the efficacy of topical intranasal corticosteroids in children and adolescents with allergic rhinitis and mild asthma. Two of these trials addressed the role of prophylactic, preseasonal treatment with nasal corticosteroids in patients with primarily seasonal symptoms. Welsh and co-workers compared the effects of intranasal beclomethasone dipropionate, flunisolide, and cromolyn versus placebo in adolescents and adults with ragweed-induced allergic rhinitis.[48] Both of the topical corticosteroids were signficantly more effective in reducing nasal symptoms than either cromolyn or placebo. Unexpectedly, in 58 of the subjects who also had mild ragweed asthma, lower airway symptoms were also significantly improved in the patients receiving intranasal corticosteroids (Figure 11.3). Corren and co-workers later examined the effects of seasonal administration of intranasal beclomethasone dipropionate on bronchial hyperresponsiveness in adolescent and adult patients with fall rhinitis and mild asthma.[49] Compared with baseline values, bronchial responsiveness to inhaled methacholine worsened significantly in the placebo group but did

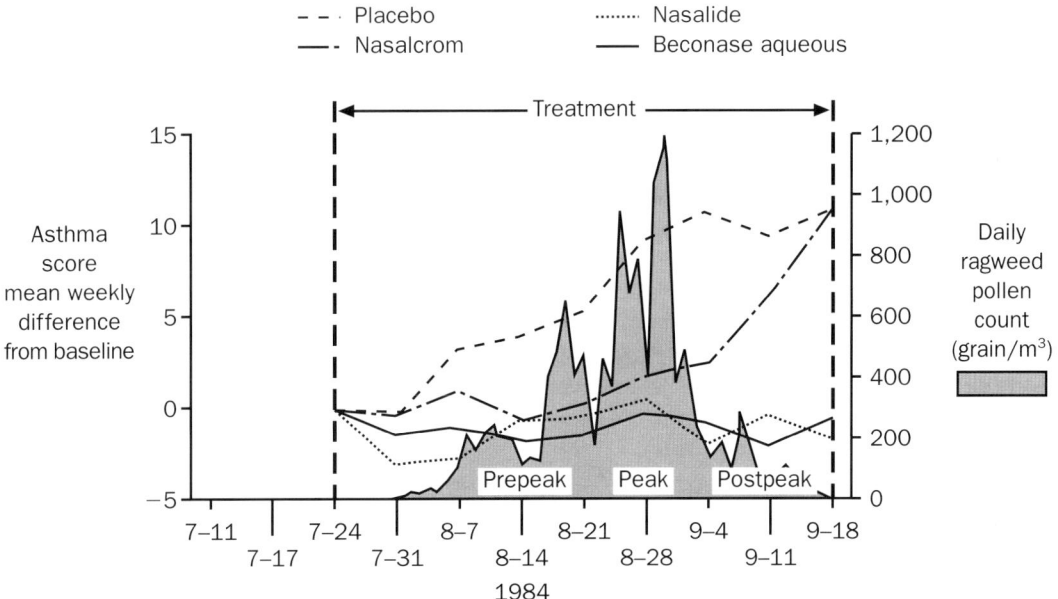

Figure 11.3 Mean weekly scores for symptoms of asthma, adjusted for baseline values in 58 patients with seasonal asthma. Daily ragweed pollen count is shown is shaded areas. Expected increase in seasonal symptoms of asthma did not occur in glucocorticoid-treated group. (Reprinted with permission from ref. 48.)

not change in the group using active treatment. Together, these two small trials suggest that prevention of seasonal nasal inflammation with topical corticosteroids reduces subsequent exacerbations of allergic asthma.

Other studies have examined the effects of intranasal corticosteroids in patients with chronic, perennial allergic rhinitis and mild asthma. The first study to document these effects employed intranasal budesonide in children with severe allergic rhinitis and concomitant asthma.[50] Four weeks of active therapy significantly reduced the objective measures of nasal obstruction as well as daily asthma symptoms and exercise-induced bronchospasm. In a subsequent study of pediatric patients with perennial rhinitis and asthma, Watson et al evaluated the effects of intranasal beclomethasone dipropionate on chest symptoms and bronchial responsiveness to methacholine.[51] Following 4 weeks of active treatment, asthma symptoms were significantly reduced as was airway reactivity to methacholine. As an adjunct to this study, the investigators performed a radiolabeled deposition study of the beclomethasone aerosol and found that less than 2% of the drug was deposited into the chest area. These studies demonstrate that intranasal corticosteroids are effective in improving lower airway symptoms and bronchial hyperresponsiveness in patients with chronic, established nasal disease and asthma. In view of the fact that the corticosteroid spray did not penetrate into the lungs, the study by Watson suggests that the reduction observed in asthma owed to improvements in nasal function rather than direct effects of the medication upon the lungs.

Antihistamines

H1-antihistamines have also been heavily studied as an adjunct treatment for asthma. Histamine is measurable in the lower airways, and serum concentrations correlate with bronchial obstruction.[52] There are a number of potential ways in which antihistaminic agents might be effective in asthma: (1) blockade of nasal histamine, leading to a reduction in neural stimulation of the lower airways;[34] (2) reduction in nasal edema and secretions, with a subsequent improvement in nasal obstruction;[53] (3) reduction in basal bronchomotor tone caused by bronchial histamine;[54] (4) reduction of allergen-induced bronchial constriction by blocking acute effects of bronchial histamine;[55] (5) possible anti-inflammatory effects (e.g. reduction in adhesion molecule expression) in both the upper and lower airways.[56]

Nearly all studies of first-generation antihistamines have shown no or minimal improvements in bronchial asthma when taken in recommended doses.[57] Lewiston compared the effects of chlorpheniramine (0.5 mg/kg per day, up to 24 mg/day) versus placebo in children with seasonal allergic rhinitis and asthma.[58] Both asthma symptoms and FEV1 were statistically better in patients treated with chlorpheniramine. However, the doses of first-generation antihistamines required to show improvements in asthma were associated with sedation and other CNS side effects, mitigating against their use as a therapeutic agent for asthma. Physicians have historically been cautioned against using these drugs in asthma because of concerns about inspissation of lower airway secretions as well as a number of case reports demonstrating acute bronchospasm following their use in young children.[59]

Initial trials of second-generation antihistamines have demonstrated inconsistent effects upon asthma symptoms and airway function in adolescents and adults.[60-64] A recent meta-analysis of antihistamines in asthmatics concluded that these agents have no significant effects on lower airway disease.[65] However, these negative results must be interpreted carefully, since available antihistamines do differ in potency. Further, patient selection in these trials varied considerably, making it difficult to combine all of these studies for analysis. More recent, large-scale trials have attempted to clarify the effects of antihistamines in asthma. Grant et al studied 193 patients with seasonal rhinitis and asthma. Comparing cetirizine 10 mg once daily versus placebo in a 6 week study, the investigators demonstated that symptoms of both rhinitis and asthma were significantly attenuated with active treatment.[66]

Neither β-agonist usage nor measures of pulmonary function were affected by treatment, most likely because of the very mild nature of asthma present in these patients.

Although amelioration of nasal obstruction appears to be mechanistically important in improving lower airway function, H1-antihistamines have only mild effects upon nasal congestion.[53] A combination of an antihistamine plus decongestant might be expected to be more effective in this regard. In another large, multicenter trial, Corren et al compared loratadine 5 mg plus pseudoephedrine 120 mg twice daily with placebo in patients with seasonal rhinitis and mild, persistent asthma.[67] Asthma symptoms, peak expiratory flow rates, and FEV_1 were all significantly improved in patients taking active therapy, with a trend toward less albuterol use. Since pseudoephedrine has not been shown to have direct bronchodilator effects in asthma,[68] these results are most likely attributable to the actions of loratadine and pseudoephedrine on nasal function.

Antileukotriene drugs

Leukotriene D4 receptor antagonists have recently been approved for use in asthma in children. In addition to their beneficial effects in asthma, these agents have also been shown to reduce symptoms of allergic rhinitis.[69,70] This class of drugs offers a promising treatment for patients who suffer from respiratory allergy affecting both the upper and lower airways.

Effects of rhinitis treatment on asthma outcomes

An important question regarding rhinitis therapy is whether individual or combinations of drugs have any effects upon acute exacerbations of asthma. A recent analysis of a large database of children (older than 12 years), adolescents, and adults showed that the combination of an oral antihistamine plus an intranasal corticosteroid was highly associated with reductions in emergency room visits for acute asthma.[71] In a second, to date unpublished, study, both emergency room utilization and hospitalizations for acute asthma were significantly associated with rhinitis therapy. These results are encouraging and may serve as a strong rationale for aggressively treating allergic rhinitis in patients with asthma.

The above studies demonstrate that treatment of rhinitis may result in modest improvements in asthma symptoms and asthma-specific quality of life, increases in FEV_1, and reductions in non-specific bronchial hyperresponsiveness. In selected patients with mild intermittent asthma, treatment of rhinitis may reduce asthma symptoms to such an extent that potential first-line, prophylactic anti-asthma drugs (such as inhaled cromolyn or nedocromil) may prove unnecessary. In addition, if recent outcome studies are validated, rhinitis therapy may also prove to be very beneficial to patients with more severe asthma as well.

Sinusitis

Early in the 20th century, surgeons observed that effective treatment of chronic sinusitis resulted in variable improvements in asthma symptoms in both children and adults. Since that time, however, there have been few controlled trials of either medical or surgical therapy of sinusitis in asthmatics.

Medical treatment

In the early 1980s a large number of studies were conducted in children to determine the effects of medical therapy for sinusitis upon asthma. In 1981, Businco et al reported that 10 of 12 children given open label treatment for sinusitis demonstrated improvements in asthma.[72] Following these observations, Rachelefsky et al performed an open label study of 48 children with a 3 month or longer history of radiographically confirmed sinusitis and wheezing.[73] After 2–4 weeks of antibiotics with or without antral lavage, 38 of the patients were able to discontinue daily bronchodilator treatments, and 20 out of 30 had normalization of pulmonary function tests. Friedman et al reported similar open label results in a series of eight children with sinusitis and chronic asthma.[74] Seven of the eight patients showed improvement in lower airway symptoms and for the group there was a significant improvement in the pulmonary response to inhaled bronchodilator. Cummings and co-workers reported the results of the first (and only) randomized, double-blind, placebo-controlled trial of sinus therapy in children with asthma.[75] Active treatment (antibiotics, nasal steroids, and oral decongestants) in children with opacification or marked mucosal thickening of the maxillary sinuses resulted in significantly fewer asthma symptoms and reduced the need for inhaled bronchodilator and oral steroid therapy. Neither pulmonary function values nor methacholine challenge test results were significantly improved in the active treatment group. A similar study was performed by Oliveira and co-workers, who demonstrated that a combination of oral antibiotics, an antihistamine-decongestant, and a short course of oral prednisone reduced bronchial hyperreactivity in children with chronic sinusitis and asthma.[76]

Surgical therapy
Over the past 65 years, there have been several observational reports about the effects of sinus surgery in pediatric and adult asthmatics. In 1936, Weille published his long-term observations on a group of 500 pediatric and adult asthmatics, nearly three-fourths of whom had chronic sinus disease.[77] Following surgery in 100 of these patients, 56 felt their chest symptoms were improved and ten experienced complete resolution of their asthma. Marked improvement in asthma symptoms, however, also occurred in 40% of the patients who did not have sinus surgery. Werth reported on a series of 22 children with severe asthma and sinusitis.[78] Following sinus surgery, 20 of 22 patients experienced a marked improvement in asthma symptoms.

To date, there have been no randomized, double-blind, controlled trials examining the effects of sinus surgery on asthma symptoms or lung function. The study by Weille[77] suggests that asthma symptoms often improve over time in the absence of surgical intervention. Controlled trials of both medical and surgical treatment of sinusitis in asthmatics is critical so that we may accurately and objectively appraise the magnitude of improvement in these patients.

CONCLUSIONS

Over the past several years there has been a growing awareness of the importance of upper airway disease in patients with bronchial asthma. Epidemiologic surveys across all age groups indicate that rhinitis is associated with more severe asthma symptoms and a greater requirement for asthma drugs. Clinical trials with a variety of rhinitis therapies have shown significant beneficial effects in mild asthma, and emerging population-based studies have shown improved asthma outcomes in patients treated for rhinitis. Although the data are less clear in the case of sinusitis, there are abundant observational data suggesting beneficial effects of medical or surgical sinus therapy in asthma. Future studies will be important in determining which patients with upper airway disease are at greatest risk of developing asthma, and whether early intervention is capable of preventing the progression to lower airway disease.

REFERENCES

1. McFadden ER. Nasal–sinus–pulmonary reflexes and bronchial asthma. *J Allergy Clin Immunol* 1986; **78**: 1.
2. Sluder G. Asthma as a nasal reflex. *JAMA* 1919; **73**: 589.
3. Gottlieb MJ. Relation of intranasal disease in the production of bronchial asthma. *JAMA* 1925; **95**: 105–8.
4. Blair H. Natural history of childhood asthma: 20 year follow-up. *Arch Dis Child* 1977; **52**: 613.
5. Smith JM. Epidemiology and natural history of asthma, allergic rhinitis and atopic dermatitis (eczema). In: Middleton E, ed. *Allergy, Principles and Practice*, 3rd edn. St Louis, C.V. Mosby, 1988.
6. Pedersen PA, Weeke ER. Asthma and allergic rhinitis in the same patients. *Allergy* 1983; **38**: 25–9.
7. Settipane GA. Allergic rhinitis—update. *Otolaryngol Head Neck Surg* 1986; **94**: 470

8. Kapsali T, Horowitz E, Diemer F, Togias A. Rhinitis is ubiquitous in allergic asthmatics. *J Allergy Clin Immunol* 1997; **99:** S138 (abstract).
9. Evans R III, Mullally DI, Wilson RW et al. National trends in the morbidity and mortality of asthma in the U.S.: prevalence, hospitalization, and death from asthma over two decades 1965–1984. *Chest* 1987; **91:** 65S–74S.
10. Arsdel PP, Motulsby KP. Frequency and hereditability of asthma and allergic rhinitis in students. *Acta Genet* 1959; **9:** 101–14.
11. Maternowski CJ, Mathews KP. The prevalence of ragweed pollinosis in foreign and native students at a midwestern university and its implications concerning methods for determining inheritance of atopy. *J Allergy* 1962; **33:** 130–40.
12. Johnstone D. A study of the natural history of bronchial asthma in children. *Am J Dis Child* 1968; **115:** 213.
13. Settipane RJ, Hagy GW, Settipane GA. Long-term risk factors for developing asthma and allergic rhinitis: a 23-year follow-up study of college students. *Allergy Proc* 1994; **15:** 21–5.
14. Madonini E, Briatico-Vangosa G, Pappacoda A, Maccagni G, Cardani A, Saporiti F. Seasonal increase of bronchial reactivity in allergic rhinitis. *J Allergy Clin Immunol* 1987; **79:** 358–63.
15. Ramsdale EH, Morris MM, Robers RS, Hargreave FE. Asymptomatic bronchial hyperresponsiveness in rhinitis. *J Allergy Clin Immunol* 1985; **75:** 573–7.
16. Townley RG, Ryo UY, Kolotkin B, Kang B. Bronchial sensitivity to methacholine in current and former asthmatic and allergic rhinitis and control subjects. *J Allergy Clin Immunol* 1975; **56:** 429.
17. Braman SS, Barrows AA, De Cotiis BA et al. Airway hyperresponsiveness in allergic rhinitis. A risk factor for asthma. *Chest* 1987; **91:** 671–4.
18. Koh YY, Lee MH, Kim CK et al. A familial predisposition in bronchial hyperresponsiveness among patients with allergic rhinitis. *J Allergy Clin Immunol* 1998; **102:** 921–6.
19. Huse DM, Harte SC, Russel MW et al. Allergic rhinitis may worsen asthma symptoms in children: the international asthma outcomes registry. *Am J Respir Crit Care Med* 1996; **153:** A860 (abstract).
20. Halpern M, Richner R, Togias A et al. Allergic rhinitis may increase asthma costs. *Am J Respir Crit Care Med* 1996; **153:** A860 (abstract).
21. Scichilone N, Sanico AM, Diemer E et al. Symptom triggers in rhinitis and asthma. *J Allergy Clin Immunol* 1999; **103:** S8 (abstract).
22. Chobot R. The incidence of sinusitis in asthmatic children. *Am J Dis Child* 1930; **39:** 257.
23. Bullen SS. Incidence of asthma in 400 cases of chronic sinusitis. *J Allergy* 1932; **4:** 402–7.
24. Berman SZ, Mathison DA, Stevenson DD et al. Maxillary sinusitis and bronchial asthma: correlation of roentgenograms, cultures, and thermograms. *J Allergy Clin Imlmunol* 1974; **53:** 311.
25. Rachelefsky GS, Goldberg M, Katz RM et al. Sinus disease in children with respiratory allergy. *J Allergy Clin Immunol* 1978; **61:** 310.
26. Schwarz HJ, Thompson JS, Sher TH et al. Occult sinus abnormalities in the asthmatic patient. *Arch Int Med* 1987; **147:** 2194.
27. Zimmerman B, Stringer D, Feanny S. Prevalence of abnormalities found by sinus x-rays in childhood asthma: lack of relation to severity of asthma. *J Allergy Clin Immunol* 1987; **88:** 268.
28. Pfister R, Lutolf M, Schapowal A. Screening for sinus disease in patients with asthma: a computed tomography-controlled comparison of A-mode ultrasonography and standard radiography. *J Allergy Clin Immunol* 1994; **94:** 804–9.
29. Crater SE, Peters EJ, Phillips CD et al. Prospective analysis of CT of the sinuses in acute asthma. *Am J Roentgenol* 1999; **173:** 127–31.
30. Hamilos DL, Leung DH, Huston DP et al. GM-CSF, IL-5 and RANTES immunoreactivity and mRNA expression in chronic hyperplastic sinusitis with nasal polyposis. *Clin Exp Allergy* 1998; **28:** 1145–52.
31. Kaufman J, Wright GW. The effect of nasal and nasopharyngeal irritation on airway resistance in man. *Am Rev Respir Dis* 1969; **100:** 626–30.
32. Kaufman J, Chen J, Wright GW. The effect of trigeminal resection on reflex bronchoconstriction after nasal and nasopharyngeal irritation in man. *Am Rev Respir Dis* 1970; **101:** 76.
33. Fontanari P, Burnet H, Zattara-Harmann MC, Jammes Y. Changes in airway resistance induced by nasal inhalation of cold dry, dry, or moist air in normal individuals. *J Appl Physiol* 1996; **81:** 1739–43.
34. Yan K, Salome C. The response of the airways to nasal stimulation in asthmatics with rhinitis. *Eur J Respir Dis* 1983; **64** (suppl): 105–8.
35. Hoehne JH, Reed CE. Where is the allergic reaction in ragweed asthma? *J Allergy Clin Immunol* 1971; **48:** 36–39.
36. Schumacher MJ, Cota KA, Taussig LM. Pulmonary response to nasal-challenge testing of

atopic subjects with stable asthma. *J Allergy Clin Immunol* 1986; **78**: 30–5.
37. Littell NT, Carlisle CC, Millman RP, Braman SS. Changes in airway resistance following nasal provocation. *Am Rev Respir Dis* 1990; **141**: 580–3.
38. Small P, Bisken N. The effects of allergen-induced nasal provocation on pulmonary function in patients with perennial allergic rhinitis. *Am J Rhinol* 1989; **3**: 17–20.
39. Corren J, Adinoff AD, Irvin CG. Changes in bronchial responsiveness following nasal provocation with allergen. *J Allergy Clin Immunol* 1992; **89**: 611–18.
40. Rolla G, Colagrande P, Scappaticci E et al. Damage of the pharyngeal mucosa and hyperresponsiveness of airway in sinusitis. *J Allergy Clin Immunol* 1997; **100**: 52–7.
41. Mullen WV, Wyder CT. Experimental lesions of lungs produced by the inhalation of fluid from the nose and throat. *Am Rev Tuberc* 1920; **4**: 6840.
42. McLaurin JG. Chest complications of sinus discase. *Ann Otol Rhinol Laryngol* 1932; **41**: 780.
43. Huxley EJ, Viroslav J, Gray WR et al. Pharyngeal aspiration in normal adults and patients with depressed consciousness. *Am J Med* 1978; **64**: 564.
44. Bardin PG, Van Heerden BB, Joubert JR. Absence of pulmonary aspiration of sinus contents in patients with asthma and sinusitis. *J Allergy Clin Immunol* 1990; **86**: 82–88.
45. Shturman-Ellstein R, Zeballos RJ, Buckley JM, Souhrada JF. The beneficial effect of nasal breathing on exercise-induced bronchoconstriction. *Am Rev Respir Dis* 1978; **118**: 65–73.
46. Griffin MP, McFadden ER, Ingram RH. Airway cooling in asthmatic and nonasthmatic subjects during nasal and oral breathing. *J Allergy Clin Immunol* 1982; **69**: 354–9.
47. Braunstahl GJ, Kleinman A, Overbeek SE, Prins JB, Hoogsteden HC, Fokkens WJ. Segmental bronchial provocation induces nasal inflammation in allergic rhinitis patients. *Am J Respir Crit Care Med* 2000; **161**: 2051–7.
48. Welsh PW, Stricker EW, Chu-Pin C et al. Efficacy of beclomethasone nasal solution, flunisolide and cromolyn in relieving symptoms of ragweed allergy. *Mayo Clin Proc* 1987; **62**: 125–34.
49. Corren J, Adinoff AD, Buchmeier AD, Irvin CG. Nasal beclomethasone prevents the seasonal increase in bronchial responsiveness in patients with allergic rhinitis and asthma. *J Allergy Clin Immunol* 1992; **90**: 250–6.
50. Henriksen JW, Wenzel A. Effect of an intranasally administered corticosteroid (budes-onide) on nasal obstruction, mouth breathing and asthma. *Am Rev Respir Dis* 1984; **130**: 1014–18.
51. Watson WTA, Becker AB, Simons FER. Treatment of allergic rhinitis with intranasal corticosteroids in patients with mild asthma: effect on lower airway responsiveness. *J Allergy Clin Immunol* 1993; **91**: 97–101.
52. Casale TB, Wood D, Richerson HB et al. Elevated bronchoalveolar lavage fluid histamine levels in allergic asthmatics are associated with methacholine bronchial hyperresponsiveness. *J Clin Invest* 1987; **79**: 1197–203.
53. Bronsky E, Boggs P, Findlay S et al. Comparative efficacy and safety of a once-daily loratadine-pseudoephedrine combination versus its components alone and placebo in the management of seasonal allergic rhinitis. *J Allergy Clin Immunol* 1995; **96**: 139–47.
54. Spector Sl, Nicodemus CF, Corren J et al. Comparison of the bronchodilatory effects of cetirizine, albuterol, and both together versus placebo in patients with mild to moderate asthma. *J Allergy Clin Immunol* 1995; **96**: 174–81.
55. Ghosh SK, DeVos C, McIlroy I et al. Effect of cetirizine on histamine- and leukotriene D4-induced bronchoconstriction in patients with atopic asthma. *J Allergy Clin Immunol* 1991; **87**: 1010–13.
56. Ciprandi G, Passalacqua G, Canonica GW. Effects of H1 antihistamines on adhesion molecules: a possible raionale for long-term treatment. *Clin Exp Allergy* 1999; **29** (suppl 3): 49–53.
57. Karlin JM. The use of antihistamines in asthma. *Ann Allergy* 1972; **30**: 342–7.
58. Lewiston NJ, Johnson S, Sloan E. Effect of antihistamine on pulmonary function of children with asthma. *J Pediatr* 1982; **101**: 458–60.
59. Schuller DE. Adverse effects of brompheniramine on pulmonary function in a subset of asthmatic children. *J Allergy Clin Immunol* 1983; **72**: 175–9.
60. Taytard A, Beaumont D, Pujet JC, Sapene M, Lewis PJ. Treatment of bronchial asthma with terfenadine; a randomized controlled trial. *Br J Clin Pharmacol* 1987; **24**: 743–6.
61. Rafferty P, Jackson L, Smith R, Holgate ST. Terfenadine, a potent H1-receptor antagonist in the treatment of grass pollen sensitive asthma. *Br J Clin Pharmacol* 1990; **30**: 229–35.
62. Wood-Baker R, Smith R, Holgate ST. A double-blind, placebo-controlled study of the effect of the specific histamine H1-antagonist, terfenadine, in chronic severe asthma. *Br J Clin Pharmacol* 1995; **39**: 671–5.

63. Bruttman G, Pedraii P, Arendt C, Rihoux JP. Protective effect of cetirizine in patients suffering from pollen asthma. *Ann Allergy* 1990; **64:** 224–8.
64. Dijkman JH, Hekking PRM, Molkenboer JF et al. Prophylactic treatment of grass pollen-induced asthma with cetirizine. *Clin Exp Allergy* 1990; **20:** 483–90.
65. Van Ganse E, Kaufman L, Derde MP et al. Effects of antihistamines in adult asthma: a meta-analysis of clinical trials. *Eur Respir J* 1997; **10:** 2216–24.
66. Grant JA, Nicodemus CF, Findlay SR et al. Cetirizine in patients with seasonal allergic rhinitis and concomitant asthma: prospective, randomized, placebo-controlled trial. *J Allergy Clin Immunol* 1995; **95:** 923–32.
67. Corren J, Harris A, Aaronson D et al. Efficacy and safety of loratadine plus pseudoephedrine in patients with seasonal allergic rhinitis and mild asthma. *J Allergy Clin Immunol* 1997; **100:** 781–8.
68. Laitinen LA, Empey DW, Bye C et al. A comparison of the bronchodilator action of pseudoephedrine and ephedrine in patients with reversible airway obstruction. *Eur J Clin Pharmacol* 1982; **23:** 107–9.
69. Donnelly AL, Glass M, Minkwitz MC, Casale TB. The leukotriene D4-receptor antagonist, ICI 204,219, relieves symptoms of acute seasonal allergic rhinitis. *Am J Resp Crit Care Med* 1995; **151:** 1734–9.
70. Meltzer EO, Malmstrom K, Lu S et al. Concomitant montelukast and loratadine as treatment for seasonal allergic rhinitis: a randomized, placebo-controlled clinical trial. *J Allergy Clin Immunol* 2000; **105:** 917–22.
71. Ronberg E, Iezzoni D, Manning B, Corren J. Treatment of allergic rhinitis is associated with lower rates of asthma-related emergency room visits and hospitalizations. *J Allergy Clin Immunol* 1998; **101:** A980.
72. Businco L, Fiore L, Frediani T et al. Clinical and therapeutic aspects of sinusitis in children with bronchial asthma. *Int J Pediatr Otorhinolaryngol* 1981; **3:** 287.
73. Rachelefsky GS, Katz RM, Siegel SC. Chronic sinus disease with associated reactive airway disease in children. *Pediatrics* 1984; **73:** 525.
74. Friedman R, Ackerman M, Wald E et al. Asthma and bacterial sinusitis in children. *J Allergy Clin Immunol* 1984; **74:** 185.
75. Cummings NP, Wood RW, Leare JL et al. Effect of treatment on rhinitis/sinusitis on asthma: results of a double-blind study. *Pediatr Res* 1983; **17:** 373.
76. Oliveira CA, Sole D, Naspitz CK, Rachelefsky GS. Improvement of bronchial hyperresponsiveness in asthmatic children treated for concomitant sinusitis. *Ann Allergy Asthma Immunol* 1997; **79:** 70–4.
77. Weille FL. Studies in asthma: nose and throat in 500 cases of asthma. *N Engl J Med* 1936; **215:** 235–9.
78. Werth G. The role of sinusitis in severe asthma. *Immunol Allergy Proc* 1984; **7:** 45.

12

Nonpharmacologic approaches to the management of asthma

Robert A Wood, Peyton A Eggleston

Introduction • Allergens and environmental control • Dust mites • Dust mite control measures • Animal allergens • Control of animal allergens • Cockroach allergens • Cockroach allergen control • Mold allergens • Indoor air pollution • Immunotherapy • Mechanisms of immunotherapy • Efficacy of immunotherapy • Safety of immunotherapy • Indications for immunotherapy

INTRODUCTION

In addition to the many pharmacologic therapies available for the treatment of asthma, there are a variety of nonpharmacologic modalities. The most important of these, allergen avoidance and immunotherapy, will be the focus of this chapter.

ALLERGENS AND ENVIRONMENTAL CONTROL

There should be no doubt that aeroallergens play a major role in the pathogenesis of asthma and allergic rhinitis. Among these, the indoor allergens are of particular importance. These principally include the allergens of house dust mites, domestic pets, cockroaches, and molds. The relative importance of these different allergens varies in different parts of the world depending on a variety of geographic and climatic factors. All studies agree, however, that children with asthma will have a high likelihood of becoming sensitized to whichever of these allergens are prominent in their local environment. Here, we will focus on the importance of allergen avoidance in the management of pediatric asthma.

DUST MITES

Dust mites are arachnids that live in the dust that accumulates in most homes, particularly the dust contained within fabrics. Favorite habitats include carpets, upholstered furniture, mattresses, pillows, and bedding materials. Their major food source is shed human skin scales, which are present in high numbers in most of these items. The major dust mite species known to be associated with allergic disease are *Dermatophagoides pteronyssinus* and *Dermatophagoides farinae*.[1,2] Other mites, including *Euroglyphus maynei* and *Blomia tropicalis*, are also important in some areas, although their distribution is considerably more limited. Dust mites grow optimally in areas that are both warm and humid and they grow very poorly when the relative humidity remains below 40%.[3] Dust mites grow from eggs to adults over the course of about 4 weeks and adult dust mites live for about 6 weeks, during which time females produce 40 to 80 eggs.[3]

Assessment of dust mite exposure has largely been accomplished through the analysis of settled dust samples. Although some studies have not been able to show a relationship between dust mite levels and allergic sensitization or disease activity, there is now general agreement that dust mite levels of greater than 2 µg of Group 1 allergen per gram of dust should be considered a risk factor for sensitization[4-7] and that levels greater than 10 µg per gram of dust are a risk factor for acute asthma.[8] Airborne sampling for dust mite has proven difficult or impossible in the absence of substantial disturbance. This is a reflection of the fact that dust mite allergens are carried on relatively large particles, most ranging from 10 to 20 µm in mean aerodynamic diameter, which settle within minutes of disturbance.[9]

The prevalence of dust mite sensitivity in asthmatic patients varies considerably from one geographic area to another. For example, studies have demonstrated prevalence rates ranging from 5% in asthmatic children in Los Alamos, New Mexico, to 66% in Atlanta, Georgia, to 91% in Papua New Guinea.[8,10,11] These differences are roughly proportional to differences in mite exposure in these different areas of the world.

At least as significant as the relationship between mite exposure and mite sensitization is the evidence that mite exposure is capable of inducing not just sensitization but the asthmatic state itself. In a prospective trial, Sporik et al demonstrated a significant increase in asthma, as well as mite sensitivity, in 11-year-old children who had experienced high mite exposure during infancy.[7] Other studies have demonstrated a striking association between asthma development and mite sensitivity,[10,12-14] although these studies lacked a prospective evaluation of mite exposure. These studies are exciting in that they indicate that allergen avoidance early in life could prevent the development of asthma in some patients, an idea that has recently been studied with encouraging results.[15]

Extensive evidence also exists to support a relationship between ongoing mite exposure and disease activity.[16-18] With regard to chronic symptoms, Vervloet et al demonstrated a significant correlation between medication requirements and current mite exposure in a group of mite-sensitive adult asthmatics.[18] Custovic et al also demonstrated a relationship between mite exposure and asthma severity as evidenced by bronchial hyperreactivity, peak expiratory flow rate variability, and FEV_1.[16] Several studies have also demonstrated mite exposure to be a risk factor for acute asthma and emergency room visits.[8,19] In a study by Call et al, inner-city children in Atlanta were evaluated after presentation to the emergency room with acute asthma.[8] Seventy-two percent of these children were found to be allergic to either dust mite alone or both dust mite and cockroach allergen. The combination of mite exposure and mite sensitization was highly associated with the development of acute asthma (21 of 35 asthmatic patients versus 3 of 22 control subjects, $P < 0.001$).

The most compelling evidence for the role of dust mites in asthma comes from studies of allergen avoidance, through either environmental control in the home or the removal of mite-allergic patients from their homes. Two classic studies from the early 1980s provided dramatic evidence as to the potential benefits of dust mite avoidance. Platts-Mills et al investigated the effects of mite avoidance by placing nine young adults with mite-induced asthma in a hospital setting for a minimum of 2 months.[20] All patients experienced reduced symptoms, seven patients had reduced medication requirements, and five patients showed at least an eight-fold reduction in bronchial reactivity, as measured by the concentration of histamine required to induce a 30% fall in FEV_1. In the second study, Murray and Ferguson studied 20 mite-allergic asthmatic children in a controlled trial of mite avoidance in the patients' homes.[21] They found significant reductions in asthma symptoms, days on which wheezing was observed, days with low peak flow rates, and bronchial hyperreactivity in the group using active mite control measures.

The vast majority of subsequent trials of mite avoidance have yielded similar results.[22-26]

Ehnert et al studied 24 children with asthma and mite sensitivity in a 1-year trial of mite avoidance.[24] The patients were divided into three groups. The first had their mattresses, pillows, and comforters covered with impermeable encasements, the second had their mattresses and carpets treated with an acaricide (benzyl benzoate), and the third had their mattresses and carpets treated with placebo. Significant reductions in dust mite allergen levels were found only in the group with mattress and pillow encasements. Similarly, a highly significant reduction in bronchial hyperreactivity was noted in that group compared with the other two. The clinical trials of mite allergen avoidance which include the use of impervious encasements on bedding have generally produced a 90% or greater reduction in mite numbers or mite allergen, and these trials have consistently been associated with a change in asthma physiology or morbidity. The evidence from these trials is well reviewed,[27,28] with the conclusion that mite allergen avoidance is effective. Recently, mite allergen clinical trials were the subject of a meta-analysis, but this approach included many trials that did not reduce mite allergen exposure or were short, lasting less than 6 weeks; these authors concluded that mite allergen avoidance was not an effective therapy for asthma.[29]

One final study of mite avoidance deserves note. It has long been recognized that dust mite levels are significantly reduced at high altitude. Peroni et al performed an extensive clinical study of mite avoidance by moving asthmatic children to a high altitude environment.[26] The study was divided into two groups, one with 22 children and the other with 23 children, who were admitted during successive years. They demonstrated significant reductions in total IgE levels, dust-mite-specific IgE levels, methacholine reactivity, and response to dust mite bronchoprovocation. These differences were first detected after 3 months in the high altitude setting and continued through the entire 9 month study. These authors were also able to study 14 of the 22 children from the first cohort 3 months after returning to their usual home environment. These children had experienced significant increases in their total IgE levels, methacholine reactivity, and response to exercise challenge. This important demonstration of reduced disease activity in the mite-free environment, followed by increased disease activity after returning to usual mite exposure, provides a remarkable demonstration of the power of both mite exposure and avoidance.

DUST MITE CONTROL MEASURES

Although there should be no doubt as to the benefits of dust mite avoidance, there is still some controversy as to the specific measures that are necessary to sufficiently reduce mite exposure to control disease (Table 12.1). This controversy arises from three major factors. First, some environmental control measures have not been adequately studied to make any accurate conclusions. Second, for some measures studies of their efficacy have yielded conflicting results. Third, in many studies a

Table 12.1 Environmental control measures for dust mites

Essential measures	Desirable measures
Encase mattresses and pillows in allergen-impermeable covers	Reduce indoor humidity to less than 50%
Wash all bedding weekly in hot water	Remove carpets from the bedroom
Minimize the number of stuffed toys in the bed	Avoid sleeping or lying on carpets or upholstered furniture

combination of environmental control measures as utilized, making it difficult to determine which measures actually led to the benefit that was observed. Specific environmental control measures will therefore be reviewed individually.

It is very clear that impermeable fabric or vinyl encasements for mattresses and pillows significantly reduce dust mite exposure.[24,30,31] In the study by Ehnert et al, polyurethane mattress encasings produced a 91% decrease in mite allergen by day 14 of treatment, which rose to 98% by month 12 of the study.[24] In another study by Owen et al, Der p I levels on encased mattresses were only 1% of those on control mattresses.[30] These encasements should therefore be recommended for all patients with mite sensitivity.

The effects of vacuum cleaning on mite levels have been extensively studied. Live mites are difficult to remove from carpeting and it is clear that vacuum cleaning in the absence of other measures will provide only limited benefit. However, regular vacuum cleaning does remove significant amounts of dust from carpets, which will at least help to reduce the allergen reservoir. Patients should also be warned that vacuuming creates considerable disturbance with transient increases in airborne mite levels. Vacuum cleaners equipped with special bags or filters to help prevent this problem are available and may be of some added benefit,[32] although it should be noted that, because dust mite allergen is carried on large particles that settle quickly, it is not clear whether these specialized vacuums are of clinical importance. There is little evidence that wet vacuum cleaning or steam cleaning provides any additional benefit. In one study, carpet shampooing was found to be no more effective than dry vacuum cleaning,[33] and in another study wet vacuum cleaning was shown to lead to a subsequent increase in mite numbers.[34] This was presumed to have occurred because of elevated humidity in the carpet after wet vacuuming.

A variety of carpet treatments have also been developed in an effort to control dust mite allergen exposure. These can be classified as either acaricides or denaturing agents. A variety of acaricides have been investigated and shown to kill house dust mites in laboratory conditions.[35–37] These range from caffeine[37] to potent and potentially toxic organophosphates.[38] Only one acaricide, benzyl benzoate, is available for use in the United States.

Although there is little doubt that benzyl benzoate is effective in killing dust mites, studies regarding the efficacy of this compound in home environments have provided varying results.[23,39–41] For example, although both Hayden et al[9] and Woodfolk et al[41] demonstrated significant reductions in dust mite allergen after treatment with benzyl benzoate, the changes were not always in a range that would be expected to produce clinical benefit and were relatively short-lived. In the Hayden et al study, mite levels were still reduced 2 months after treatment, but some increase was clearly evident compared with 1 month after treatment, suggesting that repeat applications might be required every 2–3 months to maintain effect. In another study by Huss et al, benzyl benzoate was compared with placebo in a group of 12 patients.[42] The products were applied at baseline and after 6 months and allergen levels were measured at 0, 3, 6, 9, and 12 months. The authors detected no decrease in mite allergen in the benzyl benzoate group compared with the control group. Likewise, no effect on clinical asthma was detected. It should be noted that the application of benzyl benzoate every 6 months as performed in this study was based on the manufacturer's recommendations, and that the lack of effect may have occurred simply because the product was not applied more often, or because allergen levels were not measured sooner after application.

Tannic acid is a denaturing agent that has been extensively studied for the control of dust mite allergen. This product is designed to reduce allergen levels without affecting dust mite growth or allergen production. It has also been shown in the laboratory to be highly effective. Much like benzyl benzoate, however, its efficacy in home environments is less convincing. Woodfolk et al evaluated the effects of tannic acid on 17 carpets.[43] The carpets were treated on days 0 and 28 and dust samples were collected on days 0, 1, 7, 14, 28, and 42. The treated carpets exhibited reduced mite allergen levels compared with control carpets, although the effects were not dramatic and were not maintained for long periods.

The recommendation regarding the use of benzyl benzoate and tannic acid is therefore that these products may be useful adjuncts for the control of dust mite exposure in homes where carpets, particularly bedroom carpets, cannot be removed. Especially the use of benzyl benzoate must be followed by intensive vacuum cleaning to remove residual allergen. It is likely that the combination of benzyl benzoate and tannic acid would produce the greatest effect,[44] although even this could never be a substitute for carpet removal.

Bed linens, stuffed animals, and other soft furnishings also provide excellent environments for dust mite growth. Objects such as stuffed animals should be removed whenever possible. The mite content of bedding materials and other objects that cannot be removed can typically be reduced by washing. Washing in hot water (greater than 55°C) is ideal in that it both removes allergen and kills dust mites.[45] These water temperatures, however, may not be available in many homes because of safety concerns. It is important to note, therefore, that washing in cooler water does not kill mites but does remove mite allergens very effectively. Weekly washing of all bed linens in a hot cycle is therefore recommended for all mite-allergic patients. Dry cleaning also kills dust mites,[45,46] as does tumble drying at greater than 55°C for at least 20 minutes.[30]

Dust mites are susceptible to the effects of low as well as high temperature. Freezing in a typical household freezer for 24 hours will kill most dust mites[47] although the mite allergens in the object will not necessarily be reduced. Exposing carpets to direct sun for several hours will also kill dust mites because of the high temperature, the low humidity, or both.[48] It has also been shown that electric blankets will reduce mite growth.[49] None of these methods has been established in clinical trials.

Because of the reliance of dust mites on humidity for growth, it has been suggested that methods capable of reducing relative humidity would be useful in the control of mite exposure.[50,51] Korsgaard and Iversen demonstrated that dust mite growth could be significantly reduced by keeping indoor humidity below 7 g/kg by ventilation.[51] Air conditioning and dehumidification may also help to deter mite growth and should be used whenever possible.[52] It is clear, however, that such measures will be difficult or impossible in environments with very high relative humidity. A prime example of this fact is the difficulty in eliminating dust mites from carpets over cement slab floors in basements.

Finally, air filtration devices are frequently purchased by patients for the control of their dust mite allergy. However, there is little evidence to support their use.[53–56] In addition, one would not anticipate much effect because of the fact that dust mite allergens do not remain airborne for extended periods and would therefore not be available for filtration in most instances.

In summary, effective dust mite control can be accomplished in most homes with a combination of mattress and pillow covers, hot washing of bed linen, removal of stuffed animals and other soft furnishings, and carpet removal. In the absence of carpet removal, intensive vacuum cleaning and the use of acaricides and denaturing agents may prove helpful in many homes. Because of the extraordinary benefits provided through dust mite avoidance in mite-sensitive asthmatics, these measures should be routinely recommended, and compliance with these recommendations should be reassessed at each subsequent visit.

ANIMAL ALLERGENS

Animal allergens are also potent causes of both acute and chronic asthma symptoms. Cat and dog allergens are the most important, although significant exposure to a wide variety of other furred animals is not uncommon. Sensitivity to cat and dog allergens has been shown to occur in up to 67% of asthmatic children and in some settings these are clearly the dominant indoor allergens.[11,57,58] This fact was best demonstrated in the study by Ingram et al conducted in Los Alamos, New Mexico.[11] In this environment where cat and dog allergens are common but exposure to dust mite and cockroach allergens is rare, IgE antibody to cat and dog was detected in 62% and 67%, respectively, of asthmatic children. The presence of this IgE antibody was highly associated with asthma whereas sensitivity to mite or cockroach allergen was not associated with asthma.

A number of studies have investigated the distribution of cat and dog allergens in home and other environments.[11,57-61] Using settled dust analysis, it has been shown that levels of cat and dog allergen are clearly highest in homes housing these animals. However, it is also clear from a number of studies that the vast majority of homes contain cat and dog allergen even if a pet has never lived there. This widespread distribution of cat and dog allergen has also been documented in a variety of other settings, including office buildings and schools. Although most of these non-animal-containing environments have relatively low allergen levels compared with those with a cat or dog, it is not uncommon to find high levels in some of these homes. This widespread distribution is presumed to occur primarily through passive transfer of allergen from one environment to another. The particles carrying animal allergens appear to be very sticky and, unlike dust mite allergens, can be found in high levels on walls and other surfaces within homes.[62]

The characteristics of airborne cat allergen have also been extensively studied. Cat allergen has been shown to be carried on particles that range from less than 1 μm to greater than 20 μm in mean aerodynamic diameter.[63,64] Although estimates have varied, studies agree that at least 15% of airborne cat allergen is carried on particles of less than 5 μm. Less information is available for dog allergen, but evidence to date suggests that it is distributed very much like cat allergen, with about 20% of airborne dog allergen being carried on particles less than 5 μm in diameter.[65]

Cat allergen can also be detected in air samples from all homes with cats and from many homes without cats. Bollinger et al detected airborne cat allergen in 10 out of 40 air samples from homes without cats.[66] In addition, when a subset of those homes were reinvestigated on a weekly basis for 4 weeks, all of them had detectable airborne cat allergen on at least one occasion. In an attempt to determine the clinical significance of this unsuspected cat exposure, patients were challenged in an experimental cat exposure facility to varying levels of cat allergen. It was found that allergen levels of less than 100 ng/m^3 were capable of inducing upper and lower respiratory symptoms as well as significant pulmonary function changes. These levels are similar to those found in homes with cats as well as a subset of homes without cats, suggesting that even patients without known cat exposure may be exposed to clinically significant concentrations of airborne cat allergen on a regular basis.

CONTROL OF ANIMAL ALLERGENS

At the present time, much less is known about the control of animal allergens than about the control of dust mite allergens (Table 12.2). In particular, there are still no convincing studies on the clinical benefit of environmental control measures pertaining to animal allergens. Although it is assumed that removing an animal from the home will lead to clinical improvement in patients who have disease related to their pet, even this has not been proven. Even less data are available regarding the potential benefits of methods that might be used in lieu of animal removal. Cat allergen will be specifically discussed here because the most information is available about this important allergen. Most of the information should be applicable to other allergens, although a great deal of study will need to be done before that statement can be made conclusively.

To begin, it should be stated that in any asthmatic patient who is known to be cat sensitive and whose asthma is believed to be related to any significant degree to a pet cat, the most appropriate recommendation is to remove the cat from the home. This is clearly the correct

Table 12.2 Environmental control measures for animal allergens

Remove the animal from the home if possible
If the animal cannot be removed:
- Keep the animal out of the patient's bedroom
- Keep the bedroom door closed at all times
- Place impermeable covers on the mattress and pillow
- Remove bedroom and other carpets if possible
- Use a HEPA or electrostatic air cleaner in the bedroom and elsewhere if possible

advice from a medical standpoint and we should not shy away from strenuously recommending it. A number of potential alternative measures will also be discussed, however, because of the high proportion of patients who are either reluctant or completely unwilling to remove a household pet.

Once a cat has been removed from the home, it is important to recognize that the clinical benefit may not be seen for a period of at least several months, since allergen levels fall quite slowly after cat removal.[61] In most homes, levels in settled dust will have fallen to those seen in homes without cats within 4–6 months of cat removal. Levels may fall much more quickly if extensive environmental control measures are undertaken, such as removal of carpets, upholstered furniture, and other reservoirs from the home, whereas in other homes the process may be considerably slower. This information points to the fact that thorough and repeated cleaning will be required once the animal has been removed. It has also been shown that cat allergen may persist in mattresses for years after a cat has been removed from a home,[67] so that new bedding or impermeable encasements must therefore also be recommended.

A number of studies have investigated other measures that might help to reduce cat allergen exposure without removing the animal from the home. De Blay et al demonstrated significant reductions in airborne Fel d 1 with a combination of air filtration, cat washing, vacuum cleaning, and removal of furnishings, although these results were based on a small sample size and did not include any measure of clinical effect.[68] When cat washing was evaluated separately in that study, dramatic reductions in airborne Fel d 1 were seen after cat washes. Subsequent studies, however, have presented conflicting results. Klucka et al studied both cat washing and Allerpet/c (Allerpet, Inc, New York, USA) and found no benefit from either treatment.[69] Most recently, Avner et al studied three different methods of cat washing and found transient reductions in airborne cat allergens after each.[70] There was no sustained benefit, however, with levels returning to baseline within 1 week of washing.

Information is very limited as to the clinical benefits of these environmental control measures if one or more cats are allowed to remain in the home. Three recent studies have evaluated different combinations of control measures and, although all have shown reductions in allergen levels, clinical effect was less consistent.[71–73] One study showed a clear benefit, one showed benefit only in the group in which environmental control was done along with intranasal steroid treatment, and the third showed no clinical benefit whatsoever. It therefore still remains to be seen whether allergen exposure can be sufficiently reduced to produce a clinical effect in the absence of cat removal.

In families who insist on keeping their pets the following should be recommended pending more definitive studies. The animals should be restricted to one area of the home and certainly kept out of the patient's bedroom. HEPA (high efficiency particle air) or electrostatic air cleaners should be used, especially in the patient's bedroom. Carpets and other reservoirs for allergen collection should be removed if possible, again focusing on the patient's bedroom. Finally, mattress and pillow covers should be routinely employed. Although tannic acid has been shown to reduce cat allergen levels, the effects are modest and short-lived when a cat is present, so this treatment should not be routinely recommended. Similarly, cat washing appears to be of such transient benefit that it is not likely to add significantly to the other avoidance measures.

COCKROACH ALLERGENS

The importance of cockroach allergens in asthma and allergy has been recognized only over the past 30 years. It is now clear that cockroach allergens are a major cause of asthma, particularly in urban areas. Significant cockroach exposure has been demonstrated in a number of cities and the prevalence of cockroach sensitivity in urban patients with asthma has been shown to range from 23% to 60%.[8,74,75] In addition, the combination of cockroach exposure and cockroach sensitization has been shown to be a risk factor for acute asthma exacerbations.[8,19,59]

In the most comprehensive study to date on the problem of asthma in inner-city children, 1528 children with asthma from eight major inner-city areas were extensively investigated with regard to the factors, both allergic and otherwise, that contributed to their disease.[59] Although sensitivity to cockroach, dust mite, and cat were all common (36.8%, 36.9%, and 22.7%, respectively), exposure to cockroach allergen was much more common than exposure to either dust mite or cat (50.2%, 9.7%, and 12.8%, respectively). The combination of cockroach sensitivity and high cockroach exposure was associated with significantly more hospitalizations, unscheduled medical visits for asthma, days of wheezing, missed days from school, and nights with sleep loss caused by asthma. Such a correlation was not seen for dust mite or cat allergens. These data argue persuasively that cockroach allergen is a major factor, if not the major factor, in the high degree of morbidity seen in this patient population.

Although there are at least 50 cockroach species in the United States, only four or five are domiciliary. Two species, the German cockroach (*Blatella germanica*) and the American cockroach (*Periplaneta americana*), are the most common causes of both household infestation and allergic sensitization. Several allergens from each species have been identified and characterized.[76,77] The most important among these are Bla g 1, Bla g 2, and Per a 1. There is significant cross-reactivity between *B. germanica* and *P. americana*, although most patients in the United States appear to be primarily sensitized to *B. germanica*. The source of the major cockroach allergens is still not completely clear although they do appear to be secreted or excreted, suggesting that they may also be digestive proteins.

The distribution of cockroach allergens has been studied in a number of settings. Highest levels tend to be found in kitchens, although the allergen is widely distributed through the home, including the bedroom.[59,75,77] In fact, in the inner-city asthma study noted above, the 50.2% exposure rate was found in bedroom dust samples.[59] It has been suggested that cockroach allergen levels of greater than 2 units per gram are associated with sensitization and levels greater than 8 units per gram are associated with disease activity. Cockroach allergen has also been detected at significant concentrations in schools in urban Baltimore.[78] Finally, limited study of airborne cockroach allergen has suggested that cockroach is very much like dust mite in that there is little or no measurable airborne cockroach allergen in the absence of significant disturbance.

COCKROACH ALLERGEN CONTROL

Extensive study has been performed on the chemical control of cockroach infestation, and a variety of pesticides and traps are readily available. These include chlorpyrifos (Dursban), diazanon, boric acid powder, and bait stations that contain hydranethylnon. All of these agents, with the exception of boric acid, can reduce cockroach numbers by 90% or more; boric acid reduces numbers by 40–50%. Very little is known, however, about the effects of extermination procedures on cockroach allergen levels. In one limited study, Sarpong et al did demonstrate a short-term reduction in cockroach allergen in settled dust samples after extermination in an inner-city dormitory.[79]

Other measures that should help to reduce cockroach infestation include eliminating food sources and hiding and entry points. All foods should be stored in sealed containers and the kitchen should be cleaned regularly. Finally, extensive cleaning should be performed after extermination to remove the cockroach debris as completely as possible. Even with the most aggressive measures, however, it is unlikely that cockroach exposure will be adequately reduced in some environments. This is particularly true of the older, multiple dwelling units that house a preponderance of inner-city asthma patients. It may be necessary to exterminate in the homes or apartments surrounding the patient's home to obtain maximum effect and some patients may need to find new housing altogether. No studies have been reported to date on the clinical effects of extermination or other control measures.

MOLD ALLERGENS

A wide variety of mold species can be present in both indoor and outdoor environments. *Aspergillus* and *Penicillium* species are generally regarded as the most numerous indoor molds,[60,80,81] whereas *Alternaria* is important in both indoor and outdoor environments. Several mold allergens, including Alt n 1 and Asp f 1, have been identified and characterized.

Sensitivity to *Alternaria* has been shown to be associated with asthma in Tucson, Arizona[82] and in inland regions in Australia.[6] In the Tucson study, sensitivity to *Alternaria* was demonstrated in 60.8% of 6-year-old children with persistent asthma, compared with only 11.8% for dust mite. In fact, *Alternaria* was the only allergen for which sensitivity was associated with an increased risk of asthma at ages of both 6 and 11 years.

Molds tend to grow best in warm and moist environments and mold exposure is therefore roughly correlated with these conditions. Basements, window sills, shower stalls, and bathroom carpets are common sites of mold infestation. Air conditioners and humidifiers have also been shown to be sources of significant mold exposure.[83,84] To date, the assessment of mold exposure has been more difficult than for the other indoor allergens because of the lack of readily available immunoassays to measure major allergens. The currently available methods are very time consuming, including culture and microscopic examination of air or dust samples. Airborne mold allergens have been shown to be carried on particles ranging in size from less than 2 μm to greater than 100 μm.[80]

The control of mold allergens requires a concerted approach combining fungicides, measures to reduce humidity, and the removal of mold-infested items whenever possible. A variety of fungicides are commercially available which are highly effective as long as the sites of mold growth are carefully investigated. Any measures that can be taken to reduce humidity should be recommended, including dehumidification, air conditioning, increased ventilation, and absolute abstinence from the use of humidifiers and vaporizers. Moldy items, such as a basement carpet that has suffered water damage, should be removed altogether. Although no specific data are available, air filtration devices may also assist in reducing mold exposure. No clinical studies on the efficacy of mold avoidance measures have been undertaken.

INDOOR AIR POLLUTION

Although a detailed discussion of indoor air pollution is beyond the scope of this chapter, it should be emphasized that effective environmental control cannot be achieved without attention to a variety of nonspecific irritants. The deleterious effects of passive cigarette smoke on pediatric asthma have been well documented in a number of studies.[85,86] Recently the Institute of Medicine reviewed the association of environmental tobacco smoke (ETS) and respiratory disease.[87] They found that there was a causal relationship between ETS exposure and exacerbations of asthma in preschool-aged children, and that on average exposure was associated with about a 30% risk of increased symptoms. No studies to date have assessed the clinical benefit of removal from a smoke-containing environment, but one would predict that this would have highly beneficial effects. In addition to passive cigarette smoke, a variety of other indoor pollutants such as nitrous oxide and wood smoke have been documented to exacerbate pediatric asthma. All patients must therefore be queried about their exposure to these and counseled about control of such exposure. The parents of asthmatic children who smoke need to be reminded at each visit about the ongoing damage that they are causing to their kids. The Institute of Medicine report concluded that although there was evidence that complete avoidance 'would be associated with a lower likelihood of exacerbations of asthma', there was inadequate evidence that interventions to encourage outside smoking or using air cleaners would reduce the likelihood of asthma exacerbation.

There is less evidence that exposure to indoor gaseous pollutants such as ozone, nitrogen dioxide (NO_2), volatile organic compounds (VOC), or formaldehyde affects asthma. Ozone is generated indoors by electrical appliances, but the concentration in homes averages 0.5 ppb, less than a tenth of the ambient level (0.08 ppm) that is considered hazardous by the Environmental Protection Agency (EPA). Nitrogen dioxide is generated by gas stoves and space heaters, and the use of a gas range can increase home levels above 25 ppb.[88] Although this level is lower than the ambient level that is considered hazardous by the EPA (53 ppb), it is sensible to maintain good kitchen ventilation in homes with gas ranges. There is little evidence that either volatile organic compounds or formaldehyde affects asthma.

IMMUNOTHERAPY

Another approach to the control of allergic asthma is immunotherapy. In general, allergen immunotherapy involves the administration of gradually increasing quantities of allergen(s) to which the patient is sensitive, eventually reaching a dose that is effective in reducing symptoms with subsequent exposure to the allergen(s). Immunotherapy has been shown to be effective for allergic rhinitis, allergic asthma, and allergic reactions from stinging insects. Immunotherapy is indicated only for those patients who have clear evidence of sensitivity to clinically relevant allergens. In the end the final decision about starting immunotherapy depends on the degree to which symptoms can be reduced by medication, the type and amount of medication required to control symptoms, and whether allergen avoidance is possible. Several position statements have been published recently that generally support the use of immunotherapy for the treatment of both children and adults with allergic asthma.[89–91]

MECHANISMS OF IMMUNOTHERAPY

Although immunotherapy has been used and studied for decades, its exact mechanisms of action have remained elusive (Table 12.3). Earlier work focused predominantly on circulating antibody levels, particularly IgG, whereas more recent studies suggest that the primary effects of immunotherapy owe to alterations in T-cell responses to allergen.

Serum allergen-specific IgE levels have been shown to rise initially with immunotherapy and then gradually fall over a period of months.[92] Pollen immunotherapy also typically results in a blunting of the usual seasonal increases in specific IgE levels.[93] Allergen-specific IgG levels rise with immunotherapy and it was long suggested that the production of these so-called blocking antibodies was the primary mode of action of immunotherapy.[94,95] However, it has been shown that IgG levels are unrelated to the clinical response to immunotherapy for inhalant allergens[96] and that the effects of more rapid desensitization methods, termed 'rush immunotherapy', are seen long before any changes in antibody production occur. It is now therefore presumed that IgG antibody production during immunotherapy is more likely a by-product of the effects on T-cells rather than a critical mechanism in itself.

Immunotherapy has also been shown to have

Table 12.3 Mechanisms of immunotherapy

Antibody responses
Allergen-specific IgE levels rise initially and then gradually fall
Pollen immunotherapy results in a blunting of the usual seasonal increases in specific IgE levels
Allergen-specific IgG levels rise with immunotherapy; however, this rise is unrelated to the clinical response to immunotherapy for inhalant allergens

Effector cells
Reduced mast cell numbers in the skin and respiratory tract
Reduced mediator release from mast cells and basophils
Reduced eosinophil numbers in nasal lavage fluid after allergen provocation
Reduced eosinophil cationic protein in bronchoalveolar lavage fluid

Lymphocyte responses
Downregulation of Th2 responses
Upregulation of Th1 responses
Increased in IFN-γ production
Decreased in IL-4 production

---

effects on various allergy effector cells, including mast cells and eosinophils. These effects include reductions in mast cell numbers in the skin and respiratory tract,[97] mast cell mediator release,[98] eosinophil numbers in nasal lavage fluid after allergen provocation,[99] and eosinophil cationic protein in bronchoalveolar lavage fluid.[100] Several studies have also shown that basophil histamine release is decreased after immunotherapy.

The final modes of action of immunotherapy involve a variety of effects on lymphocytes. There is evidence that Th2 responses may be downregulated whereas Th1 responses may increase with immunotherapy.[101] These changes are accompanied by increases in IFN-γ production and decreases in IL-4 production.[102] These changes may occur by several mechanisms, including the generation of allergen-specific CD4+ and CD8+ T-cell clones.[103] It is likely that these lymphocyte effects are the critical pathways to the success of immunotherapy.

EFFICACY OF IMMUNOTHERAPY

The success of immunotherapy varies depending on the disease being treated and the specific allergens involved. Its efficacy is greatest for stinging insect allergy and somewhat less so for respiratory allergy. In addition, it is critical to understand that the success of immunotherapy is dependent on the use of sufficiently high maintenance doses over an extended period of time. The quality of vaccine materials varies considerably and standardized extracts should be used whenever available. The quantitation of major allergens may be used to define the allergen doses needed for effective immunotherapy. For example, it has been shown for several common allergens, including ragweed, grass, dust mite, and cat, that maintenance doses of 5–20 μg of major allergen per injection are associated with a successful outcome.[104–109] Although benefit may initially be seen within the first 6 months of treatment, sustained improvement typically requires at least 3 years of therapy.[110]

Most immunotherapy studies have focused on a single allergen and have utilized some combination of symptom scores, medication requirements, and bronchial challenge to assess efficacy (Table 12.4). A number of double-blind, placebo-controlled studies of immunotherapy for pollen-induced asthma have provided

Table 12.4 Representative double-blind, placebo-controlled studies in immunotherapy for asthma

Reference	Allergen	Study size	Duration	Symptom/medication scores	Bronchial challenge (if done)
104	Ragweed	77	1–2 years	Drug: NS Sx: $P < 0.01$	
96	Grass	57	1 year	$P < 0.01$	
112	Grass	19	1 year	$P < 0.05$	
113	Grass	40	1 year	Improved	
105	Grass	28	3 years	$P < 0.001$	
118	Mite	91	1 year	$P < 0.02$	Improved
120	Mite	23	1 year	$P < 0.01$	$P < 0.05$
119	Mite	49	15 months	NS	
117	Mite	35	1 year	$P < 0.001$	$P < 0.05$
121	Mite	30	1 year	$P < 0.01$	
125	Cat	22	1 year		2.8-fold improvement
108	Cat	17	4 months		1.4-fold improvement
109	Cat, dog	32	1 year	Improved	Cat: 11-fold Dog: 5-fold
132	Multiple	121	18 months	NS	

NS = not significant; Sx = symptoms.

favorable results with regard to both symptoms and medication requirements.[96,105,111–114] These studies have evaluated grass and ragweed sensitive patients and have lasted for 1–3 years.

Studies of dust mite immunotherapy have also generally been positive. A number of studies have shown a reduction in mite-specific bronchial reactivity as well as an inhibition of the late phase reaction after bronchial challenge.[115,116] Immunotherapy was also shown to reduce symptoms and medication requirements in multiple controlled trials.[115,117–121] This effect is especially prominent in children. Several other studies, however, failed to demonstrate any symptomatic improvement with mite immunotherapy.[122,123]

Immunotherapy with cat and dog allergens has also been evaluated in a number of controlled studies over the past 20 years.[107,109,124–128] Most of these studies have shown a positive effect, particularly for cat allergen, and animal allergy is typically included on the list of conditions for which immunotherapy has been proven effective. However, the outcome of most of these studies has been based on challenge studies and there is still relatively little information about the benefits of animal allergen immunotherapy for the average patient with asthma. Based on the available data, which have demonstrated at best a ten-fold improvement in bronchial challenge responses after immunotherapy, it is most likely that the benefits provided will be more effective for patients with intermittent exposure rather than patients living with a cat or dog.

Less data are available on the efficacy of immunotherapy for patients with mold allergy. The quality of mold extracts has typically been less than that of pollen or mite extracts, which may significantly impact the efficacy of immunotherapy. To date, there have been three controlled studies using mold immunotherapy, each study demonstrating benefit using standardized *Cladosporium* or *Alternaria* vaccines for asthma and/or allergic rhinitis.[129–131]

As noted, the vast majority of immunotherapy studies have utilized treatment with single allergens. Although this is an ideal way to approach immunotherapy, especially for the purpose of research, it is not how immunotherapy is necessarily practiced. In fact, especially in the United States, most immunotherapy is provided as a mixture of allergens to which the patient is sensitive. One controlled study looked at the efficacy of such multi-allergen therapy in children with moderate to severe asthma.[132] The children were all closely supervised and given optimal medical management. The results demonstrated no significant differences between the active- and placebo-treated groups with regard to any variable, including medication requirements, symptom scores, peak expiratory flow readings, pulmonary function tests, or methacholine reactivity. The results of this study suggest that immunotherapy may not provide any additional benefit in patients receiving optimal medical treatment.

In 1995 a meta-analysis was published on the efficacy of immunotherapy in asthma.[133] Twenty studies were included in the analysis and outcome measures included symptoms, medication requirements, and measurements of lung function and airway hyperreactivity. In this analysis, the combined odds for an improvement in symptoms with immunotherapy for any allergen was 3.2 (95% CI 2.2–4.9). The odds for a reduction in medication after mite immunotherapy was 4.2 (95% CI 2.2–7.9) and the combined odds for a reduction in nonspecific bronchial hyperreactivity was 6.8 (95% CI 3.8–12.0). The mean effect size for immunotherapy with any allergen on all continuous outcomes was 0.71 (95% CI 0.43–1.00), which would correspond to a mean predicted improvement in FEV_1 of 7.1% from immunotherapy.

SAFETY OF IMMUNOTHERAPY

Adverse reactions to immunotherapy are common. Although most involve only local reactions that are mild and self-limited, systemic reactions with potentially devastating outcomes also occasionally occur. Local reactions can be divided into those that occur shortly after the injection and those that occur more than 30 minutes after the injection. They are uncomfortable and dosage adjustment may be necessary after a patient experiences a large local reaction. They do not, however, predict the onset of subsequent systemic reactions; in one large study of immunotherapy reactions, most systemic reactions occurred without any history of previous large local reactions.[134]

Systemic reactions typically begin within 20 minutes of the injection, although some reactions do not occur for as long as 60 minutes after the injection. Most systemic reactions are mild and can be successfully managed with antihistamines and epinephrine.[134] Several risk factors have been identified for systemic reactions. Most importantly, asthma has been shown to be a risk factor for systemic reactions[135] and poorly controlled asthma, defined as an FEV_1 of less than 70% of the predicted value, increases the risk of developing an asthmatic reaction to immunotherapy.[136] The use of high-dose, standardized vaccines[135,137] and rush immunotherapy[138] also increase the risk of systemic reactions, as do incorrect injection technique and dosing errors. Finally, treatment with beta-blocker medications may potentiate systemic reactions.

Although fatal reactions to immunotherapy are rare, they do occur.[139,140] Risk factors for fatal reactions are similar to those for systemic reactions in general and include unstable asthma, high levels of sensitivity, treatment with beta blockers, and dosing errors. In most cases deaths owed to severe respiratory compromise, which indicates the need to take special precautions in patients with asthma, especially if they are suffering from an exacerbation.

INDICATIONS FOR IMMUNOTHERAPY

In summary, there is extensive research to support the use of immunotherapy in the treatment of asthma. The real question, however, is where immunotherapy should fit into the overall asthma management plan. In general, it should be considered for all patients who have a clear allergic trigger for their asthma and who have failed standard allergen avoidance measures and pharmacotherapy. It is therefore generally considered as a third line of therapy, to be used after environmental control measures have been instituted and medications have been optimized. The role of allergic triggers in an individual patient's asthma should be evaluated by allergy testing and a detailed history. It is critical that both the presence of allergen-specific IgE and a history of symptoms related to that allergen be established before proceeding with immunotherapy.

The specific indications to proceed with immunotherapy, however, may vary from one patient to another based on a number of other factors. Patients with allergic rhinitis may experience significant relief of these symptoms as well and may therefore be better candidates for the early institution of immunotherapy. Patients with undesirable side-effects from their asthma or nasal medications may also wish to proceed more expeditiously. Patients with severe, unstable asthma, on the other hand, may be less ideal candidates because of a greater risk of adverse effects. Cost may be an issue for some patients, although in the end immunotherapy can be cost effective if money spent on medications and other treatments can be reduced. Although there is no absolute age cut-off for immunotherapy, it is generally not recommended before the age of 4 or 5 years. Finally, patients with poor compliance will also not be good candidates for immunotherapy. Although the same may apply to their pharmacologic management, it is guaranteed that immunotherapy will fail if compliance is not excellent.

REFERENCES

1. Platts-Mills TAE, De Weck A. Dust mite allergens and asthma—a world wide problem. *Bull WHO* 1989; **66**: 769–80.
2. Platts-Mills TAE, Thomas WR, Aalberse RC et al co-chairmen. Dust mite allergens and asthma: report of a 2nd international workshop. *J Allergy Clin Immunol* 1992; **89**: 1046–60.
3. Arlian LG. Biology and ecology of house dust mites *Dermatophagoides* spp. and *Euroglyphus* spp. *Immunol Allergy Clin N Amer* 1989; **9**: 339–56.
4. Kueher J, Frischer J, Meiner R et al. Mite exposure is a risk factor for the incidence of specific sensitization. *J Allergy Clin Immunol* 1994; **94**: 44–52.
5. Lau S, Falkenhorst G, Weber A et al. High mite-allergen exposure increases the risk of sensitization in atopic children and young adults. *J Allergy Clin Immunol* 1989; **84**: 718–25.
6. Peat JK, Tovey E, Mellis CM, Leeder SR, Woolcock AJ. Importance of house dust mite and *Alternaria* allergens in childhood asthma: an epidemiological study in two climatic regions of Australia. *Clin Exp Allergy* 1993; **23**: 812–20.
7. Sporik R, Holgate ST, Platts-Mills TAE, Cogswell JJ. Exposure to house-dust mite allergen (Der p I) and the development of asthma in childhood. A prospective study. *N Engl J Med* 1990; **323**: 502–7.
8. Call RS, Smith TF, Morris E, Chapman MD, Platts-Mills TAE. Risk factors for asthma in inner city children. *J Pediatr* 1992; **121**: 862–6.
9. Platts-Mills TAE, Heymann PW, Longbottom JL, Wilkins SR. Airborne allergens associated with asthma: particle sizes carrying dust mite and rat allergens measured with a cascade impactor. *J Allergy Clin Immunol* 1986; **77**: 850–7.
10. Dowse GK, Turner KJ, Stewart GA, Alpers MP, Woolcock AJ. The association between *Dermatophagoides* mites and the increasing prevalence of asthma in village communities within the Papua New Guinea highlands. *J Allergy Clin Immunol* 1985; **75**: 75–83.
11. Ingram JM, Sporik R, Rose G et al. Quantitative assessment of exposure to dog (Can f 1) and cat (Fel d 1) allergens: relationship to sensitization and asthma among children living in Los Alamos, New Mexico. *J Allergy Clin Immunol* 1995; **96**: 449–56.
12. Burrows B, Sears MR, Flannery EM, Herbison GP, Holdaway MD. Relations of bronchial responsiveness to allergy skin test reactivity, lung function, respiratory symptoms and diagnoses in thirteen-year-old New Zealand children. *J Allergy Clin Immunol* 1995; **95**: 548–56.

13. Peat JK, Tovey ER, Toelle BG et al. House-dust mite allergens: a major risk factor for childhood asthma in Australia. *Am J Respir Crit Care Med* 1996; **153:** 141–6.
14. Sears MR, Herbison GP, Holdaway MD et al. The relative risk of sensitivity to grass pollen, house dust mite, and cat dander in the development of childhood asthma. *Clin Exp Allergy* 1989; **19:** 419–24.
15. Hide DW, Matthews S, Tariq S, Arshad SH. Allergen avoidance in infancy and allergy at 4 years of age. *Allergy* 1996; **51:** 89–93.
16. Custovic A, Taggart SCO, Francis HC, Chapman MD, Woodcock A. Exposure to house dust mite allergens and the clinical activity of asthma. *J Allergy Clin Immunol* 1996; **98:** 64–72.
17. Kivity S, Solomon A, Soferman R et al. Mite asthma in childhood: a study of the relationship between exposure to house dust mites and disease activity. *J Allergy Clin Immunol* 1993; **91:** 844–9.
18. Vervloet D, Charpin D, Haddi E et al. Medication requirements and house mite exposure in mite sensitive asthmatics. *Allergy* 1991; **46:** 554–8.
19. Pollart SM, Chapman MD, Fiocco GP, Rose G, Platts-Mills TAE. Epidemiology of acute asthma: IgE antibodies to common inhalent allergens as a risk factor for emergency room visits. *J Allergy Clin Immunol* 1989; **83:** 875–82.
20. Platts-Mills TAE, Tovey ER, Mitchell EB et al. Reduction of bronchial hyperreactivity following prolonged allergen avoidance. *Lancet* 1982; **ii:** 675–8.
21. Murray AB, Ferguson AC. Dust-free bedrooms in the treatment of asthmatic children with house dust or house dust mite allergy. *Pediatrics* 1983; **71:** 418–22.
22. Carswell F, Birmingham K, Weeks J, Oliver J, Crewes A. The respiratory effects of reduction of mite allergen in bedrooms of asthmatic children—a double blind controlled trial. *Clin Exp Allergy* 1996; **26:** 386–96.
23. Dietemann A, Bessot JC, Hoyet C et al. A double-blind, placebo controlled trial of solidified benzyl benzoate applied in dwellings of asthmatic patients sensitive to mites: clinical efficacy and effect on mite allergens. *J Allergy Clin Immunol* 1993; **91:** 738–46.
24. Ehnert B, Lau-Schadendorf S, Weber A et al. Reducing domestic exposure to dust mite allergen reduces bronchial hyperreactivity in sensitive children with asthma. *J Allergy Clin Immunol* 1992; **90:** 135–8.
25. Gillies DRN, Littlewood JM, Sarsfield JK. Controlled trial of house dust mite avoidance in children with mild to moderate asthma. *Clin Allergy* 1987; **17:** 105–11.
26. Peroni DG, Boner AL, Vallone G, Antolini I, Warner JO. Effective allergen avoidance at high altitude reduced allergen-induced bronchial hyperresponsiveness. *Am J Resp Crit Care Med* 1994; **149:** 1442–6.
27. Custovic A, Simpson A, Chapman M, Woodcock A. Allergen avoidance in the treatment of asthma and atopic disorders. *Thorax* 1998; **53:** 63–72.
28. Tovey E, Marks G. Methods and effectiveness of environmental control. *J Allergy Clin Immunol* 1999; **103:** 179–91.
29. Goetsche PC, Hammarquist C, Burr M. House dust mite control measures in the management of asthma: a meta-analysis. *Brit Med J* 1998; **317:** 1105–10.
30. Owen S, Morganstem M, Hepworth J, Woodcock A. Control of house dust mite antigen in bedding. *Lancet* 1990; **335:** 396–7.
31. Tovey E, Marks G, Shearer M, Woodcock A. Allergens and occlusive bed covers. *Lancet* 1993; **342:** 126.
32. Kalra S, Owen SJ, Hepworth J, Woolcock A. Airborne house dust mite antigen after vacuum cleaning. *Lancet* 1990; **336:** 449.
33. Bohr R de. The control of house dust mite allergens in rugs. *J Allergy Clin Immunol* 1990; **86:** 808–14.
34. Wassenaar DPJ. Effectiveness of vacuum cleaning and wet cleaning in reducing house-dust mites, fungi and mite allergen in a cotton carpet: a case study. *Exp Appl Acarol* 1988; **4:** 53–62.
35. Colloff MJ. House dust mites—part II. Chemical control. *Pestic Outlook* 1990; **1:** 3–8.
36. Colloff MJ, Ayres J, Carswell F et al. The control of allergens of dust mites and domestic pets: a position paper. *Clin Exp Allergy* 1992; **22:** 1–28.
37. Russell DW, Fernandez-Caldas, Swanson MC et al. Caffeine, a naturally occurring acaricide. *J Allergy Clin Immunol* 1992; **87:** 107–10.
38. Mitchell EB, Wilkins S, Deighton J, Platts-Mills TAE. Reduction of house dust mite levels in the home: use of the acaricide, pirimiphos methyl. *Clin Allergy* 1985; **15:** 235–40.
39. Hayden ML, Rose G, Diduch KB et al. Benzyl benzoate moist powder: investigation of acaricidal activity in cultures and reduction of dust mite allergens in carpets. *J Allergy Clin Immunol* 1992; **89:** 536–45.

40. Lau-Schadendorf S, Rusche AF, Weber AK, Buettner-Goetz P, Wahn U. Short-term effect of solidified benzyl benzoate on mite-allergen concentrations in house dust. *J Allergy Clin Immunol* 1991; **87**: 41–7.
41. Woodfolk JA, Hayden ML, Couture N, Platts-Mills TAE. Chemical treatment of carpets to remove allergen. *J Allergy Clin Immunol* 1996; **96**: 325–33.
42. Huss RW, Huss K, Squire EN et al. Mite allergen control with acaricide fails. *J Allergy Clin Immunol* 1994; **94**: 27–32.
43. Woodfolk J, Hayden M, Miller J et al. Chemical treatment of carpets to reduce allergen: a detailed study of the effects of tannic acid on indoor allergens. *J Allergy Clin Immunol* 1994; **94**: 19–26.
44. Tovey ER, Marks GB, Matthews M, Green WF, Woolcock A. Changes in mite allergen *Der p* I in house dust following spraying with a tannic acid/acaricide solution. *Clin Exp Allergy* 1992; **22**: 67–74.
45. McDonald LG, Tovey ER. The role of water temperature and laundry procedures in reducing house dust mite populations and allergen content of bedding. *J Allergy Clin Immunol* 1992; **90**: 599–608.
46. Vendenhove T, Soler M, Birnbaum J, Charpin D, Vervelot D. Effect of dry cleaning on the mite allergen levels in blankets. *Allergy* 1993; **48**: 264–6.
47. Dodin A, Rak H. Influence of low temperature on the different stages of the human allergy mite *Dermatophagoides pteronyssinus*. *J Med Entomol* 1993; **30**: 810–11.
48. Tovey E, Woolcock A. Direct exposure of carpets to sunlight can kill all mites. *J Allergy Clin Immunol* 1993; **93**: 1072–4.
49. Mosbech H, Korsgaard J, Lind P. Control of house dust mites by electrical heating blankets. *J Allergy Clin Immunol* 1988; **31**: 706–10.
50. Colloff MJ. Dust mite control and mechanical ventilation: when the climate is right. *Clin Exp Allergy* 1994; **24**: 94–6.
51. Korsgaard, Iversen M. Epidemiology of house dust mite allergy. *Allergy* 1991; **46**(suppl 11): 14–18.
52. Custovic A, Taggart S, Kennaugh J, Woodcock A. Portable dehumidifiers in the control of house dust mites and mite allergens. *Clin Exp Allergy* 1995; **25**: 312–16.
53. Antonicelli L, Bilo MB, Pucci S, Schou C, Bonifazi F. Efficacy of an air-cleaning device equipped with a high efficiency particulate air filter in house dust mite respiratory allergy. *Allergy* 1991; **46**: 594–600.
54. Nelson HS, Roger Hirsch S, Ohman JL Jr et al. Recommendations for the use of residential air-cleaning devices in the treatment of respiratory diseases. *J Allergy Clin Immunol* 1988; **82**: 661–9.
55. Reisman R, Mauriello P, Davis G, Georgitis JW, DeMasi JM. A double-blind study of the effectiveness of a high-efficiency particulate air (HEPA) filter in the treatment of patients with perennial allergic rhinitis and asthma. *J Allergy Clin Immunol* 1990; **85**: 1050–9.
56. Warner JA, Marchant JL, Warner JO. Double blind trial of ionisers in children with asthma sensitive to the house dust mite. *Thorax* 1993; **48**: 330–3.
57. Sporik R, Ingram JM, Price W et al. Association of asthma with serum IgE and skin-test reactivity to allergens among children living at high altitude: tickling the dragon's breath. *Am J Res Crit Care Med* 1995; **151**: 1388–92.
58. Munir AKM, Bjorksten B, Einarsson R et al. Cat (Fel d I), dog (Can f 1) and cockroach allergens in homes of asthmatic children from three climatic zones in Sweden. *Allergy* 1994; **49**: 508–16.
59. Rosenstreich DL, Eggleston P, Kattan M et al. The role of cockroach allergy and exposure to cockroach allergen in causing morbidity among inner-city children with asthma. *N Engl J Med* 1997; **336**: 1356–63.
60. Wood RA, Eggleston PA, Ingemann L et al. Antigenic analysis of household dust samples. *Am Rev Resp Dis* 1988; **137**: 358–63.
61. Wood RA, Chapman MD, Adkinson NF et al. The effect of cat removal on allergen content in household dust samples. *J Allergy Clin Immunol* 1989; **83**: 730–4.
62. Wood RA, Mudd KE, Eggleston PA. The distribution of cat and dust mite allergens on wall surfaces. *J Allergy Clin Immunol* 1992; **89**: 126–30.
63. Wood RA, Laheri AN, Eggleston PA. The aerodynamic characteristics of cat allergen. *Clin Exp Allergy* 1993; **23**: 733–9.
64. Luczynska CM, Li Y, Chapman MD, Platts-Mills TAE. Airborne concentrations and particle size distribution of allergen derived from domestic cats (*Felis domesticus*). *Am Rev Respir Dis* 1990; **141**: 361–7.
65. Custovic A, Green R, Pickering CAC et al.

Major dog allergen Can f 1: distribution in homes, airborne levels, and particle sizing. *J Allergy Clin Immunol* 1996; **97:** 302 (abstract).
66. Bollinger ME, Eggleston PA, Wood RA. Cat antigen in homes with and without cats may induce allergic symptoms. *J Allergy Clin Immunol* 1996; **97:** 907–14.
67. Van der Brempt X, Charpin D, Haddi E, da Mata P, Vervloet D. Cat removal and Fel d 1 levels in mattresses. *J Allergy Clin Immunol* 1991; **87:** 595–6.
68. De Blay F, Chapman MD, Platts-Mills TAE. Airborne cat allergen (Fel d 1): environmental control with the cat *in situ*. *Am Rev Respir Dis* 1991; **143:** 1334–9.
69. Klucka CV, Ownby DR, Green J, Zoratti E. Cat shedding of Fel d 1 is not reduced by washings, Allerpet-C spray, or acepromazine. *J Allergy Clin Immunol* 1995; **95:** 1164–71.
70. Avner DB, Perzanowski MS, Platts-Mills TAE, Woodfolk JA. Evaluation of different techniques for washing cats: quantitation of allergen removed from the cat and effect on airborne Fel d 1. *J Allergy Clin Immunol* 1997; **100:** 357–62.
71. Bjornsdottir US, Jakobinudottir S, Runarsdottir V, Blondal Th, Juliusson S. Environmental control with cat *in situ* reduces cat allergen in house dust samples—but does it alter clinical symptoms. *J Allergy Clin Immunol* 1997; **99**(1): S389 (abstract).
72. Soldatov D, De Blay F, Greiss P et al. Effects of environmental control measures on patient status and airborne Fel d 1 levels with a cat in situ. *J Allergy Clin Immunol* 1995; **95**(1): 263 (abstract).
73. Wood RA, Johnson EF, Van Natta ML, Chen PH, Eggleston PA. A placebo-controlled trial of a HEPA air cleaner in the treatment of cat allergy. *Am J Resp Crit Care Med* 1998; **158:** 115–20.
74. Kang BC, Johnson J, Veres-Thorner C. Atopic profile of inner city asthma with a comparative analysis on the cockroach sensitive and ragweed sensitive subgroups. *J Allergy Clin Immunol* 1993; **92:** 802–11.
75. Sarpong SB, Hamilton RG, Eggleston PA, Adkinson NF. Socioeconomic status and race as risk factors for cockroach allergen exposure and sensitization in children with asthma. *J Allergy Clin Immunol* 1996; **97:** 1393–401.
76. Arruda LK, Vailes LD, Mann BJ et al. Molecular cloning of a major cockroach (*Blattella germanica*) allergen, Bla g 2. *J Biol Chem* 1995; **270:** 19563–8.
77. Pollart S, Smith TF, Morris EC et al. Environmental exposure to cockroach allergens: analysis with monoclonal antibody-based enzyme immunoassays. *J Allergy Clin Immunol* 1995; **87:** 505–10.
78. Sarpong S, Wood RA, Karrison T, Eggleston PA. Cockroach allergen (Bla g 1) in school dust. *J Allergy Clin Immunol* 1997; **99:** 486–92.
79. Sarpong SB, Wood RA, Eggleston PA. Short-term effects of extermination and cleaning on cockroach allergen Bla g 2 in settled dust. *Ann Allergy Asthma Immunol* 1996; **76:** 257–60.
80. Burge HA. Fungus allergens. *Clin Rev Allergy* 1985; **3:** 319–29.
81. Sporik RB, Arruda LK, Woodfolk J, Chapman MD, Platts-Mills TAE. Environmental exposure to *Aspergillus fumigatus* (Asp f I). *Clin Exp Allergy* 1993; **23:** 326–31.
82. Halonen M, Stern D, Wright AL, Taussig LM, Martinez FD. *Alternaria* as a major allergen for asthma in children raised in a desert environment. *Am J Respir Crit Care Med* 1997; **155:** 1356–61.
83. Burge HA, Solomon W, Boise JR. Microbial prevalence in domestic humidifiers. *Applied Environmental Microbiol* 1980; **39:** 840–4.
84. Kumar P, Lopez M, Fan W, Cambre K, Elston RC. Mold contamination of automobile air conditioner systems. *Annals Allergy* 1990; **64:** 174–7.
85. Chilmonczyk BA, Salmun LM, Megathlin KN et al. Association between exposure to environmental tobacco smoke and exacerbations of asthma in children. *N Engl J Med* 1993; **328:** 1665–9.
86. Wright AL, Holberg C, Martinez FD et al. Relationship of parental smoking to wheezing and nonwheezing lower respiratory tract illnesses in infancy. *J Pediatr* 1991; **118:** 207–14.
87. Committee on the Assessment of Asthma and Indoor Air. Exposure to indoor tobacco smoke. In *Clearing the Air: Asthma and Indoor Air Exposures*. Washington: National Academy Press, 2000, 263–97.
88. Samet JM, Lambert WE, Skipper BJ et al. Nitrogen dioxide and respiratory illnesses in infants. *Am Rev Respir Dis* 1993; **148:** 1258–65.
89. Nicklas RA, Bernstein IL, Blessing-Moore J et al. Practice parameters for allergen immunotherapy. *J Allergy Clin Immunol* 1996; **98:** 1001.
90. *Expert Panel Report 2: Guidelines for the Diagnosis*

and Management of Asthma. National Institutes of Health, 1997.
91. Bousquet, J, Lockey RF, Malling HJ eds. WHO Position Paper. Allergen immunotherapy: therapeutic vaccines for allergic diseases. *Allergy* 1998; **44:** 1–42.
92. Lichtenstein L, Ishizaka K, Norman P, Sobotka A, Hill B. IgE antibody measurements in ragweed hay fever. *J Clin Invest* 1973; **52:** 472–82.
93. Gleich GJ, Zimmerman EM, Henderson LL, Yunginger JW. Effect of immunotherapy on immunoglobulin E and immunoglobulin G antibodies to ragweed antigens. *J Allergy Clin Immunol* 1982; **70:** 261–71.
94. Van der Zee JS, Aalberse RC. The role of IgG in immediate-type hypersensitivity. *Eur Respir J Suppl* 1991; **13:** 91–6.
95. Star M, Weinstock M. Studies in pollen allergy. III. The relationship between blocking antibody levels and symptomatic relief following hyposensitization with Allpyral in hay fever subjects. *Int Arch Allergy* 1970; **38:** 514–21.
96. Bousquet J, Maasch H, Martinot B et al. Double-blind, placebo-controlled immunotherapy with mixed grass-pollen allergoids. II. Comparison between parameters assessing the efficacy of immunotherapy. *J Allergy Clin Immunol* 1988; **82:** 439–46.
97. Hedlin G, Silber G, Naclerio R et al. Comparison of the in vivo and in vitro response to ragweed immunotherapy in children and adults with ragweed-induced rhinitis. *Clin Exp Allergy* 1990; **20:** 491–500.
98. Creticos PS, Adkinson N Jr, Kagey-Sobotka A et al. Nasal challenge with ragweed pollen in hay fever patients. Effect of immunotherapy. *J Clin Invest* 1985; **76:** 2247–53.
99. Furin MJ, Norman PS, Creticos PS et al. Immunotherapy decreases antigen-induced eosinophil cell migration into the nasal cavity. *J Allergy Clin Immunol* 1991; **87:** 855–66.
100. Rak S, Lowhagen O, Venge P. The effect of immunotherapy on bronchial hyperresponsiveness and eosinophil cationic protein in pollen-allergic patients. *J Allergy Clin Immunol* 1988; **82:** 470–80.
101. Durham S, Varney V, Gaga M, Frew A, Jacobson M, Kay A. Immunotherapy and allergic inflammation. *Clin Exp Allergy* 1991; **21**(suppl 1): 206–10.
102. Renz H, Lack G, Saloga J et al. Inhibition of IgE production and normalization of airways responsiveness by sensitized CD8 T cells in a mouse model of allergen-induced sensitization. *J Immunol* 1994; **152:** 351–60.
103. Secrist H, Chelen CJ, Wen Y, Marshall JD, Umetsu DT. Allergen immunotherapy decreases interleukin 4 production in CD4+ T cells from allergic individuals. *J Exp Med/Surg* 1993; **178:** 2123–30.
104. Creticos PS, Reed CE, Norman PS et al. Ragweed immunotherapy in adult asthma. *N Engl J Med* 1996; **334:** 501–6.
105. Dolz I, Martinez-Cocera C, Bartolome JM, Cimarra M. A double-blind, placebo-controlled study of immunotherapy with grass pollen extract Alutard SQ during a 3-year period with initial rush immunotherapy. *Allergy* 1996; **51:** 489–500.
106. Haugaard L, Dahl R, Jacobsen L. A controlled dose–response study of immunotherapy with standardized, partially purified extract of house dust mite. *J Allergy Clin Immunol* 1993; **91:** 709–22.
107. Taylor WW, Ohman JL, Lowell FG. Immunotherapy in cat-induced asthma: double blind trial with evaluation of bronchial responses to cat allergen and histamine. *J Allergy Clin Immunol* 1978; **61:** 283–8.
108. Ohman JL, Findlay SR, Leitermann KM. Immunotherapy in cat-induced asthma: double blind trial with evaluation of in vivo and in vitro responses. *J Allergy Clin Immunol* 1984; **74:** 230–5.
109. Sundin B, Lilja G, Graff-Lonnevig V et al. Immunotherapy with partially purified and standardized animal dander extract: I. Clinical results of a double-blind study on patients with animal-dander asthma. *J Allergy Clin Immunol* 1986; **77:** 478–87.
110. Jacobsen L, Nuchel Petersen B, Wihl JA, Lowenstein H, Ipsen H. Immunotherapy with partially purified and standardized tree pollen extracts. IV. Results from long-term (6-year) follow-up. *Allergy* 1997; **52:** 914–20.
111. Frankland A, Augustin R. Prophylaxis of summer hay fever and asthma: a controlled trial comparing crude pollen extract with the isolated main protein components. *Lancet* 1954; **1:** 1055–8.
112. Pastorello EA, Pravettoni V, Incorvaia C et al. Clinical and immunological effects of immunotherapy with alum-absorbed grass allergoid in grass pollen-induced hay fever. *Allergy* 1992; **47:** 281–90.
113. Varney VA, Gaga M, Frew AJ et al. Usefulness

of immunotherapy in patients with severe summer hay fever uncontrolled by antiallergic drugs. *Br Med J* 1991; **302:** 265–9.
114. Reid MJ, Moss RB, Hsu YP et al. Seasonal asthma in northern California: allergic causes and efficacy of immunotherapy. *J Allergy Clin Immunol* 1986; **78:** 590–600.
115. Warner JO, Price JF, Soothill JF, Hey EN. Controlled trial of hyposensitization to *Dermatophagoides pteronyssinus* in children with asthma. *Lancet* 1978; **2:** 912–15.
116. Van Bever HP, Stevens WJ. Evolution of the late asthmatic reaction during immunotherapy and after stopping immunotherapy. *J Allergy Clin Immunol* 1990; **86:** 141–6.
117. Machiels JJ, Somville MA, Lebrun PM et al. Allergic bronchial asthma due to *Dermatophagoides pteronyssinus* hypersensitivity can be efficiently treated by inoculation of allergen-antibody complexes. *J Clin Invest* 1990; **85:** 1024–35.
118. D'Souza M, Pepys J, Wells I et al. Hyposensitization with *Dermatophagoides pteronyssinus* in house dust allergy: a controlled study of clinical and immunological effects. *Clin Allergy* 1973; **3:** 177–93.
119. Franco C, Barbadori S, Freshwater LL, Kordash TR. A double-blind, placebo-controlled study of Alpare mite *D. pteronyssinus* immunotherapy in asthmatic patients. *Allergol Immunopathol* 1995; **23:** 58–66.
120. Olsen OT, Larsen KR, Jacobsen L, Svendsen UG. A 1-year, placebo-controlled, double-blind house-dust-mite immunotherapy study in asthmatic adults. *Allergy* 1997; **52:** 853–9.
121. Pichler CE, Marquardsen A, Sparholt S et al. Specific immunotherapy with *Dermatophagoides pteronyssinus* and *D. farinae* results in decreased bronchial hyperreactivity. *Allergy* 1997; **52:** 274–83.
122. Gaddie J, Skinner C, Palmer K. Hyposensitization with house dust mite vaccine in bronchial asthma. *Br Med J* 1976; **2:** 561–2.
123. Newton D, Maberley D, Wilson R. House dust mite hyposensitization. *Br J Dis Chest* 1978; **72:** 21–8.
124. Valovirta A, Koivikko A, Vanto T. Immunotherapy in allergy to dog: a double-blind clinical study. *Ann Allergy* 1984; **53:** 85–91.
125. Van Metre TE, Marsh DG, Adkinson NF, Norman PS. Immunotherapy for cat asthma. *J Allergy Clin Immunol* 1988; **82:** 1055–62.
126. Hedlin G, Graff-Lonnevig V, Helborn H et al. Immunotherapy with cat- and dog-dander extracts: II. In vivo and in vitro immunologic effects observed in a 1-year double-blind placebo study. *J Allergy Clin Immunol* 1986; **77:** 488–96.
127. Lilja G, Sundin B, Graff-Lonnevig V et al. Immunotherapy with cat- and dog-dander extracts: IV. Effects of 2 years of treatment. *J Allergy Clin Immunol* 1989; **83:** 37–44.
128. Hedlin G, Heilborn H, Lilja G et al. Long-term follow-up of patients treated with a three-year course of cat or dog immunotherapy. *J Allergy Clin Immunol* 1995; **96:** 879–85.
129. Horst M, Hejjaoui A, Horst V, Michel FB, Bousquet J. Double-blind, placebo-controlled rush immunotherapy with a standardized *Alternaria* extract. *J Allergy Clin Immunol* 1990; **85:** 460–72.
130. Malling H-J, Dreborg S, Weeke B. Diagnosis and immunotherapy of mould allergy. V. Clinical efficacy and side effects of immunotherapy with *Cladosporium herbarum*. *Allergy* 1986; **41:** 507–19.
131. Dreborg S, Agrell B, Foucard T et al. A double-blind, multicenter immunotherapy trial in children using a purified and standardized *Cladosporium herbarum* preparation. *Allergy* 1986; **41:** 131–40.
132. Adkinson NF Jr, Eggleston PA, Eney D et al. A controlled trial of immunotherapy for asthma in allergic children. *N Engl J Med/Surg* 1997; **336:** 324–31.
133. Abramson MJ, Puy RM, Weiner JM. Is allergen immunotherapy effective in asthma. A meta-analysis of randomized controlled trials. *Am J Resp Crit Care Med/Surg* 1995; **151:** 969–74.
134. Stewart GD, Lockey RF. Systemic reactions from allergen immunotherapy. *J Allergy Clin Immunol* 1992; **90:** 567–78.
135. Hejjaoui A, Ferrando R, Dhivert H, Michel FB, Bousquet J. Systemic reactions occurring during immunotherapy with standardized pollen extracts. *J Allergy Clin Immunol* 1992; **89:** 925–33.
136. Bousquet J, Hejjaoui A, Dhivert H, Clauzel AM, Michel FB. Immunotherapy with a standardized *Dermatophagoides pteronyssinus* extract. III. Systemic reactions during the rush protocol in patients suffering from asthma. *J Allergy Clin Immunol* 1989; **83:** 797–802.
137. Hejjaoui A, Dhivert H, Michel FB, Bousquet J. Immunotherapy with a standardized *Dermatophagoides pteronyssinus* extract. IV. Systemic reactions according to the immunotherapy schedule. *J Allergy Clin Immunol* 1990; **85:** 473–9.

138. Lockey RF, Turkeltaub PC, Olive ES et al. The Hymenoptera venom study. III. Safety of venom immunotherapy. *J Allergy Clin Immunol* 1990; **86:** 775–80.
139. Lockey RF, Benedict LM, Turkeltaub PC, Bukantz SC. Fatalities from immunotherapy and skin testing. *J Allergy Clin Immunol* 1987; **79:** 660–77.
140. Reid MJ, Lockey RF, Turkeltaub PC, Platts-Mills TAE. Survey of fatalities from skin testing and immunotherapy 1985–1989. *J Allergy Clin Immunol* 1993; **92:** 6–15.

13

Indoor and outdoor allergens

L Karla Arruda, Martin D Chapman

Introduction • Association of IgE antibodies to allergens and asthma • General properties of allergens • Molecular biology • Clinical applications of recombinant allergens • Sources of allergens • Conclusions

INTRODUCTION

The history of allergens dates back to 1873, when Charles Blackley showed that pollen grains were able to induce symptoms of hay fever and that aqueous pollen extracts gave rise to immediate wheal and flare reactions when scratched into the skin of a hay fever patient (himself).[1] During the 1920s, it was appreciated that inhalation of allergens from pollens, house dust, or animals, or ingestion of allergens in foods was associated with clinical symptoms of hay fever, asthma, atopic dermatitis or food allergy, and that these conditions affected 10–20% of the population. In the 1960s, the first allergens were purified and biochemically characterized from ragweed and rye grass pollens,[2,3] and the landmark studies by the Ishizakas revealed that immediate hypersensitivity reactions were mediated by a new class of antibody, termed immunoglobulin E (IgE). During the 1960s and the 1970s, many allergens were purified; however, it was difficult to establish the nature of some of these molecules. In 1980, the house dust mite major allergen Der p 1 was purified from dust mite extract using classical immunochemistry, and subsequently shown to be concentrated in mite fecal particles.[4,5] Allergens from mites and other natural sources have since been identified, including cockroach allergens Bla g 1 and Bla g 2, and fungal allergens from *Alternaria*, *Aspergillus*, and *Trichophyton*.[6–9] By the mid-1980s a large number of allergens had been purified using biochemical techniques, but in general the yields were poor and, apart from physicochemical properties, the molecular structures of these proteins were ill defined.

The introduction of molecular biology techniques over the past 15 years has provided a new approach to the identification and characterization of allergens. In 1988, the first major allergen, Der p 1, was cloned from a house dust mite cDNA library[10] and since then over 200 allergen sequences have been reported. Important allergens form pollens, dust mite, animal danders, insects, and foods (e.g., peanut, shrimp) have been cloned and expressed as recombinant proteins. Amino acid sequence data obtained from these studies have been used to establish the structure and biological function of allergens, to identify the antigenic sites involved in IgE responses; and to investigate cellular mechanisms of inflammatory responses in asthma. Most recently, the three-dimensional structures of important allergens have been determined: birch pollen allergen, Bet v 1;[11] and mite allergens, Der p 2 and Der f 2.[12,13] Recombinant allergens are being introduced as novel tools for the diagnosis of allergic diseases and for developing therapeutic products.[14]

ASSOCIATION OF IgE ANTIBODIES TO ALLERGENS AND ASTHMA

The purification of important allergens and the production of monoclonal antibodies to allergens resulted in the development of sensitive immunoassays for the quantitation of allergen levels in the environment,[15,16] as well as for measuring allergen specific IgE from allergic patients. Techniques for measuring allergens in house dust or in the air had their greatest impact in the study of indoor allergens, because it is difficult to identify particles carrying allergens from mites, cockroach, cat or dog. On the other hand, pollens and most fungal spores can be easily identified and counted. These assays were instrumental for performing epidemiological studies worldwide, which established the strong relationship between exposure, development of specific IgE to allergens (sensitization) and asthma.[17,18] It is now well established that this correlation is very strong for indoor allergens, and weak for outdoor allergens. Although pollens are a major cause of seasonal rhinitis or hay fever, sensitization to pollens plays little role in chronic bronchial hyperreactivity. In fact, allergens from cats, dogs, house dust mites, cockroaches, and fungi consistently show the strongest association with bronchial hyperreactivity, using a variety of study designs and different population groups. Evidence that sensitization to allergens is the most important risk factor for the development of asthma has come from cross-sectional studies conducted in children and young adults, studies of children and adults presenting to the emergency room with acute attacks of asthma, and studies of populations with increased risk for allergy.[19–29] Allergen avoidance studies carried out at high altitudes or in hospital rooms have shown that reducing mite allergen exposure to <1 µg/g can result in decreased bronchial hyperreactivity and asthma symptoms. In addition, a number of studies have also suggested that allergen avoidance can reduce the prevalence of sensitization and may therefore decrease the prevalence of asthma.[18] Studies are being performed to assess whether early allergen avoidance procedures, carried out in the first 3 years of life, will reduce the prevalence of asthma. Measuring mite allergen exposure in houses using monoclonal antibody based ELISA (enzyme-linked immunosorbent assay) tests has established levels at which patients become sensitized (typically exposures of 1–2 µg of Group 1 allergens per gram of dust) and at which they are likely to develop asthma exacerbations (~10 µg/g).[18]

GENERAL PROPERTIES OF ALLERGENS

Allergens are derived from many different sources, and represent diverse groups of proteins. Inhalant allergens have common physical properties: they are usually low molecular weight proteins or glycoproteins (5000–50 000 Da), rapidly soluble in aqueous solutions, that elute promptly from the allergen source, e.g. pollen grains or mite feces.[30] These properties facilitate rapid penetration at mucosal surfaces, enabling passage through the epithelial basement membrane and subsequent transport to regional lymph nodes and triggering of the immune response. In addition, these small and rapidly soluble foreign proteins readily promote cross-linking of IgE antibodies on the mast cell surface and mediator release, to cause immediate symptoms in sensitized individuals. Another important feature of inhaled allergens is that allergic individuals become sensitized following exposure to extremely low doses of allergen. It has been estimated that 5–50 ng of allergen is inhaled per day, on airborne particles of ~5–40 µm diameter. This form of immunization appears to prime preferentially for IgE antibody production.

Many allergens have now been purified,

sequenced, cloned, and produced as recombinant proteins. Purified allergens are named according to a systematic nomenclature, developed by a subcommittee of the World Health Organization and International Union of Immunological Societies.[31] Allergens are described using the first three letters of the genus, the first letter of the species and an arabic numeral to indicate the chronological order of identification. For example, *Dermatophagoides pteronyssinus* allergen 1 is described as Der p 1. Over 200 allergens are now included in the WHO/IUIS database. To be included in this nomenclature, newly described allergens have to satisfy criteria of biochemical purity and criteria to establish their allergenic importance in a large group of allergic patients. Multiple allergenic proteins have been purified from a given source. Thus more than 10 different allergens have now been isolated or cloned from house dust mites or grass pollens.[32,33] For some allergens, such as house dust mites, the majority (80–90%) of patients makes IgE antibody responses to one or two proteins, e.g., mite allergens from *Dermatophagoides pteronyssinus*, Der p 1 and Der p 2, and these 'major' allergens are the focus of immunologic and clinical studies. Isoallergens, which are multiple molecular forms of the same allergen, sharing extensive structural and functional properties including IgE reactivity and ⩾67% amino acid sequence identity, have also been identified. Moreover, isoforms or variants, defined as sequences that are polymorphic variants of the same allergen, have been reported for several allergens (e.g., for Der p 1 and Der p 2 from mites, for Amb a 1 from ragweed and for Bet v 1 from birch).

It is important to understand the properties of the particles that carry allergens—in particular how proteins become airborne. It is assumed that free protein molecules cannot become airborne in sufficient quantities. Allergens become airborne in particles that range from <1 to 40 μm in diameter. Particles of animal dander or the spores of fungi such as *Aspergillus* and *Penicillium* are small, usually ⩽5 μm in size, whereas pollen grains, mite fecal particles, spores of *Alternaria* and particles carrying cockroach proteins are at the larger end of the range.

Mite fecal particles are about the same size as pollen grains (10–40 μm diameter) and are only transiently present in the air.[34] Airborne mite allergen cannot be detected in the air under undisturbed conditions, and even after disturbance the allergen falls rapidly and usually cannot be detected 30–40 min after disturbance. Cockroach aeroallergen particles have similar aerodynamic properties to mite allergens: they are >10 μm in diameter and detectable following disturbance.[35] On the other hand, cat and dog allergens can usually be detected in houses under undisturbed conditions.[36,37] A significant proportion (20–50%) of both Fel d 1 and Can f 1 is found on smaller particles of ~5 μm diameter, which tend to remain airborne for longer periods (2–4 hours), depending on the air exchange rate in the house. This is probably the reason why cat or dog allergic patients often present allergic symptoms within a short time of entering a house containing these pets, whereas this temporal relationship between exposure and symptoms is not usually described by mite or cockroach allergic patients. Similarly, animal handlers who are allergic to mice or rats can experience immediate symptoms upon entering a vivarium containing these animals. Rat and mouse urinary allergens become airborne in particles ~7 μm in diameter.[38]

In the past it was thought that allergens would share particular structural features as a group that would favor a particular type of immune response. This response is characterized by Th2 cells, IgE antibodies and eosinophils, and is now well studied. Sequencing of allergens has revealed the structure of these molecules and has enabled comparisons with known proteins from other sources, providing clues about the biological function of these molecules. No common chemical characteristics of allergens have become apparent. However, many allergens have sequence homology with known enzymes or have functional enzymatic activity.[39] In particular, several mite allergens are proteolytic enzymes (cysteine and serine proteases, trypsin and chemotrypsin), and the cockroach allergen Bla g 2 has homology to the aspartic protease family of enzymes.[40] Proteolytic enzymes are common components of digestion and are produced in the gastrointestinal tract in large excess. For example, the Group 1 mite allergens (Der p 1 and Der f 1) are cysteine proteases produced in the digestive tract and excreted in the feces. It has been proposed that proteolytic activity contributes to the allergenicity of mite proteins, facilitating penetration through mucosal surfaces and induction of IgE antibody responses.[41] In addition, it has been demonstrated that Der p 1 is able to cleave the low affinity IgE receptor (CD23) from the surface of B cells as well as the alpha subunit of the IL-2 receptor (CD25).[42–44] Based on this evidence, it has been speculated that these activities could increase immunogenicity.[45,46] However, to date there is no proof that allergens have enzymatic activity *in vivo*, and the idea that enzymatic activity is an important property of allergens remains a hypothesis. In keeping with this, several potent allergens have no sequence homology with enzymes and no proteolytic activity. These include binding proteins of the calycin family, proteins involved in muscular contraction such as tropomyosin and troponin, and other allergens such as Der p 2 or Fel d 1, from mite and cat, respectively.

MOLECULAR BIOLOGY

Cloning and sequencing

Allergen cloning has become the method of choice for identifying and defining important allergens. Using molecular cloning techniques, it has become possible to establish the primary structures of a number of allergens, and by screening cDNA expression libraries with human IgE new allergens have been identified and sequenced. At present, more than 200 allergen sequences are listed in protein databanks (e.g., GenBank); a partial list of major allergens is shown in Tables 13.1 and 13.2.

The purpose of cloning and sequencing is to obtain the primary structure of the allergen and to express the allergen in recombinant form. The usual approach has been to isolate mRNA from allergen source material (e.g., pollen grains, mite or cockroach bodies, fungal spores, cat salivary glands) and to use reverse transcriptase to copy the mRNA *in vitro* into complementary DNA (cDNA). The double-stranded cDNA is then introduced into bacteriophage genomic DNA (λGT11 or similar expression vectors). The result is a cDNA expression library, which can be screened with pooled IgE antibodies from allergic patients, or with polyclonal or monoclonal specific antibodies, to identify cDNA clones expressing allergen. For many major allergens, N-terminal or internal amino acid sequences, and monospecific antibodies, were available to confirm the identity of cDNA clones. In some cases, e.g., cat allergen, Fel d 1 or *Aspergillus* allergen, Asp f 1, the nucleotide sequences were obtained by polymerase chain reaction (PCR) using primers derived from the amino acid sequence.

Expression of recombinant allergens *in vitro*

The next step following cloning of allergen genes has been the development of high-level expression systems for the production of recombinant allergens. *In vitro* systems for protein expression produce high quantities (usually 10–50 mg of protein per liter of culture, but up to 1.5 g/l) of protein. The host cell may be bacteria (*Escherichia coli*), yeast (*Pichia pastoris* or *Saccharomyces cerevisiae*) or insect cells. Most recombinant allergens have been expressed in bacteria. However, prokaryotic organisms lack the post-translational modification machinery of higher organisms and are unable to glycosylate proteins or process proenzymes into their mature form. Yeast and insect cell systems can provide processing and modification steps.

Recombinant technology has made it possible to produce large quantities of allergens with a high degree of purity, and in many cases with excellent immunoreactivity as judged by skin testing and *in vitro* serum IgE antibody assays (Figure 13.1). Recombinant allergens from mite (Der p 2, Blo t 5, Der p 5), *Aspergillus* (Asp f 1), cockroach (Bla g 4, Bla g 5), grasses (Phl p 1, Phl p 5), and *trees* (Bet v 1) have good biologic activity on skin testing, and elicit posi-

Table 13.1 Structural and functional properties of indoor allergens

Source	Allergen	MW (kDa)	Homology/function	Sequence
House dust mite				
Dermatophagoides spp	Group 1	25	Cysteine protease*	cDNA
	Group 2	14	Epididymal or molting protein*	cDNA
	Group 3	30	Serine protease	cDNA
	Der p 4	60	Amylase	Protein
	Group 5	14	Unknown	cDNA
	Der p 6	25	Chymotrypsin	Protein
	Group 7	22–28	Unknown	cDNA
	Der p 8	26	Glutathione-S-transferase	cDNA
	Der p 9	24	Collagenolytic serine protease	cDNA
	Group 10	36	Tropomyosin	cDNA
Euroglyphus maynei	Eur m 1	25	Cysteine protease	PCR
Blomia tropicalis	Blo t 5	14	Unknown	cDNA
Lepidoglyphus destructor	Lep d 2	14	Epididymal or molting protein	Protein and cDNA
Cockroach				
Blattella germanica	Bla g 1	20–25	Unknown	cDNA
	Bla g 1 (Bd90K)	90	Unknown	cDNA
	Bla g 2	36	Aspartic protease	cDNA
	Bla g 4	18	Lipocalin (calycin)	cDNA
	Bla g 5	23	Glutathione-S-transferase	cDNA
	Bla g 6	18	Troponin C	cDNA
Periplaneta americana	Per a 1	20–25	Unknown	cDNA
	Per a 3	72	Arylphorin/hemocyanin	cDNA
	Per a 7	33	Tropomyosin	cDNA
Mammals				
Cat (*Felis domesticus*)	Fel d 1	36	(Uteroglobin)	PCR
Dog (*Canis familiaris*)	Can f 1	25	Cysteine protease inhibitor	cDNA
	Can f 2	27	Calycin	cDNA
Mouse (*Mus muscularis*)	Mus m 1	21	Pheromone-binding protein (calycin)*	cDNA
Rat (*Rattus norvegicus*)	Rat n 1	21	Pheromone-binding protein (calycin)*	cDNA
Fungi				
Aspergillus fumigatus	Asp f 1	18	Cytotoxin (mitogillin)	cDNA
Alternaria alternata	Alt a 1	29	Unknown	cDNA

* Allergens of known three-dimensional structure are indicated.

Table 13.2 Structural and functional properties of selected pollen and fungal allergens

Source	Allergen	MW (kDa)	Homology/function	Sequence
Grasses				
Rye (*Lolium perenne*)	Lol p 1	28	Cysteine protease	cDNA
	Lol p 2	11	Unknown	cDNA
	Lol p 3	11	Unknown	cDNA
	Lol p 10	12	Cytochrome C	cDNA
Timothy (*Phleum pratense*)	Phl p 5	31	Unknown	cDNA
Bermuda (*Cynodon dactylon*)	Cyn d 1	32	Unknown	cDNA
Weeds				
Ragweed (*Artemisia artemisifolia*)	Amb a 1	38	Pectate lyase*	cDNA
	Amb a 5	5	Neurophysins	cDNA
Parietaria (*Parietaria judaica*)	Par j 1	15	Lipid transport protein	cDNA
Trees				
Birch (*Betula verucosa*)	Bet v 1	17	Pathogenesis-related protein	cDNA
	Bet v 2	20	Profilin	cDNA
Alder (*Alnus glutinosa*)	Aln g 4	9	Calcium-binding protein	cDNA
Fungi				
Alternaria alternata	Alt a 1	29	Unknown	cDNA

* Allergens of known three-dimensional structure are indicated.

tive wheal and flare reactions at picogram doses. The major allergen rDer p 1 has been the exception. Initially produced in *E. coli*, rDer p 1 showed poor reactivity with IgE antibody, suggesting that the recombinant allergen was incorrectly folded. However, more recently, Shoji and colleagues, working with the Group 1 homologue Der f 1, have established an expression system in insect cells and have produced Der f 1 at 25 mg/l.[47] This rDer f 1 gives overlapping IgE binding curves with the natural Der f 1 and also shows comparable protease activity. The key to this success appears to be the correct processing of the proenzyme into mature protein.

CLINICAL APPLICATIONS OF RECOMBINANT ALLERGENS

Recombinant allergens could be used to standardize extracts, or in cocktails as skin test reagents, or in a mutagenized form for immunotherapy.[14,48] Traditional methods of allergy diagnosis and treatment have relied on the use of heterogeneous allergen extracts. The problems with the use of these extracts include difficulties in assessing their potency and the possible occurrence of life-threatening reaction when they are used in immunotherapy. At present, monoclonal antibody based immunoassays are used for the standardization of dust mite and cat extracts. Recombinant allergens could aid in the development of immunoassays as reproducible standards for cockroach and

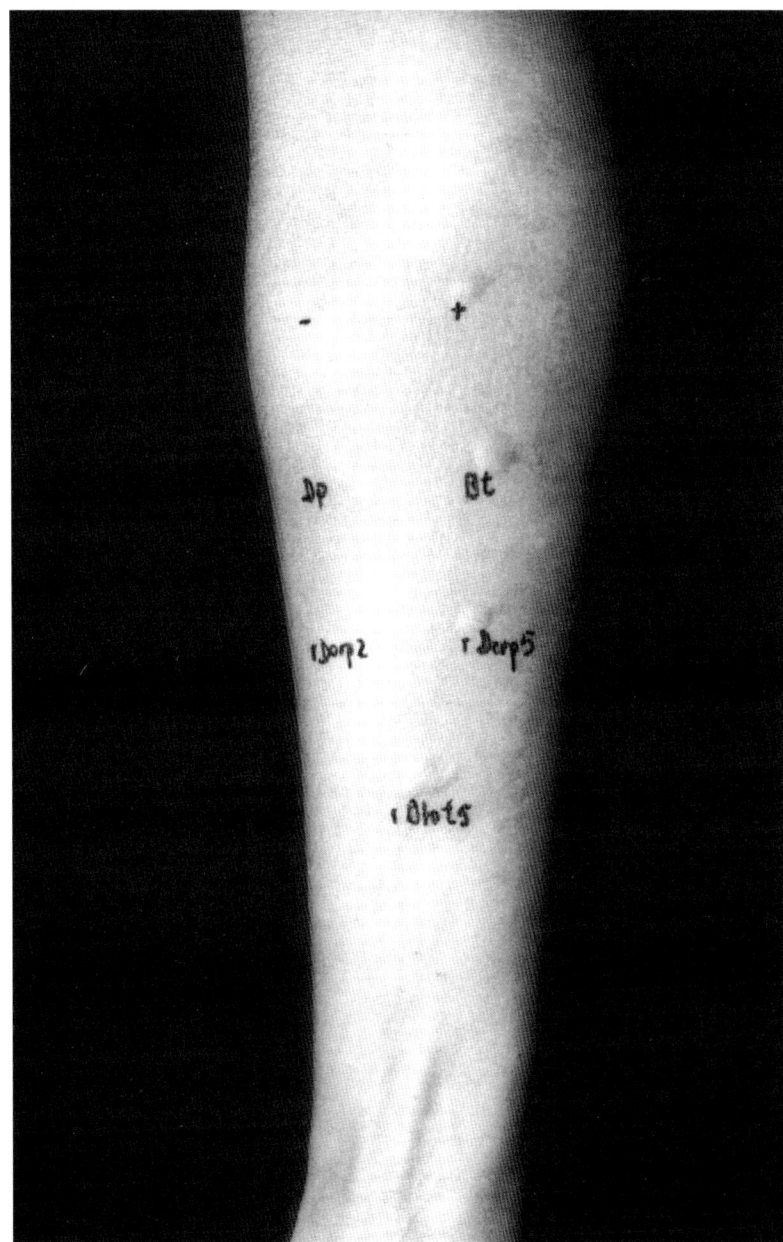

Figure 13.1 Skin tests using recombinant mite allergens. Skin prick tests were performed using *D. pteronyssinus* extract (Bayer, USA), *B. tropicalis* extract (2 mg/ml, kindly provided by Enrique Fernandez-Caldas) and recombinant (r) allergens rDer p 2 (kindly provided by Alisa Smith, University of Virginia), rDer p5 and rBlo t 5, at a concentration of 5 μg/ml. Positive (+) and negative (−) controls were histamine dihydrochloride (10 mg/ml) and sterile albumin–saline with phenol (Bayer, USA), respectively. The reaction caused by rDer p5 and rBlo t 5 was comparable to that caused by whole mite extracts. No reaction was observed with rDer p 2 in this patient.

fungal allergen assays. The objective is to provide accurate measurements, in mass units, of major allergens in a given crude extract.

Most recombinant allergens show comparable immunoreactivity to their native counterparts (Figure 13.2). *In vitro* IgE assays and skin testing of allergic individuals with recombinant allergens from mites, cockroach, pollens, and fungi have shown promising results.[49–55] It is possible to investigate whether cocktails of 3–4 allergens would be suitable for clinical purposes.

New treatment strategies have emerged as a result of cloning studies. The availability of the

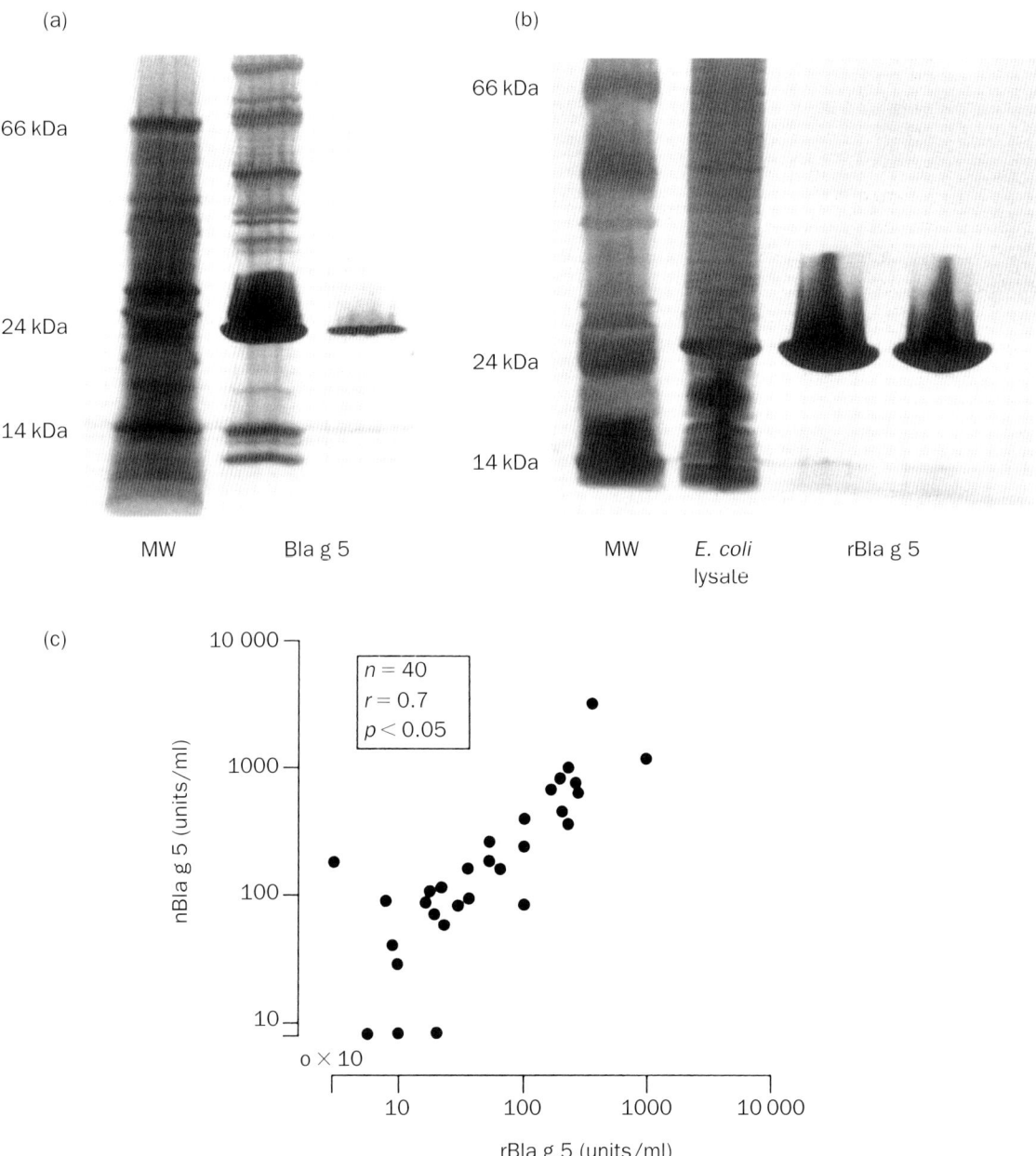

Figure 13.2 Analysis of natural and recombinant *B. germanica* allergen Bla g 5 (glutathione-S-transferase). (a) Natural Bla g 5 was purified from a whole-body *B. germanica* extract using glutathione-affinity chromatography and size exclusion HPLC. (b) Recombinant Bla g 5 produced in *E. coli*, purified from bacterial lysates over a glutathione-affinity column. Both natural and recombinant Bla g 5 migrate as a single 23 kDa band on SDS gels. The yield of natural allergen was very low (0.002% of the protein in the cockroach extract), whereas the yield of the recombinant protein was 3–4 mg protein per liter of bacterial culture. (c) Both natural and recombinant Bla g 5 showed binding to IgE from sera of a group of patients with asthma allergic to cockroach. There was a significant correlation between the levels of IgE to nBla g 5 and rBla g 5, using an antigen-binding radioimmunoassay.

primary amino acid sequence of a given allergen allows investigators to use synthetic peptides to determine T-cell epitopes. Peptide immunotherapy has gone through clinical trials for the treatment of cat-allergic subjects and also for ragweed, using peptides from Fel d 1 and Amb a 1, respectively, in concentrations up to 750 µg/dose.[56,57] The results show significant effects, but not as dramatic as expected. Another approach derived from recombinant allergens is the use of engineered hypoallergenic variants with reduced IgE reactivity but maintained T-cell epitopes. It is thought that these proteins may be more efficacious than conventional immunotherapy owing to decreased risk of side effects.[58-61] Site-directed mutagenesis has been used to eliminate disulfide bonds and generate variants of the mite allergen Der p 2 with up to 100-fold less skin reactivity, but preserving T-cell stimulatory capacity.[61] Current work on the tertiary structure of some allergens has become possible through the availability of large amounts of biologically active recombinant allergens. This work should make it possible both to define epitopes that bind IgE and to create mutagenized recombinants with modified IgE epitopes.

More recent strategies involve using plasmid DNA vaccines to act as Th1 adjuvants to elicit Th1 responses to allergens, leading to IgG1 but not IgE antibody production. Plasmid DNA vaccines have been studied in experimental animals, but there have been no trials as yet in humans. In a rat model, Hsu and colleagues[62] showed that a plasmid containing the gene for the Der p 5 mite allergen could effectively prevent the development of IgE Ab and airway hyperresponsiveness when given intramuscularly to naïve animals. In addition, treatment of previously sensitized animals with the plasmid vaccine could reduce airway hyperresponsiveness upon subsequent exposure to the allergen. Raz and colleagues[63] found similar results in a mouse model using the antigen β-galactosidase. This group characterized the bacterial DNA sequences as CpG motifs, located outside the allergen gene regions, which were responsible for an adjuvant effect eliciting IFN-g and IL-12.

These sequences were termed 'ISS' for 'immunostimulatory sequences'.[64] Subsequently, it has been shown that ISS can be administered together with a protein antigen to induce an antigen-specific Th1-type response.[65-67] It is unclear how bacterial DNA sequences interact with cells of the immune system, and this approach to treatment of allergic disease is under active investigation.

SOURCES OF ALLERGENS

Indoor

Mites
House dust mites are the most important source of allergens associated with the indoor environment. Dust mites were first recognized as a major source of allergen in house dust by Spieksma and Voohost, in 1967.[68] It is now well established from epidemiologic studies that there is a strong relationship of sensitization to mite allergens with asthma and atopic dermatitis. Mites are eight-legged relatives of spiders and ticks, measuring one-third of a millimeter in length. Optimal conditions for mite growth include a temperature between 21° and 26°C and an absolute humidity >8 g/kg, which is equivalent to a relative humidity of approximately 70%. House dust mites of the genus *Dermatophagoides* are the most common indoor mites in North America and Europe. The most common species of *Dermatophagoides* are *D. pteronyssinus* and *D. farinae*. Their primary food source is human skin scales (thus their name 'skin eating') and they are found in carpets, upholstered furniture, and bedding. Several studies revealed that the mattress contains the highest levels of mite allergen in the house. Mite feces contain high concentrations of the Group 1 allergens and become airborne following disturbance of the dust, e.g. by vacuum cleaning, bed making, etc. Allergen can be eluted from the feces within 1–2 minutes. Ten allergen groups are well defined in *Dermatophagoides*, including Group 1, which are cysteine proteases; Groups 3, 6, and 9, which are serine proteases with distinct substrate

specificities similar to trypsin, chymotrypsin, and collagenase, respectively;[32] and Group 10, which are tropomyosins.[69,70] Der p 4 is an amylase;[71] Der p 8 is a glutathione-S-transferase.[72] Der p 2 shows 25–29% sequence identity to epididymal secretory proteins from the human and chimpanzee,[73] and to a moth protein involved in molting or ecdysis.[74] Based on these homologies it has been speculated that this allergen may have a role in mite reproduction, or might be involved in shedding of the mite exoskeleton. Der p 5[75,76] and Group 7[77] allergens have no known function.

In tropical and subtropical areas of the world, the mite *Blomia tropicalis* is an important cause of asthma.[78] Previous studies carried out in regions such as the southern states of the USA, Central and South America, Singapore, Hong Kong, Taiwan, India, and Egypt have shown that *B. tropicalis* and *D. pteronyssinus* occur with high frequency and at high levels of infestation in houses. Using molecular cloning, a *B. tropicalis* allergen, Blo t 5, has been identified which shows homology to *D. pteronyssinus* Der p 5. Recombinant Blo t 5 and Der p 5 have excellent immunologic activities and induce positive skin tests in mite-allergic patients (Figure 13.1).[49]

Under certain environmental conditions, other mite species occur in house dust and can form part of the acarofauna. These include the pyroglyphid mite, *Euroglyphus maynei*, and non-pyroglyphid mites, commonly known as 'storage mites', which are primarily encountered in stored food products, grains, barns, hay, and straw.[78] Allergic reactions to non-pyroglyphic mites, including *Acarus siro*, *Lepidoglyphus destructor*, *Tyrophagus putrescentiae*, and *Glycyphagus domesticus* are usually associated with occupational asthma in grain handlers and farmers. Molecular cloning has identified allergens from *E. maynei*, *L. destructor*, and *T. putrescentiae*.[79–81]

Cockroach

Cockroach allergy has been recognized as an important cause of asthma for over 30 years. Bernton and Brown were the first to report positive skin tests to cockroach in 44% of 755 allergy clinic patients in New York.[82] Subsequently, many authors recognized that patients with asthma living in cities were commonly sensitized to this insect.[83] Kang and colleagues[84] established the causal relationship between cockroach allergy and asthma by showing early, late phase, and dual bronchoconstriction following inhalation of cockroach extract by sensitized asthmatic patients. These studies have clearly demonstrated that asthma caused by cockroach is antigen specific and that it is similar to other types of atopic asthma.

Cockroach allergy is strongly linked to socioeconomic factors and it occurs wherever living conditions sustain cockroach infestation.[83] Enzyme-linked immunosorbent assays have been developed for assessing exposure to cockroach allergens including Bla g 1, Bla g 2, Per a 1, and Per a 3, which provide a quantitative test for measuring allergen in house dust. Several studies have demonstrated that most patients sensitized to cockroach were exposed to high levels of cockroach allergens in their homes, and that cockroach allergy is an important risk factor for emergency room visits for asthma and hospital admissions.[83] More recently, the National Cooperative Inner City Asthma Study has confirmed that sensitization and exposure to cockroach allergens are a major risk factor for severity of asthma in children from large cities in the USA. A recent prospective study has demonstrated a significant association between exposure to cockroach allergens in the first 3 months of life and the development of repeated wheeze in the first year, among children from metropolitan Boston.[85] A longer follow-up of these children will reveal whether early life exposure to cockroach is a risk factor for the subsequent development of asthma.

The most common domiciliary species of cockroach are *Blattella germanica* (German cockroach) and *Periplaneta americana* (American cockroach). *B. germanica* is a small cockroach, approximately 2 cm in length, that commonly infests houses in the USA. Kitchens and bathrooms are favored sites for infestation. *P. americana* is a large cockroach, approximately 5 cm in

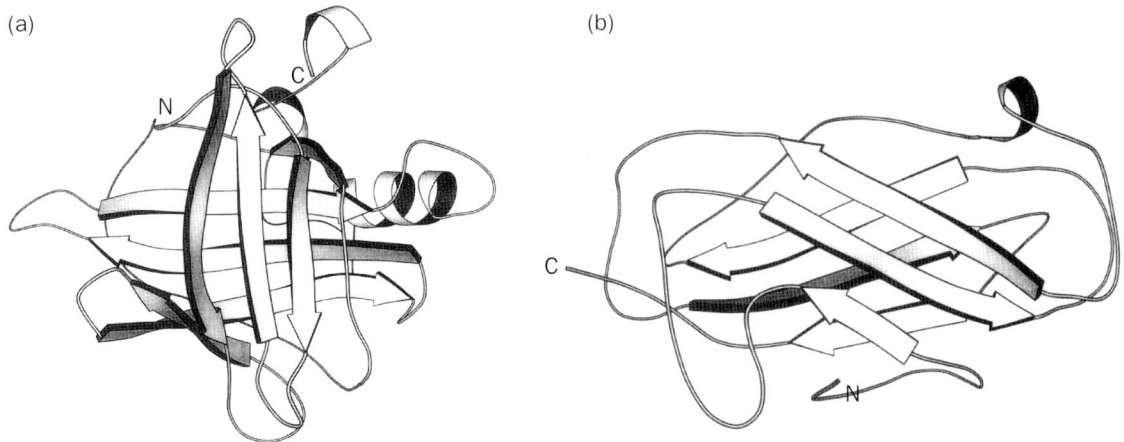

Figure 13.3 Tertiary structure of Bla g 4 and Der p 2. The tertiary structure of Bla g 4 (a) was modeled on the structures of bilin-binding protein from the butterfly and the rat urinary protein, using SYBYL (Tripos, Inc, St Louis) and CONGEN modeling programs.[90] The structure of Der p 2 (b) was solved using nuclear magnetic resonance spectroscopy.[12]

length, that infests houses, schools, hospitals, and other large buildings. American cockroaches have less fecundity than German cockroaches and require higher temperatures (~80°C) and humidity for optimal population growth.

The first cockroach allergens to be identified, using immunochemistry, were Bla g 1 and Bla g 2.[6,86] Molecular cloning techniques determined the amino acid sequence of Bla g 2 and established that it is a 36 kDa aspartic protease, found in cockroach gut tissues, which may be involved in digestion.[40] Bla g 1 has an unusual structure consisting of a series of up to seven tandem repeats, each ~100 amino acid residues in length, and includes an allergen originally reported as Bla g bd90K.[87,88] Bla g 1 is also the only *B. germanica* allergen that has a structural homologue in *P. americana* (Per a 1).[89] These cross-reactive Group 1 cockroach allergens (Bla g 1 and Per a 1) show 30% homology to a mosquito (*Anopheles gambiae*) protein precursor ANG12 which is secreted only in the female insect after a blood meal. This suggests that these allergens may have a digestive function. Previously, we have reported the cloning and expression of Bla g 4, which belongs to a superfamily of ligand-binding protein (calycins or lipocalins).[90] This family includes other important allergens such as mouse and rat urinary proteins,[91,92] dog allergens Can f 1 and Can f 2,[93] β-lactoglobulin from cows' milk,[94] and bovine and equine allergens.[95,96] The lipocalins are extracellular proteins that bind hydrophobic molecules with high affinity and selectivity. Three-dimensional models of the tertiary structure of Bla g 4 were obtained, and predicted a similar structure to other members of the calycin family (Figure 13.3). Recombinant Bla g 4 expressed in bacteria and yeast has excellent allergenic activity.[90,97] Other *B. germanica* allergens include Bla g 5, which shows sequence homology to glutathione-S-transferase enzymes,[98] and Bla g 6, a troponin. Glutathione-S-transferases (GST) are enzymes involved in the detoxification of endogenous and xenobiotic toxic compounds, and in insects GST production is associated with resistance to insecticides. Allergens from *P. americana* reactive with sera from patients living in Taiwan have been reported, including Per a 3, an insect storage protein related to arylphorin.[99]

Using sera from cockroach-allergic asthmatic children to screen a *P. americana* cDNA library,

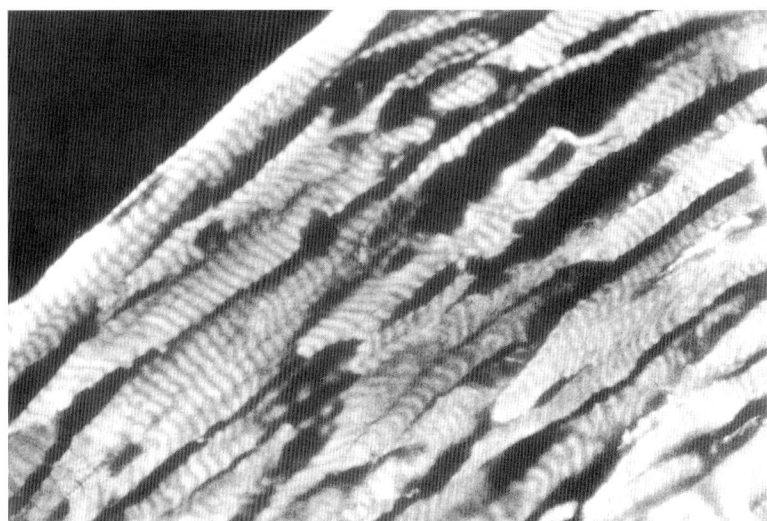

Figure 13.4 Reactivity of monoclonal antibody 1A6, directed against mite tropomyosin, with cockroach muscle tissue. Unfixed frozen sections of cockroach skeletal muscle immunostained with monoclonal antibody 1A6, anti-*D. pteronyssinus* tropomyosin, which also recognizes shrimp tropomyosin. The striations stain positive for tropomyosin.

a major cockroach allergen has been recently identified. This allergen shows a high degree of sequence identity to tropomyosins from invertebrates, particularly from mites (80% identity) and shrimp (82% identity), and has been designated as Per a 7.[100] Tropomyosins had been previously identified as important allergens in mites (*D. pteronyssinus* and *D. farinae* Der p 10 and Der f 10, respectively) and shrimp.[101] Interestingly, a monoclonal antibody raised against *D. pteronyssinus* shown previously to bind to shrimp tropomyosin also recognized cockroach tropomyosin on immunofluorescence (Figure 13.4). Our results raise the possibility that tropomyosin may be the basis for cross-reactivity among mites, cockroach, and shrimp, and that the high degree of sequence identity has clinical significance.

Although cockroach allergens are found throughout the house, including in beds, furniture, and carpets, cockroach allergen levels are highest in the kitchen. It appears that cockroach allergens derive from several sources, e.g., saliva, fecal material, debris from dead bodies.[102] Significant amounts of allergen can be recovered by washing roaches, and from the frass that accumulates in jars where cockroaches are kept in the laboratory. Cockroach aeroallergen particles have similar properties to mite allergens, in that they are relatively large (>10 μm diameter), are detectable mainly after disturbance, and are thought to fall rapidly. In keeping with this, patients are usually not aware of being allergic to cockroach and do not report symptoms of asthma on entering a house that is infested with roaches. Recently, De Lucca and colleagues[103] have used intranasal and air samplers and a sensitive immunostaining system to investigate the behavior of cockroach allergen-carrying particles. In that study, the authors could detect Bla g 1 carrying particles during quiet domestic activity or even under no disturbance, both in the air and in nasal filters, in houses containing low levels (geometric mean 1.5 U of Bla g 1/g of dust) of allergen in Australia. In agreement with previous studies, airborne particles containing cockroach allergen are associated with particles of >10 μm. These particles, described as 'flakes' or 'fibers', may contain sufficient allergen to induce sensitization and chronic inflammation upon inhalation.

Control of cockroach exposure has been considered difficult and this issue has been recently investigated in inner city houses. Although aggressive treatment of cockroach-infested houses with insecticides promptly reduces the number of roaches, allergen levels may remain elevated in the environment for up to 6 months.[104–106] It is suggested that cockroach extermination needs to be coupled with thorough cleaning measures to achieve effective control of allergen exposure.

Domestic animals

One of the most important sources of allergens in house dust is the cat (*Felis domesticus*). The major cat allergen Fel d 1 is produced on the sebaceous glands of the skin, and becomes airborne mainly in small particles.[36,107] In addition, it tends to stick to carpets, clothing, furniture, and surfaces including walls, making it difficult to decrease environmental exposure even after removal of the cat.[108] It is usually clear to cat-allergic patients that they can develop symptoms by contact with a cat or simply by entering a house that has a cat, whether the animal is present in the room or not. Recently, research carried out in Sweden has clearly demonstrated that significant exposure to cat allergen (and also to dog allergen) occurs in schools, and that clothes are a major source of spreading of cat allergen.[109,110]

The major cat allergen, Fel d 1, is composed of two polypeptide chains linked by disulfide bonds. Chain 1 is homologous to rabbit uteroglobulin; to date, no homologies have been identified for Chain 2.[107] Uteroglobulin is thought to have immunomodulatory activity based on its ability to bind steroids as well as to inhibit phospholipase A2 activity, but the significance of the homology to the function of Fel d 1 is unclear.

Dog allergen has similar properties to cat allergen, in that it can usually be detected in houses under undisturbed conditions. In addition, a significant proportion (20–50%) of both Can f 1 and Fel d 1 is found on smaller particles of approximately 5 μm diameter, which tend to remain airborne for longer periods of time (2–4 hours). The dog allergens Can f 1 and Can f 2 belong to the lipocalin family of proteins. The dog lipocalin Can f 1 is 50% identical to a human salivary protein, the von Ebner's gland protein (VEGh).[111] Can f 1 and VEGh are cysteine protease inhibitors, also known as cystatins. Recently, Chapman and colleagues[112] have reported the cDNA cloning of a cat allergen that shows homology to the cystatins. The cystatins are considered a subfamily of the lipocalins.

Rodents

Rodent proteins are potent sources of allergens, and exposure to these proteins can occur in an occupational setting in the laboratory, or when these animals are kept as pets in the household. The major allergens have been defined and are predominantly found in urine.[38] Male rat urine may contain more than 1 mg of allergen per milliliter. Mouse and rat urinary proteins Mus m 1 and Rat n 1, the major allergens, also belong to the lipocalin family and function as pheromone-binding proteins.[92,94] Rodent allergens accumulate in high quantities in the litter, which is a major source of airborne allergen. As for individuals allergic to cats or dogs, animal handlers who are allergic to mice or rats can have immediate symptoms of asthma, rhinitis, and occasionally anaphylaxis on entering a vivarium containing these animals. Rat and mouse urinary allergens occur on particles of approximately 7 μm diameter, and remain airborne in high concentrations for a long time.

Others

Other sources of allergens can be present in house dust, including arthropods such as moths, locusts, and others. The possible role of bacteria has not been experimentally proven. However, Gram-negative bacterial products such as endotoxins may have a role in exacerbating bronchial hyperreactivity or asthma symptoms in sensitized individuals. In mite-allergic asthmatic children, exposed to mite allergen Der p 1 in their homes, there was a significant correlation between exposure to endotoxin in house dust and clinical symptoms.[113]

Outdoor

Pollens

The majority of wind-pollinated plants may produce enough pollen grains to become a cause of seasonal rhinitis, provided there are sufficient plants in the area. Most pollen grains measure 10–50 μm in diameter, tend to be spherical or ellipsoid in shape, and reach concentrations of 200–300 grains/m^3 at the height of the grass pollen season, which can last from 2–3 weeks to several months.[114] Some trees produce more copious amounts of pollen, exceeding 1000 grains/m^3 (e.g., olive). Pollen grains are gametes, and they are designed to release recognition proteins in order to trigger the formation of a pollen tube after they land on the pistil. Some of the known pollen allergens are thought to be involved in recognition, but the function of other pollen allergens is not known. Pollen grains contain one or more pores (~2–10 μm in diameter), located on the outer envelope or 'excine', for transfer of genetic material, and 1–3 furrows. Pollen release by wind-pollinated (anemophilous) plants is promoted by rapidly moving air of low humidity. Once airborne, pollen grains cause allergic symptoms by impacting onto the conjunctiva, nasal mucosa, and oral cavity and rapidly releasing soluble allergens. Although pollen allergy is well recognized as an important cause of hay fever, the association with asthma is much less consistent, as compared with indoor allergens.

Currently available data fairly consistently agree that exposure to grass pollen, ragweed, or other locally relevant pollen rarely constitutes a risk factor for the development of asthma in both children and adults.[115] However, it has been well recognized that exposure to pollen allergens including those derived from grasses, ragweed, and trees (birch, parietaria) cause seasonal asthma in children and adults.[116–119] Admission of adult patients with asthma to an emergency room was strongly associated with sensitization to rye grass pollen during the pollen season in northern California.[120]

Pollen allergens have been shown to induce inflammation in the airways of asthmatic subjects. Analysis of bronchoalveolar lavage samples of pollen-sensitized asthmatic adults during the pollen season revealed increased T-cell activation, increased levels of interleukin-2 receptor, decreased number of metachromatic cells (possibly due to degranulation), and increased number of mast cells staining for secreted IL-4.[121] In addition, grass-pollen-allergic children showed a significant increase in exhaled NO during the pollen season, as compared with preseasonal levels.[122]

To date, several pollen allergens from grasses, trees, and weeds have been identified; the properties of common pollen allergens are outlined in Table 13.2. Allergenically important grasses include Bermuda grass (*Cynodon dactylon*), rye grass (*Lolium perenne*), Timothy grass (*Phleum pratense*), and orchard grass (*Dactylis glomerata*). Tree pollens of various genera are morphologically distinct and pollen identification is based on visible charateristics under light microscopy. Allergenically important genera of the Betulaceae family include birch (*Betula*), hazel (*Corylus*), and alder (*Alnus*). Other important tree pollens include Japanese cedar, oak, and maple. Weed pollens are also a major source of outdoor allergens, and vary among different geographic regions. In the eastern USA, the most important weed pollen is from short ragweed (*Ambrosia*) and the ragweed season runs from August through October. In Mediterranean regions, *Parietaria* is an important pollen source.

An interesting feature of pollen allergens is the cross-reactivity they present with certain foods.[123,124] A typical manifestation is the 'oral allergy syndrome,' characterized by symptoms including itching at the back of the throat, swelling of the lips, and facial swelling. Patients allergic to birch or grass pollen may have oral allergy syndrome after eating fruits, such as apples and pears. Likewise, ragweed-allergic patients may experience symptoms after eating watermelon. In most cases, these reactions can be explained by the existence of cross-reacting allergens present in the offending foods. Structural homologues of the birch pollen allergens, Bet v 1 and Bet v 2, occur in other trees (e.g., hazel nut), as well as in apples, pears, celery, carrots, potato, and buckwheat.

Several pollen allergens have been cloned and expressed as recombinant proteins. Genetically engineered hypoallergenic forms of Bet v 1, the major birch pollen allergen, have caused reduced reactivity on skin testing, as compared with the wild type Bet v 1.[60] It may be possible to treat birch pollen allergic patients successfully with safer immunotherapy, with a reduced risk to induce anaphylactic reactions, using these hypoallergenic derivatives of Bet v 1.

Fungi

Fungal spores range 2–100 μm in length and may be single celled or contain cross-walls giving rise to multiple cells within a single spore. Spore shape can vary from almost spherical (e.g., conidial spores of *Aspergillus*, 2 μm) to elongated, clublike spores (e.g., *Alternaria*, ~50 μm). Fungi can be important sources of indoor or outdoor allergens.[114] Common fungi involved in causing allergic disease include *Cladosporium*, *Aspergillus*, *Alternaria*, *Penicillium*, *Epicoccum*, *Fusarium*, and basidiospores. Fungal spores counts can be extremely high, up to 30 000 spores/m^3, and these can increase considerably as a result of agricultural practices, such as wheat or corn harvesting (over 10^8 spores/m^3). Similar high concentrations of fungal spores can occur as a result of occupational exposure, e.g., in the timber industry, processing of plant fibers, organic waste and sewage composting (recycling), mushroom farms, etc.

The association of exposure to fungal allergens and asthma has not been as well documented as for other indoor allergens, and a clear dose–response relationship between exposure and symptoms has not been established for most fungi. One exception is *Alternaria*. Sensitization to *Alternaria* appears to be a significant risk factor for asthma in a variety of locations worldwide,[125] although maybe not as important as sensitization to indoor allergens such as mites, cat, or cockroach.[126] Furthermore, *A. alternata* sensitivity has been associated with severe and potentially fatal attacks of asthma during the period of the year when *Alternaria* antigens are airborne.[127] However, good quantitative assays for measuring fungal allergens in the environment are not available for most fungal species. In addition to the large variety of fungal species that can be found indoors and outdoors, there is variability in the expression of allergens according to the stage of development of the fungus. One example is the major *A. fumigatus* allergen Asp f 1, which is produced only upon germination and is not present in spores.[128] The current methods of assessing exposure to fungi rely on the identification and counting of spores, but this has limitations, including the fact that some spores may not be easily distinguishable (e.g., *Aspergillus* and *Penicillium*), and hyphae and other particles of fungal origin may contain significant amounts of allergen.

Several fungal allergens from *Alternaria*, *Aspergillus*, *Cladosporium*, basiodiomycetes, and other fungal sources have recently been cloned and sequenced.[129–131] Recombinant *A. fumigatus* allergens have been used to selectively diagnose patients with allergic bronchopulmonary aspergillosis (ABPA) from *Aspergillus*-sensitive patients without ABPA.[132] Further studies should focus on developing better methods to assess exposure, in order to improve our understanding of the role of airborne molds in asthma.

CONCLUSIONS

It has been well established that asthma is an inflammatory disease and that it is associated with immediate hypersensitivity to perennial indoor allergens, rather than to those allergens that are predominantly outdoor and seasonal. Approximately 80–90% of children with asthma are sensitized to indoor allergens, and sensitization is clearly related to exposure.[18] Identifying specific sensitivities can be accomplished by skin tests or measurements of specific IgE in sera. It is accepted that the currently available methods for measuring specific IgE in serum provide results that correlate well with skin tests. Specific environmental control measures for mites have demonstrated efficacy, and these include encasement of mattresses and pillows with mite-impermeable covers, hot washing of bedding and stuffed animals, removal of carpets, and thorough cleaning of floor and surfaces with damp cloth.[18,133] For pets, removal of the animal would be the ideal approach, associated with extensive cleaning of allergen reservoirs such as carpets, furniture, and walls.

Systematic recommendations for cockroach and fungal allergens are not available. It is thought that environmental control measures play an important role in the treatment of a child with asthma, along with medication therapy.[18,133]

Over the last 20 years, there have been major advances in the characterization of allergens and the immune response to them. Molecular cloning has made it possible to obtain primary structures and, in some cases, tertiary structure of allergens, and hypoallergenic variants may be genetically engineered so that they bind less to IgE while preserving T-cell stimulatory activity. In addition, DNA vaccination or use of adjuvants are promising approaches. Clinical trials need to be conducted to investigate whether these allergen derivatives or adjuvants can be successfully used for immunotherapy. Currently, there is controversy on the efficacy of immunotherapy in childhood asthma.[134,135] Before starting a child with asthma on immunotherapy, issues such as allergen avoidance measures, appropriate pharmacologic anti-inflammatory therapy, and risk–benefit should be carefully considered. Some of the limitations of the currently available reagents for immunotherapy are the possibility of inducing severe systemic reactions, the poor standardization of some extracts, and the long time period required to achieve maintenance doses. It is possible that novel forms of immunotherapy, efficacious and safer for use in children, will be available in the future.[135]

ACKNOWLEDGEMENTS

This chapter was made possible by financial support from FAPESP and NIH grants AI 32557 and AI 34607. We are grateful to Alisa M Smith for helpful discussions, and to PC Potter for suggestions regarding outdoor allergens.

REFERENCES

1. Blackley CH. *Experimental Researches on the Causes and Nature of Catarrhus Aestivus (Hay-Fever or Hay-Asthma).* London: Bailliere, Tindall & Cox, 1873. Reprint: London: Dawson's, 1959.
2. Johnson P, Marsh DG. Isoallergens from rye-grass pollen. *Nature* 1965; **206:** 935–7.
3. King TP, Norman PS, Lichtenstein LM. Isolation and characterization of allergens from ragweed pollen IV. *Biochemistry* 1967; **6:** 1992–2000.
4. Chapman MD, Platts-Mills TAE. Purification and characterization of the major allergen from *Dermatophagoides pteronyssinus*—antigen P1. *J Immunol* 1980; **125:** 587–92.
5. Tovey ER, Chapman MD, Platts-Mills TAE. Mite faeces are a major source of house dust mite allergens. *Nature* 1981; **289:** 592–3.
6. Pollart SM, Mullins DE, Vailes LD et al. Identification, quantitation and purification of cockroach allergens using monoclonal antibodies. *J Allergy Clin Immunol* 1991; **87:** 511–21.
7. Yunginger JW, Jones RT, Nesheim ME, Geller M. Studies on Alternaria allergens. III. Isolation of a major allergenic fraction (ALT-I). *J Allergy Clin Immunol* 1980; **66:** 138–47.
8. Arruda LK, Platts-Mills TAE, Fox JW, Chapman MD. *Aspergillus fumigatus* allergen I, a major IgE binding protein, is a member of the mitogillin family of cytotoxins. *J Exp Med* 1990; **172:** 1529–34.
9. Deuell BL, Arruda LK, Hayden ML et al. *Trichophyton tonsurans* allergen I: characterization of a protein that causes immediate but not delayed hypersensitivity. *J Immunol* 1991; **147:** 96–101.
10. Chua KY, Stewart GA, Thomas WR et al. Sequence analysis of cDNA coding for a major house dust mite allergen, Der p 1: homology with cysteine proteases. *J Exp Med* 1988; **167:** 175–82.
11. Gajhede M, Osmark P, Poulsen FM et al. X-ray and NMR structure of Bet v 1, the origin of birch pollen allergy. *Nature Struct Biology* 1996; **3:** 1040–5.
12. Mueller GA, Benjamin DC, Rule GS. Tertiary structure of the major house dust mite allergen Der p 2: sequential and structural homologies. *Biochemistry* 1998; **34:** 12707–14.
13. Ichikawa S, Hatanaka H, Yuuki T et al. Solution structure of Der f 2, the major allergen for atopic diseases. *J Biol Chem* 1998; **273:** 356–60.
14. Chapman MD, Smith AM, Vailes LD, Arruda LK. Recombinant allergens. New technologies for the management of patients with asthma. *Allergy* 1997; **52:** 374–9.
15. Luczynska C, Arruda LK, Platts-Mills TAE et al.

A two site monoclonal antibody ELISA for quantification of the major *Dermatophagoides* spp. allergens *Der p* I and *Der f* I. *J Immunol Methods* 1989; **118:** 227–35.
16. Chapman MD, Smith AM, Slunt JB et al. Immunochemical methods for defining and measuring indoor allergens: in dust and in the air. *Paed Allergy Clin Immunol* 1995; **6**(suppl 7): 8–12.
17. Custovic A, Chapman MD. Indoor allergens as a risk factor for asthma. In: Barnes PJ, Grunstein MM, Leff A, Woolcock AJ, eds. *Asthma*. Philadelphia: Lippincott-Raven, 1997, pp. 1–21.
18. Platts-Mills TAE, Vervloet D, Thomas WR et al. Indoor allergens and asthma: report of the Third International Workshop. *J Allergy Clin Immunol* 1997; **100:** S3–S24.
19. Sears MR, Herbison GP, Holdaway MD et al. The relative risks of sensitivity to grass pollen, house dust mite and cat dander in the development of childhood asthma. *Clin Exp Allergy* 1989; **19:** 419–24.
20. Sporik R, Ingram JM, Orice W et al. Association of asthma with serum IgE and skin-test reactivity to allergens among children living at high altitude. *Am J Respir Crit Care Med* 1995; **151:** 1388–92.
21. Squillace SP, Sporik RB, Rakes G et al. Sensitization to dust mites as a dominant risk factor for asthma among adolescents living in central Virginia. Multiple regression analysis of a population-based study. *Am J Respir Crit Care Med* 1997; **156:** 1760–4.
22. Rosenstreich DL, Eggleston P, Kattan M et al. The role of cockroach allergy and exposure to cockroach allergen in causing morbidity among inner-city children with asthma. *N Engl J Med* 1997; **336:** 1356–63.
23. Call RS, Smith TF, Morris E et al. Risk factor for asthma in inner city children. *J Pediatr* 1992; **121:** 862–6.
24. Gelber LE, Seltzer LH, Bouzokis JK et al. Sensitization and exposure to indoor allergens as risk factors for asthma among patients presenting to hospital. *Am Rev Respir Dis* 1993; **147:** 573–8.
25. Duff AL, Pomeranz ES, Gelber LE et al. Risk factors for acute wheezing in infants and children: viruses, passive smoke, and IgE antibodies to inhalant allergens. *Pediatrics* 1993; **92:** 535–40.
26. Pollart SM, Chapman MD, Fiocco GP et al. Epidemiology of acute asthma: IgE antibodies to common inhalant allergens as a risk factor for emergency room visits. *J Allergy Clin Immunol* 1989; **83:** 875–82.
27. Sporik R, Holgate ST, Platts-Mills TAE et al. Exposure to house-dust mite allergen (*Der p* I) and the development of asthma in childhood. A prospective study. *N Engl J Med* 1990; **323:** 502–7.
28. Cookson WOCM, DeKlerk NH, Ryan GR et al. Relative risks of bronchial hyper-responsiveness associated with skin-prick test responses to common antigens in young adults. *Clin Exp Allergy* 1991; **21:** 472–9.
29. Sporik R, Squillace SP, Ingram JM et al. Mite, cat, and cockroach exposure, allergen sensitization, and asthma in children: a case–control study of three schools. *Thorax* 1999; **54:** 675–80.
30. Platts-Mills TAE, Type I or immediate hypersensitivity: hay fever and asthma. In: Lachmann PJ, Peters DK, eds. *Clinical Aspects of Immunology*. Oxford: Blackford, 1982, 579–686.
31. King TP, Hoffman D, Lowenstein H et al. Allergen nomenclature. *Int Arch Allergy Immunol* 1994; **105:** 224–33.
32. Thomas WR, Smith W. Allergy review series II. An update on allergens. House dust mite allergens. *Allergy* 1998; **53:** 821–32.
33. Wissenbach M, Holm J, van Neerven RJJ, Ipsen H. Grass pollen allergens: new developments. *Clin Exp Allergy* 1998; **28:** 784–7.
34. Tovey ER, Chapman MD, Wells CW, Platts-Mills TAE. The distribution of dust mite allergens in the houses of patients with asthma. *Am Rev Respir Dis* 1981; **124:** 630–5.
35. De Blay F, Sanchez J, Hedelin G et al. Dust and airborne exposure to allergen derived from cockroach (*Blattella germanica*) in low cost public housing in Strasbourg, France. *J Allergy Clin Immunol* 1997; **99:** 107–12.
36. Luczynska CM, Li Y, Chapman MD, Platts-Mills TAE. Airborne concentrations and particle size distribution of allergen derived from domestic cats (*Felis domesticus*): measurements using cascade impactor, liquid impinger and a two site monoclonal antibody assay for *Fel d* I. *Am Rev Respir Dis* 1990; **141:** 361–7.
37. Custovic A, Green R, Fletcher A et al. Aerodynamic properties of the major dog allergen, Can f 1: Distribution in homes, concentration and particle size of allergens in the air. *Am Rev Respir Crit Care Med* 1997; **155:** 94–8.
38. Platts-Mills TAE, Heymann PW, Longbottom JL, Wilkins SR. Airborne allergens associated

with asthma: particle sizes carrying dust mite and rat allergens measured with a cascade impactor. *J Allergy Clin Immunol* 1986; **77:** 850–7.
39. Stewart GA, Thompson PJ. The biochemistry of common aeroallergens. *Clin Exp Allergy* 1996; **26:** 1020–44.
40. Arruda LK, Vailes LD, Mann BJ, Shannon J et al. Molecular cloning of a major cockroach (*Blattella germanica*) allergen, Bla g 2: sequence homology to the aspartic proteases. *J Biol Chem* 1995; **270:** 19563–8.
41. Stewart GA, Thompson PJ, McWilliam AS. Biochemical properties of aeroallergens: contributory factors in allergic sensitization. *Pediatr Allergy Immunol* 1993; **4:** 163–72.
42. Schulz O, Laing P, Sewell HF, Shakib F. Der p 1, a major allergen of the house dust mite, proteolytically cleaves the low affinity receptor for human IgE (CD23). *Eur J Immunol* 1995; **25:** 3191–4.
43. Hewitt CRA, Brown AP, Hart BJ, Pritchard DI. A major house dust mite allergen disrupts the immunoglobulin E network by selectively cleaving CD23: innate protection by antiproteases. *J Exp Med* 1995; **182:** 1537–44.
44. Schultz O, Sewell HF, Shakib F. Proteolytic cleavage of CD-25 by Der p 1, a major mite allergen with cysteine protease activity. *J Exp Med* 1998; **187:** 271–5.
45. King C, Brennan S, Thompson PJ, Stewart GA. Dust mite proteolytic allergens induce cytokine release from cultured airway epithelium. *J Immunol* 1998; **161:** 3645–51.
46. Comoy EE, Pestel J, Duez C et al. The house dust mite allergen, *Dermatophagoides pteronyssinus*, promotes type 2 responses by modulating the balance between IL-4 and IFN-gamma. *J Immunol* 1998; **160:** 2456–62.
47. Shoji H, Shibuya I, Hirai M et al. Production of recombinant Der f 1 with the native IgE-binding activity using a baculovirus expression system. *Biosci Biotech Biochem* 1997; **61:** 1668–73.
48. Kraft D, Ferreira F, Vrtala S et al. The importance of recombinant allergens for diagnosis and therapy of IgE-mediated allergies. *Int Arch Allergy Immunol* 1999; **118:** 171–6.
49. Arruda LK, Vailes LD, Platts-Mills TAE et al. Sensitization to *Blomia tropicalis* in patients with asthma and identification of allergen Blo t 5. *Am J Respir Crit Care Med* 1997; **155:** 343–50.
50. Lynch NR, Thomas WR, Garcia NM et al. Biological activity of recombinant Der p 2, Der p 5 and Der p 7 allergens of the house-dust mite *Dermatophagoides pteronyssinus*. *Int Arch Allergy Immunol* 1997; **114:** 59–67.
51. Arruda LK, Vailes LD, Benjamin DC, Chapman MD. Molecular cloning of German cockroach (*Blattella germanica*) allergens. *Int Arch Allergy Immunol* 1995; **107:** 295–7.
52. Pauli G, Oster JP, Deviller P et al. Skin testing with recombinant allergens rBet v 1 and birch profillin, rBet v 2: diagnostic value for birch pollen and associated allergies. *J Allergy Clin Immunol* 1996; **97:** 1100–9.
53. Laffer S, Spitzauer S, Susani M et al. Comparison of recombinant timothy grass pollen allergens with natural extract for diagnosis of grass pollen allergy in different populations. *J Allergy Clin Immunol* 1996; **98:** 652–8.
54. Van Ree R, van Leeuwen WA, Aalberse RC. How far can we simplify in vitro diagnosis for grass pollen allergy? A study with 17 whole pollen extracts and purified natural and recombinant major allergens. *J Allergy Clin Immunol* 1998; **102:** 184–90.
55. Crameri R. Recombinant *Aspergillus fumigatus* allergens: from the nucleotide sequences to clinical applications. *Int Arch Allergy Immunol* 1998; **115:** 99–114.
56. Norman PS, Ohman JL, Long AA et al. Treatment of cat allergy with T cell reactive peptides. *Am J Respir Crit Care Med* 1996; **154:** 1623–8.
57. Creticos PS, Hebert J, Philip G, Allervax Ragweed Study Group. Efficacy of Allervax ragweed peptides in the treatment of ragweed induced allergy [abstract]. *J Allergy Clin Immunol* 1997; **99:** S401.
58. Smith AM, Chapman MD. Allergen specific immunotherapy: new strategies using recombinant allergens. In Bousquet J, Yssel H, eds. *Immunotherapy for Asthma*. New York: Marcel Dekker, 1998, pp. 99–118.
59. Takai T, Toyokazu Y, Yasue M et al. Engineering of the major house dust mite allergen Der f 2 for allergen-specific immunotherapy. *Nature Biotechnology* 1997; **15:** 754–8.
60. Van Hage-Hamsten M, Kronqvisy M, Zetterstrom O et al. Skin test evaluation of genetically engineered hypoallergenic derivatives of the major birch pollen allergen, Bet v 1: results obtained with a mix of two recombinant Bet v 1 fragments and recombinant Bet v 1 trimer in a Swedish population before the birch pollen season. *J Allergy Clin Immunol* 1999; **104:** 969–77.

61. Smith AM, Chapman MD. Reduction in IgE binding to allergen variants generated by site-directed mutagenesis: contribution of disulfide bonds to the antigenic structure of the major house dust mite allergen, Der p 2. *Mol Immunol* 1996; **33**: 399–405.
62. Hsu CH, Chua KY, Tao MH et al. Immunoprophylaxis of allergen induced immunoglobulin E synthesis and airway hyperresponsiveness in vivo by genetic immunization. *Nature Medicine* 1996; **2**: 540–4.
63. Raz E, Tighe H, Sato Y et al. Preferential induction of a Th1 immune response and inhibition of specific IgE antibody formation by plasmid DNA immunization. *Proc Natl Acad Sci USA* 1996; **93**: 5141–5.
64. Sato Y, Roman M, Tighe H et al. Immunostimulatory DNA sequences necessary for effective intradermal gene immunization. *Science* 1996; **273**: 352–4.
65. Roman M, Martin-Orozco E, Goodman JS et al. Immunostimulatory DNA sequences function as T helper-1-promoting adjuvants. *Nature Medicine* 1997; **3**: 849–54.
66. Broide D, Schwarze J, Tighe H et al. Immunostimulatory DNA sequences inhibit IL-5, eosinophilic inflammation, and airway hyperresponsiveness in mice. *J Immunol* 1998; **161**: 7054–62.
67. van Uden J, Raz E. Immunostimulatory DNA and applications to allergic disease. *J Allergy Clin Immunol* 1999; **104**: 902–10.
68. Voorhost R, Spieksma FThM, Varekamp H et al. The house dust mite (*Dermatophagoides pteronyssinus*) and the allergens it produces: identity with the house dust allergen. *J Allergy* 1967; **39**: 325–39.
69. Asturias JA, Arilla MC, Gomez-Bayon N et al. Sequencing and high level expression in *Escherichia coli* of the tropomyosin allergen (Der p 10) from *Dermatophagoides pteronyssinus*. *Biochim Biophys Acta* 1998; **1397**: 27–30.
70. Aki T, Kodama T, Fujikawa A et al. Immunochemical characterization of recombinant and native tropomyosin as a new allergen from the house dust mite, *Dermatophagoides farinae*. *J Allergy Clin Immunol* 1995; **96**: 74–83.
71. Lake FR, Ward LD, Simpson RJ et al. House dust mite derived amylase: allergenicity and physicochemical characterization. *J Allergy Clin Immunol* 1991; **81**: 1035–42.
72. O'Neill G, Donovan GR, Baldo BA. Identification of a major allergen of the house dust mite *Dermatophagoides pteronyssinus*, homologous with glutathione-S-transferase. *Biochim Biophys Acta* 1994; **1219**: 521–4.
73. Thomas WR, Chua KY. The major mite allergen Der p 2—a secretion of the male mite reproductive tract. *Clin Exp Allergy* 1995; **25**: 667–9.
74. Mueller GA, Smith AM, Williams DC et al. Expression and secondary structure determination by NMR methods of the major house dust mite allergen Der p 2. *J Biol Chem* 1997; **272**: 26893–8.
75. Tovey ER, Johnson MC, Roche AL et al. Cloning and sequencing of a cDNA expressing a recombinant house dust mite protein that binds human IgE and corresponds to an important low molecular weight allergen. *J Exp Med* 1989; **170**: 1457–62.
76. Kin KL, Chua KY, Thomas WR et al. Characterization of Der p V allergen. cDNA analysis and IgE mediated reactivity to the recombinant protein. *J Allergy Clin Immunol* 1994; **94**: 989–96.
77. Shen H-D, Chua KY, Lin WI et al. Molecular cloning and immunological characterization of the house dust mite allergen Der f 7. *Clin Exp Allergy* 1995; **25**: 1000–6.
78. Arruda LK, Chapman MD. A review of recent immunochemical studies of *Blomia tropicalis* and *Euroglyphus maynei* allergens. *Exp Appl Acarol* 1992; **16**: 129–40.
79. Smith W, Mills KL, Hazell LA et al. Molecular analysis of the groups 1 and 2 allergens from the house dust mite, *Euroglyphus maynei*. *Int Arch Allergy Immunol* 1999; **118**: 15–22.
80. Mills KL, Hart BJ, Lynch NR et al. Molecular characterization of the Group 4 house dust mite allergen from *Dermatophagoides pteronyssinus* and its amylase homologue from *Euroglyphus maynei*. *Int Arch Allergy Immunol* 1999; **120**: 100–7.
81. Johansson E, Eriksson TL, Olsson S et al. Evaluation of specific IgE to the recombinant group 2 mite allergens Lep d 2 and Tyr p 2 in the Pharmacia CAP system. *Int Arch Allergy Immunol* 1999; **120**: 43–9.
82. Bernton H, Brown H. Insect allergy—preliminary studies of the cockroach. *J Allergy* 1964; **35**: 506–13.
83. Chapman MD, Vailes LD, Hayden ML, Platts-Mills TAE, Arruda LK. Cockroach allergens and their role in asthma. In: Kay AB, ed. *Allergy and Allergic Diseases*. Oxford: Blackwell Science, 1996.

84. Kang B, Vellody D, Homburger H, Yunginger JW. Cockroach as a cause of allergic asthma. Its specificity and immunologic profile. *J Allergy Clin Immunol* 1979; **63**: 80–6.
85. Gold DR, Burge HA, Carey V et al. Predictors of repeated wheeze in the first year of life. *Am J Respir Crit Care Med* 1999; **160**: 227–36.
86. Schou C, Lind P, Fernandez-Caldas E, Lockey RF, Lowenstein H. Identification and purification of an important cross-reactive allergen from American and German cockroach. *J Allergy Clin Immunol* 1990; **86**: 935–46.
87. Pomés A, Melén E, Vailes LD et al. Novel allergen structures with tandem amino acid repeats derived from the German and American cockroach. *J Biol Chem* 1998; **273**: 30801–7.
88. Helm R, Cockrell G, Stanley JS et al. Isolation and characterization of a clone encoding a major allergen (*Bla g* Bd90K) involved in IgE-mediated cockroach hypersensitivity. *J Allergy Clin Immunol* 1996; **98**: 172–80.
89. Melén E, Vailes LD, Pomes A et al. Molecular cloning of Per a 1 and definition of the cross-reactive Group 1 cockroach allergens. *J Allergy Clin Immunol* 1999; **103**: 859–64.
90. Arruda LK, Vailes LD, Hayden ML et al. Cloning of cockroach allergen, Bla g 4, identifies ligand binding proteins (or calycins) as a cause of IgE antibody responses. *J Biol Chem* 1995; **270**: 31196–201.
91. Longbottom JL. Purification and characterization of allergens from the urine of mice and rats. In: Oehling A, Glazer I, Mathov E, Arbesman E, eds. *Advances in Allergology and Applied Immunology*. Oxford: Pergamon Press, 1980, 483–90.
92. Bocskei Z, Groom CR, Flower DR et al. Pheromone binding to two rodent urinary proteins revealed by X-ray crystallography. *Nature* 1992; **360**: 186–8.
93. Koneiczny A, Morgenstern JP, Bizinkauskas CB et al. The major dog allergens, Can f 1 and Can f 2, are salivary lipocalin proteins: cloning and immunological characterization of the recombinant forms. *Immunology* 1997; **92**: 577–86.
94. Flower DR, North ACT, Attwood TK. Structure and sequence relationships in the lipocalins and related proteins. *Protein Science* 1993; **2**: 753–61.
95. Mantyjarvi R, Parkkinen S, Rytkonen M et al. Complementary DNA cloning of the predominant allergen of bovine dander: a new member in the lipocalin family. *J Allergy Clin Immunol* 1996; **97**: 1297–303.
96. Gregoire C, Rosinski-Chupin I, Robillon J et al. cDNA cloning and sequencing reveal the major horse allergen Equ c 1 to be a glycoprotein member of the lipocalin superfamily. *J Biol Chem* 1996; **271**: 32951–9.
97. Vailes LD, Kinter MT, Arruda LK, Chapman MD. High-level expression of cockroach allergen, Bla g 4, in *Pichia pastoris*. *J Allergy Clin Immunol* 1998; **101**: 274–80.
98. Arruda LK, Vailes LD, Platts-Mills TAE et al. Induction of IgE antibody responses by glutathione-S-transferase from the German cockroach (*Blattella germanica*). *J Biol Chem* 1997; **272**: 20907–12.
99. Wu CH, Lee MF, Liao SC, Luo SF. Sequence analysis of cDNA clones encoding the American cockroach Cr-PI allergens. *J Biol Chem* 1996; **271**: 17937–43.
100. Santos ABR, Chapman MD, Aalberse et al. Cockroach allergens and asthma in Brazil: identification of tropomyosin as a major allergen with potential cross-reactivity with mite and shrimp allergens. *J Allergy Clin Immunol* 1999; **104**: 329–37.
101. Reese G, Ayuso R, Lehrer SB. Tropomyosin: an invertebrate pan-allergen. *Int Arch Allergy Immunol* 1999; **119**: 247–58.
102. Chapman MD, Vailes LD, Arruda LK et al. Source characterization and molecular structure of cockroach allergens. *Rev Française d'Allergol* 1998; **38**: 842–5.
103. De Lucca S, Taylor DJM, O'Meara TJ et al. Measurement and characterization of cockroach allergens detected during normal domestic activity. *J Allergy Clin Immunol* 1999; **104**: 672–80.
104. Williams LW, Reinfried P, Brenner RJ. Cockroach extermination does not rapidly reduce allergen in settled dust. *J Allergy Clin Immunol* 1999; **104**: 702–3.
105. Eggleston PA, Wood RA, Rand C et al. Removal of cockroach allergen from inner city homes. *J Allergy Clin Immunol* 1999; **104**: 842–6.
106. Gergen PJ, Mortimer KM, Eggleston PA et al. Results of the National Cooperative Inner-City Asthma Study (NCICAS) environmental intervention to reduce cockroach allergen exposure in inner-city homes. *J Allergy Clin Immunol* 1999; **103**: 501–6.
107. Morgenstern JP, Griffith IJ, Brauer AW et al. Determination of the amino acid sequence of Fel d 1, the major allergen of the domestic cat: protein sequence analysis and cDNA cloning.

Proc Nat Acad Sci USA 1991; **88:** 9690–4.
108. Ichikawa K, Iwasaki E, Baba M, Chapman MD. High prevalence of sensitization to cat allergen among Japanese children with asthma, living without cats. *Clin Exp Allergy* 1999; **29:** 754–61.
109. Perzanowski MS, Ronmark E, Nold B et al. Relevance of allergens from cats and dogs to asthma in the northernmost province of Sweden: schools as a major site of exposure. *J Allergy Clin Immunol* 1999; **103:** 1018–24.
110. Almqvist C, Larsson PH, Egmar AC et al. School as a risk environment for children allergic to cats and a site for transfer of cat allergen to homes. *J Allergy Clin Immunol* 1999; **103:** 1012–17.
111. van't Hoff W, Blankenvoorde MFJ, Veerman ECI, Nieuw Amerongen AV. The salivary Lipocalin von Ebner's gland protein is a cysteine proteinase inhibitor. *J Biol Chem* 1997; **272:** 1837–41.
112. Chapman MD, Ichikawa K, Vailes LD. Molecular cloning of a new cat allergen, cystatin, a cysteine protease inhibitor [abstract]. *J Allergy Clin Immunol* 1999; **103:** S122.
113. Rizzo MC, Naspitz CK, Fernandez-Caldas E et al. Endotoxin exposure and symptoms in asthmatic children. *Pediatr Allergy Immunol* 1997; **8:** 121–6.
114. Solomon WR, Platts-Mills TAE. Aerobiology and inhalant allergens. In: Middleton E Jr, Reed CE, Ellis EF, Adkinson NF Jr, Yunginger JW, Busse WW, eds. *Allergy: Principles and Practice* 5th edn. St Louis: Mosby Year Book, Inc, 1998, 367–403.
115. Nelson HS. The importance of allergens in the development of asthma and persistence of symptoms. *J Allergy Clin Immunol* 2000; **105:** S628–S632.
116. Hill D, Smart IJ, Knox RB. Childhood asthma and grass pollen aerobiology in Melbourne. *Med J Austr* 1979; **1:** 426–9.
117. Reid MJ, Moss RB, Hsu YP, Kwasnicki JM. Seasonal asthma in northern California: allergic causes and efficacy of immunotherapy. *J Allergy Clin Immunol* 1986; **78:** 590–602.
118. Potter PC, Cadman A. Pollen allergy in South Africa. *Clin Exp Allergy* 1996; **26:** 1347–54.
119. Charpin D, Birnbaum J, Haddi E et al. Altitude and allergy to house dust mites: a paradigm of the influence of environmental exposure on allergy sensitization. *Am Rev Respir Dis* 1991; **143:** 983–6.
120. Pollart SM, Reed M, Brown M et al. Epidemiology of emergency room asthma in northern California: association with IgE antibody to rye grass pollen. *J Allergy Clin Immunol* 1989; **82:** 224–30.
121. Djukanovic R, Feather I, Gratziou C et al. Effect of natural allergen exposure during grass pollen season on airway inflammatory cells and asthma symptoms. *Thorax* 1996; **51:** 575–81.
122. Baraldi E, Carra S, Dario C et al. Effect of natural grass pollen exposure on exhaled nitric oxide in asthmatic children. *Am J Respir Crit Care Med* 1999; **159:** 262–6.
123. Valenta R, Kraft D. Type 1 allergic reactions to plant-derived food: a consequence of primary sensitization to pollen allergens. *J Allergy Clin Immunol* 1996; **97:** 893–5.
124. Fritsch R, Bohle B, Vollman U et al. Bet v 1, the major birch pollen allergen, and Mal d 1, the major apple allergen, cross-react at the level of allergen-specific T helper cells. *J Allergy Clin Immunol* 1998; **102:** 679–86.
125. Halonen M, Stern DA, Wright A et al. Alternaria as the major allergen for asthma in children raised in a desert environment. *Am J Respir Crit Care Med* 1997; **155:** 1356–61.
126. Perzanowski M, Sporik R, Squillace SP et al. Sensitization to *Alternaria* as a risk factor for asthma in school-age children. *J Allergy Clin Immunol* 1998; **101:** 626–32.
127. O'Hollaren MT, Yunginger JW, Offord KP et al. Exposure to an aeroallergen as a possible precipitating factor in respiratory arrest in young patients with asthma. *N Engl J Med* 1991; **324:** 359–63.
128. Arruda LK, Mann BJ, Chapman MD. Selective expression of a major allergen and cytotoxin, Asp f 1, in *Aspergillus fumigatus*: implications for the immunopathogenesis of Aspergillus related diseases. *J Immunol* 1992; **149:** 3354–9.
129. Achatz G, Oberkofler H, Lechenauer E et al. Molecular cloning of major and minor allergens of *Alternaria alternata* and *Cladosporium herbarum*. *Mol Immunol* 1995; **32:** 213–27.
130. Bush RK, Sanchez H, Geisler D. Molecular cloning of a major *Alternaria alternata* allergen, Alt a 2. *J Allergy Clin Immunol* 1999; **104:** 665–71.
131. Horner WE, Helbling A, Lehrer SB. Basidiomycete allergens. *Allergy* 1998; **53:** 1114–21.
132. Hemmann S, Menz G, Ismail C et al. Skin test reactivity to 2 recombinant *Aspergillus fumigatus* allergens in *A. fumigatus*-sensitized asthmatic subjects allows separation of allergic bron-

chopulmonary aspergillosis from fungal sensitization. *J Allergy Clin Immunol* 1999; **104:** 601–7.
133. Tovey E, Marks G. Methods and effectiveness of environment control. *J Allergy Clin Immunol* 1999; **103:** 179–91.
134. Adkinson NF Jr, Eggleston PA, Eney D et al. A controlled trial of immunotherapy for asthma in allergic children. *N Engl J Med* 1997; **336:** 324–31.
135. Bousquet J, Lockey R, Malling HJ et al. Allergen immunotherapy: therapeutic vaccines for allergic diseases. A WHO position paper. *J Allergy Clin Immunol* 1998; **102:** 558–62.

14
Food allergy and asthma in children

S Allan Bock, Hugh A Sampson

Introduction • Prevalence • Differential diagnosis • Respiratory symptoms • Timing of symptoms • Mechanisms • Historical information • Laboratory testing • Management • Natural history and prevention • Future considerations

INTRODUCTION

Observations over the last three decades have markedly advanced the scientific study of food allergy. Studies from several centers have begun to shed light on the mechanisms of disease, clinical features of the illness, diagnostic tests, and the natural history of food hypersensitivity. We now have a better understanding of the role of food hypersensitivity in asthma. This chapter will explore the more recent studies in this discipline and offer the reader an approach that may be employed to determine the likelihood that food hypersensitivity is involved in the asthma process of any individual patient. The entire area of food hypersensitivity has recently been reviewed by Sampson in two excellent and detailed articles.[1,2]

PREVALENCE

How much do we really know about the prevalence of food hypersensitivity and of food hypersensitivity in asthma in particular? A large number of Americans believe that they have food hypersensitivity.[3] However, true food hypersensitivity is most prevalent in young children and individuals with atopic diseases. A study of 480 consecutively born children, followed until their third birthday, found that 28% had an adverse reaction to food.[4] Most of these occurred during the first year of life. However, only about 8% of the total group had adverse reactions that could be confirmed by food challenge. Almost all of these were gone by the third birthday and only a very few had associated IgE identified by skin testing. Other prospective studies from around the world suggest that about 2.5% of newborn children experience food hypersensitivity reactions to milk during the first year of life. In a Dutch study,[5] it was found that about 2% of the adult population had experienced adverse food reactions. A recent random digit dial survey in the US found that about 1.1% of the population (adults and children) had experienced adverse (probably allergic) reactions to peanuts and tree nuts.[6] Thus it is clear that we do not have firm numbers to assign to the prevalence of food hypersensitivity.

Homing in on the prevalence of food hypersensitivity in asthma is even more difficult. In 1986, Onorato and colleagues[7] studied 300 consecutive asthmatic subjects from 7 months to 80 years from a respiratory diseases clinic. This was a well-controlled study with the subjects undergoing double-blind, placebo-controlled food challenges (DBPCFC). Of the 300 subjects, 25 were thought to have food hypersensitivity triggering asthma, but only six (2% of the population) actually had a positive challenge. The age range of the six was 4–17 years. Half of these individuals had a reaction to at least one food in which wheezing was the only symptom, whereas the other half had additional symptoms involving the gastrointestinal tract or skin. The foods producing positive challenges were egg, wheat and corn.

Novembre et al.[8] investigated 140 children who presented histories of food-induced asthma. These children were also challenged using DBPCFC procedures. Wheezing was reproduced in eight (6%) of the children and their ages were 2–9 years. Only one of these subjects had wheezing as the sole symptom of the food reaction.

Other populations of children, primarily with atopic dermatitis, have been found to have wheezing produced during the challenges even when asthma is not a prominent part of the history. In a population of very young children, Hill et al.[9] found three different patterns of responsiveness, all based upon the timing of symptom occurrence. In the group having immediate reactions, 29% had lower airway symptoms; in the group having intermediate onset symptoms, 4% had lower airway symptoms; and in the most delayed onset group, 50% had lower airway symptoms. In this entire group the food responsible for all the reactions was milk. Exactly how these observations and percentages translate into the general population remains to be determined.

Another study examined a highly selected population of asthmatic children evaluated in a tertiary referral center.[10] There were 410 children with a history of asthma and of these 279 (68%) presented a history of one or more foods triggering asthma. All 279 underwent DBPCFC for the suspected foods; 168 (60%) had some symptom (gastrointestinal, cutaneous, respiratory) elicited during challenge. Of the 168 reacting, 67 (40%) experienced wheezing as one of the symptoms. Most of the subjects had other respiratory symptoms as well. Only five (3% of 168) subjects had wheezing as the only symptom.

What can the practitioner conclude about the prevalence of food hypersensitivity in asthma patients? Food-associated wheezing is uncommon but not rare, and therefore the history must be used to determine whether pursuit of food hypersensitivity as a trigger of asthma is warranted. The problem is more likely to occur in younger children but may occur in adults, and it is more likely to be associated with cutaneous or gastrointestinal symptoms than to occur as the sole symptom of a food-associated reaction. The precise approach to asthmatics who may have food hypersensitivity is considered in a later section.

DIFFERENTIAL DIAGNOSIS

A number of classification systems and definitions have been applied to the subject of adverse reactions to foods over the years, and a number of terms that do not have specific biochemical mechanisms have been associated with these classifications. Such terms as 'pharmacologic reaction' and 'idiosyncratic reaction' do not have precise definitions. Carbohydrate intolerance, which is very important in the differential diagnosis of adverse food reactions in the intestine, is not pertinent to the lung.

A useful classification divides adverse food reactions into toxic and non-toxic categories (Table 14.1). The non-toxic categories contain the immune-associated reactions to food, both IgE and non-IgE. It is important to have a classification scheme that includes a category to cover reactions owing to strongly held beliefs of both patients and some practitioners. It is crucial for the practitioner to understand strongly held beliefs about how foods may affect asthma, because many asthma patients alter their diets in order to avoid foods that they think trigger asthma. (The milk and mucus connection is the most notorious.) The nutritional implications of these dietary alterations and

Table 14.1 Classification of adverse reactions to food

Toxic	Non-toxic
Non-immune	Immune
Food poisoning	IgE-associated
Pharmacologic	Non-IgE-associated

exclusions need to be understood and patients should be questioned about them.

RESPIRATORY SYMPTOMS

Respiratory symptoms (Table 14.2), including wheezing and cough, are frequently attributed to food hypersensitivity. However, as noted above, asthma as the sole manifestation of an adverse food reaction is relatively unusual. More likely is the appearance of wheezing with other respiratory symptoms and with gastrointestinal and/or cutaneous symptoms.

An important presentation of food-induced lower airway symptoms is the occurrence of anaphylaxis. It is important to note that food-associated anaphylaxis can appear in the absence of any other symptoms, including urticaria and angioedema. It cannot be too strongly stressed that laryngospasm or bronchospasm may be the only manifestation of food-associated anaphylaxis. Frequently a good history of an isolated food ingestion and a positive skin test will confirm the diagnosis of food-associated anaphylaxis.

The other patterns of food-associated wheezing are less obvious and need more rigorous evaluation. In children who wheeze frequently, foods are often removed haphazardly from the diet in hopes of reducing the asthma frequency and severity. Other children with a similar problem (and an atopic constitution) often have many skin tests or radioallergosorbest tests (RASTs) performed and then all those foods for which there is a positive test are removed from the diet. Arbitrary elimination of culprit foods with no end point and no challenges are another means by which foods are removed from asthmatic individuals' diets. The problem with all of these approaches is that in the absence of clear proof that the food is causing symptoms, the diet is adhered to intermittently. Usually these diets are counter-productive and further inhibit the normal functioning of children with asthma (Table 14.3).

TIMING OF SYMPTOMS

At present, the vast majority of proven food-associated asthma episodes occur within minutes (up to a couple of hours) after ingestion of food. DBPCFC studies invariably confirm this rapid onset, but the same studies have failed to confirm delayed (hours to days) reactions.[11-14]

Table 14.2 Respiratory symptoms and signs

Nose:	rhinorrhea, congestion, sneezing, nasal pruritis
Throat:	laryngospasm, laryngeal edema
Lung:	cough, wheeze, breathlessness, chest tightness, mucus production

Table 14.3 Histories employed to exclude foods from the diet

Anaphylaxis
Immediate onset symptom
Elimination diets based upon historical observations
Elimination diets based upon skin testing and RAST
Elimination diets based upon the generic list

Some of the histories cited in the section above are clearly vague and usually unconfirmable when the details are sought. One exception to these results are the well-characterized subjects reported by Hill et al.[9] Thus far a similar population has not been reported, and these data need to be confirmed in other groups, using objective techniques.

It is not unreasonable to assume that late phase reactions in the lung could occur following food challenges. Perhaps with more sophisticated sampling techniques these reactions will be confirmed. In fact, Atkins et al.[15] probably did trigger a late phase reaction in a subject during DBPCFC with cottonseed protein. However, treatment with bronchodilators after the immediate reactions makes the data from this single subject difficult to interpret. The data from this subject are tantalizing because they appear to confirm the late phase reaction (owing to food) hypothesis during a controlled DBPCFC.

MECHANISMS

The exact mechanism by which food-allergy-associated asthma occurs has not been determined but research is moving closer to some answers providing insight into the immune processes.[1,2] During food challenges lower airway symptoms are often produced in conjunction with upper respiratory, gastrointestinal, and cutaneous symptoms. The timing of these reactions clearly suggests the activity of IgE-associated immediate hypersensitivity. However, it also seems likely that typical late phase reactions may be initiated by the immediate reaction. It is postulated that ingested food proteins are absorbed sufficiently intact to circulate through the cardiovascular system to reach immune cells that recognize these proteins.[16] James et al.[17] studied a population of 320 children with food allergy, asthma, and atopic dermatitis. Of this group 205 children exhibited reactions during 567 positive DBPCFCs. In this highly atopic population it was found that 27% of positive food challenges precipitated pulmonary symptoms. These youngsters all had strong evidence of IgE-associated responses. As mentioned earlier, Atkins[15] has demonstrated a probable biphasic reaction in an adult who reacted strongly to cottonseed protein during a double-blind placebo-controlled food challenge. Zwetchkenbaum et al.[18] sought evidence of increased bronchial responsiveness to methacholine challenge in adults following double-blind, placebo-controlled food challenge. Although there were changes in the airway reactivity following food challenges in some subjects, they were not different than in the placebo-challenged group. James et al.[19] performed a similar study in children and found significant changes in airway reactivity following methacholine challenges in some of their food-allergic asthmatic subjects. This study reported two intriguing findings. One finding was that chest symptoms (cough and/or wheezing) appeared in individuals whose forced expiratory volume in 1 second (FEV_1) did not change. The second finding was that some individuals exhibited an increase in methacholine sensitivity despite not having any chest symptoms during the double-blind placebo-controlled food challenge.

Taken together, how should these studies be viewed? It seems relatively clear that most individuals with asthma do not have food-associated symptoms. Those with food-associated asthmatic responses should be relatively easy to identify by taking a thorough history and by being concerned about subjects who have severe asthma that is difficult to control. There may be a subpopulation of subjects who have an increase in airway reactivity following ingestion of some foods. The important question is whether their asthma control is more difficult or whether they require more medication because of regular exposure to these foods. Although this remains an important question in some patients with severe asthma, it seems unlikely that there are large numbers of these individuals.

HISTORICAL INFORMATION

In order to determine, unequivocally, that a food is triggering lower airway obstruction, the

DBPCFC remains the standard against which all other tests are measured. A thorough history is required so that the challenges can be designed. The details that must be ascertained may be acquired quickly and with directed questioning. Table 14.4 presents the list of important facts. The questions must be detailed enough to determine whether the food under suspicion has actually been eaten in other forms. Often individuals who claim to be on a dairy-product-free diet are consuming dairy-containing foods in sufficient quantity to eliminate dairy as the source of reaction. The vast majority of milk-allergic youngsters will also react to goat's milk.[20] Many individuals claiming to be wheat allergic are consuming spelt, a grain that is recognized by the immune system as identical to wheat. The least amount of food which has triggered a reaction is an important piece of information so that a starting dose for a challenge may be selected and safely administered.

Table 14.4 Historical facts to be ascertained

Description of symptoms in sequence if possible
Time from ingestion of food to onset of symptoms
Most recent occurrence
Number of occasions upon which reaction to the food has occurred
Smallest quantity thought to have produced symptoms
Associated factors such as exercise

LABORATORY TESTING

In vivo testing

Skin testing
At present, skin testing for food hypersensitivity remains a very useful technique. Studies from major centers have demonstrated that prick/puncture skin testing, using allergen extracts of concentrations of 1:10 to 1:20 weight/volume, is a very accurate means of detecting IgE antibody to food.[21-23] However, it is crucial to recognize, and to explain to patients, that skin tests for food (or any allergen) do not make a diagnosis of allergy, they only detect antibody. Recognition of the fact that positive skin test responses are necessary but not sufficient to make a diagnosis of food hypersensitivity is extremely important in both understanding and explaining to patients that they may have a positive skin test but still be able to ingest some foods without experiencing symptoms.

Skin tests to be performed should be based upon the patient's histories. Rarely is a large panel of food skin tests required or desirable, especially in the evaluation of food-allergy-associated asthma. Food skin tests are primarily useful because of their high negative predictive accuracy. For the major food allergens: milk, wheat, egg, peanut, tree nuts, and usually soy, the negative skin test, in children over 3 years of age and in adults, almost always indicates that the food will not cause symptoms when placed into the diet. (Of course, skin test material, like any other reagent, must be validated by being found to detect antibody in a subject known to be sensitized to that food.) For most fruits and vegetables, skin testing with both commercial materials and fresh foods is highly desirable and will increase the utility of food skin testing.[24]

Although we have stressed the concept that food skin tests do not make a diagnosis of food allergy, there is one situation where the food skin test is almost never incorrect when it is positive. In the case of an isolated food ingestion, with prompt onset symptoms and no other possible explanations, the positive food skin test does confirm the diagnosis. It will be rare that this scenario will lead to the unnecessary removal of a food from the diet.

Labial testing/challenge
It has been suggested that foods applied to the oral mucosa and/or to the lip will be sensitive

enough to accurately diagnose food hypersensitivity and eliminate the need for food challenges.[25] Individuals experiencing oral symptoms from a food will almost always cease eating it immediately. They often remove the food from their mouths. Further research in this area may well confirm this observation. However, some individuals have been found to have oral symptoms from food contact with oral tissues, but not to react if the food is ingested when mixed with another food. (This may also be observed when food challenges are administered using capsules.) Some individuals reacting with oral symptoms may not have systemic symptoms if the food continues to be consumed.[26]

In vitro testing

For many years, the available in-vitro testing methods (radioallergosorbent testing and plasma histamine release) have been found to be about as sensitive as skin testing and much more expensive and time consuming. Now we are beginning to see the evaluation of a new type of RAST, the CAP FEIA and UNI CAP, which for the first time may allow diagnosis of food allergy without performing challenges. Sampson and Ho[27] have found that for four foods they were able to predict with high certainty whether a patient is highly likely or highly unlikely to have a food reaction. (The foods are: milk, egg, peanut, and fish. See Table 14.5.) Efforts to establish levels that are predictive (positive or negative) for other foods are underway. The major caveat, at this time, is that the levels established thus far have been observed in children with significant atopic dermatitis. Just how well these levels apply to subjects with less severe atopic dermatitis or without atopic dermatitis remains to be determined. (For peanuts, it would appear that the high cut-off levels are valid in children with less severe or no atopic dermatitis (Bock, unpublished observations).)

Table 14.5 CAP values suggesting a highly probable reaction

Food	PPV >95% kUA/l	PPV >90% kUA/l
Egg	6	2
Milk	32	23
Peanuts	16	9
Fish	20	9.5
Soy	Best PPV = 50% at 65 IU/ml	
Wheat	Best PPV = 75% at 100 IU/ml	

PPV = Positive predictive accuracy.[28]

Food challenges

In 1973, May[11] first began to systematically apply DBPCFC to the investigation of adverse food reactions in children. This technique has become the gold standard against which all other procedures and laboratory techniques are compared. No matter what the mechanism may be, the blinded food challenge will reliably and unequivocally confirm or refute the role of a food in the production of symptoms. This procedure also gives investigators a tremendously useful tool for evaluating the effectiveness of new therapies that may be applied to the treatment of food hypersensitivity. The fact that we can 'see what we eat' has been both the curse and the crutch of the study of food hypersensitivity. For difficult problems such as delayed reactions to food that patients claim as a trigger of their asthma, the arrangements require more ingenuity but the observations may still be made with a substantial degree of certainty.

Open food challenge

Open food challenges are very useful to refute vague and uncertain histories of adverse food reactions producing asthma. If an individual has stable asthma (on or off medication) and foods excluded from the diet are reintroduced without producing symptoms, the problem has been solved without additional or elaborate effort. These challenges may safely be performed in a physician's office or medical clinic. They are not used for subjects with histories suggesting severe reactions or anaphylaxis. Frequently patients report that they are avoiding certain foods but they are eating other foods that contain the incriminated food. The open challenge can quickly restore these suspected foods to the diet.

Single-blind food challenges (SBFC)

Single-blind food challenges are useful because the bias of the subject is eliminated, but the arrangements are somewhat easier to design than the double-blind placebo-controlled food challenge. SBFC may be used to document the absence of symptoms, particularly in situations where it may be desirable to refute a history of vague or subjective symptoms but where the subject has a strongly held opinion that the challenge will be positive. Single-blind challenges may also be useful in certain research protocols for selection of subjects who will then participate in the double-blind phase of a study. In many clinical settings the SBFC is a very practical technique for helping patients determine which foods from a long list are actually causing symptoms.

Double-blind, placebo-controlled food challenge

The goal of the double-blind, placebo-controlled food challenge is to reproduce the patient's history as it was presented. This is why the acquisition of an accurate history with respect to dosage and timing becomes so crucial (Table 14.4). The challenge must be designed to provide the optimal opportunity to reproduce or refute the reported symptoms. At present, there are several protocols that are used for the administration of double-blind food challenges (Table 14.6).[28] One of the best approaches is to

Table 14.6 Food challenge protocols

Single day for each active food and another day for placebo
Intersperse active food doses with placebo doses
Challenge in the morning (active food or placebo) and afternoon (placebo or active food)
Morning challenge for several consecutive days
Multiple challenge doses on multiple days (must be crossed over several times)

have a single day for the active food challenge and a separate day for administration of the placebo doses. Time constraints have resulted in protocols that administer both challenges on the same day, one in the morning (active or placebo) and the other in the afternoon (placebo or active). This is an acceptable approach for immediate onset symptoms so that the morning challenge may be consumed over a period of about 2–3 hours and then there can be an interval of more than 2 hours before the afternoon challenge commences. The afternoon challenge then follows the same procedure. The only potential limitation of this approach is that slow or delayed onset symptoms could be missed or cause confusion. If this occurs then the challenge must be repeated using separate active food and placebo days. In some instances the actual use of placebo may be omitted because multiple foods are being tested blindly and the other foods may serve as placebos as long as at least one food challenge is negative.

When evaluating subjective chest symptoms, it is useful to intersperse the active and placebo doses. This may be done randomly but the whole challenge is ingested on the same day. Thus the subject will be ingesting different numbers of challenge doses at different times in a seemingly random manner. (Using capsules as the vehicle makes this procedure relatively easy to accomplish.) Patients who complain of a tight chest or exhibit cough not accompanied by a change in lung function may be aided in drawing their own conclusions about food reactions by demonstrating to them that they feel the same whether ingesting the active or placebo substance.

As noted above, the dose and timing are determined by the history. By current convention the starting dose is usually about one-half of the amount that is thought to be the minimum amount likely to produce an immediate onset adverse reaction. Some studies use a more specific dosing protocol so that each subject ingests the same dose at the same intervals. This approach is useful for investigating immediate onset reactions; however, there are multiple approaches that may work well, depending on the reactions being investigated.

The timing of administration of each dose is scheduled so that the interval between doses is slightly longer than the time predicted by the history for a reaction to occur. The doses are doubled at the chosen interval. When the challenge is negative, up to 8–10 g dried food (single dose) or 60–100 g wet food, then the challenge is stopped, and the results are presented to the patient and/or parents. The final step is the undisguised ingestion of the food in usual portions. If this portion is consumed without symptoms then the food challenge is negative and the food is reintroduced into the diet.

The ability of the subject to ingest the incriminated food(s) without developing symptoms will eliminate many of the frequently posed questions about the effect of food preparation, digestion, and other variables upon the blinded food challenge. A positive open challenge after a negative blinded challenge is most likely to occur when the dose consumed during the blinded challenge is not high enough to trigger symptoms which then occur following a higher dose in the open challenge. Thus the dose–response threshold for a reaction is not exceeded during the blind challenge but it is surpassed during the open administration of the food. This circumstance is infrequently encountered in clinical practice or in research studies[26] (also HA Sampson, personal communication; AW Burks, personal communication).

Another major explanation for a negative blinded challenge accompanied by a positive open challenge is the subject's strongly held belief that food will cause symptoms. This concern is often not assuaged by the negative blinded challenge, and symptoms occur when the patient can see the food as it is being consumed.

A third explanation for a negative blind challenge and a positive open challenge is contact between the food and the patient's oral tissues which may not have occurred during the blinded challenge, especially if the vehicle used to hide the challenge food was capsules. Many of the earliest blinded challenge studies used capsules, which meant that local oral symptoms may not have been detected, since the capsules did not allow the food to contact the oral mucosa. The advantage of capsule use is that it allows challenges to determine whether systemic symptoms would occur in situations in which the challenge would have been halted owing to oral symptoms.

These procedures have been used successfully to study subjects with immediate onset symptoms. In fact the literature shows that very few delayed onset reactions have been confirmed except those found in the gastrointestinal tract. However, when individuals complain that chest symptoms are beginning hours to days after the ingestion of certain foods, the double-blind, placebo-controlled food challenge may be used to assess these subjects. These patients usually present one of two symptom/timing/dose patterns. The first is that a single dose of food causes symptoms hours to days after ingestion. In this situation the food is administered under observation in the morning and the subject is then asked to return when the symptoms commence. Use of the placebo is crucial and the challenge procedure should be 'crossed over' two or three times in order to ensure that the challenge is reproducible.

If the patient reports that the food must be ingested multiple times, especially over multiple days, then the only accurate means to accomplish a true double-blind, placebo-controlled food challenge is in a setting where administration of all the doses may be supervised and symptoms may be witnessed by an objective observer. For asthma subjects, the capability to check pulmonary function testing is crucial in order to scrutinize the development of subjective symptoms such as chest tightness or dyspnea. Even cough may be evaluated with increased accuracy using spirometry. It is possible to have the patient ingest challenges at home, but the food must be suitable for administration in a form that is difficult for the patient to discern or bias will not be eliminated. Frequent peak flow monitoring must be performed by the patient during these challenges. This procedure is most helpful when the challenge is negative. In the evaluation of young children thought to have food-allergy-induced wheezing/coughing, the only objective measurements for most clinicians is a stethoscope and evaluation of respiratory rates. With respect to chest complaints, it is unusual and infrequent to have to design challenges of delayed onset symptoms.

Numerous vehicles have been developed for performing food challenges. Capsules were the first regularly used vehicle and remain the best method for blinding; however, many foods are now used for masking challenges. Table 14.7 presents a list of currently used examples. At present the vehicle chosen is dependent upon the food under study and the quantity that must be administered.

MANAGEMENT

Avoidance and interval challenge

The current management of food hypersensitivity is elimination of those foods which have been found, preferably by DBPCFC, to produce symptoms. It must be stressed again that foods thought to be causing asthma must be confirmed as culprits as rigorously as possible. Unnecessary dietary elimination makes the quality of life of asthmatic subjects even more difficult than the disease itself. The importance of interval challenges must also be stressed. Unfortunately, we have not yet determined the optimal interval for all foods (see below). However, ongoing studies and the addition of quantitative in-vitro assays for specific antibodies will improve this process over time.

Different authors have proposed various time intervals for repeat challenges. These may vary from 1 to 3 months for young children with mild symptoms, up to 6–12 months for more significant reactions. Specific time intervals for individuals with food-associated asthma have not been as vigorously defined as for children with atopic dermatitis and with food-protein-induced gastrointestinal conditions.

Medication (to treat reactions, to prevent reactions)

Theoretically medication could be used to treat or to prevent food-allergic reactions triggering asthma symptoms. However, we have yet to find medication that can be safely used to allow the asthmatic individual to consume foods to which he or she is allergic. In fact, we believe that asthmatic subjects are at greater risk for severe reactions when they ingest a food to which they are allergic. In the future, molecules may be developed which are so effective at preventing allergic reactions that it may be possible for sensitized subjects to take these medications and eat foods to which they are allergic. This possibility is some years away.

It should be noted that several trials of oral

Table 14.7 Vehicles that may be useful in food challenges

Capsules	Hamburger
Infant formula	Tuna fish
Apple sauce	Ice cream (grape)
Neocate®	Popsicles
Milkshakes	Lentil soup
Chocolate pudding	Mashed potato
Tapioca fruit mixture	Cereal
Grape juice	Elecare®

disodium cromoglycate have been undertaken to test the notion that food reactions could be prevented by the regular ingestion of this medication. Unfortunately, the vast majority of these studies never demonstrated that the individuals actually had food hypersensitivity to the putative foods. The best controlled study of this hypothesis failed to detect any protective effect.[29] At present this putative approach to prevention cannot be recommended.

Similar suggestions have been made for pretreatment with antihistamines or their continuous use. No controlled studies have ever shown the efficacy of this approach. There are anecdotal reports of patients with asthma who have experienced exacerbations while taking antihistamines and ingesting dietary offenders. (All published food challenge studies have been performed when antihistamine medications have been omitted for days to weeks depending on the medication. We did elicit gastrointestinal but not chest symptoms in a child taking astemizole, during a DBPCFC.)

Oral steroids may be used in the treatment of certain food-induced reactions but not for their prevention or to allow symptom-provoking foods to be consumed. In subjects with eosinophilic gastrointestinal disease, oral steroids may be extremely helpful in gaining control of the disease and allowing time for the search for food allergens. This search should be exhaustive. In subjects with food-associated asthma who are taking oral steroids, wheezing may occur when food offenders are ingested. Thus steroids, as currently used, do not seem to be preventive.

There is a small subgroup of steroid-dependent asthmatic subjects in whom food hypersensitivity is an undiagnosed problem. Sampson and colleagues identified three steroid-dependent asthmatic individuals with multiple admission to the intensive care unit with status asthmaticus in whom food served as a trigger for their asthma (unpublished data). Identification of these patients is difficult and can only be accomplished with prolonged elimination diets. Although these patients appear to be rare, a possible food trigger should be sought when one is confronted with a patient with intractable asthma. The best starting place is probably an elimination diet. The duration necessary has not been entirely determined, but several weeks may be required. The nutritional adequacy of this elimination diet must be monitored by a nutritionist. It is an elemental diet with the addition of apples and chicken and perhaps rice. This is extremely difficult for the patient to endure and it takes a great deal of encouragement.

Medication treatment when a reaction does occur depends upon the severity of the reaction. Obviously, severe bronchospasm, laryngospasm, or anaphylaxis requires the prompt administration of intramuscular epinephrine, for which there is no good substitute at present. Adding bronchodilators, anticholinergic medication, and antihistamines will be helpful, but it appears that only epinephrine is life saving.

Vaccines for food hypersensitivity

Allergen injections for food hypersensitivity are finally on the horizon. Prototype studies with extracts of peanut have been performed. Under certain conditions they have been shown to be effective; however, they are impractical because the potential for severe side-effects means that they must be administered in an intensive care setting.[30,31]

Investigators are studying three new concepts for desensitization to food allergy (and to inhaled allergens) (Table 14.8). One approach provides a more global strategy for treating IgE-associated food allergy. This involves the use of humanized anti-IgE antibody therapy. This form of therapy has the advantage of treating multiple food sensitivities regardless of allergen specificity. Early studies of anti-IgE therapy in asthma and allergic rhinitis are showing great promise.[32–34] Using 'humanized' monoclonal antibodies specific for the Cε3 domain of IgE (portion of the IgE Fc region which binds to the Fcε receptor), investigators have shown that the anti-IgE therapy leads to a dose-dependent decrease in circulating IgE and respiratory symptoms, as well as a decrease in basophil Fcε receptor numbers.[35] However, it remains to be established whether anti-IgE therapy can reduce food-specific IgE antibody levels sufficiently over prolonged periods to prevent food-associated anaphylaxis.

A number of novel approaches for treating specific food allergies also are under investigation. One such approach involves the mutation of IgE-binding epitopes on major food proteins, i.e. Ara h1–3 in peanuts.[36–38] Mutational analyses of the immunodominant peanut protein epitopes revealed that single amino acid substitutions dramatically reduced or eliminated IgE binding to individual epitopes.[36] T-cell epitope mapping with peanut-specific T-cell lines demonstrated four immunodominant T-cell regions on the Ara h2 molecule, three of which mapped to different locations than the immunodominant IgE-binding epitopes. Similar findings have been reported for mutated *Bet v1*.[39] Since the T-cell and some IgG-binding epitopes on these peanut proteins differ from IgE-binding epitopes, the mutated recombinant proteins should desensitize peanut-allergic patients in a manner similar to standard immunotherapy without the risk of inducing anaphylactic symptoms. Studies in a peanut-allergic mouse model appear to support this hypothesis (HA Sampson, unpublished data). As more food allergens are identified and cloned, it should be possible to mutate their IgE-binding epitopes so that large numbers of food-allergen-specific vaccines will be available to re-regulate the immune response without the danger of provoking allergic symptoms.[2]

A third approach that may prove effective in treating food allergy involves using DNA-based immunization protocols, as previously suggested.[40–42] Plasmid vectors containing DNA encoding specific food proteins may be injected intramuscularly, where they are taken up by antigen-presenting cells and expressed, activating predominantly a Th1 response and downregulating the allergic response. However, recent studies in mouse models demonstrated that the type of immune response to plasmid-DNA immunization is strain dependent,[43] suggesting that interindividual variation may also occur in humans. Consequently, further studies with various plasmid constructs will be necessary before this form of therapy can be utilized in allergic patients.

Table 14.8 Vaccine approaches to treatment

DNA vaccines
Specific epitope vaccines
Anti-immunoglobulin E (IgE) vaccine

Oligonucleotide immunostimulatory sequences (ISS-ODN) containing unmethylated palindromic CpG motifs have been shown to possess immunomodulatory properties that decrease airway hyperreactivity, lung eosinophilia, and allergen-specific IgE production when administered during allergen sensitization.[44] These nucleotide sequences activate antigen-presenting cells (primarily monocytes) to secrete IFN-α,β, IL-6, IL-12, and IL-18, and NK cells to secrete IFN-γ, which promote Th1 responses. The use of ISS-ODNs as adjuvants with mutated recombinant proteins may provide a more effective form of immunotherapy for IgE-associated food allergies. Other adjuvants that induce deviation of antigen-specific Th2 responses to Th1 responses could also be utilized and include antigen-linked cytokines (e.g. IL-12, IL-18)[45] or heat-killed *Listeria monocytogenes*.[46]

All of these forms of treatment, and others that will undoubtedly be developed, offer hope that once a food allergy has been developed, it may be controlled with specific treatment and prevention measures.

NATURAL HISTORY AND PREVENTION

The natural history of food hypersensitivity encompasses both the development of food-induced symptoms and the loss of these symptoms as the individual gets older. Review of the literature on the prevention of food hypersensitivity yields conflicting results. Numerous dietary and environmental manipulations have been undertaken in attempts to prevent the onset of asthma and other atopic diseases. These studies are difficult to perform, are complex, involve many variables, and have not pointed to a clear method of prevention.[47]

In primary prevention, the diet and environment should be manipulated to prevent disease from developing. At present, no means to accomplish this goal can be recommended. Therefore, secondary prevention is currently the best approach. Secondary prevention is the identification of the problem at the earliest possible time after it commences, and institution of a treatment plan. The plan is usually avoidance with interval challenge as outlined above.

The best studies examining the loss of reactions to foods have been undertaken in children, especially children with atopic dermatitis. Unfortunately, relatively few foods have been examined in these studies. But fortunately the foods investigated are the most common food allergens. It may be stated that children lose their food hypersensitivity at a rate of about 25% per year for the common foods. In one study in adults with food hypersensitivity the subjects did lose their reactivity to food over time.[8]

There are no well-controlled studies of the loss of food hypersensitivity producing asthma symptoms. However, the guidelines for challenges and the data on loss of reactivity for other atopic conditions may be applied to asthma patients, especially in the design of studies to examine this topic.

FUTURE CONSIDERATIONS

In the nearly three decades since systematic investigation of food hypersensitivity began, substantial progress has been made in understanding it. The development of the DBPCFC brought about systematic understanding of the nature and extent of the problem. The foods most often responsible have been identified and confirmed in many studies from many centers. Skin testing was found to be of practical use if the results were properly interpreted. Recently, an in vitro test has begun to yield predictive information that has obviated the need for food challenges in specific circumstances. This progress should continue. Interval and natural history studies have demonstrated that prolonged elimination diets are unnecessary because some individuals will lose their reactivity to some foods. It is clear that a specific treatment for food hypersensitivity is on the horizon, and subjects with food-induced anaphylaxis will not have to endure a life of fear and avoidance. Ultimately it will be possible to remove the reactivity of food-allergic subjects genetically. Each of these areas has presented exciting challenges in the past and will continue to do so in the future.

REFERENCES

1. Sampson HA. Food allergy. Part 1: immunopathogenesis and clinical disorders. *J Allergy Clin Immunol* 1999; **103**: 717–29.
2. Sampson HA, Food allergy. Part 2: diagnosis and management. *J Allergy Clin Immunol* 1999; **103**: 981–9.
3. Altman DR, Chiaramonte LT. Public perception of food allergy. *J Allergy Clin Immunol* 1996; **97**: 1247–51.
4. Bock SA. Prospective appraisal of complaints of adverse reactions to foods in children during the first 3 years of life. *Pediatrics* 1987; **79**: 683–8.
5. Niestijl JJJ, Kardinall AFM, Huijbers GH, Vlieg-Boerstra BJ, Martens BPM, Ockhuizen T. Prevalence of food allergy and intolerance in the adult Dutch population. *J Allergy Clin Immunol* 1994; **93**: 446–56.
6. Sicherer SH, Munoz-Furlong A, Burks AW, Sampson HA. Prevalence of peanut and tree nut allergy in the US determined by a random digit dial telephone survey. *J Allergy Clin Immunol* 1999; **103**: 559–62.
7. Onorato J, Merland N, Terral C, Michel FB, Bousquet J. Placebo-controlled double-blind food challenge in asthma. *J Allergy Clin Immunol* 1986; **78**: 1139–46.
8. Novembre E, de Martino J, Vierucci A. Foods and respiratory allergy. *J Allergy Clin Immunol* 1988; **81**: 1059–65.
9. Hill DJ, Shelton MJ, Hosking CS. Manifestations of milk allergy in infancy: clinical and immunologic findings. *J Pediatr* 1986; **109**: 270–6.
10. Bock SA. Respiratory reactions induced by food challenges in children with pulmonary disease.

Pediatr Allergy Immunol 1992; **3:** 188–94.
11. May CD. Objective clinical and laboratory studies of immediate hypersensitivity reactions to foods in children. *J Allergy Clin Immunol* 1976; **58:** 500–15.
12. Bock SA, Lee W-Y, Remigo L, May CD. Studies of hypersensitivity reactions to foods in infants and children. *J Allergy Clin Immunol* 1978; **62:** 327.
13. Sampson HA, McCaskill CM. Food hypersensitivity and atopic dermatitis: evaluation of 113 patients. *J Pediatr* 1985; **107:** 669–75.
14. Burks AW, James JM, Hiegel A, Wilson G, Wheeler JG, Jones SM et al. Atopic dermatitis and food hypersensitivity. *J Pediatr* 1998; **132:** 132–6.
15. Atkins FM, Wilson M, Bock SA. Cottonseed hypersensitivity: new concerns over an old problem. *J Allergy Clin Immunol* 1988; **82:** 242–50.
16. Husby S, Jensenius J, Svehag S. Passage of undegraded dietary antigen into the blood of healthy adults. Quantification, estimation of size distribution and relation of uptake to level of specific antibodies. *Scan J Immunol* 1985; **22:** 83–92.
17. James JM, Bernhisel-Broadbent J, Sampson HA. Respiratory reactions provoked by double-blind food challenges in children. *Am J Respir Crit Care Med* 1994; **149:** 59–64.
18. Zwetchkenbaum JF, Skufca R, Nelson HS. An examination of food hypersensitivity as a cause of increased bronchial responsiveness to inhaled methacholine. *J Allergy Clin Immunol* 1991; **88:** 360–4.
19. James JM, Eigenmann PA, Eggleston PA, Sampson HA. Airway reactivity changes in asthmatic patients undergoing blinded food challenges. *Am J Respir Crit Care Med* 1996; **153:** 597–603.
20. Bellioni-Businco B, Paganelli R, Lucenti P, Giampietro PG, Perbom H, Businco L. Allergenicity of goat's milk in children with cow's milk allergy. *J Allergy Clin Immunol* 1999; **103:** 1191–4.
21. Bock SA, Buckley J, Holst A, May CD. Proper use of skin tests with food extracts in diagnosis of hypersensitivity to food in children. *Clin Allergy* 1977; **7:** 375.
22. Bock SA, Lee W-Y, Remigo LK, Holst A, May CD. Appraisal of skin tests with food extracts for diagnosis of food hypersensitivity. *Clin Allergy* 1978; **8:** 559.
23. Sampson HA, Albergo R. Comparison of results of skin tests, RAST and double-blind, placebo-controlled food challenges in children with atopic dermatitis. *J Allergy Clin Immunol* 1984; **74:** 26–33.
24. Rance F, Juchet A, Bremont F, Dutau G. Correlations between skin prick tests using commercial extracts and fresh foods, specific IgE, and food challenges. *Allergy* 1997; **52:** 1031–5.
25. Rance F, Dutau G. Labial food challenge in children with food allergy. *Ped Allergy Immunol* 1997; **8:** 41–4.
26. Bock SA, Atkins FM. Patterns of food hypersensitivity during sixteen years of double-blind placebo-controlled food challenges. *J Pediatr* 1990; **117:** 561–7.
27. Sampson HA, Ho DG. Relationship between food-specific IgE concentrations and the risk of positive food challenges in children and adolescents. *J Allergy Clin Immunol* 1997; **100:** 444–51.
28. Bock SA, Sampson HA, Atkins FM, Zeiger RS, Lehrer S, Sachs M et al. Double-blind, placebo-controlled food challenge (DBPCFC) as an office procedure: a manual. *J Allergy Clin Immunol* 1988; **82:** 986–97.
29. Burks AW, Sampson HA. Double blind placebo controlled trial of oral cromolyn sodium in children with documented food hypersensitivity. *J Allergy Clin Immunol* 1988; **77:** 417–23.
30. Oppenheimer JJ, Nelson HS, Bock SA, Christensen F, Leung DYM. Treatment of peanut allergy with rush immunotherapy. *J Allergy Clin Immunol* 1992; **90:** 256–62.
31. Nelson HN, Lahr J, Rule R, Bock SA, Leung DYM. Treatment of anaphylactic sensitivity to peanuts by immunotherapy with injections of aqueous peanut extract. *J Allergy Clin Immunol* 1997; **99:** 744–51.
32. Fahy JV, Fleming E, Wong HH, Liu JT, Su JQ, Reimann J et al. The effect of an anti-IgE monoclonal antibody on the early- and late-phase responses to allergen inhalation in asthmatic subjects. *Am J Respir Crit Care Med* 1997; **155:** 1828–34.
33. Boulet LP, Chapman KR, Cote J, Kalra S, Bhagat R, Swystun VA et al. Inhibitory effects of an anti-IgE antibody E25 on allergen-induced early asthmatic response. *Am J Respir Crit Care Med* 1997; **155:** 1835–40.
34. Casale TB, Bernstein IL, Busse W, LaForce CF, Tinkelman DG, Stoltz RR et al. Use of anti-IgE humanized monoclonal antibody in ragweed-induced allergic rhinitis. *J Allergy Clin Immunol* 1997; **100:** 100–10.
35. MacGlashan DW Jr, Bochner BS, Adelman DC,

Jardieu PM, Togias A, McKenzie WJ et al. Down-regulation of Fc(epsilon)RI expression on human basophils during in vivo treatment of atopic patients with anti-IgE antibody. *J Immunol* 1997; **158:** 1438–45.

36. Shin D, Compadre CM, Sampson HA, Huang SK, Maleki S, Kopper RA et al. Identification and analysis of the critical amino acids and structures necessary for specific IgE binding to Ara h 1, a major peanut allergen. *J Biol Chem* 1998; **273:** 137–59.

37. Stanley JS, King N, Burks AW, Huang SK, Sampson H, Cockrell G et al. Identification and mutational analysis of the immunodominant IgE binding epitopes of the major peanut allergen Ara h 2. *Arch Biochem Biophys* 1997; **342:** 244–53.

38. Rabjohn P, Helm R, Stanley J, West C, Sampson HA, Burks AW et al. Molecular cloning and epitope analysis of the peanut allergen, Ara h3. *J Clin Invest* 1999; **103:** 535–42.

39. Ferreira F, Ebner C, Kramer B, Casari G, Briza P, Kungl AJGR et al. Modulation of IgE reactivity of allergens by site-directed mutagenesis: potential use of hypoallergenic variants for immunotherapy. *FASEB J* 1998; **12:** 231–42.

40. Seder RA, Gurunathan S. DNA vaccines—designer vaccines for the 21st century. *N Engl J Med* 1999; **341:** 277–8.

41. Hsu C, Chua K, Tao M, Lai Y, Wu H, Huang S et al. Immunoprophylaxis of allergen-induced immunoglobulin E synthesis and airway hyperresponsiveness in vivo by genetic immunization. *Natur Med* 1996; **2:** 540–4.

42. Spiegelberg H, Orozco ER, Roman M, Raz E. DNA immunization: a novel approach to allergen-specific immunotherapy. *Allergy* 1997; **52:** 964–8.

43. Li XM, Huang CK, Schofield B, Burks AW, Bannon GA, Kim KH et al. Strain-dependent induction of allergic sensitization caused by peanut allergen DNA immunization in mice. *J Immunol* 1999; **162:** 3316–20.

44. Broide D, Schwarze J, Tighe H, Gifford T, Nguyen M, Malek S et al. Immunostimulatory DNA sequences inhibit IL-5, eosinophilic inflammation, and airway hyperresponsiveness in mice. *J Immunol* 1998; **161:** 7054–62.

45. Kim TS, DeKruyff RH, Rupper R, Maecker HT, Levy S, Umetsu DT. An ovalbumin-Il-12 fusion protein is more effective than ovalbumin plus free recombinant IL-12 in inducing a T helper cell type—dominated immune response and inhibiting antigen-specific IgE production. *J Immunol* 1997; **158:** 4137–44.

46. Yeung VP, Gieni RS, Umetsu DT, DeKruyff RH. Heat-killed Listeria monocytogenes as an adjuvant converts established murine Th-2-dominated immune responses into Th1-dominated responses. *J Immunol* 1998; **161:** 4146–52.

47. Zeiger RS, Heller SH. The development and prediction of atopy in high-risk children; follow-up at age seven years in a prospective randomized study of combined maternal and infant food allergen avoidance. *J Allergy Clin Immunol* 1995; **95:** 1179–90.

15

Psychosocial factors mediating asthma treatment outcomes

Bruce G Bender

Knowledge and skill • **Treatment adherence** • **Psychosocial factors affecting health care behavior** • **Future directions**

With an adequate treatment program, most asthma can be effectively controlled, thus avoiding hospitalizations and emergency room visits. However, numerous factors influence the success of any asthma treatment program. Prominent among these influences are psychological, social, and behavioral characteristics of the patient and other family members.

In order for asthma to be well controlled, a number of conditions must be present. The patient must have (1) access to appropriate medical care, (2) a strong working relationship with a qualified care giver, (3) an understanding of the disease and its treatment and the skills to carry out the treatment plan, and (4) motivation and competence to care for the asthma. If the patient is a child, the parents must be motivated and competent. A significant portion of these requisites are affected by psychosocial factors. Although the core treatment may consist of medications and various environmental control measures, the success of the treatment is largely determined by the patient's health care behavior. Appropriate knowledge and skill will enable the patient to respond effectively to changing symptoms. Motivation to adhere to the treatment plan will be the single most potent behavioral factor affecting treatment outcome. A host of psychosocial factors will impact on adherence motivation, including belief in the treatment plan and one's own self-efficacy, trust in the physician, social support, stress, the presence of psychopathology and family dysfunction, and socioeconomic conditions in the life of the patient and his or her family.

Psychosocial factors affecting asthma treatment outcomes will be examined in this chapter, with the objective of understanding how these factors, individually and collectively, impact on the disease and the treatment process. Discussion will focus on four areas of investigation: knowledge and skill; treatment adherence; psychosocial factors affecting health care behavior; and future directions.

KNOWLEDGE AND SKILL

Educating patients

Asthma management involves a constellation of sometimes complex patient health care behaviors. Multiple medications are often prescribed for patients with asthma. Many of these are administered by metered dose inhaler (MDI), requiring a series of actions and coordination of inhaler actuation and inhalation. New dry-powder inhalers, each involving its own inhaler-specific technique, are being rapidly introduced. Patients are asked to adapt their environment and to avoid particular allergens. When symptoms change, patients may be expected to change their behavior, including altering their medication use and communicating key information to their care giver. For many patients, these activities require daily action. Where the patient is a child, the coordinated efforts of two parents are frequently necessary, and many family plans must be structured around management of the child's asthma. In addition to the time and energy expended, numerous sacrifices may come into play, including asking a parent to cease smoking, or the family to give up a cherished pet, and committing financial resources to health care.

In short, much is asked of patients to maintain control of their asthma. Not surprisingly, many patients do not engage in the complete and consistent sets of behaviors necessary to maintain health. Lack of knowledge or skill is the first barrier to good asthma self-management. Logically, patients who do not understand the nature of their illness or the purpose of the medication prescribed for them cannot be expected to adhere diligently to the treatment regimen. Furthermore, the technology of asthma treatment requires skill that must be taught to patients. Proper MDI technique is essential for optimally effective drug delivery. One study of 59 adults with asthma revealed that only 25% of the patients met study criteria of correct MDI technique, including correct timing of actuation and inhalation, deep inhalation, and adequate breath-holding time.[1] In another study of 501 patients, 89% made at least one error in their MDI technique, most commonly improper timing of actuation.[2] Health care givers poised to educate patients about proper MDI technique may themselves be ill equipped to instruct; 59% of emergency room housestaff, attending physicians, and nurses at five Midwestern community hospitals were unable to demonstrate correct technique.[3]

Numerous asthma education programs have been developed to provide necessary information to patients and parents.[4] Guidelines for new asthma education programs have been developed; most visible among these are those of the National Asthma Education and Prevention Program.[5] Despite these well-directed efforts, however, providing patients with information about the management of their asthma does not invariably lead to better self-management. One meta-analysis examining 11 asthma education trials concluded that in aggregate the asthma education programs had little impact on asthma outcome measures such as school absenteeism, asthma attacks, hospitalizations, hospital days, or emergency room visits.[6] Although other patient education studies have reported more effective outcomes,[7,8] transmitting information does not automatically translate into improved health care behavior.[9]

Symptom perception

If knowing *what* to do is an important step towards effective asthma self-management, knowing *when* to take action is the next key component. Effective management requires patients to respond quickly and appropriately to changes in their disease. Timely response to changes in asthma symptoms can occur only after the patient correctly perceives a change in their airways. Blunted symptom perception can contribute to poorly controlled asthma.[10] Delayed and insufficient response can, in the worst of scenarios, contribute to asthma-related death.[11] Conversely, overperception of symptoms is associated with excessive illness behavior including overuse of medication and hospitalization.[12] Recent investigations have focused upon symptom perception, or the perceptual processes constituting awareness of airway obstruction and the sensation of breathlessness. In signal detection studies, a series of resistive loads are introduced as the patient breathes through a mouthpiece connected to a set of resistive elements. During a predetermined sequence of breaths, patients are asked to judge breathing changes as resistive loads are varied.[13] The 'threshold' of perception is the point of resistance detected by the patient. Alternatively, the discrepancy between patient-estimated and measured peak expiratory flow rates is utilized as a measure of perceptual accuracy.[14] The science of respiratory perception is clearly young and there is no standardized definition of what differentiates 'accurate' from 'inaccurate' respiratory perception. Still, some interesting associations are emerging. Approximately 15% of adult asthmatics were unable to perceive a 50% lung function reduction.[15] Children with asthma were less perceptive of lung function changes than were well control children.[16] In another study of children with asthma, higher perceptual accuracy was related to less functional morbidity. After controlling for asthma severity, perceptual accuracy was correlated with both days of school absence and emergency room visits.[17] Patients with 'near-fatal' asthma sometimes have blunted perception of breathlessness[18] and dyspnea,[19] which presumably contributes to delayed response to deteriorating symptoms.

Still, the frequency and degree of perceptual inaccuracy in these studies is not dramatic, and there is no clear evidence that the absence of physiologic perception underlies the near-fatal episodes. Failure to respond to symptom changes may occur not because the patient cannot perceive changes, but because of avoidance or denial of symptoms possibly secondary to psychological problems. Attempts to provide relaxation training to asthma patients have resulted in small and temporary changes, and have no impact on inflammatory processes.[20] A group of 11 adults with near-fatal asthma episodes involving either mechanical ventilation or acute severe hypercapnic respiratory insufficiency demonstrated poor adherence and increased psychologic disturbance compared with age, sex, and disease-matched controls.[21] Disregard of symptoms, inadequate self-care, and history of psychological problems were among the factors associated with asthma-related deaths in a case study of 21 children in which 'a major factor in their fatal attacks was a delay in seeking medical care.'[11] In short, it is the failure to respond appropriately to symptom changes, rather than failure to perceive them, which appears to be the most significant contributor to treatment failure.

TREATMENT ADHERENCE

Treatment adherence is the fundamental link between the medical process and treatment outcome. Patients are not passive recipients of asthma care. Disease control depends upon consistent adherence to health care behaviors, the most central of these being appropriate use of prescribed medications. Numerous studies have found that a remarkable proportion of prescribed medication is not taken by patients. Utilizing microchip-equipped metered dose inhalers, investigators have reported that on average less than half of prescribed medication is used,[22] and that adherence sufficient to reach consistent pharmacologic benefit occurs only in 26–52% of adult patients.[23,24] Despite parental involvement, treatment adherence in children with asthma is little better. In a 3 month study of 24 8–12-year-old children with asthma, median inhaled corticosteroid use was 58.4%.[25] Adherence was only slightly higher in a Scottish study of preschool children in which a median of 77% of prescribed doses were taken.[26]

The consequences of treatment non-adherence can be measured in personal suffering, health care cost, and compromised clinical trial outcomes. Non-adherent adults had more airway obstruction than adherent patients.[27] Children who did not adhere to their asthma treatment regimen had poorer asthma control[28] and required more urgent care visits, steroid bursts, and hospitalizations.[25] The cost of asthma treatment is impacted by non-adherence. In 1990 dollars, the direct and indirect cost of asthma treatment in the US was US$6.2 billion. Almost US$3 billion resulted from emergency room visits and hospitalizations.[29] When health care behaviors improve, these costs decrease. Intensive pediatric adherence-intervention programs resulted in dramatic decreases in rates of hospitalization and emergency room visits, reducing the average annual asthma care costs by US$105 to US$1642 for each participating patient.[30,31] In clinical trials, undetected non-adherence can lead to erroneous conclusions about a drug's effectiveness.[32] In some cases, partial adherence results in diminished apparent efficacy. Consequently, drugs may enter the market with recommended doses that are much higher than necessary for therapeutic effect.[33]

The influence of non-adherence on asthma treatment outcome is only partially understood. The measurement of adherence to asthma medications is improving, in large part because of the introduction of electronic monitoring devices, but is still at best an inexact science.[34] Most studies collapse adherence data into single, summary quotient scores which average adherence over weeks and months by dividing the number of doses taken by the number prescribed. This approach provides a convenient, single adherence index that allows for easy comparison across subjects groups, and informative correlation with associated disease, demographic, and psychosocial factors. However, the single-index approach frequently embraces two assumptions: (1) the degree of adherence remains static and consistent over time; and (2) all adherence is good adherence. Neither assumption is correct. Patients with a 50% adherence rate seldom take every other dose of their medication. Rather, adherence fluctuates widely, often with periods of drug 'holiday' during which patients take no medication for several days at a time.[33] Depending upon the duration of action and side-effects profile, such holidays may have several potential consequences, including waning drug action, hazardous rebound effects when administration stops abruptly, and overdose effects when administration of full-strength drugs suddenly resumes.[33] In studies of MDI use among children with asthma, no use of inhalers occurred on 42% and 48% of study days,[35,36] and abandonment of medication frequently occurred for several consecutive days. The implications of such start-and-stop adherence patterns are unknown. Time to onset of the effectiveness of inhaled corticosteroids in the treatment of mild to moderate asthma is about 3 weeks, with faster impact (3 days) on morning peak expiratory flow in patients with severe asthma.[37] It remains to be determined whether abandonment of medication for ≥3 consecutive days in erratically adherent patients will expose patients with severe asthma to rapid deterioration of symptoms. If this is the case, then patients with relatively high adherence who fail to use their medication for a week at a time may have more poorly controlled asthma than those who use less total medication but use it with better regularity.

Non-adherence can involve overuse as well as underuse of medication. Asthmatic adults overused their inhaler bronchodilator on 10% of days.[23] Children with asthma overused their inhaled corticosteroid on 22% of study days.[36] Such overuse is significant, both because patients may be receiving too much medication, and because overuse confounds data interpretation. Specifically, averaging overuse and underuse usually results in overestimating adherence because overuse artificially raises the mean score.[34] Before the impact of adherence on clinical outcomes can be accurately evaluated, a comprehensive assessment of adherence must be made including an accurate adherence measure and data analysis strategies sufficient to account for varying patterns of behavior.

In the treatment of asthma, as with the treatment of other diseases such as diabetes,[38] non-adherence can be a particularly pronounced problem among adolescent patients.[11] In this age group, shedding signs of dependence upon one's parents and increasing identification with an adolescent peer group may conflict with any indications of chronic illness. Symptom denial and resistance toward asthma medications are self-defeating attempts to be normal. As conflict with parents or care givers increases, adolescents with asthma become more willing to defiantly refuse parental wishes, including the use of asthma medications.[11] Conversely, a strong working alliance with the medical care giver is associated with improved treatment adherence in adolescents with asthma.[39]

PSYCHOSOCIAL FACTORS AFFECTING HEALTH CARE BEHAVIOR

Aside from skill and knowledge, a variety of psychosocial factors may affect patients' adherence to their asthma treatment protocol. Although adherence often refers to consistent use of medications, other health care behaviors are involved in asthma management. These include prevention strategies such as avoiding precipitants, attack management behaviors, a crisis action plan, and appropriate communication with care givers. All of these asthma management behaviors can be affected by stress, family functioning, personality attributes, psychopathology, social support, socioeconomic status, and self-efficacy.

Stress and emotions

Stress can be a significant factor for patients and their families, and can in multiple ways undermine good asthma control. The many stressors experienced by patients can include obviously traumatic events, such as being in a serious accident, experiencing the loss of a relationship, being the victim of a crime, and living through a natural disaster such as an earthquake or tornado. Additionally, the experience of stress is a subjective phenomenon. An event that is only mildly disruptive for one individual, such as losing a job or taking a final exam, may be severely distressing for another. Further, some stressors, such as marital discord, can be chronic and thus exercise a long-term and progressive effect on the individual. Different kinds of stress may have different impact on the individual and upon disease states. In some cases, a measurable physiologic change may occur following stress which alters the course of the asthma; in other cases, stress may trigger other behavioral changes that impede disease control.

Stress can produce immunologic and endocrinologic changes that may impact on asthma.[40] These changes can affect asthma either directly (e.g. through changes in the production of cytokines or granula leukocytes) or indirectly (e.g. through heightened susceptibility to respiratory infection).[41] Increased respiratory illness has been associated with psychological stress.[42] Although little clear evidence exists to demonstrate that long-term stress alters asthma, some data support the immediate effects of acute stress on asthma symptoms. When exposed to violence, inner-city children have been shown to have increased asthma symptoms and use of bronchodilator medication.[43] A subgroup of patients with asthma may have heightened susceptibility to stress, with the result that stress can have a more profound effect on their asthma than among other patients. About 25% of patients with asthma respond with increased bronchoconstriction when watching intensely sad films,[44] listening to interactions involving conflict,[45] or performing difficult computations.[46]

A subset of patients have a particular psychological profile affecting treatment outcome. Kinsman and colleagues identified a 'panic–fear' personality based upon results from the Minnesota Multiphasic Personality Inventory.[47] Patients who scored high on this dimension were characteristically anxious, emotional, and fearful,[48] tended to overuse their asthma rescue medication,[49] and required more health care including physician visits, medication prescriptions, and hospitalizations.[50] Conversely, patients scoring low on the panic–fear dimension[48] or who expressed greater optimism[51] were more adherent and less likely to require hospitalization.

Another group of asthma patients has been found to be susceptible to the effects of suggestion on airway sensitivity. Nineteen of 40 adults with asthma exhibited bronchoconstriction in response to inhalation of saline that was described as either an allergen or respiratory irritant.[52] These findings were replicated in other studies which additionally demonstrated that bronchoconstriction in the form of reduced forced expiratory volume occurred only when patients were told that the saline was an irritant, and not in a control group given saline without suggestion. Further, the suggestion-induced bronchoconstriction was reversed with administration of ipratropium bromide, indicating the possibility of a cholinergic-mediated response.[53,54] Relaxation training or hypnosis have been shown to produce a significant, if modest, positive effect on air flow.[20] Whether the subset of patients who are susceptible to suggestion are also those who are susceptible to the effects of stress on their asthma is unclear. Nonetheless, results from studies of stress, emotions, and susceptibility to suggestion indicate that asthma symptoms and health care behaviors may be influenced by emotional factors, and that these factors are particularly potent for some patients.

Stress and emotions may also influence asthma treatment outcome through an entirely different set of mechanisms. Aside from the direct effect of stress on physiological pathways, stress impacts the psychological environment around the patient, which in turn alters the patient's capacity to care for their asthma. Patients with chronic emotional disorders often have difficulty with the management of their asthma. Emotionally unstable patients are less adherent.[55–57] Such individuals may be distressed and distracted, and may approach many elements of their life in a disorganized and haphazard manner. Feelings of helplessness and hopelessness, about both their life in general and their illness, may immobilize them. Personal conflicts, financial problems, frequent moves, sleep disorders, unemployment, and erratic daily schedules may accompany serious emotional disorders and preclude the development of regular health care behaviors. For such individuals, treatment of the emotional disorder must occur before improvement in self-management skills can be expected.[58]

Family functioning

A relationship between emotional disturbance and non-adherence is also seen in families of children with asthma. A healthy, emotionally supportive, well-organized family system is likely to be capable of (1) understanding the needs of the child with asthma, (2) structuring household routines to care for asthma, (3) creating strategies and action plans for employment during periods of acute illness severity, (4) acting out these plans when they are required, (5) communicating important and timely information to the child's physician, (6) coordinating parental responsibilities for asthma care to allow each adult to attend to other commitments, and (7) providing an emotionally nurturing environment that can counter the emotional distress experienced by the child during periods of disease exacerbation. One study demonstrated that families with good child–parent communication, including discussion about important asthma management decisions, were more effective in their management of the illness.[59]

Conversely, a dysfunctional family may be less able to care for the child's asthma, and significantly less capable of responding effectively to changing disease or other stressful and distressing events. Family dysfunction has been repeatedly associated with severe, poorly controlled pediatric asthma, usually because such families have difficulty adhering to a treatment regimen.[60] Decreased communication, organization, and emotional support were associated with medication non-adherence in two studies of asthmatic children and their families.[35,61] In one of these studies, inhaled corticosteroids were taken only on 42% of study days; adherence was even lower in families with lower scores on a measure of family functioning, although it was unrelated to a measure of child psychological adaptation.[35] Thus, whereas adherence is associated with the psychological health of adult patients with asthma, for children it is the psychological climate of the family, not the adaptation of the individual child, which predicts adherence. In another study, family conflict signaled non-adherence and poorly controlled asthma.[62] When asthma severity, family dysfunction, and poor adherence are increased, risk of asthma-related death also increases.[11]

The psychological functioning of the parent is a major determining factor influencing family stability and management of the child's illness. Distressed or psychologically unstable parents may not provide the structure and support necessary to ensure adherence of the child. A parent's psychological functioning affects how well a family monitors a child's symptoms and makes decisions about home management of symptoms and appropriate timing for involving the medical expertise of health care providers.[60] Increased psychiatric symptoms among the mothers of children with chronic illness, including asthma, were associated with increased functional limitations in their children.[63] In a study of asthma risk factors, parenting problems—including psychiatric difficulty and poor knowledge of child care practices—were associated with increased probability of a young child developing asthma, particularly when combined with frequent illness and elevated serum IgE levels.[64] In some instances, the parent may expect the child to assume responsibility for their own asthma management beyond the child's developmental capacity to do so.[22] Stressful events in the life of a family, such as frequent moves or parental unemployment, add to a negative emotional climate and diminish the family's capacity to maintain the energy and organization necessary to care for a chronically ill child. The child care burden is increased when the child has more than one physical illness[65] or physical disability,[66] further taxing the family system.

Family poverty and membership in urban minority groups are associated with greater asthma morbidity and mortality. Asthma mortality and hospitalization rates are greater among non-whites[67] and low-income patients.[68] Medication adherence rates have been reported to be relatively lower in non-white adult[69] and pediatric patients.[70] In a study of 50 adult asthma patients, non-adherence was linked to non-white ethnicity, low income, lower level of formal education, and poor provider–patient communication; 62% of African-American and Hispanic patients were non-adherent, in contrast to 24% of white patients.[71] For these patients, barriers to good asthma care may include decreased access to health care, presence of other crises requiring immediate attention, failure to recognize illness severity, and greater exposure to respiratory infections and environmental conditions that tend to exacerbate asthma, such as air pollution, dust mites, indoor molds, and cigarette smoke.[72] Additionally, these families may be less trustful of the long-term safety of medications prescribed for their children.[73] Studies of inner-city patients in East St Louis revealed lack of regular care, reliance on self-treatment with over-the-counter medications, delay in seeking treatment,[74] and perception of the health care system as insensitive.[75]

Processes that bolster healthy family functioning can enhance the family's capacity to care for the child with asthma. One of these is social support. Social support has been shown to be important to a variety of health outcomes. Socially isolated families have more frequent days and nights with asthma symptoms, poorer asthma management practices, and more urgent-care visits than those of less isolated families with an asthmatic child.[76] Greater social networks have been linked to positive health behaviors, such as improving diet and exercise,[77] and decreased psychological distress.[78] In general, families who have multiple relationships outside their nuclear family, including both friends and extended family members, can cope better with chronic illness and counter its disruptive and stressful influence. A community program designed to increase neighborhood organizational strategies and social networking among asthmatic families resulted in reductions in acute care for asthmatic children.[76]

Self-efficacy

Self-efficacy has been increasingly identified as a key element in treatment outcome success. Self-efficacy is the patient's belief that they can carry out the behaviors necessary to good asthma management, and that their illness will be improved as a result. If the patient, or the patient's family, does not have this fundamental belief about their own self-efficacy, treatment adherence is likely to be incomplete and to diminish over time.[78] Self-efficacy thus makes an important distinction between knowledge and expectation. Many asthma education programs impart information to patients about the care of their asthma, but without a firm belief in a probable outcome the patient is less likely to respond to the new information with a commitment to behavior change. Hence, many patient education programs have successfully improved patients' understanding of their asthma, but failed to elicit the behavior changes necessary to alter treatment end points such as hospitalization or absence from work or school.[6] Patients who reported lower levels of 'perceived control' of their asthma had poorer illness outcomes.[79] Measured self-efficacy was found to account for a significant portion of outcome success in studies of exercise,[80,81] breast cancer screening,[82] addictive behavior,[83] and treatment for heart disease.[80]

The concept of self-efficacy overlaps with several other psychological constructs that have been proposed and studied in relationship to chronic illness management. Positive 'coping styles' among adults with asthma were associated with optimism, greater social contact, and increased capacity to manage asthma.[51] Becker's 'health belief model'[84] proposes that patients' adherence to a treatment regimen is largely determined by their beliefs about their illness, the competence of their health care giver, and the relative benefits of behavior change. 'Locus of control' or 'perceived control' theories focus on the degree to which patients perceive that events in their lives, including those influencing poverty, safety, and control of illness, are under their own control.[85] Similarly, 'learned helplessness' models recognize that some individuals, particularly those trapped in the lower socioeconomic strata, see themselves as the passive victims of the adverse events of their lives and unable to alter the course of their misfortune.[86] All of these psychosocial models—coping styles, self-efficacy, health belief model, locus of control, and learned helplessness—highlight the underlying perceptions that help determine whether patients will demonstrate the motivation and determination to work at adhering to a prescribed treatment plan.

Evidence of the importance of health beliefs, motivation, and self-efficacy emerge from unlikely sources—two placebo-controlled clinical trials. In a study of post-myocardial infarction recovery, 1103 men were assigned to either active clofibrate or placebo treatment.[87] After 5–8 years of study participation, patients who had adhered well to the clofibrate medication had a 15% mortality rate, whereas those with less than 80% adherence had a 25% mortality rate. Remarkably, the mortality rates were almost identical in the placebo group; good adherence resulted in an average mortality of 15% and poor adherence resulted in an average mortality of 28%. Clofibrate was not associated with decreased mortality following myocardial infarction, but adherence to a drug regimen, active or placebo, was. Although no other information was provided to differentiate the behavior of good and poor adherers, the outcome suggests that patients who take their medication conscientiously may also work to take care of their health in other ways, including participating in diet and exercise programs and avoiding behaviors such as smoking which are detrimental to health. In a second study, 22 071 physicians who had experienced myocardial infarction were assigned randomly to either aspirin or placebo treatment.[88] At the end of 60 months, the death rate for participants with low adherence was over four times that for patients with high adherence in both medication conditions. A significant correlation between low adherence and baseline characteristics including cigarette smoking, obesity, lack of exercise, and history of angina supports the conclusion that medication adherence is associated with other behaviors that reflect a positive drive toward improved health. Patients who want to be well, and have developed the belief that they can engage in behaviors that will help them restore health, are more likely to do so than patients lacking self-efficacy.

Patient–physician relationship

The above discussion has focused upon problems and perceptions within the patient, or the patient's family, which interfere with treatment outcome. The relationship between the health care giver and the patient is also influential in determining whether the patient will develop a sense of self-efficacy and engage in health care behaviors sufficient to insure successful treatment of the disease. The *Guidelines for the Diagnosis and Management of Asthma*[5] emphasizes that patient education must occur within this care-giver–patient partnership. This relationship has a more powerful influence on adherence than any other factor.[89] The strength of the physician–patient treatment alliance, as rated by the physician, predicted treatment adherence and nonroutine office visits in the year after hospitalization of 60 adolescents with severe, chronic asthma.[90] In the realm of psychotherapy, stronger therapeutic alliance has similarly been positively related to better outcomes.[39] In some cases, the behavior and attitude of the patient prevent the health care giver from developing an optimal working relationship. However, there is considerable evidence that the behavior of the physician plays a significant role in defining the strength of the treatment alliance. Patients are more adherent to their treatment regimen when their physician has answered all the patient's questions[91] and communicated clearly[92] and positively.[93] The physician's interest in spending time with a patient, attempting to understand his or her beliefs and perceptions about the illness, signals the desire to developing a partnership that will result in treatment success.[94]

FUTURE DIRECTIONS

In the last decade, the combination of advances in the availability of new and highly effective anti-inflammatory medications and the development of practitioner guidelines for the care of asthma has greatly increased our capacity to control asthma effectively. The pathway that connects judiciously prescribed treatments and successful outcomes, however, passes through the psychosocial fabric of the patient. Although asthma treatments have improved, patient adherence to these treatments has not. Adherence to inhaled anti-inflammatory medications is no better than was adherence to theophylline 10 years ago.[22] Treatments fail when the patient does not understand the nature of the illness and its treatment, does not perceive airway changes, is overwhelmed by life's other demands, struggles with or has a parent with a psychological disorder, or is shackled by fundamental doubts about his or her ability to bring about change in the disease. Given the large number of factors that interact to determine patient health care behavior, it follows that solutions must necessarily be multifaceted. No single intervention can resolve the myriad of human problems that prevent treatment adherence. Programs that have banked on a singular approach to behavior change—typically through education—have met disappointment.[6]

Despite the large number of published studies addressing adherence and compliance with asthma treatment, much remains to be learned about patient behavior, underlying causes, and interventions. Even the methods of adherence measurement are a work in progress which, with improvement, will lead to increased understanding of this problem. With increased ability to assess the psychosocial factors that prevent a particular patient from engaging in effective self-management, specific interventions may be applied. The patient without sufficient knowledge about the disease and treatment may require only a brief asthma education program. Where insufficient symptom perception prevents a timely response, training in ability to achieve airway changes may result in earlier and hence more effective intervention. As the psychosocial roadblocks become more complex, however, the solutions become more elusive. Patients and families demonstrating psychological dysfunction require psychological interventions. When these interventions are provided by mental health practitioners knowledgeable about the disease and working in concert with the medical team, the interventions are more likely to result in a change in asthma management behavior.[58] However, psychological interventions do not invariably result in improvement in the psychological disorder or treatment outcome. Further, other correlates of treatment non-adherence, including poverty, parental psychopathology, and stressful life events, are often the result of complex causal factors and beyond the reach of the individual health care provider. Large-scale programs such as the National Cooperative Inner-City Asthma Study, sponsored by the National Institutes of Health, represent attempts to discover broad solutions to these difficult problems. Results from such investigations will add insight into potential solutions but may not provide immediate, pervasive answers to the problem of high morbidity and mortality among inner-city children with asthma. There is as yet no indication that this troubling trend is changing.

While the search for large-scale solutions to poorly controlled asthma continues, there are three strategies in place which show promise for improving treatment adherence and outcomes. Although these may not provide nationwide or even citywide solutions, they represent interventions that can have a positive impact on the adherence of groups of patients with asthma. Further, these programs may achieve partial success in patient populations that include those who have experienced poorly controlled asthma and are frequent users of high-cost medical care.

Self-management training

Discussion of patient education programs frequently includes a variety of education-based interventions, some effective and others not. A distinction is drawn here between traditional patient education approaches and asthma self-management training. 'Educational programs' refers here to efforts to impart information. Many books, videos, and other materials contain valuable information for patients with asthma and their families. Additionally, educational classes are sometimes offered to patients, although less frequently than other take-home materials. The content of most of these materials and programs is similar to that recommended by the NHLBI Expert Panel Report[5] and includes (1) basic facts about asthma, (2) medications, (3) skills such as inhaler and spacer use, (4) environmental control measures, and (5) rescue actions.

'Self-management training' also concerns itself with imparting information, but goes further in its attempts to change beliefs, expectations, and behavior. Creer and Bender[95] concluded that self-management training includes three components: (1) patients are helped to integrate new information about asthma with their personal beliefs, abilities, experiences, and expectations; (2) patients are helped to make decisions about which behaviors and skills they will adopt, and to begin to practice those skills; (3) patients are encouraged to utilize their new knowledge and skill over time to maintain long-term asthma control. Self-management training is often individualized for patients, occurs over a number of visits, and should include instruction by the physician and other care providers as an ongoing component of the partnership between care giver and patient.[20,96] Using this approach, self-management training programs have demonstrated success in improving adherence and symptom control while decreasing health care costs.[97–99]

In the case of preschool children, non-adherence remains a problem even though responsibility for medication administration is typically placed entirely in the hands of parents. In two studies of children 15 months to 5 years of age, full medication adherence was documented with electronic metered dose inhalers on only 50% of study days.[100] The parent's health beliefs and sense of efficacy impact on administration of their child's medication—as they do on their own. Further, parental discomfort over the struggle to convince a young child to take a medication they are resisting, greatly complicated in the case of MDI-administered medications, and concerns about medication safety[59] further erode parental commitment to daily medication adherence. Whereas developmentally targeted education is helpful for increasing adherence in older children, for preschool children it is the parents who must be educated, receive comprehensive asthma management training, and be the recipients of efforts to establish a strong caregiver–patient alliance. The Family Asthma Management System[101,102] includes a structured interview designed to assess the family's current management of their child's asthma and a strategic approach to increase the family's management skills.

Physician training

Self-management training is most effective when conducted by the care giver in the setting where routine health care is obtained.[5,22] The alliance between care giver and patient yields the best opportunity both to provide basic asthma information and to enhance the patient's belief in their ability to self-manage. Training physicians to educate and motivate patients can change adherence, patient satisfaction, and treatment outcomes.[98,99,103] Clark and colleagues[72] examined the impact on asthma outcomes of education for physicians in a trial in which 74 general practice pediatricians were assigned to either an education program or a control group. The education intervention group received 5 hours of training in communication skills aimed at creating a supportive atmosphere in which information about asthma self-care could be conveyed and positive health care behaviors reinforced. Pediatric asthma patients treated by this intervention group subsequently reported more satisfaction with their physician, were more informed about self-management, and made fewer non-emergency office visits. The intervention also resulted in more frequent prescribing of inhaled anti-inflammatory medications; patients who received these prescriptions had significantly less symptoms, emergency room visits, and hospitalizations. The Bayer Institute for Health Care Communication has conducted health-behavior-enhancing workshops for more than 20 000 clinicians in the United States and Europe, emphasizing the importance of the physician–patient relationship and teaching specific skills which include use of open-ended questions, reflective listening, and active empathizing with the patient.[104]

Intensive, hospital-based adherence interventions

More intensive interventions may be needed in cases where asthma is poorly controlled, life threatening, and undermined by family dysfunction and non-adherence. In one such program, pediatric patients were invited to participate when the previous year had seen three or more hospitalizations, four or more emergency room visits, four or more corticosteroid bursts, corticosteroid dependence, hypoxic seizures, or 30 days or more of school absence.[30] The program included medical assessment and management, physical exercise, asthma education with the child and family, and a sequence of family interviews designed to improve the family's home management of the illness. The program continued with outpatient follow-up and resulted in significant reductions in asthma care and cost in the 4-year follow-up.

Patients with both severe asthma and psychological difficulty—a population with marked non-adherence and high health care utilization—are treated in the Day Treatment Program at the National Jewish Medical and Research Center.[105] The partial hospitalization program provides a daily treatment milieu that integrates medical appointments, asthma education, psychological interventions, and ancillary services such as art therapy, rehabilitation therapy, speech therapy, and dietitian services. In the 12 month period following this treatment program, functional severity, oral steroid requirements, hospitalization, and cost of medical care were significantly reduced.[106]

Patient self-management training, physician training, and intensive hospital-based interventions represent three different approaches to improving patients' ability to manage their asthma. Each makes a specific contribution to asthma care; all three may be used in various combinations. Even though these approaches show promise, it is unlikely that they will soon reverse national trends of increasing morbidity. Significant, large-scale changes in asthma outcomes will occur when information from these and other innovative interventions are subject to objective assessment, the successful elements from these programs are separated from those with little impact, and new behavioral approaches are developed and applied on an increasingly large scale.

REFERENCES

1. Goodman DE, Israel E, Rosenberg M. The influence of age, diagnosis, and gender on proper

use of metered-dose inhalers. *Am J Respir Crit Care Med* 1994; **150:** 1256–61.
2. Larsen JS, Hahn M, Ekholm B, Wick KA. Evaluation of conventional press-and-breathe metered-dose inhaler technique in 501 patients. *J Asthma* 1994; **31:** 193–9.
3. Jones JS, Holstege CP, Riekse R. Metered-dose inhalers: do emergency health care know what to teach? *Ann Emerg Med* 1995; **26:** 308–11.
4. Hanson JE. Patient education in pediatric asthma. In: Murphy S, Kelly HW, eds. *Pediatric Asthma*. New York: Marcel Dekker, 1999, 183–210.
5. National Heart, Lung and Blood Institute. *Guidelines for the Diagnosis and Management of Asthma. Highlights of the Expert Panel Report II.* National Institutes of Health, 1997. Publication no. 97–4051.
6. Bernard-Bonnin A, Stachenko S, Bonin D, Charette C, Rousseau E. Self-management teaching programs and morbidity of pediatric asthma: a meta-analysis. *J Allergy Clin Immunol* 1995; **95:** 34–41.
7. Clark NM, Feldman CH, Evans D, Levison MJ, Wasilewski Y, Mellins RB. The impact of health education on frequency and cost of health care use by low income children with asthma. *J Allergy Clin Immunol* 1986; **78:** 108–15.
8. Bailey WC, Richards JM, Brooks CM, Soong S, Windsor RA, Manzella BA. A randomized trial to improve self-management practices in adults with asthma. *Arch Intern Med* 1990; **150:** 1664–8.
9. Blessing-Moore J. Does asthma education change behavior? To know is not to do. *Chest* 1996; **109:** 9–19.
10. Barnes PJ. Poorly perceived asthma. *Thorax* 1992; **47:** 408–9.
11. Strunk RC, Mrazek DA, Wofson GS, Fuhrmann J, LaBrecque JF. Physiological and psychological characteristics associated with deaths from asthma in childhood: a case-controlled study. *J Am Med Assoc* 1985; **254:** 1193–8.
12. Rietveld S. Symptom perception in asthma: a multidisciplinary review. *J Asthma* 1998; **35**(2): 137–46.
13. Harver A, Mahler DA. Perception of increased resistance to breathing. In: Kotses H, Harver A, eds. *Self-Management of Asthma*. New York: Marcel Dekker, 1998, 147–93.
14. Fritz GK, Wamboldt MZ. Pediatric asthma: psychosomatic interactions and symptom perception. In: Kotses H, Harver A, eds. *Self-Management of Asthma*. New York: Marcel Dekker, 1998, 195–230.
15. Rubinfeld AR, Pain MC. Perception of asthma. *Lancet* 1976; **2:** 882.
16. Rietveld S, Prins PJM, Kolk AMM. The capacity of children with and without asthma to detect external resistive loads on breathing. *J Asthma* 1996; **33**(4): 221.
17. Fritz GK, McQuaid EL, Spirito A, Klein RB. Symptom perception in pediatric asthma: relationship to functional morbidity and psychological factors. *J Am Acad Child Adolesc Psychiatry* 1996; **35:** 1033–41.
18. Ruffin RE, Latimer KM, Schembri DA. Longitudinal study of near fatal asthma. *Chest* 1991; **99:** 77–83.
19. Kikuchi Y, Okabe S, Tamura G et al. Chemosensitivity and perception of dyspnea in patients with a history of near-fatal asthma. *N Engl J Med* 1994; **330:** 1329–34.
20. Kotses H. Individualized asthma self-management. In: Kotses H, Harver A, eds. *Self-Management of Asthma*. New York: Marcel Dekker, 1998, 309–28.
21. Boulet LP, Deschesnes F, Turcotte H, Gignac F. Near-fatal asthma: clinical and physiologic features, perception of bronchoconstriction, and psychologic profile. *J Allergy Clin Immunol* 1991; **88:** 838–46.
22. Bender B, Milgrom H, Rand C. Nonadherence in asthmatic patients: is there a solution to the problem? *Ann Allergy Asthma Immunol* 1997; **79:** 177–86.
23. Mawhinney H, Spector SL, Heitjan D et al. As-needed medication use in asthmatic usage patterns and patient characteristics. *J Asthma* 1993; **30:** 61–71.
24. Tashkin DP, Rand C, Nicles M et al. A nebulizer chronolog to monitor compliance with inhaler use. *Am J Med* 1991; **91:** 335–65.
25. Milgrom H, Bender B, Ackerson L et al. Noncompliance and treatment failure in children with asthma. *J Allergy Clin Immunol* 1996; **98:** 1051–7.
26. Gibson NA, Ferguson AE, Aitchison TC, Paton JY. Compliance with inhaled asthma medication in preschool children. *Thorax* 1995; **50:** 1274–9.
27. Horn CR, Clark TJH, Cochrane GM. Compliance with inhaled therapy and morbidity from asthma. *Respir Med* 1990; **84:** 67–70.
28. Cluss PA, Epstein LH, Galvis SA et al. Effects of compliance for chronic asthmatic children. *J Consult Clin Psychol* 1984; **52:** 909–10.
29. Weiss K, Gergen P, Hodgson T. An economic

30. Weinstein AG, Faust D. Maintaining theophylline compliance/adherence in severely asthmatic children: the role of psychologic functioning of the child and family. *Ann Allergy Asthma Immunol* 1997; **79**: 311–18.
31. Greineder DK, Loane KC, Parks P. Reduction in resource utilization by an asthma outreach program. *Arch Pediatr Adolesc Med* 1995; **149**: 415–20.
32. Lasagna L, Hutt PB. Health care, research, and regulatory impact of noncompliance. In: Cramer JA, Spilker B, eds. *Patient Compliance in Medical Practice and Clinical Trials*. New York: Raven Press, 1991, 393–403.
33. Urquhart J. Role of patient compliance in clinical pharmacokinetics. *Clin Pharmacokinet* 1994; **27**: 202–15.
34. Bender B. Adherence assessment: is there any way to tell what patients are really doing? Presented at the Annual Meeting of the American Academy of Allergy, Asthma and Immunology, Orlando, February 1999.
35. Bender B, Milgrom H, Rand C, Ackerson L. Psychological factors associated with medication nonadherence in children with asthma. *J Asthma* 1998; **353**: 347–53.
36. Bender BG, Milgrom H, Rand C, Wamboldt FS. Measurement of treatment nonadherence in children with asthma. In: Drotar D, ed. *Adherence in Chronic Childhood Illness*. Mahwah, NJ: Lawrence Erlbaum, in press.
37. Szefler SJ, Boushey HA, Pearlman DS et al. Time to onset of effect of fluticasone propionate in patients with asthma. *J Allergy Clin Immunol* 1999; **103**: 780–8.
38. Anderson B, Ho J, Brackett J, Finkelstein D, Laffel L. Parental involvement in diabetes management tasks: relationships to blood glucose monitoring adherence and metabolic control in young adolescents with insulin-dependent diabetes mellitus. *J Pediatr* 1997; **130**: 257–65.
39. Krupnick JL, Sotsky SM, Simmens S et al. The role of the therapeutic alliance in psychotherapy and pharmacotherapy outcome: findings in the National Institute of Mental Health treatment of depression collaborative research program. *J Consult Clin Psychol* 1996; **64**: 532–9.
40. Wright RJ, Rodriguez M, Cohen S. Review of psychosocial stress and asthma: an integrated biopsychosocial approach. *Thorax* 1998; **53**: 1066–74.
41. Busse WW, Kiecolt-Glaser JK, Coe C et al. Stress and asthma. *Am J Respir Crit Care Med* 1995; **151**: 249–52.
42. Cohen S, Tyrrell DAJ, Smith AP. Psychological stress and susceptibility to common cold. *N Engl J Med* 1991; **325**: 606–12.
43. Wright RJ, Hanrahan JP, Tager I et al. Effect of the exposure to violence on the occurrence and severity of childhood asthma in an inner-city population. *Am J Respir Crit Care Med* 1997; **155**: A972.
44. Miller B, Wood B. Psychophysiologic reactivity in asthmatic children: a cholinergically mediated confluence of pathways. *J Am Acad Child Adolesc Psychiatry* 1994; **33**: 1236–45.
45. Tal A, Miklich D. Emotionally induced decrease in pulmonary flow rates in asthmatic children. *Psychosom Med* 1976; **38**: 190–200.
46. Miklich DR, Rewey HH, Weiss JH et al. A preliminary investigation of psychophysiological responses to stress among different subgroups of asthmatic children. *J Psychosom Res* 1973; **17**: 1–8.
47. Kinsman RA, O'Banion K, Resenikoff P et al. Subjective symptoms of acute asthma within a heterogeneous sample of asthmatics. *J Allergy Clin Immunol* 1973; **52**: 284–329.
48. Dirks JF, Horton DJ, Kinsman RA et al. Patient and physician characteristics influencing medical decisions in asthma. *J Asthma Res* 1978; **15**: 171–7.
49. Baron C, Veilleux P, Lamarre A. The family of the asthmatic child. *Can J Psychiatry* 1992; **37**: 12–16.
50. Brooks CM, Richards JM, Bailey WC. Subjective symptomatology of asthma in an outpatient population. *Psychosom Med* 1989; **51**: 102–8.
51. Staudenmayer H, Kinsman RA, Jones NF. Attitudes towards respiratory illness and hospitalization in asthma. *J Nerv Ment Dis* 1978; **166**: 624–34.
52. Luparello T, Lyons HA, Bleecker ER, McFadden ER. Influences of suggestion on airway reactivity in asthmatic subjects. *Psychosom Med* 1968; **30**: 819–25.
53. McFadden ER, Luparello T, Lyons HA, Bleecker E. The mechanism of action of suggestion in the induction of acute asthma attacks. *Psychosom Med* 1969; **31**: 134–43.
54. Neild JE, Cameron JR. Bronchoconstriction in response to suggestion: its prevention by an inhaled anticholinergic agent. *Br Med J* 1985; **290**: 674.

55. Besch CL. Compliance in clinical trials. *AIDS* 1995; **9:** 1–10.
56. Lewinsohn PM, Haberman H, Terri L, Hautzinger M. An integrative theory of depression. In: Reiss S, Bootzin R, eds. *Theoretical Issues in Behavior Therapy.* New York: Academic Press, 1985, 331–59.
57. Bosley CM, Fosbury JA, Cochrane GM. The psychological factors associated with poor compliance with treatment in asthma. *Eur Respir J* 1995; **8:** 899–904.
58. Bender B. Tertiary care respiratory medicine: is there a place for psychology in the managed care world? *Health Psychologist* 1996; **18:** 10–26.
59. Clark NM, Levison MJ, Evans D et al. Communication within low income families and management of asthma. *Pat Educ Couns* 1990; **15:** 191–210.
60. Bender BG, Klinnert MD. Psychological correlates of asthma severity and treatment outcome in children. In: Kotses H, Harver A, eds. *Behavioral Contributions to the Management of Asthma.* New York: Marcel Dekker, 1998, 63–84.
61. Christiannse MD, Lavigne JV, Lerner CV. Psychosocial aspects of compliance in children and adolescents with asthma. *Dev Behav Pediatr* 1989; **10:** 75–80.
62. Wamboldt FS, Wamboldt MZ, Gavin LA et al. Parental criticism and treatment outcome in adolescents hospitalized for severe chronic asthma. *J Psychosom Res* 1995; **39:** 995–1005.
63. Jessop DJ, Riessman CK, Stein REK. Chronic childhood illness and maternal mental health. *J Dev Behav Pediatr* 1988; **9:** 147–56.
64. Mrazek DA, Klinnert M, Mrazek PJ et al. Prediction of early-onset asthma in genetically at-risk children. *Pediatr Pulmonol* 1999; **27:** 85–94.
65. Kopp CB, Krakow JB. The developmentalist and the study of biological risk, a view of the past with an eye toward the future. *Child Dev* 1983; **54:** 1086–108.
66. Cadman D, Boyle M, Szatmari P, Offord DR. Chronic illness, disability, and mental and social well-being: findings of the Ontario Child Health Study. *Pediatrics* 1987; **79:** 805–13.
67. Sly RM. Mortality from asthma, 1979–1984. *J Allergy Clin Immunol* 1988; **82:** 705–17.
68. Wissow LS, Gittelsohn AM, Sazklo M et al. Poverty, race, and hospitalization for childhood asthma. *Am J Public Health* 1988; **78:** 777–82.
69. Apter AJ, Reisine AT, Affleck G et al. Adherence with twice-daily dosing of inhaled steroids. *Am J Respir Crit Care Med* 1998; **157:** 1810–17.
70. Marder D, Targonski P, Orris P et al. Effect of racial and socioeconomic factors on asthma mortality in Chicago. *Chest* 1992; **101:** 426S–429S.
71. Vargas PA, Rand CS. A pilot study of electronic adherence monitoring in low-income, minority children with asthma. *Am J Respir Crit Care Med* 1999; **159:** A260.
72. Clark NM, Gong M, Schork MA et al. Impact of education for physicians on patient outcomes. *Pediatrics* 1998; **101:** 831–6.
73. Haire-Joshu D, Fisher EB, Munro J, Wedner HJ. A comparison of patient attitudes toward asthma self-management among acute and preventive care settings. *J Asthma* 1993; **30:** 359–71.
74. Munro JF, Haire-Joshu D, Fisher EB, Wedner HJ. Articulation of asthma and its care among low-income emergency care recipients. *J Asthma* 1996; **33:** 313–25.
75. Fisher E, Sussman L, Shannon W et al. Neighborhood asthma coalition impacts among low income, African-American children. *Am J Respir Crit Care Med* 1997; **155:** A728.
76. Cohen S. Psychosocial models of the role of social support in the etiology of physical disease. *Health Psychol* 1988; **7:** 269–97.
77. Cohen S, Wills TA. Stress, social support and the buffering hypothesis. *Psychol Bull* 1985; **98:** 310–57.
78. Clark NM, Dodge JA. Exploring self-efficacy as a predictor of disease management. *Health Educ Behav* 1999; **26:** 72–89.
79. Katz PP, Yelin EH, Smith S, Blanc PD. Perceived control of asthma: development and validation of a questionnaire. *Am J Respir Crit Care Med* 1997; **155:** 577–82.
80. Sorenson M. Maintenance of exercise behavior for individuals at risk for cardiovascular disease. *Perceptual Motor Skills* 1997; **85:** 867–80.
81. Calfas KJ, Sallis JF, Oldenburg B, French M. Mediators of change in physical activity following an intervention in primary care: PACE. *Prev Med* 1997; **26:** 297–304.
82. Lechner L, de Vries H, Offermans N. Participation in a breast cancer screening program: influence of past behavior and determinants on future screening participation. *Prev Med* 1997; **26:** 473–82.
83. Moore PJ, Turner R, Park CL, Adler N. The impact of behavior and addiction on psychological models of cigarette and alcohol use dur-

ing pregnancy. *Addictive Behav* 1996; **21:** 645–58.
84. Becker MH. Patient adherence to prescribed therapies. *Med Care* 1985; **23:** 539–55.
85. Stein MJ, Wallston KA, Nicassio PM et al. Correlates of a clinical classification schema for the arthritis helplessness index. *Arthritis Rheum* 1988; **31:** 876–81.
86. Peterman C. Learned helplessness and health psychology. *Health Psychol* 1982; **1:** 153–68.
87. Coronary Drug Project Research Group. Influence of adherence to treatment and response of cholesterol on mortality in the coronary drug project. *N Engl J Med* 1980; **303:** 1038–41.
88. Glynn RJ, Buring JE, Manson JE et al. Adherence to aspirin in the prevention of myocardial infarction. *Arch Intern Med* 1994; **154:** 2649–57.
89. Cromer BA. Behavioral strategies to increase compliance in adolescents. In: Cramer JA, Spilker B, eds. *Patient Compliance in Medical Practice and Clinical Trials.* New York: Raven Press, 1991, 99–105.
90. Gavin LA, Wamboldt MZ, Sorokin N et al. Treatment alliance and its association with family functioning, adherence, and medical outcome in adolescents with severe, chronic asthma. *J Pediatr Psychol* 1999; **24:** 355–65.
91. DiMatteo MR, Sherbourne CD, Hays RD et al. Physicians' characteristics influence patients' adherence to medical treatment: results from the medical outcomes study. *Health Psychol* 1993; **12:** 93–102.
92. Armstrong D, Glanville T, Bailey E, O'Keefe G. Doctor-initiated consultations: a study of communication between general practitioners and patients about the need for reattendance. *Brit J Gen Pract* 1990; **40:** 241–2.
93. Hall JA, Roter DL, Katz NR. Meta-analysis of correlates of provider behavior in medical encounters. *Med Care* 1988; **26:** 1–19.
94. Spilker B. Methods of assessing and improving patient compliance in clinical trials. In: Cramer JA, Spilker B, eds. *Patient Compliance in Medical Practice and Clinical Trials.* New York: Raven Press, 1991, 37–56.
95. Creer TL, Bender BG. Asthma. In: Gatchel RJ, Blanchard EB, eds. *Psychophysiological Disorders: Research and Clinical Applications.* Washington: American Psychological Association, 1993, 151–203.
96. Kotses H, Bernstein IL, Bernstein DI et al. A self-management program for adult asthma. Part I: development and evaluation. *J Allergy Clin Immunol* 1995; **95:** 529–40.
97. Bailey WC, Davies SL, Kohler CL. Adult asthma self-management programs. In: Kotses H, Harver A, eds. *Self-Management of Asthma.* New York: Marcel Dekker, 1998, 293–308.
98. Davis DA, Thomson MA, Oxman AD, Haynes RB. Evidence for the effectiveness of CME: a review of 50 randomized controlled trials. *JAMA* 1992; **268:** 1111–17.
99. Maiman LA, Becker MH, Liptak GS et al. Improving pediatricians' compliance-enhancing practices: a randomized trial. *Am J Dis Child* 1988; **142:** 773–9.
100. Gibson NA, Ferguson AE, Aitchison TC, Paton JY. Compliance with inhaled asthma medication in preschool children. *Thorax* 1995; **50:** 1274–9.
101. Klinnert M, Bender B. Psychological implications of pediatric asthma. In: Kaptein A, Creer T, eds. *Behavioral Sciences and Respiratory Disorders.* New York: Harwood Academic Publishers, in press.
102. Klinnert M, McQuaid E, Gavin L. Assessing the Family Asthma Management System. *J Asthma* 1997; **34:** 77–88.
103. Roter DL, Hall JA, Kern DE et al. Improving physicians' interviewing skills and reducing patients' emotional distress: a randomized clinical trial. *Arch Intern Med* 1995; **155:** 1877–84.
104. Keller VF, White MK. Choices and changes: a new model for influencing patient health behavior. *J Clin Outcomes Manage* 1997; **4:** 33–6.
105. Gavin LA, Roesler TA, Brenner AM. Day treatment for pediatric patients with medical and psychiatric needs. *Continuum* 1996; **3:** 95–102.
106. Gavin L, Klinnert M, Glenn K et al. Cost saving and outcome following attendance of a multidisciplinary day program for pediatric patients with severe asthma. *J Allergy Clin Immunol* 1998; **101:** S45.

16
Education programs

Virginia S Taggart

Introduction • What are the basics for asthma education? • What educational methods are best? • What asthma management behaviors are reasonable to expect at different ages? • Conclusion

INTRODUCTION

Asthma creates a significant burden for children and their families. Worldwide, asthma is increasing, ranging from about 3% in Greece, China, and India to over 15% in Australia, Ireland, New Zealand, and the United Kingdom.[1] Asthma disproportionately affects children. In the United States, asthma hospitalization rates are highest among persons aged 0–4 years; for this age group, the rates have increased by more than 28% in the last 15 years. Mortality rates have increased faster among children aged 5–12 years than among those aged 15–34 years.[2] Nearly one third of children with asthma restrict their activities because of the disease.[3,4] Asthma is a leading cause of school absences, resulting in a loss of over 11 million school days in 1 year.[5] Yet much of this burden is unnecessary: medical treatments that can enable most children with asthma to participate fully in all childhood activities are available. The challenge is to ensure that children around the world have access to these treatments. Education is a critical component of treatment because medications alone have no value if the child and his or her family are not willing and able to use them correctly.

All published asthma clinical practice guidelines stress that patients who become active participants in their care have an improved likelihood for well-controlled asthma.[6–8] Optimal education builds a therapeutic alliance between the clinician and patient (and family) through which the patient acquires self-management skills to become active in his or her care, and the patient (and family) and clinician work together to develop a tailored treatment plan and regularly review it to identify and overcome barriers to managing the patient's asthma.[9] A wide spectrum of asthma education programs has been developed for use in different settings (e.g., clinics, hospitals, schools, community centers, and homes) and for people of different cultures and ages. But their effectiveness varies widely. Are there essential ingredients to educational programs with demonstrated benefit that comprise a core for asthma education regardless of setting? What asthma management behaviors are reasonable to expect for children of different ages, and what educational methods are most likely to help children adopt these behaviors? This chapter addresses these questions.

WHAT ARE THE BASICS FOR ASTHMA EDUCATION?

Key information

Published clinical practice guidelines consistently list the following essential information for asthma patients, including children and their families:

(a) Asthma is a chronic inflammatory condition with recurrent exacerbations.
(b) Exacerbations are prevented through anti-inflammatory medication and reducing exposure to environmental factors that make asthma worse.
(c) There are two types of medications. One is taken daily for providing long-term control of symptoms and preventing exacerbations, and the other is taken only intermittently for prompt relief of symptoms and treatment of exacerbations.
(d) Self-monitoring of symptoms and peak flow helps patients and their families recognize exacerbations and take prompt action to keep them from being severe. Self-monitoring also helps the patient (and family) and clinician adjust the asthma management plan to provide optimal long-term asthma control with minimal side effects.

This basic information provides an important rationale for the treatment plan, but it is seldom sufficient to promote a patient's implementation of the plan. Furthermore, too many educational programs stop with the provision of information – or they give more information than is needed. Understanding elaborate descriptions of lung function is no more necessary to managing asthma than understanding the structure and mechanics of a bicycle is necessary to riding one. Indeed, one study has demonstrated that teaching patients about inflammation and when asthma medications should be used improved patient outcomes, but giving additional information about lung physiology had no effect.[10]

Key behaviors

The emphasis of education must be asthma management behaviors and helping patients incorporate them into their daily lives. Essential asthma management behaviors for children and their families include:

(a) Taking medications correctly;
(b) Monitoring symptoms, activity tolerance, and (for moderate to severe asthma) peak flow;
(c) Recognizing early signs of worsening asthma and following a recommended action plan;
(d) Seeking help appropriately and communicating effectively with the clinician providing care
(e) Instituting environmental control strategies to reduce exposure to relevant allergens and irritants.

Asthma self-management programs for children that focus on teaching and reinforcing these behaviors have proved to be effective through randomized controlled trials. Documented impacts include increases in self-management skills, symptom scores, and school performance and attendance, as well as reductions in urgent care visits and hospitalizations.[11-21] In looking at the long-term impact of asthma self-management programs, some studies note continued impact 2 years after the intervention,[22] other studies show short-lived impact,[23] and still other studies show that asthma management develops slowly[24] and actually improves over time.[25] Although more study is needed, these findings clearly support the educational principles of continual education and repetition of messages over time.

Key behavior change principles: the five R's of asthma teaching

Numerous factors predispose a child's and his or her family's motivation to adopt a recommended health behavior – most notably their perceptions about the seriousness of the condition, the effectiveness of treating it, and the economic and social costs of taking the treatment.[26] Behavior change also requires a basic ability and confidence to perform the behaviors successfully.[27] Successful asthma management depends as well on a child's and his or her family's ability to adjust the asthma management plan according to different circumstances and exposures because asthma severity varies over time and in different situations. It is impossible for clinicians to prescribe for every situation children with asthma must face, so these children and their parents must develop the decision-making skills necessary to allow them to independently refine their asthma management plan as needed, using the general guidelines given by the doctor.

Asthma education programs based on the self-regulation model of behavior change promote decision-making skills by teaching a process of observing, making judgments, and reacting realistically and appropriately to the child's own efforts to manage a task. Children with asthma and their parents determine what they will do given their specific goals, social context, and perception of capability. The program helps them identify and practice handling situations in which they have to recognize when the disease interferes with their goals, judge what might improve the situation, make practical judgments, test management strategies by trying out new behaviors, and draw conclusions. Through this, the children with asthma and their parents develop confidence to carry out appropriate behaviors in future situations. This model posits that neither information, confidence (self-efficacy), nor specific management techniques and skills are sufficient alone, but that all fit together to promote effective asthma management behavior.[28,29]

Behavior change depends on knowing what to do, believing it is worth doing, being able to do it, and being reinforced for doing it. The five R's of asthma education that are described here and listed in Table 16.1 provide a succinct framework for incorporating these behavioral change principles into educational programs.

Table 16.1 The five R's for teaching

Reach agreement on goals for treatment
    Tailor treatment to the patient's routine; keep it simple
    Set priorities
    Specify actions for handling exacerbations
Rehearse asthma management skills
    Taking medication
    Monitoring symptoms and, if appropriate, peak flow
    Decision making
Repeat messages
Reinforce appropriate behavior
Review results

Reach agreement on goals and the treatment plan

Goals for treatment and for evaluation of treatment outcomes should be mutually agreed upon by both the clinician and the child with asthma and his or her parents. Goals for therapy promoted by published guidelines include freedom from symptoms day and night, near normal pulmonary function, normal activity including exercise, pharmacology to control asthma with the fewest side effects, no emergency department visits or hospitalizations for asthma, and satisfaction with asthma care. These goals need to be personalized to increase the likelihood of the treatment plan being followed. For example, many parents accept sleepless nights and persistent cough as something that just has to be lived with, and children often adapt their choices of activities to accommodate their disease. Children with asthma and their parents often need to be encouraged to raise their expectations for what can be accomplished with therapy. However, some parents may be fearful of medication or overwhelmed by a lengthy list of recommendations, such that the goals offered by the clinician seem impractical or not worthwhile.

A crucial first step in helping patients listen to the clinician's advice and reach agreement on treatment is to elicit and address patient concerns about asthma.[30] Open discussion about concerns often convinces the child and parents that the recommended treatments will actually help the child with asthma reach his or her personal goals, which is a prerequisite for adherence to the treatment.[31]

Once goals are identified, a realistic treatment plan can be developed by the clinician, child, and parents together. Treatment plans have two parts:

(1) a plan for daily management of asthma that delineates recommended daily medications, prophylactic treatment for exercise if indicated, and environmental control measures to reduce exposure to allergens or irritants known to worsen the child's asthma;
(2) an action plan specifying actions to take for prompt relief of symptoms and exacerbations. Writing the plans down is strongly associated with increased adherence.[32–36] Written plans serve as a reference point that helps children and their parents be active participants in care by delineating conditions for adjusting the treatment plan; this responsibility is often an incentive for adhering to the plan[37] (see resources listed in Table 16.2 for sample written plans, especially National Asthma Education and Prevention Program).

Rehearse asthma management skills

Necessary skills include medication-taking skills, monitoring skills, and decision-making skills. Treatment failures can often be traced to inadequate inhaler technique. Over 50% of patients do not use inhalers correctly; many are never shown how.[38,39] It is essential for clinicians to demonstrate correct technique and have the child demonstrate back, and to review technique at every patient visit.

Self-monitoring by the child with asthma and his or her parents helps evaluate clinical asthma control over time and detect exacerbations and initiate early rescue treatment to prevent symptoms from becoming severe. To accomplish this, children with asthma and their families need to know the signs and symptoms of worsening asthma: waking at night with asthma symptoms, increased need for rescue inhaled beta-agonist medication, shortened duration of medication effect or tolerance for daily activities, and escalating symptoms of shortness of breath, wheezing, chest tightness, and progressive coughing.

Peak flow monitoring is useful for children over the age of 4 years who have difficulty recognizing or reporting symptoms, or who have moderate or severe asthma.

Repeat messages

Patients often have difficulty recalling messages given in the context of a brief medical care visit, or given as a part of a lengthy educational program. Repeating key messages at least three times significantly increases patient recall.[40] This can easily be accomplished by giving a verbal message, giving written or video materials to support the message, and having the child and parents repeat back the message in their own words.

Reinforce appropriate behavior

Reinforcement shapes and maintains behavior: behavior that is rewarded is repeated. Reinforcement for children can range from praising asthma management behaviors verbally, to offering token prizes for completing self-management tasks (such as keeping a diary or taking daily medication), and to telephoning children or their parents to inquire about any problems and discuss ways to address them. People who are important to the child should be recruited to help give support and reinforcement. Social support is a predictor of adherence and more positive health outcomes.[41] Mothers of children with asthma frequently express a sense, for both themselves and their children,

Table 16.2 Education resources for children with asthma

Asthma Education and Prevention Program
Information Center
PO Box 20105
Bethesda, MD 20824-0105
USA
Tel: +1-301-592-8573
www.nhlbi.nih.gov

Allergy and Asthma Network
Mothers of Asthmatics, Inc.
2751 Prosperity Avenue, Suite 150
Fairfax, VA 22031
USA
Tel: +1-703-641-9595

Allergy and Asthma Federation
Sibeliuksenkatu 11 A 2
Helsinki
Finland
Tel: +358-0-9-441-911
allergia.asthmaliitto@aal.pp.fi

Asthma and Allergy Foundation of America
1233 20th Street, N.W., Suite 402
Washington, DC 20036
USA
Tel: +1-202-466-7643
www.aafa.org

American Academy of Allergy, Asthma, and Immunology
611 East Wells Street
Milwaukee, WI 53202
USA
Tel: +1-800-822-2762

American Lung Association
American Thoracic Society
1740 Broadway
New York, NY 10019-4374
USA
Tel: +1-212-315-8700
www.lungusa.org

Global Initiative for Asthma (GINA)
MCR, Inc. 8316 86th Ave., NW
Gig Harbor, WA 98332
USA
www.ginasthma.com
**An August 1998 GINA newsletter includes an Asthma Association Directory listing organizations around the world that have patient education and support groups.

National Asthma Campaign – Australia
Level 1, 1 Palmerston Crescent
South Melbourne, VIC3205
Australia
Tel: +61-03-92-14-1400
nac@ozonline.com.au

National Asthma Campaign – United Kingdom
Providence House, Providence Place
London, N1 0NT
United Kingdom
Tel: +44-020-7226-2260
www.asthma.org.uk

National Jewish Medical and Research Center
Lung LINE
1400 Jackson St.
Denver, CO 80206
USA
Tel: +1-800-222-LUNG

Pedipress, Inc.
125 Redgate Lane
Amherst, MA 01002
USA
Tel: +1-800-344-5864

that they are alone in facing this condition. Support groups provide emotional support and help people share and hence lighten the burden of asthma.

Review

Asthma is a chronic, dynamic condition that varies considerably over time for patients, especially children. Thus continual review is necessary to assess whether therapeutic goals have been met and whether the treatment plan needs to be adjusted or further education is needed. Open-ended questions can elicit accurate information on, for example, how many sleep interruptions the child has experienced since the last visit, how much rescue inhaler treatment was used, in what way the child's asthma has interfered with daily activities, and what problems the child and parents have had following the treatment plan. Of course, review also includes observation of the child's and parents' medication and monitoring techniques. Through this review, joint decision making can identify and address problems.

Key communication strategies for behavior change

Incorporate cultural beliefs and use the appropriate language

Cultural and language differences may present barriers to communication and education by preventing accurate understanding and acceptance of recommended treatments. Wherever possible, supplementing clinician instruction with instruction by an educator who speaks the same language as the child with asthma and his or her family is helpful. Further, cultural beliefs can often be incorporated into the treatment plan and thus boost acceptance and provide reassurance that the clinician is trying to tailor recommendations to patient lifestyles as much as possible. For example, in one community, because diseases like asthma were considered cold and thus needed hot treatment, taking asthma medication along with a warm drink was recommended. Some cultural practices can be detrimental. Open-ended questions, such as 'What else have you tried to help your asthma?', 'What local home remedies are recommended in your community?', 'Have any of these things helped?', can help reveal relevant cultural practices. The clinician can negotiate with the child's family to change those practices that must be changed and work around those that cannot be changed. This will strengthen the partnership and increase the likelihood of the child and family accepting the medical recommendations.

Enhance the clinician–patient relationship

The clinician–patient relationship has a greater influence on treatment adherence than any other factor.[31,42,43] Communication strategies that enhance this relationship as well as increase patient satisfaction with medical care and improve patient adherence and problem solving[9,22,30] are listed in Table 16.3 and include:

(a) Showing attentiveness. Friendliness, smiling, making eye contact, sitting at the same level as the patient, and leaning forward slightly are positively associated with patient satisfaction.
(b) Addressing immediate concerns and expectations for the visit. Ask open-ended questions, such as 'What would you like from this visit?'

Table 16.3 Communication strategies for behavior change

- Show attentiveness
- Address immediate concerns and expectations for the visit
- Elicit underlying fears
- Give reassuring messages
- Talk with the child and parents in an open, interactive dialog
- Provide verbal and nonverbal encouragement

(c) Eliciting underlying fears. Fears about asthma or asthma treatments distract patients from either listening to or adopting new recommendations. Ask open-ended questions, such as 'What does asthma mean to you?', 'What bothers you about it?', 'What concerns do you have about asthma medications?' Common fears – such as fear of addiction to medication, fear of medication side effects, fear of loss of effect over time, and fear of engaging in physical activity – may need to be addressed.

(d) Giving reassuring messages. Expressing empathy and providing reassuring information will help to allay patient fears and boost renewed attempts to follow the asthma management plan. For example, many parents are reluctant to continue chronic daily medications, and they will try to reduce either the doses or the number of administrations without realizing that stopping daily therapy altogether will probably result in a recurrence of symptoms. Reassurance that efforts will be made to reduce therapy carefully and gradually depending on the child's progress will encourage the parents to continue with the treatment, and monitor the child's asthma to help make decisions about adjusting treatment.

(e) Talking with the child and parents in an open, interactive dialogue. Use simple language and analogies to make information about asthma more meaningful to the child. Ask open-ended questions; recruit the child and parents into a joint problem-solving effort to address difficulties in following the asthma management plan; encourage the child to use decision-making skills and talk through how different situations might be handled (e.g., a school field trip or an overnight visit to a friend's house). An open discussion will also help the parents and child set realistic priorities.

(f) Giving both verbal and nonverbal encouragement. That is, give verbal praise for using effective management strategies and nod agreement or smile as the child and parents talk.

The teaching skills and communication strategies listed in Tables 16.1 and 16.3 can serve as a checklist reminder for each clinical visit.

Involve the child directly in the communication
This involvement is essential during medical care visits and educational programs. Many clinicians assume that 'asthma partnership' means working with parents, and reasonably so because numerous studies document that children's compliance is affected by parental beliefs and motivations. But the child should be included as well – even the young child. A researcher in primary care medicine described a scenario in which a father brought his 7-year-old daughter for follow-up after treatment for otitis media. The physician asked the father four sequential questions about the treatment and the father responded incorrectly; the daughter interjected with the correct information. Not once in the exchange did the physician break eye contact with the father or acknowledge the daughter's comments, even when the medication had to be changed.[44] This is not an isolated observation: studies of communications between physicians and children reveal that very little goes on between them in a medical encounter. Even those studies in which 45% of the physician communication was directed at the child, most of it was in the form of directives (such as 'Take off your shirt') or of humoring the child. Only 6% of the communication was focused on medical information.[45] The incongruity of this is disconcerting. Young children, even as young as 2 years, are expected to follow complex instructions at home, day care, or at school; and young children make many decisions that influence asthma outcomes (including whether to cooperate with the medical treatment, play with the cat, or report symptoms to their caregivers). But they are seldom viewed as capable of receiving medical instructions or of being actively involved and responsible in the treatment of their condition[44,46] – which is the ultimate goal of asthma management for all patients. Recruiting young children early into the asthma partnership provides an important foundation for them to become active participants in their own care as

young adults. Moreover, a study among children found that parent satisfaction and cooperation with medical care increased when the physician talked directly and extensively with the child.[47]

WHAT EDUCATIONAL METHODS ARE BEST?

The superiority of any one teaching method or setting is not yet established. Research evaluations have been conducted in many settings, including outpatient clinics or medical offices, hospitals, emergency rooms, schools, and community centers, but no studies have compared one setting or teaching method directly to another. Nor is it clear whether a particular teaching method is superior.

Group programs

Group educational classes may be more cost effective than individual education because more people can be taught at one time. Group learning strategies have widespread acceptance in elementary and high school classroom settings, and they have proved to be effective in teaching children with chronic diseases about their condition. Group programs can be a valuable source of social support and peer training in which members of the group can exchange tips on coping with the day-to-day challenges of juggling asthma care with daily routines and the competing needs within the child's family. Group education has, on the one hand, yielded equal and more efficient results on some outcome measures compared to individual education;[48] on the other hand, group programs are often not related in any meaningful way with the child's source of medical care. Further, many children and parents cannot arrange the time or transportation to attend extended functions that are separate from the medical encounter. Another concern is that educators may shorten the published programs in order to appeal to more patients and use fewer staff resources, but these abbreviated classes may seriously compromise the validity and effectiveness of the original, evaluated program. For example, educational strategies employed in group classes such as group problem-solving tasks and homework assignments are particularly effective in motivating children with asthma to make behavior changes and should not be deleted.[49]

Individualized programs

Individualized programs delivered by clinicians during medical care visits have the distinct and substantial advantage of integrating the educational messages with the medical treatment, which is a powerful intervention.[31,50,51] Involving the entire staff in giving consistent messages (receptionists, nurses, respiratory technicians) is desirable, and has resulted in long-standing changes in children attending public health clinics.[52] However, the direct involvement of the principal clinician is essential.

A potential limitation of individualized education is that it may take more time than clinicians perceive they have to give during a medical visit – even though the entire visit may be wasted without appropriate education. But extensive time expenditure by the clinician may not be necessary: one study in which physicians were instructed to be more effective educators found that the children with asthma had sustained reductions in the need for urgent care two years following the intervention and these physicians spent no more time with patients than did physicians who had not received the instruction.[22]

Innovative strategies have been developed to help clinicians deliver education efficiently. Among these are published guidelines that recommend an incremental approach to education in which different topics are taught on sequential visits, in addition to the key every-visit reviews of the treatment plan and of any difficulties the patient may have with it, and observations of the child's (or parent's) patients' medication technique.[6,53] Some strategies encourage clinicians to offer brief instruction by simply talking about whatever activity they are performing in the visit, reviewing asthma status since the last visit, and giving a nebulizer treatment or a peak flow measurement.[54,55] Recruiting the whole health care professional team to take advantage of such opportunities enhances the education. Having questionnaires at the reception area to ask about patient asthma status since the last visit and questions for the current visit, placing written and video materials in the waiting and examination rooms, reviewing adherence and inhaler techniques while taking a history, flagging the patient record to focus the clinician's discussion time on areas needing most attention, and making referrals to group education all provide valuable instruction and reinforcement.

Other formats

Additional educational formats can also be useful. Videos giving instruction on inhalation technique produced better performance scores than did personal instruction,[56] perhaps because patients could take the video home for repeated instruction. However, videos are not necessarily preferred, or successful in improving adherence.[57] Pamphlets, books, and workbooks can introduce topics to patients or reinforce messages delivered by the clinician. They are in high demand by patients and enhance patient satisfaction,[9] but they are not a replacement for education delivered directly by the clinician. One study found that patients given pamphlets about their condition along with nurse instruction did worse than with nurse instruction alone,[58] presumably because the nurse instructors relied too heavily on the written material to do the job for them. Computer and video games are recent advances in reaching children, and they may have similar benefits,[56,59,60] but more extensive evaluation of this newer technology is needed.

The variety of educational media and approaches gives clinicians the opportunity to tailor their educational approaches to the preferences and learning styles of individual children and their parents, and educational principles stress that multiple strategies are often necessary to accomplish the complex behavior changes required for adequate asthma management. According to a recent Cochrane collaborative review of adult education programs (which is likely to apply equally to childhood programs), the most successful asthma management education is integrated into the medical care routine – by coupling training in asthma self-management, which involves self-monitoring by either peak expiratory flow or symptoms, with regular medical review and a written action plan.[36] Whatever the method of delivering the education, effective programs are those that focus on teaching and reinforcing asthma behaviors.

WHAT ASTHMA MANAGEMENT BEHAVIORS ARE REASONABLE TO EXPECT AT DIFFERENT AGES?

Because the goal is to teach children skills for managing their asthma well on a daily basis, it is essential to approach children's asthma education in the same way that children's education in the skills of daily living are approached: start early, gradually increase responsibility, and foster personal decision making and independence as soon as the child is ready. Table 16.4 shows asthma management behaviors that can be expected at different ages, depending on individual variations in maturity among children.[61–63] To adapt expectations and educational messages to suit different age groups, it is helpful to consider perceptions about illness and learning styles that are typical of the different age groups. These considerations (for ages 2–5, 6–12, and 13–18 years) are based on principles from developmental psychology[64] and the behavioral and social learning theories discussed earlier.

Ages 2–5 years

This is the age of magical thinking. Children often think that they have asthma because they have been bad. Ninety percent of children in one study interpreted their hospitalization as punishment or rejection.[65] Preschoolers, then, need reassurance and simple explanations that asthma 'just happens' – that, just as some children have curly hair, freckles, or brown eyes, they have asthma. They need simple reassurance that when asthma makes them feel bad, they will be taken care of and not left alone. They also need to be helped to adopt an attitude that asthma is a part of life and to take pride in mastering steps toward handling it. Children this age are at a 'pre-operational' stage in which thinking is dominated by the child's perceptions rather than by logic. However, although it is often difficult for the child to see things in a larger context, the child watches, listens, and asks questions. A study of children aged 4–7 years found that 92% could repeat advice given to the mother during a visit to the doctor, and that all of the children had specific questions related to the reason for the visit but none was given the chance to talk.[47] Thus children should be included in the conversation, and should be given an opportunity to ask questions and receive concrete, simple answers, even though the clinician may direct most of the medical instruction to the parents.

Asthma education at this age should include asking the children what asthma means to them, and what they think the medicine will do to them, with simple demonstrations of how the children can cooperate with treatment, identify body signs and symptoms of asthma, and report these to an adult.[19] Because young children learn by imitating behaviors of their caregivers, giving demonstrations with dolls or stuffed toys and allowing the child to manipulate the treatment objects will be helpful. Storytelling, song, and play activities are successfully used to teach specific asthma skills.[66] Some preschools have an asthma corner in which children can play house with asthma equipment. Booklets about the feelings of having asthma and videos about recognizing and reporting symptoms provide entertaining and reassuring lessons about accepting asthma and taking care of it (see resource list, Table 16.2, especially American Lung Association and Mothers of Asthmatics).

Children aged 4–5 years enjoy trying out different roles, and thus they respond well to stories and comic books depicting superhero-like characters taking charge of asthma. This provides important modeling of desired behaviors. Children at age 4 years can begin carrying out many daily medication routines, with adult supervision. They can gradually assume more responsibility for remembering when to take the medications, preparing the medications, and taking the medication themselves. Most 4-year-olds can use a peak flow meter and help mark symptom diaries, which reinforces accurate reporting of asthma signs and symptoms. Asthma education at this age, then, must provide opportunities to practice different asthma management behaviors and must reinforce children for performing them.

Ages 6–12 years

Children in this age range are in a 'concrete operational' stage in which they still learn from observing and interacting but can also use symbols to organize thought and represent experiences. They can apply general rules of causality, and like to learn about the connection between events. Indeed, 6–12-year-olds are eager to understand 'why,' and many think asthma can be caught like a cold. These children can classify things and events into meaningful categories. They can start understanding the viewpoints of others. Common fears about asthma at this age concern help being there when they need it and worry about being teased or perceived to be different from other children. Children at this stage can look at others who manage asthma successfully and want this for themselves.

Simple explanations about the key features of asthma – inflammation and bronchoconstriction – and what causes symptoms and more severe exacerbations are important at this stage. This is an ideal time to introduce the concept of 'asthma triggers' (exposure to certain allergens and irritants that make asthma worse) and to recruit the child into dealing with them. The child can learn to identify and classify things around the house or school that make his or her asthma worse, and to take action with the family to reduce exposure. Symptom and peak flow

Table 16.4 Asthma management behaviors for children

Age range (years)	Management behaviors
1.5–2	Cooperates with treatment Develops body awareness: labels symptoms
3	Reports symptoms to adult
4–5	Takes routine medications with supervision Uses inhaler with spacer Uses peak flow meter Recognizes and reports signs and symptoms of worsening asthma Begins communicating with others about asthma Talks about fears and concerns with parents and clinician

6–12	Learns medication schedule
	Avoids asthma triggers
	Recognizes and responds to symptoms of worsening asthma
	Monitors asthma with parents
	Keeps symptom and peak flow diaries (even if just 2 weeks before clinician's office visit)
	Reports asthma status to clinician:
	  – frequency of beta agonist use
	  – limitations of daily activities
	  – night-time awakenings
	Recognizes and reports side-effects
	Talks with clinician about barriers to following the asthma management plan and how to overcome them
	Communicates with others about asthma (e.g. peers, teachers)
	Begins problem solving to make decisions:
	    Stop and figure out what the problem is
	    Think about all the possible ways to solve the problem
	    Ask what would happen with each choice
	    Respond by making a choice and testing it out

13–17	Takes medication independently Remembers when it is time to take medication Brings medication when away from home Decides when it is necessary to take medications to relieve symptoms (called 'quick relief', 'reliever', or 'rescue' medications) Monitors asthma independently Reports to parents when medications need to be refilled Avoids asthma triggers Uses decision-making skills to handle contingencies Decides when to seek medical attention Helps family make and keep medical appointments for routine care

diaries, even if kept for limited intervals, can help children see the connection between daily medication and improved ability to participate in daily childhood activities. A simplified action plan for handling asthma symptoms that can be kept on prominent display in the house, taken to school, and kept in the child's book bag will provide reassurance to the child that asthma can be handled wherever he or she goes.

Most evaluated asthma educational programs are for this age group. Many use group instruction, which provides the additional benefits of helping children with asthma to learn they are not alone and of practicing communicating with peers about their asthma. Some individual education programs accomplish this objective through video.[67,68] All programs incorporate the instructional methods of modeling desired behaviors, providing opportunities to practice and receive feedback about performance, and teaching asthma decision-making skills.

Educational programs that teach decision-making skills for asthma management and that appeal to this age group include a variety of teaching methods. Because children learn best by 'doing,' the education must include ample opportunities to practice decision-making skills. Analogies are useful. One program uses the analogy of cars and traffic signals and puts children in the driver's seat to teach them which conditions mean 'go' (green light), 'slow down' (yellow light), or 'stop' (red light).[16] Stories about sports figures or community leaders with asthma can provide inspiration and help a child discover that asthma need not be the defining factor in his or her life. Board, video, or computer games improve knowledge about basic asthma facts and management strategies. Remembering the 'STAR' is an attractive and easy way for children to figure out what to do:

- **S**top (figure out what the problem is)
- **T**hink (think about all the possible ways to solve the problem)
- **A**sk (ask what would happen with each choice)
- **R**espond (respond by making the best choice and testing it out)[62]

Role-playing scenarios depicting different situations a child could expect to be in are helpful. Clinician and family discussions with the child about such anticipated events as overnight visits away from home and school field trips will also prepare a child to handle them responsibly. Small playing cards with 'What would you do if...' scenarios on one side and recommended actions on the flip side can be used in waiting rooms both to reinforce decision-making skills and to prompt discussion with the clinician and parent.

The settings for educational programs targeted to this age group vary widely. Education in the ambulatory and hospital setting have demonstrated benefit, both through group instruction[13,16] and individual patient counseling.[48,68,69] School-based programs are increasingly popular as an opportunity to reach more children with asthma because many children do not have medical care providers who offer education, and because not all families can afford the time or additional travel to classes. School programs range from one-day events that increase awareness about asthma and expectations for normal play,[70] to formal classes that teach children with asthma some specific management skills and improve overall asthma management and school performance and reduce the frequency and severity of asthma episodes.[15] However, these programs have so far not involved school personnel in changing the school environment, so it is often difficult for children to follow their asthma management plans at school, have access to their medication, get assistance during an episode, or get encouragement or support for participating in physical education activities.[71] A school nurse intervention that did not result in any changes[72] underscores the importance of targeting school efforts at a demonstrated need (e.g. high levels of absences due to asthma) and providing continuing support to the school staff and students. Efforts to address these issues are currently being evaluated, and focused on programs designed to include school personnel and change school policies, to train school nurses to be more proactive,[73] and to offer materials such as a 'How Asthma Friendly Is Your School' checklist and prototype curricula for classroom teachers to teach all children in the school about asthma and how to help a student who has it (see resource list in Table 16.2, especially National Asthma Education and Prevention Program).

Summer camps for this age group of children with asthma as well as other chronic medical conditions have proliferated. Such camps offer these children the benefits of camping as well as of learning about their own condition and of practicing putting their condition into a healthy perspective – all within a safe environment with medical experts nearby.[74]

Ages 13–17 years

Adolescents are in a 'formal operations' stage in which they use reason, think logically, and are interested in theoretical possibilities. Self-reflection is strong. Teens have the developmental task of accomplishing greater individuation and separation from their family, and may choose noncompliance as a measure of assuming control and testing the boundaries – both of their asthma and their parents. Peers have a substantial influence in shaping the adolescent's perception of themselves, health practices, and choices about daily activities.

Educational strategies for teens promote the balance between parents and peers that is necessary to help them take positive responsibility for their asthma care. Negotiating about treatment options, dosing times, and schedules is important. Opportunities must be provided for the teen to have control. Written asthma management plans that serve as contracts are highly effective tools for making the asthma management plan clearer, more objective, and accountable for all concerned. Clarification of roles is important, as demonstrated in a study that found higher levels of non-adherence and morbidity among African American adolescents when parents decreased their involvement in asthma management activities because they overestimated the adolescents' assumption of responsibility.[63] The clinician can be a valuable resource for helping teens and parents be explicit about dividing family responsibilities for asthma management.

Support groups such as SAY (Support for Asthmatic Youth) in the United States (see resource list in Table 16.2, especially Asthma and Allergy Foundation of America) play a critical role because they provide opportunities for teens to observe desired behaviors, rehearse these behaviors, and be reinforced for performing the behaviors by their peers. 'Inoculation' role-playing can stimulate appropriate cognitive development of foreseeing and planning for consequences – essential in asthma management. Games and get-togethers allow teens to learn through play (still the 'job' of childhood). Special projects that can be designed to meet a group's perceived needs and involve all group members in learning about and caring for their asthma include not only developing games about asthma, but also creating videos to teach young children about asthma, arranging visits to group members who have to be hospitalized, and organizing parties and performances for parents.

Educational videos, interactive computer games, and internet web-sites[75] also offer promising opportunities for reaching adolescents. Clinicians report that e-mail has enhanced communication with older children and young adults.[76] However, research to evaluate the impact of such methods on changing asthma management behavior is needed.

Parents

Asthma management programs have frequently been called 'self-management programs', presumably to emphasize the importance of actively engaging patients in taking care of their condition. Unfortunately, this may discount the partnership among patient, family, and clinician that is essential for effective asthma management. Asthma self-management education for children is not meant to leave children by themselves to manage the condition on their own, but rather to teach skills for gradually increasing responsibility and independence within a partnership.

Teaching asthma management behaviors to children is just part of the effort. Many group educational programs include sessions for parents about asthma, and school programs send information home to parents about what the children have learned. An innovative hospital program in which a nurse visited the home for discussion about adequate home management and prevention of exacerbations both strengthened the link between medical recommendations and the realities of daily living, and resulted in significantly fewer re-admissions.[69]

In addition to learning about asthma, parents may need help appreciating those parenting behaviors that will foster effective asthma management skills among their children, such as those listed in Table 16.5. Children's feelings of self-confidence and self-esteem are influenced strongly by parents' attitudes about what the child can do to manage asthma, and teenagers' adherence to medical recommendations is strongly predicted by parental involvement.[77] Children with highly critical parents, limited demonstration of affection, conflict between family members, denial of symptoms by the parent, or no clear expectations and consequences for their behavior have significantly lower rates of adherence to medical regimens and higher morbidity caused by their condition.[31]

The clinician can help set the tone of respect for the child's capabilities, the goal of greater independence, and the expectation for parental support every step of the way. Written asthma management plans can be a helpful tool for delineating expectations about who should be doing what task. This may be especially important where multiple caregivers are involved and there can be tension among caregivers about how best to handle things. The clinician can help the primary caregivers agree on who is responsible for the child's asthma care, on a clear plan for handling attacks and notifying the appropriate people, and on how to provide consistency in managing asthma. The written plan can help maintain objectivity, consistency, and a clear focus on the priority asthma behaviors. At routine follow-up medical care visits, the clinician can conduct developmental updates to adjust family-based treatment plans according to the child's maturity. Families may need assistance in determining when it is appropriate to shift the distribution of responsibility for management tasks.[63]

Table 16.5 Parent behaviors to promote asthma management

- Deals with asthma in a straightforward manner
- Encourages age-appropriate independence in the child
- Teaches age-appropriate asthma management skills to the child
- Sets expectations for adherence behavior and consequences for nonadherence
- Does not use asthma as an excuse for the child
- Does not use asthma as an excuse to deny the child

(Adapted with permission from Wilson S, Fish L, Page A, Starr-Schneidkraul N. *Wee Wheezers: An educational program for parents of children with asthma under the age of seven.* Instructor's Manual. Palo Alto, CA: American Institutes for Research, 1994)

CONCLUSION

Well-organized education programs to teach children asthma management have proven effectiveness in reducing illness owing to asthma and in improving school performance and participation in a wide range of childhood activities. The ultimate vision is for education to be in every setting meaningful to children, including the clinician's office, the home, and school. In this comprehensive approach, education starts very early in life and helps the child learn asthma management skills alongside other skills for daily living. Clinicians talk directly to children about their asthma as soon as the child experiences symptoms, whether he or she is 1 year old or 11 years old; education for asthma management behaviors is integrated into all medical care visits; and parents supplement the messages at home and reinforce the child's performance of appropriate asthma management behaviors. Children attend 'asthma friendly' schools that allow prompt access to medications, minimize exposure to known irritants, encourage participation in all school activities, and foster peer support; asthma education and support groups are available to help children (and parents) feel accepted and to discover ways to put asthma into a healthy life perspective. Information and reassurance about asthma are readily available to children through attractive media, including computers, the internet, video, and books. Each type of program has a role. Programs with proven success are those that focus on asthma behavior, not knowledge. Key elements to that success are incorporation of effective communication strategies and the educational principles of the R's: reaching agreement on goals, rehearsing skills, repeating educational messages, reinforcing appropriate behavior, and reviewing asthma management results. Including these elements in education programs for children helps children of all ages accomplish the goal of learning lifelong skills to work in partnership to manage asthma.

REFERENCES

1. ISAAC Steering Committee. Worldwide variation in prevalence of symptoms of asthma, allergic rhinoconjunctivitis, and atopic eczema: ISAAC. The international study of asthma and allergies in childhood. *Lancet* 1998; 25; **351**(9111): 1225–32.
2. Mannino DM, Homa DM, Pertowski CA, et.al. Surveillance for Asthma-United States, 1960–1995. In CDC Surveillance Summaries April 24, 1998. MMWR 1998; 47 (No. SS–1): 1–28.
3. Department of Health and Human Services, USA. Action against asthma: a strategic plan for the Department of Health and Human Services. Washington (DC): Office of Science Policy, May 2000.
4. Department of Health and Human Services, USA. *Healthy People 2010: Objectives for improving health*. Washington (DC), 2000, chapter 24.
5. Weiss K, Sullivan S, Lyttle C. Trends in the cost of illness for asthma in the United States, 1985–1994. *J Allergy Clin Immunol* 2000; **106**: 493–9.
6. National Heart, Lung, and Blood Institute. Global initiative for asthma. Global strategy for asthma management and prevention. NHLBI/WHO workshop report. National Institutes of Health Publication No. 95–3659, 1995.
7. British Thoracic Society et al. The British guidelines on asthma management 1995 review and position statement. *Thorax*, 1997; **52**(Suppl) 51–521.
8. Ernst P, Fitzgerald JM, Spier S. Canadian Asthma Consensus Conference Summary of Recommendations. *Can Resp J* 1996; **3**(2): 89–100.
9. Partridge MR, Hell SR. Enhancing care for people with asthma: The role of communication education, training and self management. *Eur Resp J* 2000; **16**: 333–48.
10. Takakura S, Hasegawa T, Ishihara K et al. Assessment of patients' understanding of asthmatic condition established in an outpatient clinic. *Eur Respir J* 1998; **12:** (suppl) 29, 24S.
11. Staudenmayer H, Harris PS, Selner JC. Evaluation of a self-help education-exercise program for asthmatic children and their parents: Six-month follow-up. *J Asthma* 1981; **18**: 1–5.
12. Clark NM, Feldman CH, Evans D et al. Managing better: Children, parents and asthma. *Patient Educ Counsel* 1986; **8:** 27–38.
13. Clark NM, Feldman CH, Evans D et al. The impact of health education on frequency and cost of health care use by low income children with asthma. *J Allergy Clin Immunol* 1986; **78**(1): 108–15.
14. Clark NM, Gotsch A, Rosenstock IR. Patient, professional, and public education on behavioral aspects of asthma: a review of strategies for change and needed research. *J Asthma*, 1993; **30**(4) 241–55.
15. Evans D, Clark NM, Feldman CH et al. A school health education program for children with asthma aged 8–11 years. *Health Educ Q* 1987; **14**(3): 267–79.
16. Lewis CE, Rachelefsky G, Lewis MA et al. A randomized trial of ACT (asthma care training) for kids. *Pediatrics* 1984; **74**: 478–86.
17. Creer TL, Wigal JK, Kotses H, Lewis P. A critique of 19 self management programs for childhood asthma: comments regarding the scientific merit of the programs. *Pediatr Asthma Allergy Immunol* 1990; **4**: 41–55.
18. Fireman P, Friday G, Gira C et al. Teaching self-

management skills to asthmatic children and their parents in an ambulatory care setting. *Pediatrics* 1981; **68:** 341–8.
19. Mesters I, Meertens R, Kok G et al. Effectiveness of a multi disciplinary education protocol in children with asthma (0–4 years) in primary health care. *J Asthma* 1994; **31:** 347–59.
20. Hughes DM, McLeod M, Garner B et al. Controlled trial of a home and ambulatory program for asthmatic children. *Pediatrics* 1991; **87:** 54–61.
21. Wilson SR, Starr-Schneidkraut N. State of the art in asthma education: The US experience. *Chest* 1994; **106:** 197S–205S.
22. Clark NM, Gong M, Schork MA et al: Impact of education for physicians on patient outcomes. *Pediatrics* 1998; **101:** 831–6.
23. Bolton MB, Tilley BC, Kuder J, Reeves T, Schultz LR. The cost and effectiveness of an education program for adults who have asthma. *J Gen Intern Med* 1991; **6**(5): 401–7.
24. Wilson S, Starr-Schneidkraut NJ, Austin DM et al. Early intervention with parents of very young children reduces nocturnal symptoms and improves overall control. *Am Rev Respir Dis* 1993; **147**(suppl 4): A774.
25. Toelle BG, Peat JK, Salome CM et al. Evaluation of a community-based asthma management program in a population sample of schoolchildren. *Med J Aust* 1993; **158**(11): 742–6.
26. Rosenstock IM. The health belief model: explaining health behavior through expectancies. In: Glanz K, Rimer B, Lewis F, eds. *Health Behavior and Health Education: Theory Research and Practice*. San Francisco (CA): Jossey Bass, 1990.
27. Parcel GS, Baronowski T. Social learning theory and health education. *Health Educ Monogr* 1981; **12:** 14–18.
28. Clark NM, Janz NK, Dodge JA, Sharpe PA. Self-regulation in health behavior: The "Take PRIDE" program. *Health Educ Q* 1992; **19:** 341–54.
29. Clark NM, Gong M. Management of chronic disease by practitioners and patients: are we teaching the wrong things? *BMJ* 2000; **320:** 572–5.
30. Korsch BM, Gozzi EF, Francis V. Gaps in doctor-patient communications: Doctor–patient interaction and patient satisfaction. *Pediatrics* 1968; **42:** 855–71.
31. Bender B, Milgrom H, Rand C. Nonadherence in asthmatic patients: is there a solution to the problem? *Ann Allergy Asthma Immunol* 1997; **79:** 177–84.
32. Woolcock AJ, Yan K. Salome CM. Effect of therapy on bronchial hyper responsiveness in the long term management of asthma. *Clin Allergy* 1988; **18:** 165–76.
33. Charlton I, Charlton G, Broomfield J. Mullee MA. Evaluation of peak flow and symptoms- only self management plans for control of asthma in general practice. *BMJ* 1990; **301:** 1355–9.
34. Boulet LP, Chapman KR, Green LW, Fitzgerald JM. Asthma Education. *Chest* 1994; **106** (4)supp: 184S–196S.
35. Kolbe J, Vamos M. Fergusson W, Elkind G, Garrett J. Differential influences on asthma self-management knowledge and self-management behavior in acute severe asthma. *Chest* 1996; **110**(6): 1463–8.
36. Gibson PG, Coughlan J, Wilson AJ et al. Self-management education and regular practitioner review for adults with asthma. (Cochrane Review). *The Cochrane Library* 2000.
37. Mellins RB, Evans D, Clark N et al. Developing and Communicating a Long Term Treatment Plan for Asthma. *Am Fam Physician* 2000; **61:** 2419–28, 2433–4.
38. Manzella B. Brooks C, Richard J, et al. Assessing the use of metered dose inhalers by adults with asthma. *J Asthma* 1989; **25**(4): 223–30.
39. King D, Earnshaw SM, Delaney J. Pressurized aerosol inhalers. The cost of misuse. *Br J Clin Pract* 1991; **42:** 48–9.
40. Doak C, Doak L, Root J. Teaching patients with low literacy skills. Philadelphia (PA): JB Lippincott, 1985.
41. Janson-Bjerklie S. Ferketich S, Benner P. Predicting the outcomes of living with asthma. *Rese Nurs Health* 1993; **6**(4): 241–50.
42. Becker MH. Patient adherence to prescribed therapies. *Med Care* 1985; **23:** 539–55.
43. Cromer BA. Behavioral strategies to increase compliance in adolescents. In: Cramer JA, Spilker B, eds. *Patient Compliance in Medical Practice and Clinical Trials*. New York: Raven Press, 1991: 89–105.
44. Pantell R. Improving the process and outcomes of medical care for children: how effective communication impacts children taking medicine. In United States Pharmacopeia Conference Proceedings: Children and Medicines. September 29, 1996, Reston, Virginia.
45. Pantell R, Stewart T, Dias JK et al. Physician communication with children and parents. *Pediatrics* 1982; **70**(3): 396–402.
46. Bush PJ, Iannotti RJ. A children's health belief model. *Med Care* 1990; **28:** 69–86.

47. Perlman N, Abramovitch R. Visit to the pediatrician: children's concerns. *J Pediatr* 1987; **110**(6): 988–90.
48. Wilson SR, Scamagas P, German DF et al. A controlled trial of two forms of self-management education for adults with asthma. *Am J Med* 1993; **94**: 564–76.
49. Thapar A. Educating asthmatic patients in primary care: a pilot study of small group education. *Fam Pract* 1994; **11**(1): 39–43.
50. Mayo PH, Richman J, Harris HW. Results of a program to reduce admissions for adult asthma. *Ann Intern Med* 1990; **112**: 864–71.
51. Ignacio-Garcia JM, Gonzales-Santos P. Asthma self-management education program by home monitoring of peak expiratory flow. *Am J Resp Crit Care Med* 1995; **151**: 353–9.
52. Evans D, Mellins R, Lobach K et al. Improving care for minority children with asthma: professional education in public health clinics. *Pediatrics* 1997; **99**: 157–66.
53. National Heart, Lung, and Blood Institute. Expert Panel Report 2. Guidelines for the diagnosis and management of asthma. National Institutes of Health Publication No 97–4051, 1997.
54. Plaut T. *One Minute Asthma*. Amherst (MA): Pedipress Inc., 1991.
55. Li J, Sheeler R. Getting the most out of a 15-minute asthma visit. *J Resp Dis* 1997; **18**(2): 135–41.
56. Van der Palen J, Klein JJ, Kerkoff AHM, van Herwaarden CLA, Seydel ER. Evaluation of the long-term effectiveness of three instruction modes for inhaling medicine *Pat Educ Couns* 1997; **32**: S87–S95.
57. Powell KM, Edgren B. Failure of educational videotapes to improve medication compliance in a health maintenance organization. *Ann J Health Syst Pharm* 1995; **52**: 2196–9.
58. Maiman LA, Green LW, Gibson G, MacKenzie EJ. Education for self-treatment by adult asthmatics. *JAMA* 1979; **241**: 1919–22.
59. Rubin DH, Leventhal JM, Sadock RT et al. Educational intervention by computer in childhood asthma: a randomized clinical trial testing the use of a new teaching intervention in childhood asthma. *Pediatrics* 1986; **77**: 1–10.
60. Osman LM, Abdalla MI, Beattie JAG et al. Reducing hospital admission through computer supported education for asthma patients. *BMJ* 1994; **308**(6928): 568–71.
61. Wilson S, Latini D, Starr N et al. Education of infants and very young children with asthma: a developmental evaluation of the Wee Wheezers Program. *J Asthma* 1996; **33**: 239–54.
61A. Wilson SR, Mitchell JH, Rolnick S, Fish L. Effective and ineffective management behaviors of parents of infants and young children with asthma. *J Pediatr Psychol* 1993; **18**: 63–81.
62. Asthma and Allergy Foundation of America. *You Can Control Asthma*. Washington (DC), 1991.
63. Walders N, Drotar D, Kercsmar C. The allocation of family responsibility for asthma management tasks in African-American adolescents. *J Asthma* 2000; **37**(1), 89–99.
64. O'Brien R, Bush PJ. Helping children learn how to use medicines. *Office Nurse* 1993; **6**(3): 14–19.
65. Perrin EC, Gerrity S. There's a demon in your belly: children's understanding of illness. *Pediatrics* 1981; **67**: 841–9.
66. Mathews B, Dickinson A, Cram F. Establishment and evaluation of a preschool asthma program: a pilot study. *Nurs Pract NZ* 1998; **13**: 25–34.
67. Taggart V, Zuckerman A, Sly R et al. You can control asthma: Evaluation of an asthma education program for hospitalized inner-city children. *Patient Educ Counsel* 1991; **17**: 35–47.
68. Taggart V, Zuckerman A, Lucas S, Acty-Lindsey A. Adapting a self-management education program for use in an outpatient clinic. *Ann Allergy* 1987; **58**: 173–8.
69. Madge P, McColl J, Paton J. Impact of a nurse-led home managment training programme in children admitted to hospital with acute asthma: a randomised controlled study. *Thorax* 1997; **52**: 223–8.
70. Meurer JR, McKenzie S, Mischler E et al. The awesome Asthma School Days Program: educating children, inspiring a community. *J. Sch Health* 1999; **69**(2): 63–8.
71. Sander N, Boyer J. The National Allergy and Asthma Network Report: The Impact of asthma and allergies on school children and their families. *Am J Asthma Allerg Ped* 1991; **4**: 225–7.
72. Hill R, William J, Britton J, Tattersfield A. Can morbidity associated with untreated asthma in primary school be reduced? A controlled intervention study. *BMJ* 1991; **303**: 1169–74.
73. Calabrese BJ, Nanda JP, Huss K et al. Asthma knowledge, roles, functions, and educational needs of school nurses. *J Sch Health* 1999; **69**(6): 233–8.
74. Sosin, Allen. Asthma Camp/Education for Living. *J Asthma* 1991; **28**(5), 357–68.
75. Neville RG and Colin McCowan. Asthma and the Internet. *Asthma J* 1998; **3**: 47–50.

76. Neill RA, Mainous AG III, Clark JR, Hagen MD. The utility of electronic mail as a medium for patient-physician communication. *Arch Fam Med* 1994; **3:** 268–71.

77. Cromer BA, Tarnowski KJ. Noncompliance in adolescents: a review. *J Dev Behav Pediatr* 1989; **10**(4): 207–15.

17

Delivery of aerosols to children: devices and inhalation techniques

Myrna B Dolovich, Mark L Everard

Introduction • Factors affecting delivery of aerosol to children • Aerosol delivery systems for treating children • The choice of drug/device combinations • Class of drug • What is the correct dose of inhaled drug for a child? • What have we learned? • Future considerations

INTRODUCTION

Considerations for delivering inhalant therapy to infants and children are similar to those for adults, that is, ease of use, production of therapeutic aerosol within the size range for optimal deposition in the lung, minimal oropharyngeal deposition and reliable, and reproducible device performance. However, with infants and young children, the breathing parameters are a prime influence in determining how much aerosol is inhaled into the lung. Children have lower tidal volumes, which translates into reduced delivery,[1,2] and breathing patterns vary widely,[3,4] with inspiratory flow rates (IFR) ranging from near 0 to approximately 40 l/min. Higher flow rates mean deposition on more proximal airways. Furthermore, a crying child will have higher IFRs, with the result that decreased amounts of drug are inhaled into the lung.[5] Inhaling aerosol through the nose, or nasal breathing in addition to mouth-breathing during treatment, also reduces the dose to the lung.[6]

Most aerosol delivery systems currently on the market have been designed for use by adults and have subsequently been used to treat children simply because they were available. There are two principal reasons for this. One is that manufacturers recognize that, although the prevalence of asthma is at its highest in school-age children, there are many more adults with asthma than children with asthma. More importantly, until very recently, aerosol delivery systems have been marketed on the basis that a *pharmacodynamic* effect has been observed – that is, the use of a device to deliver a particular drug has resulted in a therapeutic response. The 'science' has been added later. Jet nebulizers were first developed in the 1930s to deliver bronchodilator agents, and pressurized metered dose inhalers (pMDIs) were developed in the 1950s to replace the hand-held portable glass nebulizers. Although these devices were clearly able to produce a pharmacodynamic effect – that is, the delivery of beta-agonists resulted in bronchodilation and relief of dyspnoea in asthmatic patients – it was many decades before some understanding of the performance of these devices in terms of the dose of drug delivered to the lungs was achieved. These devices were introduced because a clinical effect could be obtained, and similar logic lead to their adoption or adaptation for children.

Most of the basic principles influencing the delivery of airborne particles to the lungs were described by workers in the field of industrial hygiene interested in occupational lung disease. From this work it was appreciated that particles of approximately 1–7 μm would deposit reasonably effectively in the lungs. Current devices employ an energy source (CFC or HFC propellants for pMDIs, compressed gas for jet nebulizers and the patient's inspiratory effort for current DPIs) to generate such particles capable of penetrating beyond the upper airway and depositing in the lungs. Over the past 15–20 years there has been a vast amount of research undertaken in order to understand how these devices perform in terms of drug delivery to the lungs and some addressing issues that influence the therapeutic index of various drug combinations. In general such studies have been *in vitro* bench-top studies or have been undertaken in adults, frequently using well-trained healthy volunteers closely supervised on a given day. More recently, some groups have used pharmacokinetic techniques or gamma scintigraphy to determine lung doses in children and infants. Although not numerous, such studies have provided very valuable data on which to base recommendations for the use of aerosol therapy in children; however, it should be remembered that the only guide to the dose prescribed remains the principle of using the lowest dose that works.

FACTORS AFFECTING DELIVERY OF AEROSOL TO CHILDREN

When considering the specific needs of children, we must remember that early childhood is a period of great change, with enormous changes in physical, intellectual and social development occurring in the pre-school years. Although there has been considerable speculation regarding the effects of physical size on the pattern of deposition when delivering drugs to young children, it is the effect (as in the elderly) of competence that has the most profound impact on drug delivery. Very young children do not have the intellectual ability (competence) to master complex inhalation manoeuvres. In progressing from the newborn period to late pre-school age, a child's weight may increase five-fold while at the same time the child may progress from simply inhaling an aerosol passively during tidal breathing through to mastery of the complex inhalation manoeuvres required to operate current dry-powder inhalers and pMDI. The mastery of more controlled breathing manoeuvres permits delivery of drug through the mouth rather than the nose which will in itself have a profound influence on the pattern of deposition in the airways.[6]

Anatomical changes

The effects of anatomical changes in the early years of life are unclear. Airways will, in absolute terms, be smaller than those in an adult, but they may be relatively larger than those of adults in comparison to body size while inspiratory flows tend to be much lower. These lower flow rates tend to reduce the likelihood of impaction in the upper and central airways.[7] A variety of mathematical models have suggested that under conditions of regular tidal breathing, the nose may be more or less efficient at excluding foreign material from the airways than in adults.[8] Once particles reach the lower airways, most models predict relatively greater central airways deposition than for the adult due to the narrower airways in small children.[9,10] These predictions have been verified in a study using mouth inhalation of solid, stable particles of 1, 2, and 3 μm in children up to age 13 years of age (Figure 17.1),[11] which showed greater total deposition in the children compared to the adults. One study using jet nebulizers in older children with cystic fibrosis did suggest a striking increase in upper-airways deposition as a percentage of the total deposition in younger children and has been used to argue that upper-airways deposition is relatively greater in young children.[12] However, the data can be better explained by the greater lung deposition observed in the older patients with more severe lung disease. The absolute doses of activity deposited in the upper airway were greater in the older children.

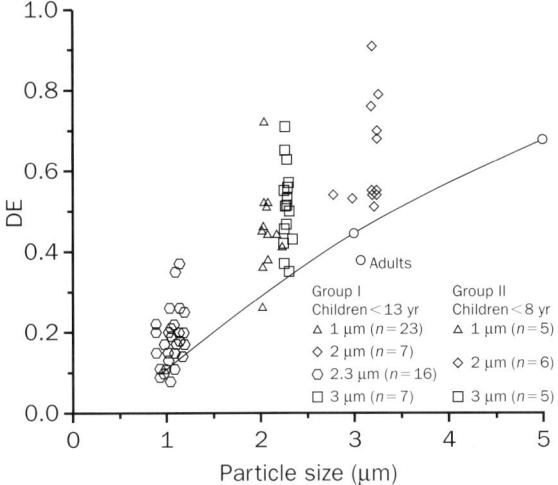

Figure 17.1 Total deposition fraction (DE) measured as a function of particle size in children and young adults breathing spontaneously. As the particle size increased, deposition increased and was greater than for the adult population (solid line).[11]

Competence

All current portable devices have been designed for subjects with sufficient cognitive ability to learn how to inhale through the mouth while performing a complex inhalation manoeuvre. School-age children can generally master the maximal inspiratory effort required to use DPIs but, as with adults, few can use pMDIs effectively. In order to treat pre-school children we must provide an aerosol cloud that can be inhaled using less sophisticated manoeuvres. Currently, the two devices available are the jet nebulizers and pMDI with holding chamber. These devices generate aerosol clouds and do not require careful co-ordination. Infants and young toddlers can use tidal breathing, while older children using pMDIs with holding chambers can learn to 'pant'. Dry-powder holding chambers have been proposed but are not yet in clinical use.[13]

The issue of competence has profound effects on aerosol delivery in young children since they are unable both to perform complex inhalation manoeuvres and to master inhaling reliably through the mouth. These factors, rather than any anatomical factor, are of prime importance when considering drug delivery to the lungs of young children.

Nose vs mouth-breathing

The anatomical design of the upper airway forms the most important defence protecting the lower airway from inhaled foreign material. The nose is particularly effective at trapping inhaled particulate matter. Turbulence created as inspired air passes through the internal ostium results in impaction of airborne particles against the sides of the nasal cavity. The mouth is also very effective in trapping inhaled particles though less so than the nose. The very narrow aperture created between tongue and the roof of the mouth together with the 90° change in direction of the airflow at the nasopharynx is also very efficient at trapping airborne particles. Particles less than 6 μm do penetrate these defences relatively well, although the efficiency depends upon the inspiratory flow and resultant momentum of the particles. Finer aerosols containing particles less than 1 μm traverse the nasal passages very effectively and do reach the lungs.[8] However, because of their lower mass and settling velocity, a higher percentage will be exhaled even when using a breath hold. Thus a window of opportunity exists for delivering drug to the lower airways which employs particles with a mass median aerodynamic diameter (MMAD) in the range 1–6 μm in which particles are relatively efficiently deposited in the lungs.[14]

Studies in adults and young children have indicated that upper airways deposition is significantly less when inhaling through the mouth than the nose.[6] Consequently, when attempting to deliver drug to the lungs using the inhaled route, mouth-breathing is desirable. However, mouth-breathing has to be learned and it normally takes between two and a half and three years before children can master a 'panting' technique when using a holding chamber,[15] although a few can manage this technique early in the third year of life, while others are well into their fourth year of life. As a result, most infants and young toddlers inhale via their nose, which is likely to significantly increase upper airways deposition and reduce delivery of particles to the lungs. In children younger than 6 months of age, it is quite possible that drug delivery is greater via the nose owing to the pharyngeal anatomy which is adapted to breast-feeding.

Breathing patterns

As noted above, we have little control over the breathing patterns of young children and therefore tidal breathing must be relied on. To do this we must generate a standing cloud using a pMDI and holding chamber, or a jet nebulizer. One of the problems with using mathematical modelling is that an assumption is made that the respiratory cycle is regular, yet data indicate that in young children breathing patterns can be very irregular[3,16] (Figure 17.2), again emphasizing the need for a standing cloud that permits the infant to access drug over a period of some seconds or longer. We have little control over this, although it is possible that sophisticated breath-active systems could enhance the efficiency of drug delivery by timing boluses of aerosol to the inspiratory phase of the infant's inspiratory cycle.[17] Greater efficacy would, however, be highly dependent on the design of the system, including low-resistance valves that open easily on inhalation and the use of a mask with a good seal to the face to prevent leakage of aerosol around the mask.[18,19]

Some school-age children can, when properly instructed, master complex inspiratory techniques and generate high inspiratory flows when using DPIs, although the maximum PIF generated through a given device tends to increase with age.[20,21] However, a study by Kamps et al. of 60 children with newly diagnosed asthma, boys and girls ranging 1–14 years of age, showed the opposite, despite the children receiving prior instruction as to how to use their inhalers.[22] Improvement in the children's technique was seen, particularly following further instruction at the pharmacy. Thus it is necessary to check and re-check how children are using the inhalers to ensure proper delivery of the drug; in addition, it would be wise to ensure that parents and caregivers also practice with the devices that are prescribed to their children.

Crying/distress

The most important parameter in terms of breathing pattern in young children is whether they are co-operative or distressed. Although it has been suggested that crying may enhance drug delivery as a result of the increased inspiratory volume and the use of mouth-breathing, there is now overwhelming evidence that administering aerosol to a distressed child achieves little other than causing the child and their carer distress.[22–24] The two principal reasons for this reduced delivery are failure to achieve a seal with a facemask and the very short, rapid inspiration associated with crying.[19]

When using a facemask, failure to achieve a good seal will greatly diminish drug delivery. When using a jet nebulizer even a very small gap of 1–3 cm between facemask and face will significantly reduce the drug inhaled.[17] For a pMDI and holding chamber, failure to obtain a good seal will have a profound effect on drug delivered, far outstripping any effect of chamber design.[23] In addition, the very short rapid inhalations of crying infants result in a reduction in total inhaled dose and, more importantly, a marked reduction in lung dose.[5,24] The issue of device acceptance is particularly a problem from the latter part of the first year of life through to the third year of life, by which time the normal maturational event of wishing to demonstrate more autonomy acts in favour to improve co-operation and effective drug delivery.

AEROSOL DELIVERY SYSTEMS FOR TREATING CHILDREN

Choosing devices for children should not be difficult. Issues of competence limit the choice

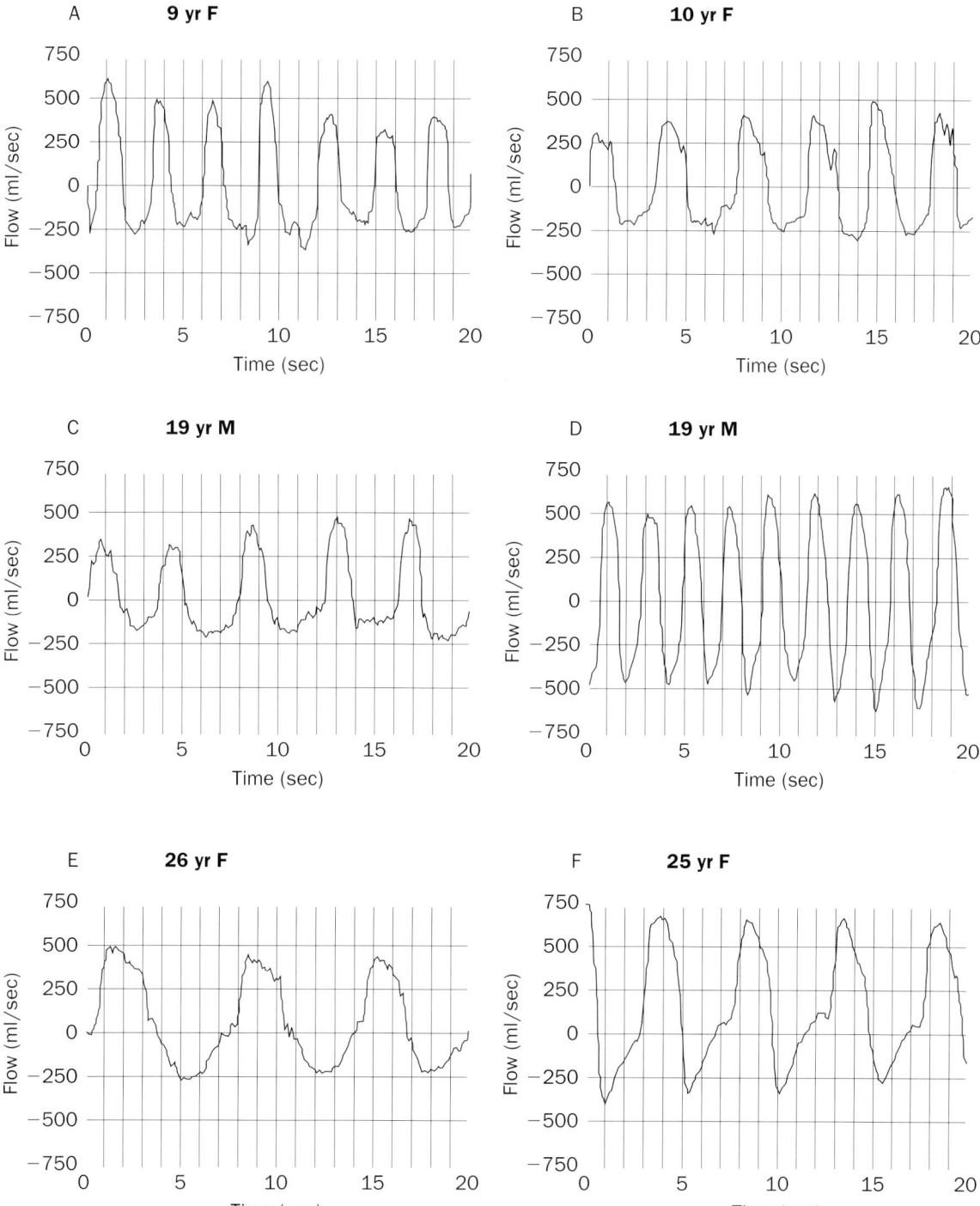

Figure 17.2 Examples of breathing patterns in age-matched healthy (A, C, E) and cystic fibrosis (B, D, F) subjects obtained with a Pari Breath Monitor.[81]

in younger children to pMDIs with holding chambers or in some cases, jet nebulizers. In older children the choice would include DPIs and, in some cases, breath-actuated pMDIs.[25–27]

The pMDI was developed in the 1950s to provide a multi-dose portable delivery system for beta-agonists. Although the developers considered using the device for other drug classes, such as the peptide insulin, they abandoned the idea because of the high intra-subject variability in drug delivery. A historical accident a decade later led to the adoption of this system for delivering inhaled steroids. The contrast in drug classes could not be greater. Beta-agonists need to be accessible whenever and wherever patients require symptomatic relief. Inhaled corticosteroids (ICS) must be administered regularly for prolonged periods with no direct feedback relating administration to therapeutic efficacy. Subsequently, spacers and holding chambers were developed to address the difficulties many patients experienced when trying to use pMDIs effectively and to improve the therapeutic ratio of ICS delivered using pMDIs.

Dry-powder delivery systems were developed initially for sodium cromoglycate in the 1960s, and subsequently devices using similar principles were developed for beta-agonists and ICS. The perceived wisdom that it was desirable to have both beta-agonists and ICS in the same device was driven largely by marketing considerations, rather than through consideration of the type of device appropriate for each class of drug.

'CFC' replacement

Following the establishment of the Montreal Protocol setting the guidelines and timetables for the phasing-out of CFC propellants,[28] the pharmaceutical industry chose, for some corticosteroids formulations using non-CFC propellants, to produce an aerosol that was the 'same as' the CFC inhaler being replaced – the so called 'seamless transition'. These decisions followed the transition strategies for the new pMDI delivery systems outlined by the various governments and were applied even though the numerous shortcomings for pressurized ICS inhalers were well known. The process has taken much longer and has been far more costly than anticipated. For some CFC-free steroid pMDIs, the label claim or the emitted dose per actuation has been reduced to meet clinical and regulatory requirements. The resultant devices do have a number of advantages over their predecessor, including reduced 'cold Freon' effect,[29] greater dose uniformity and less variability with temperature; however, in terms of efficacy, lung dose and therapeutic index they are, with a few exceptions, essentially the same as their CFC predecessors.

Several companies have elected to totally reformulate their steroid inhalers, manufacturing solution aerosols rather than suspension aerosols. For some drugs, this also included a redesign of the pMDI hardware, specifically valves and seals, both to accommodate the HFC formulations but also to improve inhaler performance. Solution aerosols produce finer aerosols that result in increases to the total lung dose with changes to the pattern of deposition within the lungs. QVAR, a beclomethasone dipropionate HFA solution aerosol from 3M Pharmaceuticals, UK, releases a slower-moving cloud of drug and propellant droplets on actuation which may make inhaling the dose easier for some children. The finer droplets and lower velocity reduce impaction in the oropharynx compared with the conventional CFC pMDI.[29] Children should still use a holding chamber to take the doses though, not only for co-ordination of actuation with inhalation, but to minimize the total body dose from the inhaled steroid.[29] Even though the spray temperature of the HFA formulations are above freezing in contrast to the CFC aerosols, there is still the opportunity to hesitate during inhalation. Holding chambers help overcome this problem that many children experience when taking pressurized aerosols. Because of its aerosol characteristics, lung deposition from QVAR is approximately 53% and appears to be similar across ages.[30] This value reported for lung deposition is a three-fold greater dose from HFA beclomethasone dipropionate (BDP) compared to 16.4% for the same asthmatic adults inhaling the BDP CFC aerosol.[31] Comparative data is not yet available for infants, but the lung doses to children have also been measured at 55% of the emitted dose from the pMDI.[32]

HFA 134a salbutamol has been trialed in children with mild-to-moderate asthma. In a randomized, double-blind, parallel group study, children, aged 5–17 years and using a large-volume valved spacer to inhale the doses, showed no significant difference in response as measured by changes in spirometry ten minutes after inhaling two puffs of the HFA pMDI or CFC salbutamol.[33] This finding is not unexpected as the aerosol size characteristics of the HFA salbutamol are very similar to the CFC formulation.[34] Thus, for the standard dose of this bronchodilator, the HFA formulation can be substituted for its CFC counterpart without a decrease in efficacy.

pMDIs and spacers

In delivering pMDI therapy to children and infants, it is well understood that the components of the inhalation manoeuvre – that is, inspiratory volume, inspiratory flow rate and breath-hold at end-inspiration – are difficult or impossible to control. Furthermore, as synchronization of actuation with inhalation of the pressurized aerosol is difficult for all children, the use of holding-chamber devices or tube spacers with pMDIs will eliminate many of these problems, allowing tidal breathing for inhaling the medication rather than deep breaths – a technique very young children and infants cannot master.

Holding chambers and tube spacers effect a reduction in MMAD of the original spray through evaporation and impaction of the larger particles on the walls or valves of the device.[35] Thus, a finer aerosol is provided for inhalation with, potentially, a higher degree of success in getting the therapy into the child's lungs. Oropharyngeal deposition is also markedly decreased, reducing the total body dose of drug.[36,37] Also, with the retention of the larger droplets in the holding chamber, the 'cold Freon' effect from both CFC and HFA pMDIs, although less in the latter formulations, and which causes many children to stop inhaling, is eliminated. This is the same outcome for drugs which have a foul taste. The larger droplets contain more drug and propellant, and by collecting this portion of the dose in the holding chamber, the overall taste sensed with these formulations becomes more palatable. The use of a valved holding chamber should be viewed as a necessary accessory to the pMDI for pediatric and neonatal delivery of these aerosol therapies.

The presence of a one-way valve between the body of the spacer and the mouthpiece is the design feature that allows aerosol to be contained within the holding chamber for a finite period of time. The resistance of the inhalation valve is important to the ability easily to inhale aerosol from the holding chamber.[38] The valve must be able to withstand the initial pressure from the pMDI on firing to minimize loss of aerosol, but have a sufficiently low resistance to open readily on inhalation, particularly when the device is used by children and infants.[39] The requirement for low resistance would similarly apply to the exhalation valve in the facemask attached to a spacer device used for infants and children. Too high a resistance may prevent the valve from opening on exhalation, contributing to a re-breathing of aerosol accumulated in the face mask area.

The volume of the spacer and presence of a low-resistance valve are important considerations when recommending spacers for infants and children. Studies investigating the effect of inhalation technique and spacer use have shown that young children can derive similar benefit taking multiple tidal breaths through a holding chamber fitted with a facemask, as when taking a full inspiratory breath.[40] This inhalation method is easier to perform and of practical use, particularly when the volume of the spacer device is greater than the inspiratory capacity of the child; it may also be a useful practice in the emergency room, when breathing rates are increased owing to acute shortness of breath.[41] Despite the gravitational loss of some aerosol to the walls of the spacer, which will occur between tidal breaths, sufficient drug can be obtained to provide a bronchodilator effect. However, the emptying time for large holding chambers may be too long at very low tidal volumes (< 50 ml). It would thus be preferable to use a small-volume holding chamber spacer, particularly for infants, as this will initially provide a more concentrated aerosol and allow a greater mass of drug to be inhaled with each inspiratory breath.[42]

Additional considerations surrounding the use of valved spacers with pMDIs include the actuation of multiple doses of the pMDI into the spacer, the time interval between spraying into the spacer and taking a breath, and the effect of electrostatic charge on drug available from a spacer. While seemingly practical for those children reluctant to take their therapy, if more than one drug dose is actuated into a spacer or if there is too long a delay prior to initiating the inhalation, both the total dose and respirable dose of drug available for inhalation are reduced.[43] The extent of these losses will vary for different drugs and spacer designs. Drug output from plastic spacers is reduced in the presence of electrostatic charge.[43] Use of a metal spacer[44] or washing the plastic spacer in light detergent and allowing it to air-dry[45] can overcome this loss, increasing delivery ex-spacer[44] and somewhat reducing the variability in the inhaled dose.[45,46] It should be noted that with use, the interior walls of the plastic spacer become coated with a thin layer of surfactant and drug. This will lessen the charge effect and reduce drug losses within the spacer, increasing output.[23,47] The issue of charge appears to be less of a problem with HFA propellant pMDIs and drug available ex-spacer seems to be less a function of spacer volume, at least within the range tested of 145–700 ml.[48] Thus, smaller-volume spacers can be used to inhale HFA pMDI aerosols with comparable delivery to large-volume spacers. Electrostatic charge is also eliminated in humidified circuits in the ICU.[49] Plastic spacers can be used in ventilator circuits for patients receiving inhalant therapy while on mechanical ventilation without loss of drug due to static charge.

pMDI aerosols in acute asthma and in the neonatal intensive care unit

There are a number of published clinical studies supporting the use of pMDIs with spacers as an alternative to nebulizers for delivering aerosolized bronchodilator therapy to children with acute asthma and older infants with recurrent wheeze. All demonstrated equivalent or better response with the use of valved spacers and fewer side-effects.[50–55] Equivalent responses have been obtained either at equal doses given by either delivery method or at dose ratio equivalents ranging up to 6:1 for nebulizer:pMDI.[56]

Support for the use of ICS in pre-term intubated infants with RDS or early bronchopulmonary dysplasia is mixed. In several trials, late administration, after day 14 of life, using a pMDI and valved holding chamber, appeared to improve lung function and reduce symptoms, increase rates of extubation and reduce or eliminate the need for systemic steroids.[57–59] However, benefit in trials where similar treatment was started earlier, from day 3 of life, is less clear.[60–62] While the use of ICS in this group may be indicated, the time of intervention may be the key factor.[63] Whether more efficient delivery devices or aerosols with improved deposition in ambulatory patients, such as the HFA steroid solution pMDI aerosols, can provide better dosing and outcomes is not yet known. Clearly, these are options that need to be explored in the neonatal population.

Dry powder inhalers

Dry powder systems have the great advantage of being breath actuated, obviating the need for co-ordinating actuating the device and inhaling. However, because of their inherent resistance to airflow, a function of their design, they do display varying degrees of 'flow dependence', that is, the inspiratory effort of patients using DPIs influences the effectiveness of aerosol dispersal.[64] The greater the energy imparted by the patient the more effectively is the powder aerosolized resulting in an increase in the 'respirable doses'.[65] Some of the more recent DPIs

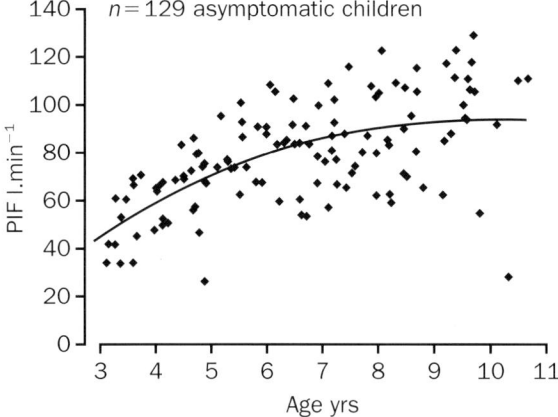

Figure 17.3 Relationship between peak inspiratory flow rate and age measured when using the Diskus DPI (GlaxoSmithKline, UK). PF below the age of 6 years appears to vary with age to a greater extent than for the older child. However, children in this age group are able to achieve a PF of 40–80 l/min, sufficient to dispense the drug dose from the inhaler.[21]

are relatively flow independent at clinically relevant flows appearing to operate nearly as efficiently at low flows as at high flows. Predictably, older children are able to generate higher inspiratory flows compared to younger children[21] (Figure 17.3) and in the few studies to date, this translates into significantly greater lung dose with increasing age. The improved aerosol dispersion not only results in a greater lung dose but also an increased lung to upper airways ratio, improving the therapeutic index for drugs absorbed from the GI tract. Whether this is of any clinical significance or not is unclear. Though this effect of improved drug delivery with age may appear to argue against the use of DPIs, it should be noted that if the lung dose is considered as µg/kg body weight, drug delivery from the Turbuhaler was relatively constant from 6 to 16 years of age.[66] The effects of inspiratory flow on dispersal vary between DPIs and some with relatively less flow dependence are likely to deliver relatively more drug to the lungs per kg body weight when used by young children than when used by older children and adults.

Numerous clinical trials have demonstrated that DPIs can be used to treat children successfully with asthma. The issue of a reduced emitted dose from the DPI if a less than optimal inspiratory flow rate is used may affect response in both adults and children.[67] A recent study in children with exercise-induced asthma, inhaling salmeterol from the Diskus DPI (GlaxoWellcome, UK) with a low (30 l/min) inspiratory flow rate (IFR) or a high (90 l/min) IFR indicated flow independence in bronchoprotection from the drug.[21] The emitted dose from the Diskus has been shown to be consistent over the flows 30–90 l/min, but an approximately 30% decrease in the fine particle dose at these two flow rates has been measured.[65] From this information, one should expect a reduced dose deposited in the peripheral lung. At the higher IFR, deposition would be more proximal, with more impaction of drug in the oropharynx. However, these differences do not appear to have affected the clinical outcome in the above study.

THE CHOICE OF DRUG/DEVICE COMBINATIONS

The choice of device (in all age groups) as outlined in Table 17.1 should be based on the following:

- the class of drug to be delivered
- the patient's competence in using a delivery device
- the likelihood that if competent, the patient will continue to use the device effectively.

CLASS OF DRUG

Inhaled steroids

For inhaled steroids, patients require a device that will reliably, safely and reproducibly deliver drugs to the lungs. The device must be simple to use effectively, and the vast majority of steroid reaching the systemic circulation should do so via the lungs. For drugs that are

Table 17.1 Recommendations for aerosol delivery systems to be used with pediatric patients

Age (yrs)	Short acting β-agonists	ICS Long-acting β-agonists
0–3	pMDI/holding chamber with facemask Nebulizer*	pMDI/holding chamber with facemask Nebulizer*
3–5†	pMDI/holding chamber ('panting') Nebulizer*	pMDI/holding chamber ('panting') Nebulizer* ?DPI‡
5+	pMDI/holding chamber Breath actuated pMDI DPI‡ Nebulizer*	pMDI/holding chamber DPI‡

* Jet nebulizers are rarely required; may have a role to treat very young children who will not accept holding chamber and facemask and in severe acute asthma.
† Age at which toddlers can use holding chambers without a facemask vary considerably and may occur between 24 and 48 months of age, though generally occurs at 30–36 months of age.
‡ DPIs are appropriate for inhaled corticosteroids providing the systemic effects of steroids absorbed from the gastrointestinal tract are minimized using an ICS with low first pass metabolism or using a device with low upper airways depostion.

only partly metabolized as they pass through the liver from the GI tract (e.g. beclomethasone), upper-airways deposition should be minimized, whereas this is less of a concern for rapidly metabolized steroids. Currently, the options consist of a pMDI with holding chamber (provided the patient will use the holding chamber) or an 'efficient' DPI or a DPI delivering steroids with very low GI availability. These options will help maximize the therapeutic ratio by ensuring that what drug does reach the systemic circulation does so via the lungs, and so contributes to the therapeutic effect. Minimizing upper-airways deposition will also tend to minimize upper-airways side-effects, such as oropharyngeal candida and hoarseness.

Short-acting beta-agonists

Much more flexibility is available for beta-agonists and here patients' preference for the delivery device is important, as they frequently need to carry the device around with them. Feedback that drug delivery is inadequate permits patients to repeat doses to compensate when necessary, although within limits.

Other drug classes

A variety of other drugs are delivered to the lungs of children using aerosol delivery systems. For most, such as inhaled antibiotics, the lack of any alternative ensures that standard jet nebulizers must be used,[68,69] although it is clear that the technology is available to deliver these drugs with greater efficiency to the lung and using more convenient delivery systems. However, the market is generally small and of little interest to large pharmaceutical companies.

Competence and contrivance

It is frequently stated that patients should be

given a device they like and that is simple to use. There is no evidence that liking a device influences either effective use of the device or compliance. The phrase 'simple to use' should be replaced with *simple to use effectively*. pMDIs are perceived to be simple to use, yet they are very difficult to use *effectively*, and indeed the majority of patients, doctors, nurses and pharmacists are unable to use them effectively.[22,70] Unfortunately, this problem is compounded by the falsely reassuring feedback that patients receive using beta-agonists. Poor technique is compatible with bronchodilation as these drugs are used in supra-maximal doses and even very inefficient delivery can result in a therapeutic effect. If the response is insufficient to cause complete relief of symptoms, further doses are taken. Such titration compensating for poor technique is not possible with inhaled steroids.

There is increasing evidence that as many as two-thirds of patients are prescribed a holding chamber to use when inhaling ICS, regularly use the pMDI alone. These patients and their parents are generally competent and choose or contrive to use the delivery system in a way that it is likely to prevent or minimize effective delivery of drug to the lungs.

In summary, the patient should be supplied with a drug device combination that has a good therapeutic index, can be used effectively by the patient and will be used effectively by the patient.

WHAT IS THE CORRECT DOSE OF INHALED DRUG FOR A CHILD?

The lung dose for a child may vary 60-fold depending upon the device chosen, the child's age and, most importantly, their competence with the device. It is clear that difficulties using current devices (patient competence) along with compliance are the major impediments to ensuring that all children benefit maximally from the potent drugs that are currently available.

As with adults, the only current guide to prescribing is to use *the lowest dose that produces a given therapeutic effect*.[27] This will ensure that a clinical improvement can be achieved, while minimizing the risk of adverse events and maximizing the therapeutic index.

Assessment of aerosol delivery systems

As noted above, the vast majority of delivery systems were originally developed for adults, and only subsequently used for children, as they were the only delivery systems available. Pediatricians have been able to influence the process to some extent. For example, Friegang[71] developed a spacer and facemask based on a plastic vinegar bottle some years before the first large-volume holding chamber was developed[72] and more than a decade before a North American manufacturer added a facemask to a commercially available valved holding chamber.[73] However, the input of paediatricians has been largely to assess marketed devices and define the numerous problems associated with them.

Methods for assessing devices include the following:

- *in vitro* assessment
- assessment of dose delivered (filter studies)
- pharmacodynamic studies
- assessment of lung dose (imaging and pharmacokinetic studies).

All these techniques have strengths and weaknesses. Performing studies in children can be difficult, and compromises are necessary to accommodate the poor inhalation technique and the inability to measure spirometry in the very young child. The vast majority of studies relating to aerosol therapy in children must be interpreted with considerable caution.

In vitro assessment of dose/*in vivo* confirmation of response to the dose

A great number of *in vitro* studies have been published over the years. These range from simple bench-top studies assessing the particle size characteristics of the aerosol cloud through simple pump systems to mimic the respiratory patterns of children, to very sophisticated studies using computer-controlled pumps to simulate recorded patient breathing patterns[74-76] combined with sophisticated casts of upper airways obtained in a variety of ways.[77-79] The former are very easy to undertake, are relatively quick and cheap, but only give an indication of maximum drug available at the mouth from the delivery system. Arguably, for metered doses that can be inhaled with a single inspiratory capacity breath by an adult or older child, the total drug collected on a filter would be similar over a wide range of inspiratory flow rates. However, the amount on the filter cannot differentiate dose to the lung from dose ex-lung, and in particular, dose to the oropharynx.[46] Although the vast majority of these types of filter studies are of little consequence clinically, they are useful in the development of new devices to determine whether the project is on the correct track and for quality control during manufacturing. They may have a role in the early assessment of currently available devices but the information cannot accurately predict lung doses in adults, and certainly we cannot achieve this in children with their low and variable breathing parameters.

An illustration of this is the large number of *in vitro* studies assessing static charge in holding chambers. Such studies have varied the device, the drug, the sizing technique and so on but have all come to the same conclusion: plastic spacers are prone to holding a static charge and this may decrease drug delivery.[45,46] Details have been discussed earlier in this chapter. Despite all this, a recent filter study has indicated that the effect of static on reproducibility of drug delivery is negligible in very young children and small in school age children.[23] *In vivo* measurements of lung deposition using radio-labeled salbutamol inhaled from detergent-coated spacers in children was found to be greater compared to other measurements of salbutamol inhaled through non-treated spacers.[47] But a recent study using HFA134a salbutamol has demonstrated that clinical effects are unchanged using static-free devices.[80] The lack of a clinical difference however, may be the result of testing for effects using a bronchodilator; subjects could well have been on the plateau of their dose–response curves with the test doses. In this same study, the authors also showed similar peak flows when static or static-free holding chambers of different volumes (145–750 ml) were used, supporting the *in vitro* measurements of emitted doses from these same types of holding chambers.[79]

More sophisticated *in vitro* measurement techniques to establish lung dose in children are likely to provide more information. However, in spite of complex and expensive equipment used to make these measurements, the results still tend to reflect idealized situations. Trends though can be seen and comparison of device performance may be useful in guiding the physician in choosing an inhaler.

Assessment of dose delivered

Collecting drug onto filters interposed between the subject and the inhaler is another type of *in vitro/in vivo* study and may provide more relevant information about drug delivery than when using a breathing simulator.[81] By assaying the quantity of drug on the filter one can obtain an idea of the dose likely to have been inhaled. A comparison of budesonide inhaled via a pressurized aerosol through a holding chamber versus the powder formulation from the Turbuhaler showed that children under the age of 4 years derive better clinical benefit from a pMDI with valved spacer than a DPI.[82] For children older than 5 years, treatment could be successfully provided by a DPI (Figure 17.4). Although this technique may give an estimate of the dose reaching the lungs, the results must be interpreted with caution. Another example is with a standard jet nebulizer producing aerosol continuously. Up to 60% of the reservoir dose may be lost while the patient is exhaling. This is in addition to the 25% of the inhaled dose that can be exhaled during tidal breathing, whereas with a pMDI or DPI less than 1% of the nominal dose is commonly exhaled after a breath hold.[66] Delivery of aerosols to very young children can be very difficult if they are distressed by the experience. There are a number of studies indicating that the lung dose is greatly reduced in

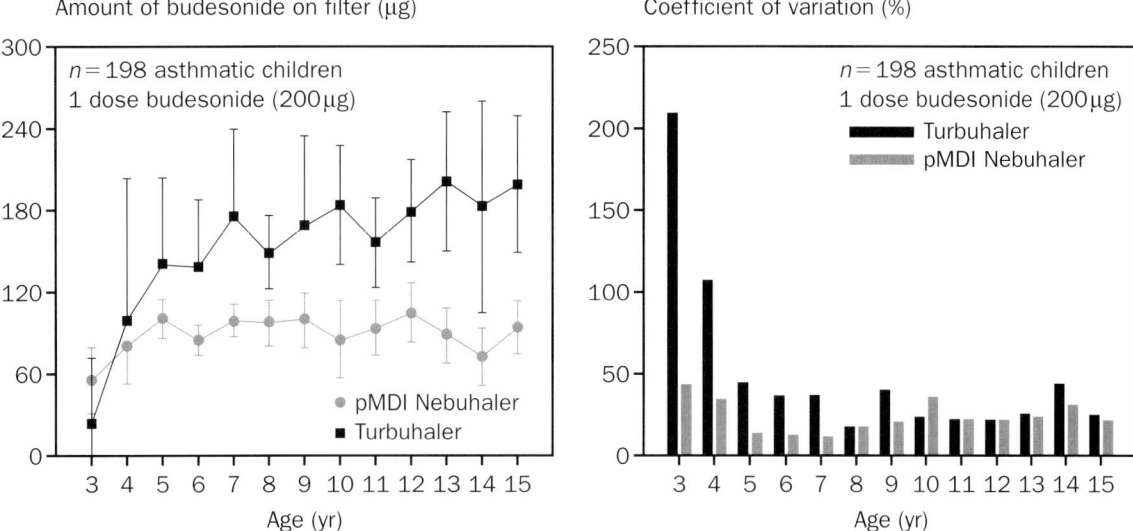

Figure 17.4 *In vitro* filter study comparing budesonide 'inhaled' via the Turbuhaler with the pMDI and Nebuhaler. This cross-over study in 198 children with asthma showed better delivery of drug and less variability in the dose of drug collected onto the filter with the pMDI+VHC in children 5 years of age and younger.[82] Children older than 5 years had better delivery to the filter from the Turbuhaler with comparable variability in the dose to the pMDI+VHC. However, the higher amount of budesonide with the Turbuhaler reflects that portion of the dose that would be deposited in the oropharynx, approximately 60%, whereas with the VHC, this contribution would be about 10–15%.[37] Correcting the differences in oropharyngeal dose will provide a better estimate of the dose inhaled into the lung for these two delivery methods.

upset and crying toddlers when compared to quiet and relaxed tidal-breathing children.[83] This is due to the alteration in the breathing pattern. Although the inhaled dose is often reduced, deposition in the upper airways increases significantly and so changes in the total inhaled dose will not be reflected in the lung dose collected onto a filter. Only direct measurements using radiotracers can differentiate the distribution of the dose within the respiratory tract.

Again, useful information can be provided by such studies but the results must be interpreted in light of limitations that include the potential for altering respiratory patterns such as if a significant dead space is introduced by the use of an inappropriate filter.

Pharmacodynamic studies

Pharmacodynamic studies are the basis for the licensing of new drug/device combinations. Regulatory authorities need to know that a device/drug combination is able to produce a therapeutic effect and that the safety profile is acceptable. For devices delivering beta-agonists, evidence that the delivery system can result in bronchodilation, or can block bronchoconstriction in response to stimuli such as exercise or methacholine, has long been the gold standard. Side-effects can be assessed by measuring heart rate, tremor, or indeed fall in serum K^+ when using very large doses of beta-agonists.

For inhaled steroids demonstration of efficacy is more of a problem. Most studies find it difficult to demonstrate a dose–response curve, owing to factors including the variability in lung dose between and within patients. Studies outcomes can include FEV_1, peak flow, diurnal variability, symptoms, beta-agonist use and quality of life. Most of these are very poor at discriminating between devices, and therefore 'equivalence' data are relatively easy to obtain. Side-effect outcomes would include assessment of growth, adrenal function and bone metabolism. Again, the choice of outcome measure can influence the likelihood or otherwise of detecting a clinically significant difference.

The issues surrounding the assessment of devices delivering inhaled steroids are complex, and a full exploration is beyond the scope of this chapter. However such studies are vital, and issues surrounding the therapeutic ratio (efficacy vs. side-effect profile) cannot be inferred simply by reviewing *in vitro* and deposition data, as illustrated by the intense debate regarding the benefits or otherwise of adopting solution-based pMDI delivery systems.

Deposition studies

Assessment of lung dose can be achieved in one of two ways:

- imaging (planar gamma scintigraphy, SPECT, PET);
- pharmacokinetic (direct and indirect).

Imaging
Planar gamma scintigraphy is the most popular approach with an increasing number of studies involving children being published. The majority have involved patients with cystic fibrosis but neonates and patients with asthma or HIV have also been studied.[1,66,84–88] The ethical issues surrounding such studies have been reviewed.[89] The advantage of this approach is that it is relatively simple. The greatest difficulty is in achieving accurate labeling of drug which ensures that the characteristics of the aerosol are not altered and that the label follows the drug to provide an accurate representation of drug deposition. There are also significant technical issues in quantifying the activity; failure to standardize approaches means that it is difficult to compare results from different centres.

Concerns regarding the use of radioactivity to study young children persist, but doses are generally low and the risk associated with participation in such studies is perceived to be minimal. The ability to obtain informed consent in children remains an issue.

SPECT scanning uses the same methods for labeling drugs but the use of two or more imaging heads permits the creation of a 3-D image that can produce more accurate data regarding localization of drug than 2-D planar imaging.[90] However, the need to use higher doses of radioactivity along with increased technical difficulties, including long acquisition times that require the use of non-absorbable tracers, has limited the adoption of this approach.[91]

Positron emission tomography (PET) scanning offers many potential advantages, not least because the drug can be directly labeled.[92,93] However, because this approach is very expensive and requires access to a cyclotron, few centres are able to undertake such studies. Studies in children are limited,[94] although animal studies used to model disease states in neonates have been very useful.[95] A disadvantage is the higher doses used compared to planar imaging.

In vivo deposition studies in children
There are relatively few studies measuring *in vivo* deposition of aerosol in children. An early study in children with cystic fibrosis, showed that lung deposition was patchy, increased in the central airways and varied with the severity of the disease.[84] Total deposition was found to be greater in the older patients (Figure 17.5),[66] a finding confirmed by Wildhaber[87] and Chua.[88] The rationale for using adult doses in pediatric patients becomes obvious when *in vivo* measurements such as those obtained from Fok et al[86] demonstrate how little drug is deposited in the lungs of young children. These investigators showed that less than 1% of salbutamol aerosol generated either by nebulizer or MDI was deposited in the lungs of 9–36-month-old asthmatic children. Recent studies using radiolabeled budesonide powder in children ranging from 3–16 years of age showed a trend towards increased drug deposition in the lung with increasing age and inspiratory flow rate.[87]

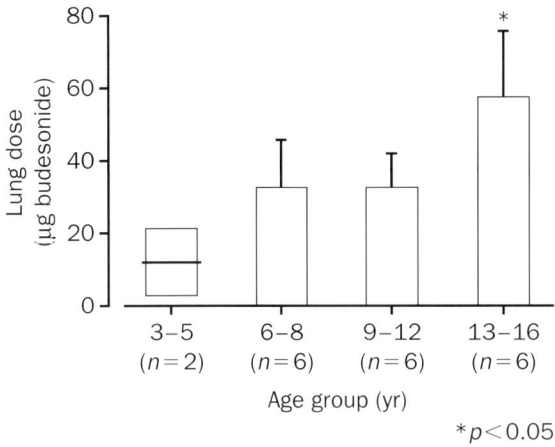

Figure 17.5 Lung deposition from the Turbuhaler in children with cystic fibrosis. There is less of a dose dependency with age in these subjects. Children in the oldest age group received close to adult doses.[66]

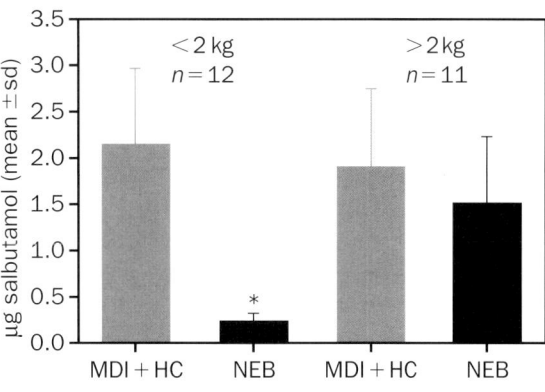

Figure 17.6 Lung deposition data for salbutamol obtained in 23 ventilated and spontaneously breathing non-ventilated infants with bronchopulmonary dysplasia. Infants <2 kg birth weight received significantly more radioabeled pMDI using the Aerochamber® compared to jet nebulizer; delivery was similar from both systems in those infants >2 kg birth weight.[96]

Increased deposition can be related to tidal volume and inspiratory flow rate, with a plateau reached as the inhalation of the total drug dose metered is inhaled with a single inspiratory breath. Not surprisingly, deposition was more variable in the youngest group. Values obtained for the deposited lung dose, corrected for body weight, were within or greater than adult levels, supporting the effectiveness of using powder inhalers for delivering therapy in young children.

In studies referred to earlier, delivering aerosol therapy to newborns, whether spontaneously breathing or mechanically ventilated, is more complex. A deposition study in babies with bronchopulmonary dysplasia (age 37–417 days, birth weight 0.9–4 kg, at time of study) has shown that <2% of salbutamol nebulizer solution or pMDI aerosol was deposited in the lungs.[96] Deposited doses varied between infants, but delivery correlated with body weight for the nebulizer but not the pMDI plus valved spacer (Figure 17.6).[97] These differences are likely due to the use of a continuously generated aerosol compared to a metered dose captured into a holding chamber. With the latter delivery system, the infant inhales a more concentrated aerosol for a finite time (30 s); with the nebulizer, the dose is less concentrated and, while inhaled until dryness, not enough of the dose is inhaled, particularly with the low-weight infants. Similar observations reported from an *in vivo* filter study also showed that deposition was weight-dependent for nebulizer delivery of drug, but not for pMDI with spacer. These measurements were carried out in wheezy infants (aged 4–12 months, and 6–10 kg birth weight), approximately the same age as the neonates studied, but heavier.[46]

Pharmacokinetic studies in children
Direct pharmacokinetic studies involve quantifying the amount of drug reaching the systemic circulation via the lungs. Some drugs such as sodium cromoglycate are effectively not absorbed from the GI tract. For others, drug absorption can be blocked by drinking activated charcoal, but this would not be an option in pediatric studies. Generally, multiple blood samples are required and injection of a known dose is also needed to obtain an internal

reference value. Because of difficulties in assaying very low quantities of drug in the circulation, relatively few such studies have been undertaken in children, although the sensitivity of detection is improving.

Indirect pharmacokinetic studies have been undertaken in adults but as yet no pediatric studies have been published. This approach involves measuring levels of drug in plasma or urine 30 minutes after inhalation, before significant quantities of drug have been absorbed from the GI tract.[98,99] The results provide only an indirect assessment of dose that can be used to compare devices or inhalation techniques but will not provide an absolute value of lung dose.

Limitation of deposition studies

Most deposition studies have used small groups of trained subjects on a single occasion, and since all the techniques involve potential errors, the results obtained are ball-park figures rather than absolute values. These studies have provided invaluable information regarding the performance of delivery systems when used to treat infants and children, but the performance of devices in the general population may be very different.

Differences have been noted in adult studies between results obtained using planar imaging and pharmacokinetic techniques. In some studies, the imaging produces a higher figure than the pharmacokinetic techniques and it has been claimed that this may be attributed to removal of drug from the lung by mucociliary clearance.[100] Drug cleared from the lungs before it is absorbed will not be identified in pharmacokinetic studies but will appear to be pulmonary on gamma scintigraphy. However, this does not fully explain the differences as there have been other pharmacokinetic studies which have found higher lung doses from pharmacokinetic results than from gamma scintigraphy measurements.

WHAT HAVE WE LEARNED?

The studies discussed in this chapter have indicated that the dose to the lungs is influenced by choice of device, anatomical differences and, most importantly of all, inhalation technique and competence. The choice of spacer or nebulizer may influence lung dose in infants and toddlers but any influence of device on lung dose will disappear if the child is upset when inhaling. The least variable results in older children have been obtained with dry-powder delivery systems, which are relatively less prone to user error than pMDIs.

Although factors such as upper airways geometry are important, it is still unclear whether upper airways deposition is relatively greater in younger children. For infants and older children using facemasks, upper airways is significantly greater than when mouth-breathing because of deposition in the nose. Drugs such as steroids are rapidly absorbed into the systemic circulation and much of the drug deposited in the nasal cavity will be absorbed before being cleared by mucociliary clearance and swallowed.[101]

In the mouth-breathing child, the likelihood of impaction in the upper airways may increase due to the smaller geometry in younger children; however, the smaller airways are accompanied by lower inspiratory flows, and this will tend to reduce the likelihood of impaction. To date, deposition studies have not resolved this issue. In studies with DPIs, upper-airways deposition is greater but this can be attributed, in large part, to lower inspiratory flows with more drug remaining in large 'non-respirable' particles.

The best device for a child is one that can be used effectively, and this is influenced by age and cognition. For example, there is evidence that some 3- and 4-year-olds can used DPIs[20] effectively while there are others who still cannot use a spacer with a mouthpiece.[22] It is to be hoped that future generations of inhalers will serve the needs of the asthmatic child in that they will be intuitive to use, deliver drug reliably and reproducibly to the lungs, and be designed to ensure that pediatric patients use them optimally.

FUTURE CONSIDERATIONS

Lung deposition data in children is difficult to obtain for a variety of reasons, as discussed in this chapter. A comparison of *in vivo* delivery efficiencies for inhalers with specific drugs, coupled with efficacy parameters in the same children, would provide data to help guide the physician and healthcare provider in recommending a drug/delivery system for a particular age group and possibly for a specific disease. In the last several years, we have gained greater accuracy in the measurement of aerosol characteristics and can determine how clinical factors influence these characteristics or vice versa. This has led to a better understanding of the quality of the aerosol inhaled from the various types of delivery systems and that portion of the aerosol which contributes to clinical benefit as opposed to side effects.

In the laboratory, using breath simulators and breath monitors to more accurately apply realistic breathing patterns for children of different ages for *in vitro* measurements should lend greater precision to the measurements of the drug available at the mouth for inhalation. However, a major limitation of most *in vitro* models is that they do not incorporate the effects of airways disease on the deposition of aerosol. Changes in airway geometry profoundly affect the dose and distribution of inhaled therapies in the upper and lower respiratory tract. These changes in distribution impact on the rate of absorption and/or clearance of deposited drug from the lung and nasal cavity, influencing efficacy and systemic side effects. As a start, future work in this area could attempt to build these abnormalities into *in vitro* protocols by using lung casts with dimensions reflecting deviations in airway calibre from normal. Much work has been done in trying to address basic questions regarding inhaled drug delivery in infants and children. This research has provided a solid foundation for future studies.

REFERENCES

1. Everard ML, Clark AR, Milner AD. Drug delivery from holding chambers with attached facemask. *Arch Dis Child* 1992; **67:** 580–5.
2. Collis GC, Cole CH, LeSoeuf PN. Dilution of nebulised aerosols by air entrainment in children. *Lancet* 1990; **336:** 341–3.
3. Bisgaard H. Patient-related factors in nebulized drug delivery to children. *Eur Respir Rev* 1997; **7:** 376–7.
4. Nikander K, Bisgaard H. Impact of constant and breath-synchronized nebulization on inhaled mass of nebulized budesonide in infants and children. *Pediatr Pulmonol* 1999; **28:** 187–93.
5. Iles R, Lister P, Edmunds AT. Crying significantly reduces absorption of aerosolised drug in infants. *Arch Dis Child* 1999; **81:** 163–5.
6. Everard ML, Hardy JG, Milner AD. Comparison of nebulised aerosol deposition in the lungs of healthy adults following oral and nasal inhalation. *Thorax* 1993; **48:** 1045–6.
7. Becqueim MH, Swift DL, Bouchikhi A, Roy M, Teillac A. Particle deposition and resistance in the nose of adults and children. *Eur Respir J* 1991; **4:** 694–702.
8. Morrow PE, Yu CP. Models of aerosol behavior in airways and alveoli. In: Morén F, Dolovich MB, Newhouse MT, Newman SP, eds. *Aerosols in Medicine: Principles, Diagnosis and Therapy* 2nd edn. Amsterdam: Elsevier Science, 1993: 157–93.
9. Xu JB, Yu CP. The effects of age on deposition of inhaled aerosols in the human lung. *Aerosol Sci Technol* 1986; **5:** 349–57.
10. Hofmann W, Martonen TB, Graham RC. Predicted deposition of nonhygroscopic aerosols in the human lung as a function of subject age. *J Aerosol Med* 1989; **2:** 49–68.
11. Schiller-Scotland ChF, Hlawa R, Gebhart J. Experimental data for total deposition in the respiratory tract of children. *Toxicol Lett* 1994; **72:** 137–44.
12. Diot P, Palmer LB, Smaldone A et al. RhDNase I: aerosol deposition and related factors in cystic fibrosis. *Am J Respir Crit Care Med* 1997; **156:** 1662–8.
13. Bisgaard H. Future options for aerosol delivery to children. *Allergy* 1999; **54**(Suppl. 49): 97–103.
14. Martonen T, Musante CJ, Segal RA et al. Lung models: strengths and limitations. *Respir Care* 2000; **45:** 712–36.
15. Gleeson J, Price J. Nebuhaler technique. *Br J Dis Chest* 1988; **82:** 172–4.
16. Nikander, K. Adaptive aerosol delivery: the principles. *Eur Respir Rev* 1997; **7:** 385–7.
17. Nikander K, Turpeinen M, Wollmer P. Evaluation of pulsed and breath-synchronized nebulization of budesonide as a means of reducing nebulizer wastage of drug. *Pediatr Pulmonol* 2000; **29:** 120–6.

18. Lowenthal D, Kattan M. Facemask versus mouthpieces for aerosol treatment of asthmatic children. *Pediatr Pulmonol* 1992; **14:** 192–6.
19. Nikander K, Agertoft L, Pedersen S. Breath-synchronized nebulization diminishes the impact of patient-device interfaces (face mask or mouthpiece) on the inhaled mass of nebulized budesonide. *J Asthma* 2000; **37:** 451–9.
20. Goren A, Noviski N, Avital A et al. Assessment of the ability of young children to use a powder inhaler device (Turbuhaler). *Pediatric Pulmonol* 1994; **18:** 797–802.
21. Nielsen KG, Auk IL, Bojsen K et al. Clinical effect of Diskus dry-powder inhaler at low and high inspiratory flow-rates in asthmatic children. *Eur Respir J* 1998; **11:** 350–4.
22. Kamps AWA, van Ewijk B, Roorda RJ, Brand PLP. Poor inhalation technique, even after inhalation instructions, in children with asthma. *Pediatr Pulmonol* 2000; **29:** 39–42.
23. Janssens HM, Heijnen EMEW, de Jong VM et al. Aerosol delivery from spacers in wheezy infants: a daily life study. *Eur Respir J* 2000; **16:** 850–6.
24. Murakami G, Igarashi T, Adachi Y. Measurement of bronchial hyperreactivity in infants and preschool children using a new method. *Ann Allergy* 1990; **64:** 383–7.
25. Bisgaard H. Delivery of inhaled medication to children. *J Asthma* 1997; **34:** 443–67.
26. Pedersen S. Inhalers and nebulizers: which to choose and why. *Respir Med* 1996; **90:** 69–77.
27. Everard ML. Guidelines for devices and choices. *J Aerosol Med* 2001; **14:** S1–6
28. Hayman GD. CFCs and the ozone layer. *Br J Clin Pract* 1997; **89**(Suppl): 2–9.
29. Dolovich M, Leach C. Drug delivery devices and propellants. In: Busse W, Holgate S, eds. *Asthma & Rhinitis*, 2nd edn. Oxford: Blackwell Science, 2000: 1719–31.
30. Dolovich MB, Conway JH, Le Souef P, Leach CL. Lung deposition >50% consistently demonstrated for hfa-beclomethasone dipropionate (bdp) extrafine aerosol. 2000; ACAAI abstract no. 46, p. 14.
31. Dolovich MB, Rhem R, Gerrard L, Coates G. Lung deposition of coarse CFC vs fine HFA pMDI aerosols of beclomethasone dipropionate (BDP) in asthma. 2000; **161**(3 Part 2): A33.
32. Devadason SG, Huang T, Turner SW et al. Distribution of ^{99m}Tc-labelled HFA-BDP inhaled via Autohaler® in children. *Eur Respir J* 2000; **16**(Suppl 31): P540S.
33. Desager KN, Van Bever HP, Vermeire PA. Comparison of non-chlorofluorocarbon containing salbutamol and conventional inhaler. *Lancet* 1996; **348:** 200–10.
34. Dolovich M. New delivery systems and propellants. *Can Respir J* 1999; **6:** 290–5.
35. Dolovich M. Characterization of medical aerosols: physical and clinical requirements for new inhalers. *Aerosol Sci Technol* 1995; **22:** 392–9.
36. Dolovich M, Ruffin R, Corr D, Newhouse M. Clinical evaluation of the Aerochamber: a simple demand inhalation MDI aerosol delivery device. *Chest* 1983; **84:** 36–41.
37. Thorsson L, Kenyon C, Newman SP, Borgstrom L. Lung deposition of budesonide in asthmatics: a comparison of different formulations. *Int J Pharm* 1998; **168:** 119–21.
38. Sennhauser FH, Sly PD. Pressure flow charcteristics of the valve in spacer devices. *Arch Dis Child* 1989; **64:** 1305–7.
39. Buchdahl R, Ward S, Summerfield A. Letter to the Editor: Spacer devices in asthma. *Thorax* 2000; **55:** 1070.
40. Gervais A, Begin P. Bronchodilatation with a metered-dose inhaler plus an extension, using tidal breathing vs jet nebulization. *Chest* 1987; **87:** 822–4,
41. Closa RM, Ceballos JM, Gomez-Papi A. Efficacy of bronchodilators administered by nebulizers versus spacer devices in infants with acute wheezing. *Pediatr Pulmonol* 1998; **26:** 344–8.
42. Campbell R, Dolovich M, Chambers C, Newhouse M. Effect of holding chamber volume on MDI albuterol dose delivered in vitro through an endotracheal tube at low tidal volumes. *Am Rev Respir Dis* 1993; **147**(Part 2): A267.
43. Barry PW, O'Callaghan C. The effect of delay, multiple actuations and spacer static charge on the in vitro delivery of budesonide from the Nebuhaler. *Br J Clin Pharmacol* 1995; **40:** 76–8.
44. Janssens HM, Devadason SG, Hop WCJ. Variability of aerosol delivery via spacer devices in young asthmatic children in daily life. *Eur Respir J* 1999; **13:** 787–91.
45. Pierart F, Wildhaber JH, Vrancken I, Devadason SG, Le Souef PN. Washing plastic spacers in household detergent reduces electrostatic charge and greatly improves delivery. *Eur Respir J* 1999; **13:** 673–8.
46. Wildhaber JH, Devadason SG, Hayden MJ et al. Aerosol delivery to wheezy infants: a comparison between a nebulizer and two small volume spacers. *Pediatr Pulmonol* 1997; **23:** 212–16.
47. Wildhaber JH, Janssens HM, Pierart F et al. High-percentage lung delivery in children from detergent-treated spacers. *Pediatr Pulmonol* 2000; **29:** 389–93.
48. Dubus JC, Rhem R, Dolovich M. In vitro characterization of salbutamol generic MDIs:

delivery via small spacers. *Eur Resp J* 1998; **12**: 65S (Abstract).
49. Wildhaber JH, Hayden MJ, Dore ND, Devadason SG, LeSouef PN. Salbutamol delivery from a hydrofluoroalkane pressurized metered-dose inhaler in pediatric ventilator circuits: an in vitro study. *Chest* 1998; **98**: 186–91.
50. Chou KJ, Cunningham SJ, Crain EF. Metered dose inhalers with spacers vs nebulizers for pediatric asthma. *Arch Pediatr Adolesc Med* 1995; **149**: 201–5.
51. Parkin PC, Saunders NR, Diamond SA, Winders PM, Macarthur C. Randomised trial spacer v nebuliser for acute asthma. *Arch Dis Child* 1995; **95**: 239–40.
52. Dewar AL, Stewart A, Cogswell JJ, Connett GJ. A randomized controlled trial to assess the relative benefits of large volume spacers and nebulizers to treat acute asthma in hospital. *Arch Dis Child* 1999; **80**: 421–3.
53. Ploin D, Chapuis FR, Stamm D et al. High dose albuterol by metered dose inhaler plus a spacer device versus nebulization in preschool children with recurrent wheezing: a double blind, randomized equivalence trial. *Pediatrics* 2000; **106**(2): 311–17
54. Fuglasang G, Pedersen S. Comparison of nebuhaler and nebuliser treatment for acute severe asthma in children. *Eur J Resp Dis* 1986; **69**: 109–13.
55. Cates CJ. Comparison of holding chamber and nebulisers for beta-agonists in acute asthma. In: Cates CJ, Ducharme FM, Gibson P et al, eds. Airways module of the Cochrane Database of Systematic Review. The Cochrane Collaboration, Issue 2. Oxford: Update Software, 1997.
56. Rubin BK, Nakanishi A, Smith E, Lamb B. Salbutamol by metered dose inhaler plus holding chamber is more effective than salbutamol by jet nebulizer for the treatment of acute childhood asthma. *Eur Resp J* 1995; **8**(Suppl 19): 13s.
57. LaForce WR, Brundo DS. Controlled trial of beclomethasone dipropionate by nebulization in oxygen-dependent and ventilator-dependent infants. *J Pediatr* 1993;**122**: 285–8.
58. Arnon S, Grigg J, Silverman M. Effectiveness of budesonide aerosol in ventilator-dependent preterm babies: a preliminary report. *Pediatr Pulmonol* 1996; **21**: 231–5.
59. GiepT, Raibble P, Zuerlein T, Schwartz ID. Trial of beclomethasone dipropionate by metered-dose inhaler in ventilator-dependent neonates less than 1500 grams. *Am J Perinatol* 1996; **13**: 5–9.
60. Cole CH, Colton T, Shah BL et al. Early inhaled glucocorticoid therapy to prevent bronchopulmonary dysplasia. *N Engl J Med* 1999; **340**: 1005–10.
61. Fok TF, Lam K, Dolovich M et al. Randomised controlled study of early use of inhaled corticosteroid in preterm infants with respiratory distress syndrome. *Arch Dis Child Fetal Neonatal Ed* 1999; **80**: F203–8.
62. Merz U, Kusenbach G, Hausler M, Peschgens T, Hornchen H. Inhaled budesonide in ventilator-dependent preterm infants: a randomized, double-blind pilot study. *Biol Neonate* 1999; **75**: 46–53.
63. Shah V, Ohlsson A, Halliday HL, Dunn MS. Early administration of inhaled corticosteroids for preventing chronic lung disease in ventilated very low birth weight preterm neonates (Cochrane Review). In: The Cochrane Library, Issue 1, 2000. Oxford: Update Software.
64. Dolovich M. Changing delivery methods for obstructive lung diseases. *Curr Opin Pulm Med* 1997; **3**: 177–89.
65. Prime D, Grant AC, Slater AL, Woodhouse RN. A critical comparison of the dose delivery characteristics of four alternative inhalation devices delivering salbutamol: pressurized metered dose inhaler, Diskus inhaler, Diskhaler inhaler, and Turbuhaler inhaler. *J Aerosol Med* 1999; **12**(2): 75–84.
66. Devadason SG, Everard ML, MacEarlan C et al. Lung deposition from the TurbuHaler® in children with cystic fibrosis. *Eur Respir J* 1997; **10**: 2023–8.
67. Pedersen S, Hansen OR, Fuglsang G. Influence of inspiratory flow rate upon the effect of a Turbuhaler. *Arch Dis Child* 1990; **65**: 308–10.
68. Geller DE. Choosing a nebulizer for cystic fibrosis. *Curr Opinion Pulm Med* 1997; **3**: 414–19.
69. Standaert TA, Vandevanter D, Ramsey BW et al. The choice of compressor effects the aerosol parameters and the delivery of tobramycin from a single model nebulizer. *J Aerosol Med* 2000; **13**: 147–53.
70. Hanania NA, Wittman R, Kesten S, Chapman KR. Medical personnel's knowledge of and ability to use inhaling devices. Metered-dose inhalers, spacing chambers, and breath-actuated dry powder inhalers. *Chest* 1994; **94**: 111–16.
71. Friegang L. New method of beclomethasone administration to children under 4 years of age. *CMA J* 1977; **117**: 1308–9.
72. Morén F. Drug deposition of pressurized inhalation aerosols I. Influence of actuator tube design. *Int J Pharm* 1978; **1**: 205–12.
73. Conner WT, Dolovich MB, Frame RA, Newhouse MT. Reliable salbutamol administration in 6- to 36-month-old children by means of a metered dose inhaler and Aerochamber with mask. *Pediatr Pulmonol* 1989; **8**: 263–7.

74. Smaldone GC, Cruz-Rivera M, Nikander K. In vitro determination of inhaled mass and particle distribution for budesonide nebulizing suspension. *J Aerosol Med* 1998; **11:** 113–25.
75. Pelkonen AS, Nikander K, Turpeinen M. Jet nebulization of budesonide suspension into a neonatal ventilator circuit: Synchronized versus continuous flow. *Pediatr Pulmonol* 1997; **24:** 282–6.
76. Finlay WH. Inertial sizing of aerosol inhaled during pediatric tidal breathing from an MDI with attached holding chamber. *Int J Pharm* 1998; **168:** 147–52.
77. Avent ML, Gal P, Ransom JL, Brown YL, Hansen CJ. Comparing the delivery of albuterol metered-dose inhaler via an adaptor and spacer device in an in vitro infant ventilator lung model. *Ann Pharmacother* 1999; **33:** 141–3.
78. Janssens HM, Krijgsman AM, Verbraak TFM et al. Fine particle size improves lung deposition of inhaled steroids in infants: a study in an upper airway model. *Am J Respir Crit Care Med* 2000; **161** (Part 2): A32.
79. Borgstrom L. In vitro, ex vivo, in vivo veritas. *Allergy* 1999; **54**(Suppl 49): 88–92.
80. Dompeling E, Oudesluys-Murphy AM, Janssens HM et al. Randomised controlled study of clinical efficacy of spacer therapy in asthma with regard to electrostatic charge. *Arch Dis Child* 2001; **84:** 178–82.
81. Dolovich M, Mistry J, Rhem R. Modelling drug output of nebulized cationic lipid:plasmid complexes based on simulated breathing patterns. *Am J Resp Crit Care Med* 2001; **163**(Part 2): (Abstract).
82. Agertoft L, Pedersen S, Nikander S. Drug delivery from the Turbuhaler and Nebuhaler pressurized metered dose inhaler to various age groups of children with asthma. *J Aerosol Med* 1999; **12:** 161–9.
83. Tal A, Golan H, Grauer N et al. Deposition pattern of radiolabeled salbutamol inhaled from a metered-dose inhaler by means of a spacer with mask in young children with airways obstruction. *J Pediatr* 1996; **128:** 479–84.
84. Ilowite JS, Gorvoy JD, Smaldone GC. Quantitative deposition of aerosolized gentamicin in cystic fibrosis. *Am Rev Respir Dis* 1987; **136:** 1445–9.
85. Mallol J, Rattray S, Walker G, Cool D, Robertson CF. Aerosol deposition in infants with cystic fibrosis. *Pediatr Pulmonol* 1996; **21:** 276–81.
86. Fok TF, Monkman S, Dolovich M G et al. Efficiency of aerosol medication delivery from a metered dose inhaler versus jet nebulizer in infants with bronchopulmonary dysplasia. *Pediatr Pulmonol* 1996; **21:** 301–9.
87. Wildhaber JH, Devadason SG, Wilson JM et al. Lung deposition of budesonide from Turbuhaler in asthmatic children. *Eur J Pediatr* 1998; **157:** 1017–22.
88. Chua HL, Collis GG, Newbury AM et al. The influence of age on aerosol deposition in children with cystic fibrosis. *Eur Respir J* 1994; **7:** 2185–91.
89. Everard ML Studies using radiolabelled aerosols in children. *Thorax* 1994; **49:** 1259–66.
90. Fleming JS, Halson P, Conway J et al. Three-dimensional description of pulmonary deposition of inhaled aerosol using data from multimodality imaging. *J Nucl Med* 1996; **37:** 873–7.
91. Dolovich M, MacIntyre NR, Anderson PJ et al. Consensus statement: aerosols and delivery devices. *Respir Care* 2000; **45:** 589–96.
92. Dolovich M, Nahmias C, Coates G. Unleashing the PET: 3D imaging of the lung. In: Byron P, Dalby R, Farr SJ, eds. *Proceedings of Respiratory Drug Delivery* VII. NC: Serentec Press, 2000: 215–30.
93. Berridge MS, Heald DL. In vivo characterization of inhaled pharmaceuticals using quantitative positron emission tomography. *J Clin Pharmacol* 1999; **39:** 25S–29S
94. Andersen C, Kent A, Schmidt B et al. Early activity of imflammatory cells in the lungs of very low birth weight (VLBW) infants. *Pediatr Res* 2000; (submitted).
95. Kirpalani H, Abubakar K, Nahmias C, Desa D, Coates G, Schmidt B. [18F]Fluorodeoxyglucose uptake in neonatal acute lung injury measured by positron emission tomography. *Pediatr Res* 1997; **41:** 892–6.
96. Dolovich M, Fok TF, Monkman S et al. Relationship between infant weight and lung deposition of aerosol. *Eur Resp J* 1995; **8**(Suppl 19): 201S.
97. Dolovich M. Rationale for spacer use. *Pediatr Pulmonol* 1997; Suppl 16: 184–5.
98. Hindle M, Chrystn H. Determination of the relative bioavailability of salbutamol to the lung following inhalation. *Br J Clin Pharmacol* 1992; **34:** 311–15.
99. Derendorf H, Hochhaus G, Rohatagi S et al. Pharmacokinetics of triamcinolone acetonide after intravenous, oral and inhaled administration. *J Clin Pharmacol* 1995; **35:** 302–5.
100. Borgstrom L, Newman S, Weisz A, Morén F. Pulmonary deposition of inhaled terbutaline: comparison of scanning gamma camera and urinary excretion methods. *J Pharm Sci* 1992; **81:** 753–5.
101. Lipworth BJ, Seckl JR. Measures for detecting systemic bioactivity with inhaled and intranasal corticosteroids. *Thorax* 1997; **52:** 476–82.

18
Economics in pediatric asthma

Sean D Sullivan, Paula Lozano, Kevin B Weiss

Introduction • Foundations of health economic analysis • Types of economic evaluation methods • Economic evaluation studies of asthma pharmacotherapy • Controller medication • Economic studies of asthma patient education and consultation programs • Linking cost-effectiveness analysis with the development of clinical practice guidelines • Conclusion

INTRODUCTION

Public and private health care systems are developing methods to minimize the cost of managing chronic diseases while maintaining a high quality of care for their member populations. The goals of minimizing cost and ensuring quality often are in conflict, particularly in an era of budget constraints. Tension arises because public and private coverage of health care creates incentives for patients (and often providers) to consume care with little regard for the unit price of that care. As a consequence, decision makers are finding themselves in new roles as managers of disease management strategies that balance the need for fiscal responsibility with patients' desire to obtain the most technologically advanced and beneficial care that is available. Because the process of allocating scarce resources among competing medical treatments can be emotional and politically charged, decision makers prefer to adopt rational, standardized tools for economic evaluation which are designed to maximize health for a given level of medical care expenditure. Health economics provides a set of tools to serve this need.

The rising cost of asthma care, however, is at odds with moves to tighten health care budgets. Asthma has been the target of intense activity in the areas of clinical practice guidelines, disease management, drug formulary design and other efforts that are at least in part aimed at reducing medical expenditures and increasing quality for asthma care. Because asthma has become such an important topic to the public, decision makers must be mindful of the social as well as clinical aspects of this disease in their efforts to control the costs of asthma care. Since economic evaluations combine a societal perspective with analysis of clinical and economic effectiveness, this methodology holds great promise as an aid to therapeutic decision making for populations of patients with asthma.

The purpose of this chapter is to briefly define the discipline and uses of economic evaluation studies, to review the literature on the cost-effectiveness of asthma interventions, and to suggest best practices for conducting economic evaluations of therapies for asthma all in the context of the pediatric patient.

FOUNDATIONS OF HEALTH ECONOMIC ANALYSIS

Cost-effectiveness analysis can be defined as a set of research methods to assess and quantify the costs and clinical consequences of medical care interventions in order to estimate the value of the intervention in relation to alternative uses for the same resources.[1] Pharmacoeconomic analysis is cost-effectiveness analysis as it is applied to pharmacological therapies. A cost-effectiveness analysis of alternative medical interventions should incorporate evidence about the clinical consequences (efficacy and safety) and the total costs of treatment alternatives.[2]

Essential concepts

Cost-effectiveness analysis is derived from a single equation that integrates costs and outcomes:

$$\text{Incremental cost-effectiveness ratio} = \frac{\text{Cost}_A - \text{Cost}_B}{\text{Effectiveness}_A - \text{Effectiveness}_B} \quad (1)$$

The equation shows a cost-effectiveness comparison of two interventions, A (usually the new or proposed intervention) and B (the established or usual care intervention). The incremental cost-effectiveness is the attributable health benefit of A and the level of health care expenditure for A when compared with the health benefits and costs of B.

From this equation one can readily see that there are only four possible cost and outcome combinations that can result. These are illustrated in Figure 18.1.[3] Quadrant B illustrates a treatment that is less beneficial or more harmful and costs more than the comparator treatment. Quadrant C depicts a dominant intervention — one that improves health outcome and achieves cost savings. Results B and C are unambiguous from a decision-making standpoint, indicating that the new intervention should be rejected (B) or accepted (C) for payment or coverage by the health care system.

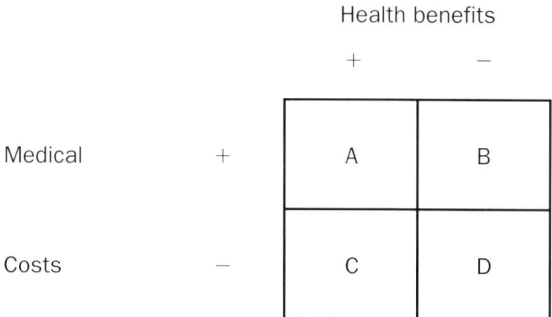

Figure 18.1 Depiction of possible results of economic evaluation studies.

Quadrant D represents a less expensive treatment with a reduced health outcome compared to standard therapy. Quadrant A shows the cost–outcome relationship of most new medical technology. Here, health benefits improve, but at an additional expense to the health care system. For cost-effectiveness evaluations that fall within quadrant A, clinicians, patients, and payers must decide whether the improvement in health benefit from the new intervention is worth the additional costs of using the new intervention. Note that in a health care system with a fixed budget, additional expenditure on new treatments reduces the amount of resources that are available for other interventions and patients with other disease states. Presently, health plans and government payers implicitly make trade-off decisions in much the same way as described above, although with less rigor and specificity of incremental outcomes and costs. In this chapter, we describe the results and implications of cost and cost-effectiveness studies targeted at pediatric asthma patients.

TYPES OF ECONOMIC EVALUATION METHODS

Cost identification and cost-of-illness studies

Cost-of-illness studies seek to estimate the economic burden of a disease to society. Cost-of-illness studies are not cost-effectiveness analyses, since they do not compare alternative interventions. Still, they are commonly performed as a way to raise awareness about the economic consequences of illnesses, particularly those whose impact on society may be undervalued by health care policy makers and the public. For example, the often cited study by Weiss and colleagues on the economic impact of asthma in the United States found that this 'mild' chronic illness accounted for US$6.2 billion in societal costs during 1990.[4] Furthermore, more than US$1 billion of these costs were as a consequence of lost days of school in children affected with the disease.[4] The literature is now replete with papers characterizing the cost of asthma for adults and children in various countries.[5–9]

Several studies have now described the economic costs of pediatric asthma nationally and in special populations and care delivery settings.[10–17] A variety of population-based surveys — including the National Health Interview Survey, the National Hospital Discharge Survey, the National Ambulatory Medical Care Survey, and others—have been used to assess the magnitude of health care utilization and cost among children with asthma. In 1988, children with asthma had an additional 12.9 million contacts with physicians and 200 000 hospitalizations compared with children without asthma.[18] Direct expenditure for children with asthma in 1985 was estimated to be US$465 million.[4] However, because none of these national surveys collects both diagnostic and expenditure data, per capita costs cannot be estimated for an individual child or family.

More recently, managed care data systems have been used to describe the epidemiology of pediatric asthma and the associated utilization and cost within specified enrollee populations.[11,13] However, these populations cannot be considered to be nationally representative.

A population-based national probability survey, the National Medical Expenditure Survey (NMES), was conducted in 1987 to determine the use and cost of health care services in the United States. Responses for all children aged 1–17 with ($n = 667$) and without ($n = 6911$) asthma were evaluated in order to estimate the societal burden of pediatric asthma. Children were identified with asthma using a population-based screening question. Frequency and cost of medications, ambulatory visits, emergency department (ED) care, and hospitalizations for all reasons (including asthma) were assessed.

The period prevalence of childhood asthma was estimated at 8.8% and the treated prevalence (any asthma medications) was 4.0%. Forty-one percent of families with asthmatic children were identified as having no primary insurance. Children with asthma used substantially more services in all categories of care: 3.1 times as many prescriptions, 1.9 times as many ambulatory provider visits, 2.2 times as many ED visits, and 3.5 times as many hospitalizations. Only 10.7% of children with asthma were defined as chronic users of medications. Children with asthma incurred an average of US$1129 (standard deviation US$5310) per child per year in total health care expenditure compared with US$468 (standard deviation US$2960) for children without asthma, a 2.4-fold difference.

In two of these studies, the data show an important age effect related to both utilization and expenditure among children with asthma.[12,13] Very young children (<5 years old) and adolescents (12–17 years old) have higher rates of expenditures for asthma (and all disease) when compared with children aged 5–11 years.

Comparative health economic analyses

The most common comparative health economic evaluation technique is cost-effectiveness analysis. The measure of effectiveness (denominator in equation 1) in a cost-effectiveness study is an ad hoc measure of benefit which is most suitable to the study. Here, health outcomes of treatments are expressed in predefined clinical units such as symptom-free time or quality-adjusted years of life saved. Ad hoc denominators have the advantage of being readily identifiable and unambiguous aspects of a disease which are clearly affected by the treatments in question. However, important outcomes beyond the selected effectiveness measure that may also be affected by the treatment (e.g. quality of life) are sometimes ignored.

ECONOMIC EVALUATION STUDIES OF ASTHMA PHARMACOTHERAPY

There are a number of economic analyses of asthma interventions, but to date few of these have met the agreed standards for economic evaluation in health care.[19] Health economic evaluation is an evolving science. Still, there are several reasons to establish standard methods of economic evaluation for interventions such as asthma treatment. Drummond and colleagues give the following rationale for establishing standards: (1) to maintain high methodological standards; (2) to facilitate the comparison of the results of economic evaluations for different health care interventions; and (3) to facilitate interpretation of study findings from health care setting to setting.[20,21] The latter issue arises both within countries with diverse health delivery systems (such as the US) and in international interpretation of studies.

Tables 18.1 and 18.2 summarize the important observational and randomized health economic evaluations of asthma pharmacotherapy in pediatric patients. All of the published studies evaluate controller therapy in combination with rescue medication.

CONTROLLER MEDICATION

There is substantial evidence of the positive clinical benefits and minimum safety risks of combining controller medications with as-needed rescue therapy for the management of asthma.[22,23] The therapeutic management guidelines of the US National Asthma Education and Prevention Expert Panel Report (NAEPP), the International Consensus Report (ICR), the Global Initiative for Asthma Report (GINA), and the British Thoracic Society Guidelines recommend as initial treatment such combination therapy for people with moderate to severe asthma. However, adding expensive controller medications to an existing regimen of inhaled or oral bronchodilator therapy contributes significantly to the overall cost of treating asthma. An important question for health economists and medical resource decision makers is whether the added costs of controller therapy are justified in terms of added health benefit to patients.

Ross and co-workers made use of patient and health services records in one large group practice to estimate the economic consequences of including cromolyn sodium in the treatment regimen of asthma patients.[24] A total of 53 patients were retrospectively identified from medical records and categorized into two groups: those who received cromolyn sodium for at least 1 year ($n=27$) and those who received no cromolyn sodium as part of the treatment regimen ($n=26$). Patients receiving cromolyn sodium provided an average of 3.2 years of health service utilization data, and those in the comparison group provided 3.8 years of data. Medication costs for patients on cromolyn sodium were slightly higher (US$27.90 per month) than for the control group (US$25.20 per month). However, emergency department and hospital costs declined significantly for cromolyn sodium patients; after the change in medication, they experienced a 96% reduction in the rate of emergency department visits and a 92% reduction in the rate of hospital admissions.

Gerdtham and colleagues constructed a pooled, time-series economic model to determine the association between greater use of inhaled corticosteroids and asthma-related hospital days in 14 counties over an 11 year period using a non-experimental design.[25] More than 80% of inhaled corticosteroid use during this time was with budesonide. Although not a cost-effectiveness analysis, the study did indicate a strong negative association between use of inhaled corticosteroids and hospital-bed-days for asthma. An approximate cost–benefit ratio was developed from the multivariate models suggestive of positive economic benefits in

Table 18.1 Nonrandomized health economic studies of asthma pharmacotherapy in pediatric and adolescent patients

Study	Study method used	Sample size	Perspective	Treatments studied	Length of study	Costs measured	Health outcomes measured	Economic outcomes
Ref. 24	Retrospective; pre/post quasi-experimental design	53	Health system	2 groups: cromolyn users and non-users	3.2–3.8 years*	Direct	None	Estimated 92–96% reduction in health services use
Ref. 25	Retrospective; econometric model	†	Societal	All inhaled corticosteroids	11 years	Direct	Reduction in hospital bed days and discharges for asthma	Estimated benefit:cost ratio of between 1.5:1 and 2.8:1
Ref. 37	Prospective; pre/post quasi-experimental design	86	Societal	2 groups: various doses of beclomethasone and budesonide	4 years	Direct	Reduction in acute severe attacks, hospital admissions, breakthrough wheezing, missed school days, and treatment satisfaction	Estimated 83% reduction in total costs of care; US$0.04 per unit increase in patient satisfaction with treatment

*Cromolyn users contributed 3.2 years of data and non-users of cromolyn contributed 3.8 years of data.
†Unit of analysis is counties and not persons. The study represents a total of 71% of the Swedish population.

Table 18.2 Randomized health economic studies of asthma pharmacotherapy in pediatric and adolescent patients

Study	Study method used	Sample size	Perspective	Treatments studied	Length of study	Costs measured	Health outcomes measured	Economic outcomes
Ref. 28	Randomized controlled trial	40	Societal	2 groups: budesonide compared with placebo	26 weeks	Direct and indirect	Lung function (FEV_1), symptoms, symptom-free days	Budesonide is dominant therapy; saved US$9.43 for each symptom-free day gained
Ref. 31	Randomized controlled trial	116	Societal	2 groups: budesonide and salbutamol, salbutamol alone	3 years*	Direct and indirect	Lung function (FEV_1), symptom-free days, school absences	Budesonide is cost-effective; US$83 per 10% improvement in FEV_1, US$4.75 per symptom-free day gained
Ref. 30	Randomized controlled trial	225	Societal	2 groups: sodium cromoglycate 20 mg qid compared to fluticasone 50 µg bid	8 weeks	Direct	Lung function (PEFR), symptom scores, and the probability of successful treatment	Fluticasone is cost-effective compared to sodium cromoglycate; cost-effectiveness ratios vary according to outcome measure selected
Ref. 32	Randomized controlled trial	353	Societal	2 groups: budesonide 800 µg bid compared with fluticasone/salmeterol combination bid	24 weeks	Direct	Lung function (FEV_1), symptom-free days, and the probability of successful treatment	The combination of fluticasone and salmeterol bid is more cost effective than budesonide bid

*The study had a planned 3 year follow-up but only 39 patients reached a follow-up period of 22 months.

excess of costs on the order of between 1.5:1.0 and 2.8:1.0, depending on the analytic model. Similar associations between medication use and outcome have been reported in the United States.[26,27]

Several recent studies have employed experimental research designs to investigate the cost effectiveness of controller therapy. Connett and colleagues studied the cost-effectiveness of inhaled budesonide compared with placebo in a 6 month randomized trial of 40 children aged 1–3 years with persistent asthma.[28] The outcome results indicated that budesonide produced a favorable clinical response, increasing the frequency of symptom-free days when compared with placebo (195 versus 117 days). Direct medical costs (including the cost of budesonide) and indirect costs were tabulated for the numerator of the cost-effectiveness ratio. The results suggested that budesonide is a dominant therapy, that is, compared with placebo, budesonide increases overall effectiveness and reduces overall costs by £6.33 (about US$9.45) per symptom-free day gained.

Rutten-van Mölken and associates reported on the cost-effectiveness of adding inhaled corticosteroid to as-needed bronchodilator compared with as-needed bronchodilator alone in a 12 month randomized trial of 116 children with asthma 7–16 years of age.[29] The investigators evaluated FEV_1 as the primary outcome. Frequency of symptom-free days and the number of school absences were included as secondary outcome measures. Patients randomized to inhaled corticosteroid plus as-needed bronchodilator experienced significantly increased lung function (FEV_1) and symptom-free days and reduced days missed from school relative to as-needed bronchodilator alone. Compared with bronchodilator alone, bronchodilator plus inhaled corticosteroid increased FEV_1 by 10% at an additional total cost of about US$83. The additional cost of bronchodilator plus inhaled corticosteroid was about US$4.75 per symptom-free day gained. Thus, inhaled corticosteroid plus bronchodilator was more effective than bronchodilator alone but at an additional cost. The relative value differed depending on whether one focused on improved lung function (FEV_1) or better symptom control.

The cost-effectiveness of fluticasone was studied in a group of 4–12-year-old children who required inhaled prophylactic treatment for asthma.[30] Over an 8 week study period, 115 patients received sodium cromoglycate 20 mg four times daily and 110 patients received fluticasone propionate 50 μg twice daily. The effectiveness of both treatments was determined by morning and evening PEFR, daily symptom control, safety, proportion of successfully treated patients, and incidence of adverse consequences. The authors concluded that over an 8 week period fluticasone was cost-effective when compared with sodium cromoglycate for prophylactic treatment using treatment success rates as the primary cost-effectiveness outcome measure.

Other cost-effectiveness studies in mixed populations of adults and children have shown (1) no clinical and economic difference between similar inhaled long-acting bronchodilators and (2) that a combination of salmeterol and fluticasone is more cost-effective than budesonide alone.[31,32]

Based on the Chochrane Airways Group review of anticholinergics, several investigators evaluated the cost-effectiveness of ipratropium bromide when used in combination with rescue bronchodilator therapy.[33] Using an economic modeling approach, the authors concluded that the addition of ipratropium bromide to inhaled β-agonists in children with severe acute asthma would result in cost savings to the British National Health Service.

The results from these studies suggest a favorable economic impact from the use of controller therapy when added to short-acting bronchodilator treatment. Similarly, other studies have demonstrated that controller therapy reduces hospitalization rates in people with chronic asthma,[34-37] although they did not include formal economic evaluation.

While each of the studies has its own merits, the ability of decision-makers to compare results across studies is hampered by the lack of standardization in study design.

ECONOMIC STUDIES OF ASTHMA PATIENT EDUCATION AND CONSULTATION PROGRAMS

Several reports document the clinical and economic impact of patient-oriented asthma education programs for both pediatric and adult populations. Educational interventions for asthma have included formal classroom-based medication compliance programs and asthma self-management programs for adults and children and their parents.[38] Since the mid-1980s several models of asthma education for children and adults, well designed and based on behavioral theory, have been evaluated and shown to achieve the desired outcomes, such as reduced use of health services and better quality of life.

Economic evaluations of these programs have been quite favorable, in particular when the programs have been directed at high-risk patients or those with documented resource-intensive care needs such as a prior hospitalization, frequent unscheduled visits, or frequent dispensings of rescue medication.[39–57] Unfortunately, most of these studies were not conducted on pediatric or adolescent asthmatic populations and thus there is little to learn by way of information for resource allocation from this literature.

Other analyses have examined the economic impact of referrals of moderate to severe asthmatics to specialists.[58] In retrospective chart reviews, these studies find significant reductions in sick office visits, ED visits, hospital days, and costs of care for patients. Most of these analyses, however, suffered from poor design and evaluation methods. Flaws included: failing to include the cost of the intervention; inadequate specification of the time horizon for treatment, lack of adjustment for potential confounding in patient selection.

LINKING COST-EFFECTIVENESS ANALYSIS WITH THE DEVELOPMENT OF CLINICAL PRACTICE GUIDELINES

Ideally, health economic evidence should be weighed along with clinical data when creating clinical practice guidelines for asthma management. Since much of the drive for guidelines has been the growing economic importance of asthma, it makes sense to bring formal economic analysis into the guideline development process using methods that are agreed upon by leaders in the field. Economic data can then be linked with clinical data as part of the evidence that justifies the management strategy that is outlined in the guideline.

To date, health economic data have not been explicitly factored into clinical practice guidelines for asthma. This owes in part to the fact that health economic studies have varied widely in quality, and partly because the outcomes measures vary widely from study to study. Two issues must be addressed before health economic data can be effectively integrated into the clinical practice guideline process. First, the methodologic quality of the studies must improve substantially. Second, meaningful and relevant outcome variables must be selected for inclusion in all analyses to facilitate comparison of different interventions. A recent report by the National Heart, Lungs and Blood Institute (NHLBI) Workshop on Asthma Outcome Measures for Research Studies provides a useful review of the many end points available to researchers who study asthma.[59] The National Asthma Education and Prevention Program Task Force on the Cost-effectiveness, Quality and Financing of Asthma Care has recommended the use of symptom-free days as the standard outcome measure for cost-effectiveness evaluation of asthma treatments, in part because the measure reflects aggregate disease morbidity.[60]

CONCLUSION

Health care decision makers are interested in employing rational approaches to allocating resources among the populations they serve. Many embrace economic evaluation as a set of tools to assess the value of asthma interventions, given the conflicts generated by constrained health budgets and a rising demand for medical care. There is reasonably solid evidence of the positive health economic benefits of controller therapy for children, particularly with inhaled corticosteroids when used in moderate to severe disease. Education and self-management interventions in targeted 'at risk' populations also have been shown to represent good value for money. However, before health economic data can be integrated into the decision-making process the methodologic standards of these studies must improve and common measures of outcome must be incorporated into all evaluations. High standards will ensure that the internal and external validity of these studies is apparent to decision makers and researchers. Common measures of outcome will ensure the comparability of data on the economic value of different treatments, particularly as new therapies are introduced into practice. When methods and outcomes for economic evaluations of the most commonly used therapies are standardized, this important information can then be made part of the process of creating clinical practice guidelines for asthma.

REFERENCES

1. Drummond MF, Stoddart GL, Torrance GW. *Methods for the Economic Evaluation of Health Care Programmes*. New York: Oxford University Press, 1987.
2. Banta HD, Luce BR. *Health Care Technology and Its Assessment*. New York: Oxford University Press, 1993.
3. Ellwood P. Outcomes management: a technology of patient experience. *NEJM* 1988; **318:** 1549–56.
4. Weiss KB, Gergen PJ, Hodgson TA. An economic evaluation of asthma in the United States. *N Engl J Med* 1992; **326:** 862–6.
5. Sullivan SD. Cost and cost-effectiveness in asthma: use of pharmacoeconomics to assess the value of asthma interventions. *Immunology and Allergy Clinics of North America* 1996; **16:** 819–39.
6. Szucs TD, Anderhub H, Rutishauser M. The economic burden of asthma: direct and indirect costs in Switzerland. *Eur Respir J* 1999; **13:** 281–6.
7. Graf von der Schulenburg JM, Greiner W, Molitor S, Kielhorn A. Cost of asthma therapy in relation to severity. *Med Klin* 1996; **91:** 670–6.
8. Smith DH, Malone DC, Lawson KA, Okamoto LJ, Battista C, Saunders WB. A national estimate of the economic costs of asthma. *Am J Respir Crit Care Med* 1997; **156:** 787–93.
9. Chew FT, Goh DY, Lee BW. The economic cost of asthma in Singapore. *Aust N Z J Med* 1999; **29:** 228–33.
10. Lozano P, Connell FA, Koepsell TD. Use of health services by African-American children with asthma on Medicaid. *JAMA* 1995; **274:** 469–73.
11. Lozano P, Fishman P, VonKorff M, Hecht J. Health care utilization and cost among children with asthma who were enrolled in a health maintenance organization. *Pediatrics* 1997; **99:** 757–64.
12. Lozano P, Sullivan SD, Smith DH, Weiss KB. The economic burden of asthma in US children: estimates from the National Medical Expenditure Survey. *J Allergy Clin Immunol* 1999; **104:** 957–63.
13. Stempel DA, Hedblom EC, Durcanin-Robbins JF, Sturm LL. Use of a pharmacy and medical claims database to document cost centers for 1993 annual asthma expenditures. *Arch Fam Med* 1996; **5:** 36–40.
14. Coventry JA, Weston MS, Collins PM. Emergency room encounters of pediatric patients with asthma: cost comparisons with other treatment settings. *J Ambulatory Care Manage* 1996; **19:** 9–21.
15. Hoskins G, McGowan C, Neville RG, Thomas GE, Smith B, Silverman S. Risk factors and costs associated with an asthma attack. *Thorax* 2000; **55:** 19–24.
16. Meurer JR, Kuhn EM, George V, Yauck JS, Layde PM. Charges for childhood asthma by hospital characteristics. *Pediatrics* 1998; **102:** E70.
17. Nash DR, Childs GE, Kelleher KJ. A cohort study of resource use by Medicaid children with asthma. *Pediatrics* 1999; **104:** 310–12.
18. Taylor WR, Newacheck PW. Impact of childhood asthma on health. *Pediatrics* 1992; **90:** 657–62.
19. Gold MR, Siegel JE, Russell LB, Weinstein MC. *Cost-effectiveness in Health and Medicine*. New York: Oxford University Press, 1996.
20. Drummond MF, Brandt A, Luce B, Rovira J. Standardizing methodologies for economic evaluation in health care: practice, problems, and potential. *Int J Technol Assess Health Care* 1993; **9:** 26–36.

21. Drummond MF, Richardson WS, O'Brien BJ, Levine M, Heyland D. Users' guides to the medical literature: XIII. How to use an article on economic analysis of clinical practice: A. Are the results of the study valid? *JAMA* 277: 1552–7.
22. Barnes PJ, Pedersen S. Efficacy and safety of inhaled corticosteroids in asthma. *Am Rev Resp Dis* 1993; **148**: S1–S26.
23. Plotnick LH, Ducharme FM. Should inhaled anticholinergics be added to beta-agonists for treating acute childhood and adolescent asthma? A systematic review. *BMJ* 1998; **317**: 971–7.
24. Ross RN, Morris M, Sakowitz SR, Berman BA. Cost-effectiveness of including cromolyn sodium in the treatment program for asthma: a retrospective, record-based study. *Clin Ther* 1988; **10**: 188–203.
25. Gerdtham UG, Hertzman P, Boman G, Jonsson B. Impact of inhaled corticosteroids on asthma hospitalization in Sweden. *Applied Economics* 1996; **28**: 1591–9.
26. Donahue JG, Weiss ST, Livingston JM, Goetsch MA, Greineder DK, Platt R. Inhaled steroids and the risk of hospitalization for asthma. *JAMA* 1997; **277**: 887–91.
27. Vollmer WM, Markson LE, O'Connor E, Sanocki LL, Fitterman L, Berger M et al. Association of asthma control with health care utilization and quality of life. *Am J Respir Crit Care Med* 1999; **160**: 1647–52.
28. Connett GJ, Lenney W, McConchie SM. The cost-effectiveness of budesonide in severe asthmatics aged one to three years. *Br J Med Econ* 1993; **6**: 127–34.
29. Rutten-van Mölken MP, Van Doorslaer EK, Jansen MC et al. Cost-effectiveness of inhaled corticosteroid plus bronchodilator therapy versus bronchodilator monotherapy in children with asthma. *PharmacoEconomics* 1993; **4**: 257–70.
30. Booth PC, Wells NEJ, Morrison AK. A comparison of the cost effectiveness of alternative prophylactic therapies in childhood asthma. *PharmacoEconomics* 1996; **10**: 262–8.
31. Rutten-van Molken M, van Doorslaer EK, Till MD. Cost-effectiveness analysis of formoterol versus salmeterol in patients with asthma. *PharmacoEconomics* 1998; **14**: 671–84.
32. Lundback B, Jenkins C, Price MJ, Thwaites RM. Cost-effectiveness of salmeterol/fluticasone propionate combination product 50/250 microg twice daily and budesonide 800 microg twice daily in the treatment of adults and adolescents with asthma. *Respir Med* 2000; **94**: 724–32.
33. Lord J, Ducharme FM, Stamp RJ, Littlejohns P, Churchill R. Cost effectiveness analysis of anticholinergics for acute childhood and adolescent asthma. *BMJ* 1999; **319**: 1470–1.
34. Karalus NC, Harrison AC. Inhaled high-dose beclomethasone in chronic asthma. *N Z Med J* 1987; **100**: 306–8.
35. Wennergren G, Kristjasson S, Strannegard I. Decrease in hospitalization for treatment of childhood asthma with increased use of anti-inflammatory treatment, despite an increase in prevalence. *J Allergy Clin Immunol* 1996; **97**: 742–8.
36. Suissa S, Dennis R, Ernst P, Sheehy O, Wood-Dauphinee S. Effectiveness of the leukotriene receptor antagonist zafirlukast for mild-to-moderate asthma. A randomized, double-blind, placebo-controlled trial. *Ann Intern Med* 1997; **126**: 177–83.
37. Perera BJC. Efficacy and cost effectiveness of inhaled steroids in asthma in a developing country. *Arch Dis Child* 1995; **72**: 312–16.
38. Clark NM, Gong M. Management of chronic disease by practitioners and patients: are we teaching the wrong things? *BMJ* 2000; **320**: 572–5.
39. Green L. Toward cost–benefit evaluations of health education: some concepts, methods and examples. *Health Edu Monog* 1974; **2**: 34–64.
40. Boulet L, Champan K, Green L, FitzGerald J. Asthma education. *Chest* 1994; **106**: 184S–196S.
41. Windsor R, Bailey W, Richards JJ, Manzella B, Soong S, Brooks M. Evaluation of the efficacy and cost effectiveness of health education methods to increase medication adherence among adults with asthma. *Am J Public Health* 1990; **80**: 1519–21.
42. Muhlhauser I, Richter B, Kraut D, Weske G, Worth H, Berger M. Evaluation of a structured treatment and teaching program on asthma. *J Intern Med* 1991; **238**: 157–64.
43. Trautner C, Richter B, Berger M. Cost-effectiveness of a structured treatment and teaching programme on asthma. *Eur Respir J* 1993; **6**: 1485–91.
44. Bolton M, Tilley B, Kuder J, Reeves T, Schultz I. The cost and effectiveness of an education program for adults who have asthma. *J Gen Intern Med* 1991; **6**: 401–7.
45. Sondergaard B, Davidsen F, Kirkeby B et al. The economics of an intensive education program for asthmatic patients: a prospective controlled trial. *PharmacoEconomics* 1992; **1**: 207–12.
46. Kauppinen R, Sintonen H, Vilkka V, Tukiainen H. Long-term economic evaluation of intensive

patient education for self-management during the first year in new asthmatics. *Respir Med* 1999; **93:** 283–9.
47. Fireman P, Friday G, Gira C, Vierthaler W, Michaels L. Teaching self-management skills to asthmatic children and their parents in an ambulatory care setting. *Pediatrics* 1981; **68:** 341–8.
48. Lewis C, Rachelefsky G, Lewis M, De la Soto A, Kaplan M. A randomized trial of ACT (asthma care training) for kids. *Pediatrics* 1984; **74:** 478–86.
49. Clark N, Feldman C, Evans D, Levison M, Wasilewski Y, Mellins R. The impact of health education on frequency and cost of health care use by low income children with asthma. *J Allergy Clin Immunol* 1986; **78:** 108–15.
50. Greineder DK, Loane KC, Parks P. Reduction in resource utilization by an asthma outreach program. *Arch Pediatr Adolesc Med* 1995; **149:** 415–20.
51. Levenson T, Grammer LC, Yarnold PR, Patterson R. Cost-effective management of malignant potentially fatal asthma. *Allergy & Asthma Proc* 1997; **18:** 73–8.
52. Higgins JC, Kiser WR, McClenathan S, Tynan NL. Influence of an interventional program on resource use and cost in pediatric asthma. *Am J Manag Care* 1998; **4:** 1465–9.
53. Windsor R, Bailey W, Richards J et al. Evaluation of the efficacy and cost-effectiveness of health education methods to increase medication adherence among adults with asthma. *Am J Public Health* 1990; **80:** 1519–21.
54. Deter H. Cost–benefit analysis of psychosomatic therapy in asthma. *Psychosom Res* 1986; **30:** 173–82.
55. Folgering H, Rooyakkers J, Herwaarden C. Education and cost/benefit ratios in pulmonary patients. *Monaldi Arch Chest Dis* 1994; **49:** 166–8.
56. Sondergaard B, Davidsen F, Kirkeby B et al. The economics of an intensive education programme for asthmatic patients. *PharmacoEconomics* 1992; **1:** 207–12.
57. Neri M, Migliori GB, Spanevello A et al. Economic analysis of two structured treatment and teaching programs on asthma. *Allergy* 1996; **51:** 313–19
58. Westley C, Spiecher R, Starr L et al. Cost effectiveness of an allergy consultation in the management of asthma. *Allergy and Asthma Proc* 1997; **18:** 15–18.
59. National Heart, Lung, and Blood Institute. Asthma outcome measures. *Am J Respir Crit Care Med* 1994; **149:** S1–S90.
60. Sullivan SD, Elixhauser A, Buist AS, Luce BR, Eisenberg J, Weiss KB. National Asthma Education and Prevention Program working group report on the cost effectiveness of asthma care. *Am J Respir Crit Care Med* 1996; **154:** S84–S95

19

Prediction and prevention of asthma

John O Warner

Allergic sensitization • Ontogeny of allergic sensitization • Pregnancy as an allergic phenomenon • The route of fetal antigen exposure and sensitization • Modification of antenatal allergen-specific immune responses • Maternal nutrition and fetal susceptibility to allergy and asthma • Environmental tobacco smoke and wheezing illness in childhood • Genetic and environmental diversity • The hygiene hypothesis • Gut microbial flora • Tertiary prophylaxis

It is clear that although pharmacological intervention to treat established asthma is highly effective in controlling symptoms and improving quality of life, this approach does not modify the natural course of the disease. Hitherto, no cure of the condition has been identified. This must focus the attention particularly of paediatricians on the potential for prevention, which must be the ideal approach to any chronic disease.

Taking the analogy of the prophylaxis for tuberculosis, preventive strategies might be considered at three levels. Primary prophylaxis would be introduced before there was any evidence of sensitization to factors that might subsequently induce disease. With increasing evidence that allergic sensitization, which is a common prelude to the development of asthma, can occur antenatally, much of the focus of primary prophylaxis will be on preconceptual and antenatal interventions. Secondary prophylaxis is employed after evidence of sensitization is apparent but before there is any evidence of disease. This will focus very specifically on the first year or so of life. Tertiary prophylaxis is introduced when there is already evidence of atopic disease, such as eczema or allergic rhinitis, but not yet any evidence of asthma. Finally, it will also be necessary to consider early therapeutic intervention when the first signs of asthma have occurred but before the immunopathology of the disease has been fully established. Whether or not this latter strategy is either possible or effective remains to be established. Furthermore, at all levels of prevention, many of the issues remain speculative and have yet to be put to the test in proper long-term controlled clinical studies, though many studies are in progress at the present time.

A prerequisite for establishing any form of preventive strategy is to have reliable markers that will predict progression to disease. Limited progress has been made in identifying such markers, though it is clear that no single marker will suffice, nor is any combination of markers sufficiently sensitive and specific to justify, yet, the introduction of a population-wide strategy for asthma prevention.

ALLERGIC SENSITIZATION (Figure 19.1)

There is a strong association between allergy and asthma, particularly among genetically

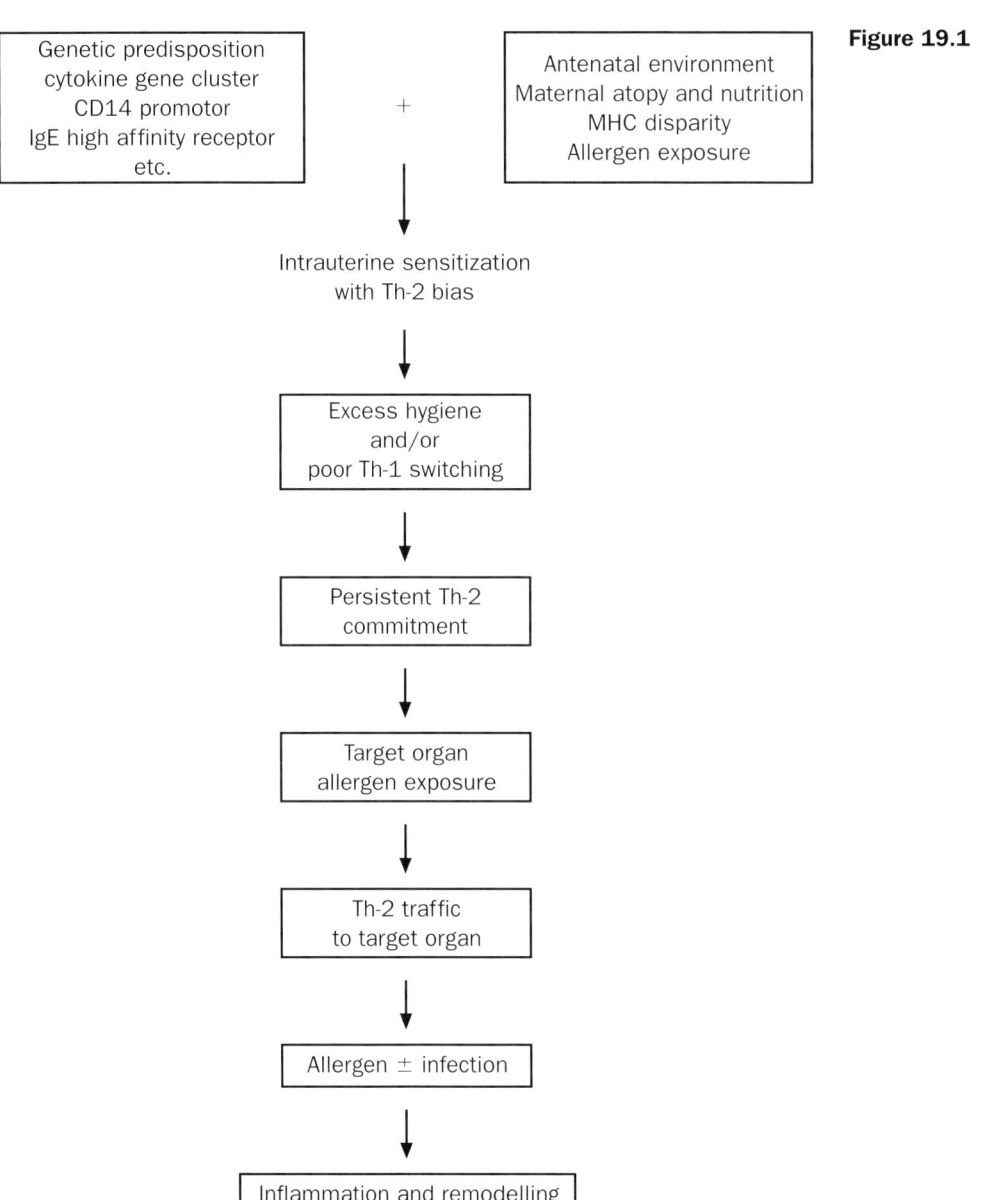

Figure 19.1

predisposed children. Thus early allergic sensitization, particularly to indoor allergens, plays an important role in the development of asthma. This has best been established in relation to early sensitization to the house dust mite, to which high levels of exposure in early life are associated with an over four-fold greater risk of having continuing asthma at the age of 11.[1] More recently, sensitization to cockroach allergens has been recognized as an important risk factor for asthma in many regions of the world and particularly in North American inner-city dwellers.[2] High level exposure to indoor allergens is strongly associated with allergic sensitization in the first 3 years of life according to a German birth cohort study.[3]

Table 19.1 Factors increasing or decreasing allergic sensitization

Timing		Increase	Decrease
Pregnancy	3–6 months	Placental IL-4, IL-13 Maternal IgE MHC disparity Low dose allergen exposure	Fetal IFN-γ Maternal IgG via amniotic fluid
	6–9 months	Programmed rapid fetal growth with nutritional compromise Maternal IL-10	High dose allergen exposure Maternal IgG across placenta
	0–3 years	High dose allergen exposure Gram-negative gut colonization RSV infection	Gut colonization with lactobacillin Severe infections—e.g. measles, tuberculosis—in absence of immunization

RSV = respiratory syncytial virus

Furthermore, chronic asthma with persisting symptoms and bronchial hyperresponsiveness through adolescence is associated with early allergic sensitization in Australia.[4] The risk of sensitized children developing airway hyperresponsiveness doubles with every doubling of exposure to the house dust mites.[5,6]

With the above compelling evidence that allergy is an important precursor for the development and persistence of asthma, understanding the ontogeny of the allergic sensitization process is an important prerequisite for identifying targets for prevention.

THE ONTOGENY OF ALLERGIC SENSITIZATION (Table 19.1)

It is now clear that the neonate is not immunologically naïve but is capable of mounting significant immune responses to environmental antigens. This can have occurred only as a result of antenatal sensitization. A number of studies have shown that peripheral blood mononuclear cell sensitivity to allergens in neonatal blood samples has predicted the subsequent development of allergic disease.[7–9] Indeed in the Prescott et al. study,[8] proliferative responses of cord blood cells occurred to house dust mite in 46% of samples, to the purified major allergen of house dust mite in 73%, and to ovalbumin from hen's egg in 42%. The group was also able to establish that this was not a consequence of maternal cross-contamination of the neonatal blood sample by genotyping T-cell clones from the blood samples and demonstrating that they were definitely of fetal origin. By studying the peripheral blood mononuclear cell responses from fetuses through gestation, it has been possible to establish that specific allergen-induced responses can occur from as early as 22 weeks' gestation.[10]

It should not be surprising that fetal sensitization occurs. Stem cells are present in the human yolk sac at 21 days of gestation with the first lymphocyte seen in the thymus at the end of the ninth week of gestation. B-lymphocytes can be seen in a range of organs, including the lungs and gut from 14 weeks, and by 19–20 weeks circulating B-cells have detectable surface immunoglobulin M. This implies that the full sensitization process must have occurred from antigen presentation through T-cell proliferation to B-cell stimulation and antibody production. Paediatricians are most familiar with the antenatal immune response in relation to the detection of IgM rubella antibodies in fetuses infected by their mothers with this virus.

However, there remains a commonly held prejudice that the neonate is immunologically naïve.[11] Evidence would now suggest that this is not true immunological naïveté owing to lack of sensitization but more to a late gestation suppression of immune responses. Indeed, one study has been able to demonstrate that birch and timothy grass pollen exposure via the mother only sensitizes fetuses if it takes place in the first 6 months of pregnancy. Exposure in later pregnancy appears to result in either immune suppression or tolerance.[12]

Thus, it is clear that on the one hand there is virtually universal priming to environmental antigens occurring before birth, but in those infants destined to be allergic and to develop diseases such as asthma the responsiveness is altered. At its most extreme, a small percentage of infants destined to have allergic disease already have raised cord blood total and specific IgE. This has proved to be a highly specific but very insensitive marker of later disease.[13–17] Other studies have demonstrated differences in cytokine profiles from allergen and mitogen stimulated peripheral blood mononuclear cells in neonates destined to be allergic.[7–9,18] All of these studies suggest that there is a disturbance of the balance between cytokines which suppress an allergic response as characterized by T-helper 1 (Th-1) phenotypic responses compared with allergy-promoting Th-2 responses. In the former, the characteristic cytokines are interleukin-12 (IL-12) and interferon-gamma (IFN-γ), and in the latter IL-4, IL-5, IL-10 and IL-13.

PREGNANCY AS AN ALLERGIC PHENOMENON

In animal models, it is well known that the fetoplacental unit produces Th-2 cytokines such as IL-4, IL-5 and IL-10 throughout pregnancy.[19] It is felt that these cytokines are instrumental in inhibiting maternal Th-1 activity where factors such as IFN-γ, IL-2 and tumor necrosis factor β would compromise continuation of the pregnancy.[20] IL-2 promotes proliferation of uterine large granular lymphocytes, creating lymphokine-activated killer cells with enhanced cytotoxic activity.[21] Furthermore, IL-2 in vitro increases the lymphocyte expression of CD16, which in turn is associated with increased killing of cultured trophoblast cells. This may compromise the invasiveness of trophoblasts during implantation and placental growth.[22] IFN-γ is an abortifactant with an effect mediated by activation of NK cells and this in turn is inhibited by IL-10.[23]

In human pregnancy, rather less information is available. However, IL-4 has been shown to be produced by human amnion epithelium in both the first and third trimesters of pregnancy.[24] Furthermore, mRNA coding for IL-10 has been demonstrated in term human placental tissue,[25] and my own group has recently demonstrated IL-13 production by the placenta predominantly during the second trimester of pregnancy.[26]

Obviously the markedly biased exposure of mother to Th-2-promoting, Th-1-suppressing, cytokines manufactured by decidual tissues will also affect the fetus. It is, therefore, perhaps not surprising that there is a universal bias of the fetus towards a Th-2, allergy promoting immune response that can be detected at birth but under normal circumstances rapidly downregulates postnatally.[8,27] However, it is not all one-way traffic in relation to a Th-2-biased fetal immune response. Our own preliminary investigations have shown that most fetuses spontaneously release IFN-γ from cultured unstimulated peripheral blood mononuclear cells during the second trimester of pregnancy. Furthermore, another group has shown that fetal plasma concentrations of IFN-γ are higher in the first trimester and slowly subside as pregnancy proceeds.[28] One might expect that such IFN-γ production would to some extent counterbalance the effects of the Th-2 cytokines from the placenta, thereby protecting the fetus from overcommitment to an allergic response. Furthermore, IFN-γ does have additional roles in stimulating the expression of HLA-G by trophoblasts, which allows these cells to avoid cytolysis by decidual large granular lymphocytes. Trophoblasts do not express MHC class II or class I antigens and HLA-G is a non-classical, non-polymorphic product which, therefore, does not activate maternal immune responses.

The Th-2 cytokines probably have additional functions in stimulating cell growth and differentiation. This is certainly a role of IL-4, which will, in addition, upregulate MHC class II molecules, thereby assisting activation of antigen-presenting cells and promoting the fetal ability to respond to antigens.[29] Granulocyte macrophage colony stimulating factor GMCSF has a critical effect on surfactant homeostasis by stimulating differentiation and proliferation of type 2 pneumonocytes, thereby having profound effects on lung function.[30]

There is, therefore, a remarkably fine balance of cytokine production between mother, placenta, and fetus, orchestrating a downregulation of maternal-immune responses to feto-paternal antigens at the same time as encouraging normal fetal growth and immunological responsiveness. It is perhaps not surprising that relatively minor perturbations can have an impact either decreasing or increasing the risk of subsequent allergic disease.

THE ROUTE OF FETAL ANTIGEN EXPOSURE AND SENSITIZATION

The cytokines generated by decidual tissues are present in significant quantities in amniotic fluid.[31] Furthermore, we have also found significant levels of IgE proportionate to maternal IgE levels in amniotic fluid. Thus those mothers with higher levels who are themselves atopic expose their fetuses to higher quantities of IgE through the amniotic fluid even though this IgE does not cross the placenta into the fetal circulation.[32] More recently, we have also been able to detect allergens such as Der p1 of house dust mite and ovalbumin from hen's egg in some amniotic fluids. The protein turnover in amniotic fluid occurs at a rate of 70% each day with much of this removal being via fetal swallowing.[33] Clearly, the fetus also aspirates amniotic fluid into the respiratory tract and in addition has a highly permeable skin through which direct exposure might occur. However, the fetal gut has been established as containing the most mature immune-active tissues during gestation.

We have found many human leucocyte antigen-DR (HLADR)-positive cells including macrophages, B-cells and dendritic cells in lymphoid follicles of the rudimentary Peyer's patches from fetuses very early in the second trimester of pregnancy. Surface markers on these cells suggest that they have all the necessary co-stimulatory signals available to facilitate antigen presentation to T-lymphocytes, which can also be detected from as early as 16 weeks' gestation. The antigen-presenting cells also have high and low affinity IgE, as well as IgG, receptors. Therefore, there is the potential not only for sensitization to occur but also for IgE to facilitate this process to occur by so-called antigen focusing, which allows sensitization to remarkably low concentrations of allergen.[34]

We have hypothesized that this sophisticated gut immunological response early in pregnancy could well have evolved to facilitate neonatal host responses to obligate exposure to maternal helminths.[32] Certainly infants born to helminth-infected mothers have specific Th-2-biased immune responses to helminth antigen and IgE antibodies to these antigens.[35] Now that we have very low parasite exposure, it is likely that molecules present in sensitizing allergens have molecular counterparts in parasites, leading to stimulation of the same immune response.[36]

MODIFICATION OF ANTENATAL ALLERGEN-SPECIFIC IMMUNE RESPONSES

A number of studies have suggested that IgG may have a role in modulating the fetal immune response to allergen. Thus we have shown that proliferative responses to house dust mite by cord blood peripheral mononuclear cells are inversely correlated with the level of cord blood house dust mite specific IgG.[37] High levels of cord blood IgG antibodies to cat dander and the major allergen of birch pollen were associated with less atopic symptoms in children during the first 8 years of life, with an inverse relationship between cat IgE antibodies in children and their levels of IgG cat antibodies at birth.[38] This very much mirrors older murine studies in which maternal IgG was found to suppress IgE responses in neonates.[39]

The levels of IgG in the cord blood clearly are a reflection of maternal IgG, which in turn is likely to reflect maternal allergen exposure. Thus high exposure will increase the IgG levels. Therefore, children of mothers who had undergone rye grass immunotherapy during pregnancy and consequently have high IgG antibody levels, compared with children born to untreated mothers, had been followed postnatally and had fewer positive skin test responses to the grass 3–12 years later.[40] This was an open observational study but is certainly consistent with other observations, and this would also be consistent with the observation that birch pollen exposure during the last 2–3 months of pregnancy, when IgG transfer across the placenta is maximal, is associated with much less birch pollen reactivity in the offspring than occurs if the exposure were between 3 and 6 months' gestation.[12] It would also provide an explanation for the so-called horoscope effect in relation to month of birth and seasonal allergen sensitization. Several studies have shown an increased risk for allergy to seasonal allergens in children born shortly before the relevant pollen season. Birth at this time of year would be associated with the lowest maternal, and thus fetal, levels of IgG antibody.[38]

IgG antibodies might be considered to have a blocking effect by antigen neutralization preventing access to IgE and therefore IgE antigen focusing. However, it is also possible that the IgG antibody directly confers an inhibitory signal via immunoreceptor tyrosine based inhibition motifs on FcγRIId receptors that specifically bind IgG1 and IgG3, which are preferentially transported across the placenta rather than IgG2 and IgG4.[41] This implies that the major downregulatory effect of IgG antibody will be systemic and relate to transport directly across the placenta. However, before 20 weeks' gestation, the major IgG exposure of the fetus will occur via the amniotic fluid. Certainly levels can be detected in amniotic fluid, and epithelial cells in the human fetal gastrointestinal tract express neonatal IgG receptor (FcRn).[42] Thus mechanisms may exist to inhibit the initial sensitizing events in early gestation in the fetal gut.

These latter observations indicate one of the first potential primary prophylactic therapeutic targets. High dose allergen exposure of the mother at critical stages during pregnancy to raise her IgG antibody levels may be a significant primary preventive measure. The only other alternative in relation to allergen exposure is complete avoidance, which has proved to be virtually impossible for most major allergens.

MATERNAL NUTRITION AND FETAL SUSCEPTIBILITY TO ALLERGY AND ASTHMA

The demographic trends in asthma prevalence, which has increased in parallel with increasing affluence, have generated a number of hypotheses, one of which relates to the influence of changing diet. There has been a declining rate of consumption of fresh fruit and vegetables, particularly in the UK, which has paralleled the rise in atopic disease.[43] Such foods are associated with antioxidant activity and could be implicated in protecting against the development of airway inflammation. Retinoids, for instance, have been shown to inhibit IL-4-dependent IgE production by murine B-cells.[44] It is possible that this latter effect will have its major impact antenatally rather than postnatally. Nevertheless, a recent British survey suggested that once the confounding effects of cigarette smoking had been excluded, low fresh fruit intake had an influence only on severity of disease rather than its prevalence.[45]

The other nutrients that have been shown to have some influence on established asthma, namely fatty acids, may also have an effect in the genesis of disease. There has been an increased consumption of polyunsaturated fatty acids (PUFA) in recent decades. Diets rich in linolenic acid promote prostaglandin E_2 production which, in turn promotes production of IL-4, which is a Th-2 cytokine.[46] It is well established that fish oil supplementation produces a decrease in production of pro-inflammatory mediators such as tumor necrosis factor α and leukotrienes.[47] The effects on clinical features of the condition are modest or non-existent.[48] Under such circumstances, one might consider that fatty acid dietary supplementation would have a greater impact if introduced at an early stage in the evolution of the disease.

There are some remarkable observations that suggest that fetal nutrition may have a profound influence on outcome in relation to the development of atopy and asthma. There is an intriguing association between a large head circumference at birth and the levels of total IgE at birth,[49] in childhood[50] and in adulthood.[51] Perhaps more importantly, large head circumference at birth is also strongly associated with asthma and particularly severe symptomatic asthma.[50] A large neonatal head size in the presence of normal body weight has been associated with a rapid fetal growth trajectory. It has also been associated with increased prenatal exposure to long-chain PUFA, which again is associated with promotion of Th-2 responses.[46] It is proposed that good maternal nutrition programmes the fetus in the first trimester to grow rapidly. Towards the end of pregnancy, neither maternal nutrient intake nor the placental capacity to deliver nutrients to the fetus can sustain the rapid growth. At this stage, a head and brain sparing reflex facilitates continuing head growth at the expense of the body. This results in the disproportionate newborn baby. The poor nutrition to the body will affect rapidly growing tissues such as those in the immune system, which could subtly alter the balance between Th-1 and Th-2 activity and thereby increase the risk of atopy. Trials are urgently required to investigate various forms of supplementation, of which those related to fatty acids may be particularly relevant. They may provide another strategy for primary prophylaxis.

It is also relevant to consider the ways in which nutrients might have an impact on lung growth and thereby increase susceptibility to airway disease. It has long been known that vitamin A plays a major role in lung development, with severe deprivation resulting in major disturbances of lung organogenesis, including a predisposition to pulmonary atresia.[52] More recently, at least in murine models, it has been shown that mild vitamin A deficiency can have effects on airways branching and lung epithelial cell differentiation.[53] Furthermore, vitamin A levels between 30 and 60% of normal can result in abnormalities of surfactant protein production, which in turn regulates phospholipid release.[54] Abnormalities of surfactant protein production will affect host defence as well as phospholipid generation, because they serve an opsonizing role in the airways. Thus, a deficiency of a single nutrient has been shown to have an impact on airway geometry and immune function simultaneously. Many would favour a concept of asthma which incorporates these two underlying abnormalities. It is very likely that other nutrients and combinations of nutrients will also have such effects.

ENVIRONMENTAL TOBACCO SMOKE AND WHEEZING ILLNESS IN CHILDHOOD

No discussion of the prevention of asthma would be complete without consideration of the impact of exposure to environmental tobacco smoke. The health effects of passive smoking have been extensively reviewed and re-reviewed by Cook and Strachan.[55] These authors have published a series of literature reviews on passive smoking. The conclusion relating parental smoking to lower respiratory illness in early life up to 3 years of age indicated a direct causal relationship between parental smoking and lower respiratory illnesses in infancy. Based on epidemiological studies, however, it was impossible to distinguish the independent contributions of prenatal and postnatal maternal smoking.[56] However, in-depth studies of lung function immediately after birth have shown that maternal pregnancy smoking clearly has a direct influence on lung development.[57,58] Indeed, a very recent study of lung function in over 3000 southern California schoolchildren highlighted an independent association between decreased small airway flow and *in utero* exposure to maternal smoking.[59] One latter study demonstrated increased airway resistance, in full-term delivered infants, at a mean of 8 weeks of age whose mothers smoked, compared with infants of mothers who did not smoke. Furthermore, the infants of smoking mothers were four times more likely to develop wheezing illnesses in the first year of life.[58] Similar effects on lung function have been found by a number of other groups,[60,61] and the latter study (by Lødrup Carlsen et al.[61]) subsequently demonstrated an association with later recurrent wheezing.[62] Thus the combination of epidemiological and detailed respiratory physiological studies points very strongly to an effect of maternal smoking in pregnancy on reduced lung function at birth and a higher risk of wheezing illnesses in infancy. However, the effect of early passive environmental tobacco smoke exposure on wheezing illnesses diminishes progressively with increasing age of the child. Indeed the long-term prognosis for early wheezing illnesses associated with maternal smoking is good. There is, in fact, little evidence based on meta-analyses that maternal pregnancy smoking has an effect on allergic sensitization.[63] However, a review of the literature on the effect of environmental tobacco smoke exposure on severity of established asthma strongly suggests that smoking in the household has a significant impact on disease severity.[63]

The conclusion from smoking studies, therefore, is that pregnancy smoking has an impact on lung development, which in turn increases the frequency of non-atopic wheezing illnesses in infancy, but that there is little impact of this exposure on later atopic asthma. Later passive environmental tobacco smoke exposure in established atopic asthmatics, however, will increase the severity of the disease. There is little doubt, therefore, that avoidance of environmental tobacco smoke exposure, both antenatally and postnatally, will have an appreciable impact on the prevalence of wheezing illnesses in infancy and the severity of asthma. Thus if there was a single measure to be recommended for the primary and tertiary prevention of asthma, it certainly would be banning cigarette smoking.

GENETIC AND ENVIRONMENTAL DIVERSITY

It is remarkable that the highest prevalences of allergic disorders worldwide are among English-speaking communities.[64] As environmental conditions are very similar in many non-English-speaking European communities that have lower prevalences of atopic disease, it is understandably difficult to identify extrinsic factors that might explain this difference.

English-speaking communities in general have a far broader genetic diversity in terms of ethnic backgrounds than many other north European affluent communities. With greater genetic diversity, there is a far wider range of major histocompatability complex genes, which in turn leads to a far wider capacity to present antigens in the first step towards sensitization. Thus, with the combination of far more diverse exposure to environmental antigens which characterizes affluent populations, together with the wider genetic diversity characterizing English-speaking communities, there is perhaps an underlying immunological explanation for the greater prevalences of atopic disorders.

It is also possible that this genetic diversity will have its effects *in utero*. It has been shown that women with rheumatoid arthritis (a Th-1-mediated disease) often improve appreciably during pregnancy only to relapse or indeed develop the disease for the first time in the postpartum period.[65] Direct measurement of Th-1 cytokines from stimulated peripheral blood mononuclear cells of healthy pregnant women has demonstrated a reduction in Th-1

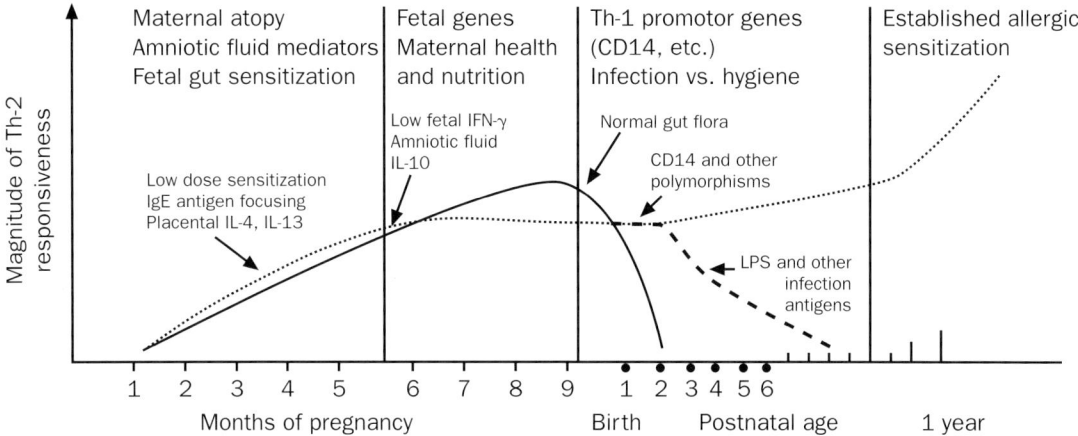

Figure 19.2 The four phases of allergen sensitization. (LPS = lipopolysaccharide)

function, which has been proposed as the mechanism for improvement in rheumatoid arthritis during pregnancy.[66] However, not all women with rheumatoid arthritis improve during pregnancy and one study has suggested that improvement is dependent on the degree of mismatching in major histocompatibility complex genes. Thus the materno-fetal disparity in alleles for HLA DR and DQ antigens is greater (26 of 34 pregnancies) in cases where rheumatoid arthritis remits or improves compared with those who have continuing active disease (three of 12 pregnancies).[67] This would suggest that the Th-2 bias of pregnancy is switched on by genetic disparity between the mother and fetus. It would, therefore, be equally credible to suggest that greater genetic disparity between mother and fetus would produce an increased drive towards the development of allergy. Thus genetic diversity in English-speaking communities could have created an intrauterine immunological environment that affected the risks for an increased polarization towards allergic sensitization. This hypothesis could be easily investigated, though no studies have yet been published.

All the data that have accumulated in relation to antenatal immune mechanisms and fetal sensitization point to an opportunity to consider immunomodulatory strategies as a primary prophylaxis for allergic disease. However, before such strategies are considered, it is important to be aware that if the subtle balance in immune responsiveness is upset in order to achieve a reduction in allergic disorders, there may be potential to increase risks of autoimmune disease. Thus it is more likely that, in the short term, preventive strategies will focus on secondary prophylaxis.

THE HYGIENE HYPOTHESIS (Figure 19.2)

In 1989, Strachan demonstrated an inverse relationship between birth order in families and the prevalence of hay fever. He proposed that infections in early infancy brought home by older siblings might prevent sensitization.[68] There is clearly a highly credible biological explanation to support this hypothesis. Early infection, whether with viruses or bacteria, will tend to stimulate a Th-1 immune response, which, if it occurs early enough postnatally, will switch any Th-2-biased allergic immune responses to common allergens to a Th-1-immunizing pattern.[69]

Subsequent studies have all tended to support this hypothesis. Thus in Japan, an inverse relationship was found between tuberculin responsiveness and allergy.[70] In the murine model, it has been possible to demonstrate that BCG can suppress local Th-2 immune responses.[71] Additional inverse relationships have been found between allergy and hepatitis A[72] and measles infection in early childhood.[73] These observations have promoted research into the development of Th-1 immunoadjuvants as a treatment for allergic disease. BCG and heat-killed *Listeria* monocytogenes are currently the main focuses of work, though in the longer term DNA vaccines may prove to be more effective.[74] Thus immunomodulation perinatally may become an important strategy for secondary prophylaxis.

There are, however, some paradoxes that still need to be reconciled in relation to the hygiene hypothesis. It is likely that not all infections are generically likely to produce the same end result. Thus respiratory syncytial virus (RSV) bronchiolitis has been clearly associated with higher subsequent prevalence of recurrent wheezing disorders and, though controversially, perhaps, even greater risk of atopy.[75] The unresolved issue in relation to these observations is whether RSV actually predisposes to atopic disease or whether atopically predisposed individuals are more likely to get severe RSV bronchiolitis. It is, however, clear that a Th-2 response to the virus is associated with more severe outcomes.[69] Furthermore, as distinct from murine studies, some human observational studies have failed to show any effect of either BCG[76] or measles immunization.[77] These observations have led to the proposal that perhaps only a major kick to switch the immune system from Th-2 to Th-1 will reduce atopy and this is only likely to occur with active infection rather than immunization.[78]

GUT MICROBIAL FLORA

It is perhaps more credible to consider that infant gut colonization by microbial flora might have the most important immunizing effects. It is improbable that a mechanism for downregulating Th-2 responsiveness postnatally would require active infection (in other words, kill or cure).[79] The proposers of the 'gut flora' hypothesis have now shown that children from a country with a low prevalence of atopy, Estonia, have very different intestinal bacteria to infants from a country with higher atopy prevalence, namely Sweden. Furthermore, the group have shown that in both Estonia and Sweden allergic children were less often colonized with lactobacilli as compared with non-allergic children. The allergic children had higher counts of aerobic microorganisms such as coliforms and *Staphylococcus aureus*.[80] A number of groups have questioned whether this might explain the remarkable observation that there is a much lower risk of asthma among children of farmers who have been born on farms. Ingestion of higher quantities of raw and sometimes unpasteurized milk containing a higher microbial load, particularly of lactobacilli, may well be protective.[81,82] This observation may, however, also be explained by a greater exposure to infecting organisms and particularly their products such as lipopolysaccharide (LPS), which would be consistent with the earlier hygiene hypothesis.[83]

Lipopolysaccharide-induced immune responses are primarily mediated via the receptor CD14. A possible role for this antigen-presenting cell membrane bound molecule in relation to allergy has recently come into focus with the identification of a polymorphism in the flanking region of the CD14 gene associated with allergy.[84] It has now become clear that the signalling pathway for CD14 ligation with LPS to effect immune responsiveness is via Toll-like receptor 4. There are polymorphisms described in the gene for this molecule which hitherto have been associated with susceptibility to Gram-negative infections. The key product of stimulation of this pathway is IL-12, which in turn promotes IFN-γ production. Thus it is clear that further work will focus on polymorphisms in relation to allergy and asthma.[85]

Studies of the evolution of the postnatal

immune response have shown that the Th-2 bias to antigenic stimulus at birth very rapidly downregulates postnatally in those destined not to have atopic disease. However, the ultimate atopics consolidated their neonatal pattern of Th-2 polarized allergen-specific responses.[86] Interestingly a study in Perth (Australia) has demonstrated that ultimately atopic infants not only have reduced production of IFN-γ with a Th-2-biased response but in fact in some respects are more immunologically 'immature' in having reduced levels of production of many other cytokines compared with ultimately non-atopic infants.[8,27] To what extent this is true, immaturity or the effect of a suppressive factor operative late in pregnancy remains to be established. We have shown that IL-10 levels are particularly higher in the amniotic fluid of atopic compared with non-atopic mothers. IL-10 can have a downregulatory effect on many immune responses. This might explain the neonatal observations, in that the atopic mother is more likely to confer an atopic tendency on her infant.[37]

It is likely that the early switch from Th-2 to Th-1 biased response postnatally is a consequence of postnatal microbial exposure as described in the preceding sections. Thus those infants with an intact response to microbial antigens such as LPS will have a very rapid switch orchestrated through the CD14 molecule once the gut becomes colonized with organisms. Those infants with abnormalities in this response and, indeed, those who have already had significant overcommitment to a Th-2 response as a result of antenatal factors will not be so easily switched and will have a higher probability of having a persistent response go on to atopic disease. It is, however, possible that some of these individuals will at a later stage switch as a result of significant infection. Since the measles study from Guinea-Bissau[73] demonstrated that measles occurring at a mean age of 3 years reduced subsequent atopy, there is clearly a fairly broad time frame in which such switching can be orchestrated. This will undoubtedly be a focus for immunomodulatory secondary prophylactic interventions which might include Th-1 immunoadjuvants, DNA vaccines, antigen IL-12 and/or IFN-γ or oral administration of relevant gut organisms. Although all these strategies remain in the realm of hypothesis and require appropriate investigation, the potential rewards are considerable.[87]

TERTIARY PROPHYLAXIS

Pharmacotherapy

Once allergic sensitization has begun to manifest, there are additional opportunities to prevent evolution through to asthma. Atopic dermatitis is a very high-risk predisposition for the development of asthma. This has prompted two studies to investigate a pharmacotherapeutic intervention to prevent the development of asthma in infants with atopic dermatitis. The first employed ketotifen or placebo for 1 year in 110 infants in a double-blind study and showed a considerable reduction in the prevalence of asthma over that 1 year period in those on active treatment.[88] The second much larger study on similar infants compared cetirizine with placebo. This study also demonstrated a significant reduction in prevalence of asthma over 18 months of active treatment compared with placebo but only in those with evidence of house dust mite and/or grass pollen sensitivity, who constituted 20% of the total population recruited.[89] This study also showed that house dust mite and pollen sensitivity as well as sensitivity to cats were the strongest predictors of subsequent asthma in the population of atopic dermatitis infants. These latter observations are quite consistent with the former trial using ketotifen, in which only those infants with a significantly raised total serum IgE achieved benefit.[88] One other study has used ketotifen in infants with a family history of allergy and raised total IgE levels. This also showed a significant reduction in the subsequent prevalence of asthma.[90] The proposed mechanism by which relatively 'mild' medications, such as antihistamines, might have a prophylactic effect is through inhibition of allergen-mediated eosinophil trafficking into the airway.[91] It will be intriguing to see whether other drugs having more potent similar effects will have a role in prophylaxis—drugs such as leukotriene receptor antagonists.

Allergen avoidance

It seems appropriate to suggest that allergen avoidance is a reasonable strategy for both secondary and tertiary prophylaxis. However, the main difficulty in employing such a strategy is that techniques to reduce exposure to the commonest allergen, the house dust mite, are far from satisfactory. Indeed, a recent heavily criticized meta-analysis of trials suggested that it was not likely to be effective.[92] There is, however, a good correlation between early high level exposure to house dust mite and the subsequent increase in prevalence and severity of asthma.[1] Similar associations have been found in relation to cockroach exposure.[2] Indeed, high level exposure to a number of indoor allergens is strongly associated with sensitization in the first 3 years[3] and early sensitization is associated with greater probability of persistence of bronchial hyperresponsiveness and symptoms of asthma in late childhood and adolescence.[4] Furthermore, the precedence created by studying occupational allergic asthma suggests that early removal from exposure to offending allergens can achieve total resolution of symptoms in situations where more continued exposure will eventually lead to chronic irreversible changes and ongoing disease even in the absence of continuing allergen exposure.[93]

Review of the studies that have attempted allergen avoidance in high risk infants with or without pre-existing evidence of sensitization but not yet with disease have yielded very disappointing outcomes. Some interventions have even commenced antenatally. The attitude to antenatal dietary avoidance has been formed on the basis of one study in which elimination of egg, milk, fish and nuts from the maternal diet in the last trimester of pregnancy had no impact on outcome in relation to disease. Furthermore, the mothers gained less weight during pregnancy as a consequence of the diet.[94] However, one might argue that the intervention was started too late, since we now have evidence that sensitization might have occurred at an earlier stage in the pregnancy. Nevertheless, it also sounds a note of warning about potential adverse nutritional consequences of antenatal dietary manipulation.

Postnatal avoidance has again tended to focus on diet with the promotion of breast feeding. Many studies have been performed, with very diverse results extending from reduced prevalence of food-associated atopic disease, through no effect, to some studies showing a higher prevalence of atopy in intervention groups. Importantly, however, only one of many studies has demonstrated any long-term effects of early dietary manipulation on the prevalence of asthma.[95] Most studies, if they have demonstrated any benefits at all, have been to reduce the period prevalence of food-associated atopic disease in infancy but with no long-term impact on any atopic problems and certainly not on asthma.[96,97] One of the studies also employed house dust mite avoidance measures.[97] However, the degree of reduction in house dust mite levels was probably not enough to achieve any meaningful benefits. A number of trials are now in progress to attempt to reduce aeroallergen exposure to a far greater extent from early in pregnancy and it remains to be seen whether these strategies will be truly effective in reducing the prevalence of disease.

Immunotherapy as tertiary prophylaxis

Allergen immunotherapy has been employed for the treatment of allergic disorders for nearly 90 years. However, it still remains a highly controversial therapy which has not necessarily gained a clear place in the management of asthma, as evidenced by the lack of clear recommendations in recently published consensus reports.[98] However, a meta-analysis of 20 randomized controlled trials of allergen immunotherapy for asthma provided good evidence that this approach to treatment decreased asthma symptoms and requirements for asthma medication and improved allergen-specific bronchial hyperresponsiveness by comparison with placebo.[99] A subsequent published trial, however, has muddied the waters by suggesting that there was no benefit in allergic perennially asthmatic children.[100] One concern has been that immunotherapy might enhance nonspecific bronchial hyperresponsiveness. However, recent studies suggest that the opposite is true and that immunotherapy will decrease the nonspecific response as well as that specific to the allergen in question.[101]

The mechanism of action of immunotherapy has recently been elaborated and has been shown to orchestrate an immunological switch from a predominant Th-2 pattern of response with generation of IL-4, to a Th-1 response with a generation of more IFN-γ.[102] Furthermore, this immunological switching can be sustained even after discontinuation of therapy provided this has previously been sustained for 3–4 years.[103] This being the case, it is important to consider whether early employment of such therapy will have any long-term prophylactic effect. It has long been felt that the earlier such therapy is employed, the more effective the outcome.[104]

One study has investigated the effect of specific immunotherapy on the prevention of development of new sensitizations over a 3 year follow-up in a non-randomized study on 6-year-old asthmatic children. When they commenced the study, they were allergic only to house dust mite. 45% of those on active therapy did not develop any new sensitizations, whereas all those in the control group had a wider range of sensitivities.[105] This study suggests that specific immunotherapy might truly alter the natural course of allergy and have a role in tertiary prophylaxis.

This latter concept is currently under further investigation. A trial is being conducted in Europe known as the Preventive Allergy Treatment study (PAT). Hitherto, only conference abstracts are available on the outcomes of this study but they do suggest that after 2 years of pollen allergen immunotherapy in children with pure allergic rhinitis, fewer have subsequently developed asthma than in an untreated control group.[106]

Although the above observations suggest that allergen immunotherapy might have a preventive role, sadly at present the recommendations for the use of this therapy exclude children under the age of 5 years. Thus for all practical purposes, it will have little role, since most asthma begins long before age 5 years.

Targets for prophylaxis (Table 19.2)

It is apparent that for primary prophylaxis the target is the fetus. Much sensitization will have already occurred by birth. This raises the question of whether there should be a whole-population strategy for modifying outcome or whether the focus should be on high risk populations such as where a first-degree relative already has atopic disease. However, this latter approach would pick up only about 40% of the ultimately atopic population. Over half come from families where neither parent has any atopy themselves.[107] Thus, if strategies are to be employed for the whole population, they would need to be cheap, non-invasive and without any potential for inducing side-effects. In this category would certainly come avoidance of maternal smoking during pregnancy. Optimized nutrition, particularly in the third trimester of pregnancy, may be an additional strategy with perhaps lipid, antioxidant and vitamin A supplementation. Any other strategies at this stage will have to await trials of whether either avoidance of allergen or exposure to high doses has any efficacy.

Secondary prophylaxis, after sensitization has occurred but before there is any disease, will focus on the newborn infant and young child up to 2–3 years of age. The high risk group may be identified by a persistent Th-2-biased response to allergen between birth and 6 months. However, the sensitivity and specificity of such assays have yet to be established. Raised cord blood IgE is highly specific but extremely insensitive. Strategies will include the use of Th-1 immunoadjuvants, DNA vaccines, seeding the gut with appropriate intestinal flora, allergen avoidance and the avoidance of environmental tobacco smoke.

Tertiary prophylaxis, which is introduced after allergic disease has manifest but before any symptoms of asthma, will occur at some age between 6 months and 3–4 years. Targets will be infants with

Table 19.2 Targets for prophylaxis

	Primary	Secondary	Tertiary
Definition	Before allergic sensitization	Before disease but after sensitization	Before asthma but after sensitization and disease
Timing	Prenatal	0–3 years	6 months – 4 years
Targets	Whole population or allergic first-degree relatives	Th-2-biased allergen response 0–6 months Raised cord IgE	Atopic eczema Allergic rhinitis Allergy prick skin test or RAST positivity
Strategies	Avoid maternal smoking Optimize nutrition High or no allergen exposure	Immunomodulation Th-1 immunoadjuvants Gut bacteria Allergen avoidance ETS avoidance	Pharmacotherapy Immunotherapy Immunomodulation Allergen and ETS avoidance

RAST = radio-allergo-sorbent test; ETS = environmental tobacco smoke

atopic eczema or allergic rhinitis and perhaps those who have developed a positive skin prick test or raised IgE antibody to common aeroallergens. The forms of therapy that might be considered include antihistamines (and perhaps in the future leukotriene receptor antagonists), inhaled cortico-steroids, cromones, allergen immunotherapy, immunomodulation with Th-1 immunoadjuvants or anti-IgE antibodies, allergen avoidance and the avoidance of environmental tobacco smoke. For most, trials are required.

REFERENCES

1. Sporik R, Holgate ST, Platts-Mills TAE et al. Exposure to house dust mite allergen (Der p 1) and the development of asthma in childhood. *New Engl J Med* 1990; **323**: 502–7.
2. Platts-Mills TAE, Vervloet D, Thomas WR et al. Indoor allergens and asthma. Report of the Third International Workshop. *J Allergy Clin Immunol* 1997; **100**: S1–24.
3. Wahn U, Lau S, Bergmann R et al. Indoor allergen exposure is a risk factor for sensitization during the first 3 years of life. *J Allergy Clin Immunol* 1997; **99**: 763–9.
4. Peat JK, Salome CM, Woolcock AJ. Longitudinal changes in atopy during a 4-year period. *J Allergy Clin Immunol* 1990; **85**: 65–74.
5. Peat JK, Tovey ER, Toelle BG et al. House dust mite allergens: a major risk factor for childhood asthma in Australia. *Am J Respir Crit Care Med* 1996; **153**: 141–6.
6. Sherril D, Stein R, Curzius-Spencer M, Martinez F. On early sensitization to allergens and development of respiratory symptoms. *Clin Exp Allergy* 1999; **29**: 905–11.
7. Warner JA, Miles EA, Jones AC et al. Is deficiency of interferon-gamma production by allergen triggered cord blood cells a predictor of atopic eczema? *Clin Exp Allergy* 1994; **24**: 423–30.
8. Prescott SL, Macaubas C, Holt BJ et al. Transplacental priming of the human immune system to environmental allergens: universal skewing of initial T cell responses towards the Th-2 cytokine profile. *J Immunol* 1998; **160**: 4730–7.
9. Kondo N, Cubiyashi Y, Shinoda S et al. Cord blood lymphocyte responses to food antigens

for the prediction of allergic disease. *Arch Dis Child* 1992; **67**: 1003–7.
10. Jones AC, Miles EA, Warner JO et al. Fetal peripheral blood mononuclear cell proliferative responses to mitogenic and allergenic stimulae during gestation. *Pediatr Allergy Immunol* 1996; **7**: 109–16.
11. Hayward AR. Ontogeny of the immune system. In: Ulijaszek SJ, Johnston FE, Preece MA, eds. *The Cambridge Encyclopaedia of Growth and Development*. Cambridge: Cambridge University Press, 1998, 166–9.
12. Van Duren-Schmidt K, Pichler J, Ebner C et al. Prenatal contact with inhalant allergens. *Pediatr Research* 1997; **41**: 128–31.
13. Michel FB, Bousquet J, Greillier P et al. Comparison of cord blood immunoglobulin E and maternal allergy for the prediction of atopic diseases in infancy. *J Allergy Clin Immunol* 1980; **65**: 422–30.
14. Croner S, Kjellman N-IM. Development of atopic disease in relation to family history and cord blood IgE levels—11 year follow-up in 1,654 children. *Pediatr Allergy Immunol* 1990; **1**: 14–21.
15. Edenharter G, Burgmann RL, Burgmann KE et al. Cord blood IgE as risk factor and predictor of atopic diseases. *Clin Exp Allergy* 1998; **28**: 671–8.
16. Ruiz RGG, Richards D, Kemeny DM, Price JF. Neonatal IgE: a poor screen for atopic disease. *Clin Exp Allergy* 1991; **21**: 467–72.
17. Hide DW, Arshad SH, Twiselton R, Stevens M. Cord serum IgE: an insensitive method for prediction of atopy. *Clin Exp Allergy* 1991; **21**: 739–43.
18. Tang MLK, Kemp AS, Thorburn J, Hildy J. Reduced IFN-γ and subsequent atopy. *Lancet* 1994; **344**: 983–5.
19. Wegmann T, Lin H, Guilbert L, Mosmann T. Bi-directional cytokine interactions in the maternal fetal relationship: is successful pregnancy a Th-2-like phenomenon? *Immunol Today* 1993; **14**: 353–6.
20. Raghupathy R. Th-1-type immunity is incompatible with successful pregnancy. *Immunol Today* 1997; **18**: 478–82.
21. Shohat B, Shohat M, Faktor JH et al. Soluble interleukin-2 receptor and interleukin-2 in human amniotic fluid of normal and abnormal pregnancies. *Biol Neonates* 1993; **63**: 281–4.
22. King A, Loky YW. Human trophoblast and JEG chorio-carcinoma cells are sensitive to lysis by IL-2 stimulated decidual NK cells. *Cell Immunol* 1990; **129**: 435–8.
23. Di Andrea A, Aste-Amezaga M, Valiante NM et al. Interleukin-10 inhibits human lymphocyte interferon-gamma production by suppressing natural killer cell stimulatory factor/IL-10 synthesis in accessory cells. *J Exp Med* 1993; **178**: 1041–8.
24. Jones CA, Williams KA, Finlay-Jones JF, Hart HA, Harty PH. Interleukin-4 production by human amnion epithelial cells and regulation of its activity by glycosa amino glycan binding. *Biol Reprod* 1995; **52**: 839–47.
25. Cadet P, Rady PL, Tyring SK et al. Interleukin-10 messenger ribonucleic acid in human placenta: implications for the role of IL-10 in fetal allograph protection. *Am J Obstet Gynaecol* 1995; **173**: 25–9.
26. Williams TJ, Jones CA, Miles EA, Warner JO, Warner JA. Fetal and neonatal interleukin-13 production during pregnancy and at birth and subsequent development of atopic symptoms. *J Allergy Clin Immunol* 2000; **105**: 951–9.
27. Prescott SL, Macaubas C, Smallacombe T et al. Development of allergen specific T cell memory in atopic and normal children. *Lancet* 1999; **353**: 196–200.
28. Abbas A, Thiliginathan B, Buggins AGS et al. Fetal plasma IFN-γ concentration in normal pregnancy. *Am J Obstet Gynaecol* 1993; **168**: 1414–16.
29. Rupert J, Friedrichs D, Xu H, Peters JH. IL-4 decreases the expression of the monocyte differentiation marker for CD14, paralleled by an increased accessory potency. *Immuno Biol* 1991; **182**: 449–52.
30. Whitsett JA, Wert SE. Molecular determinants of lung development. In: Chernik U, Boat TF, eds. *Kendig's Disorders of the Respiratory Tract in Children*, 6th edn. Philadelphia: WB Saunders, 1998, 1–19.
31. Jones CA, Holloway JA, Warner JO. Does atopic disease start in foetal life? *Allergy* 2000; **55**: 2–10.
32. Jones CA, Warner JA, Warner JO. Fetal swallowing of IgE. *Lancet* 1998; **351**: 1859.
33. Bloomfield FH, Harding JE. Experimental aspects of nutrition and fetal growth. *Fetal Mat Med Rev* 1998; **10**: 91–107.
34. Warner JO, Jones CA. Fetal origins of lung disease. In: Barker DJF, ed. *Fetal Origins of Cardiovascular Lung Diseases*. Monographs from Lung Biology and Health and Disease. National Heart Lung & Blood Institute, Marcel Dekker, 2000, 297–321.

35. Melhotra I, Ouma J, Wamachi A et al. In utero exposure to helminth and microbial antigens generates cytokine responses similar to that observed in adults. *J Clin Invest* 1997; **99:** 1759–66.
36. Stewart GA, Thompson PJ. The biochemistry of common aeroallergens. *Clin Exp Allergy* 1996; **26:** 1020–44.
37. Warner JA, Jones CA, Jones AC, Miles EA, Francis T, Warner JO. Immune responses during pregnancy and the development of allergic disease. *Pediatr Allergy Immunol* 1997; **8**(suppl 10): 5–10.
38. Jenmalm MC, Bjorksten B. Cord blood levels of immunoglobulin G subclass antibodies to food and inhalant allergens in relation to maternal atopy and the development of atopic disease during the first 8 years of life. *Clin Exp Allergy* 2000; **30:** 34–40.
39. Jarrett EEE, Hall E. IgE suppression by maternal IgG. *Immunology* 1983; **48:** 49–58.
40. Glovsky MM, Ghekiere L, Rejzek E. Effect of maternal immunotherapy on immediate skin test reactivity, specific rye IgG and IgE antibody and total IgE of the children. *Ann Allergy* 1991; **67:** 21–4.
41. Gergely J, Sarmay G. FcγRII regulation of human B cells. *Scan J Immunol* 1996; **44:** 1–10.
42. Israel EJ, Taylor S, Wu Z et al. Expression of the neonatal Fc receptor FcRn on human intestinal epithelial cells. *Immunology* 1997; **92:** 69–74.
43. Seaton A, Godden DJ, Brown KM. Increase in asthma: a more toxic environment or a more susceptible population? *Thorax* 1994; **49:** 171–4.
44. Tokuyama H, Tokuyama Y, Nakanishi K. Retinoids inhibit IL-4 dependent IgE and IgG1 production by LPS stimulated murine splanchnic B cells. *Cell Immunol* 1995; **162:** 153–8.
45. Butland BK, Strachan DP, Anderson HR. Fresh fruit intake and asthma symptoms in young British adults: confounding or effect modification by smoking. *Europ Respir J* 1999; **13:** 744–50.
46. Langley-Evans S. Fetal programming of immune function and respiratory disease. *Clin Exp Allergy* 1997; **27:** 1377–9.
47. Arm JP, Horton CE, Spurr BW et al. The effects of dietary supplementation with fish oil lipids on the airways response to inhaled allergen in bronchial asthma. *Am Rev Respir Dis* 1989; **139:** 1395–400.
48. Hodge L, Salome CM, Hughes JM et al. Effect of dietary intake of omega-3 and omega-6 fatty acids on severity of asthma in children. *Europ Respir J* 1998; **11:** 361–5.
49. Orysz Oryszczyn MP, Annesi-Maesano I, Campagna D et al. Head circumference at birth and maternal factors related to cord blood total IgE. *Clin Exp Allergy* 1999; **29:** 334–41.
50. Gregory A, Doull I, Pearce N et al. The relationship between anthropometric measurements at birth: asthma and atopy in childhood. *Clin Exp Allergy* 1999; **29:** 330–3.
51. Godfrey KM, Barker DJP, Osmond C. Disproportionate fetal growth and raised IgE concentration in adult life. *Clin Exp Allergy* 1994; **24:** 641–8.
52. Wilson JGC, Roth CB, Warkany J. An analysis of the syndrome of malformations induced by maternal vitamin A deficiency: effects of restoration of vitamin A at various times during gestation. *Am J Anat* 1953; **92:** 181–217.
53. Cardoso Cardoso WV, Williams MC, Mitsialis SA et al. Retinoic acid induces changes in the pattern of airway branching and alters epithelial cell differentiation in the developing lung *in vitro*. *Am J Respir Cell Mol Biol* 1995; **12:** 464–76.
54. Chailley-Heu B, Chelly N, Lelievre-Pegorier M et al. Mild vitamin A deficiency delays fetal lung maturation in the rat. *Am J Respir Cell Mol Biol* 1999; **21:** 89–96.
55. Cook DG, Strachan DP. Summary of effects of parental smoking on respiratory health of children and implications for research. *Thorax* 1999; **54:** 357–66.
56. Strachan DP, Cook DG. Parental smoking and lower respiratory illness in infancy in early childhood. *Thorax* 1997; **52:** 905–14.
57. Martinez FD, Wright AL, Taussig LM et al. Asthma and wheezing in the first 6 years of life. *New Engl J Med* 1995; **332:** 133–8.
58. Dezateux C, Stocks J, Dundas I, Fletcher ME. Impaired airway function and wheezing in infancy: the influence of maternal smoking and a genetic predisposition to asthma. *Am J Respir Crit Care Med* 1999; **159:** 403–10.
59. Gilliland FD, Berhane K, McConnell R et al. Maternal smoking during pregnancy, environmental tobacco smoke exposure and childhood lung function. *Thorax* 2000; **55:** 271–6.
60. Young S, Le Souef PN, Geelhoed GC et al. The influence of a family history of asthma and parental smoking on airway responsiveness in infancy. *New Engl J Med* 1991; **324:** 1168–73.
61. Lødrup Carlsen KC, Jaakkola JJ, Nafstad P, Carlsen K-H. *In utero* exposure to tobacco

smoke influences lung function at birth. *Europ Respir J* 1997; **10**: 1774–9.
62. Lødrup Carlsen KC, Carlsen K-H, Nafstad P, Bakketeig L. Perinatal risk factors for recurrent wheeze in early life. *Pediatr Allergy Immunol* 1999; **10**: 89–95.
63. Strachan DP, Cook DG. Parental smoking and childhood asthma: longitudinal and case control studies. *Thorax* 1998; **53**: 204–12.
64. International Study of Asthma and Allergies in Childhood (ISAAC) Steering Committee. Worldwide variation in prevalence of symptoms of asthma, allergic rhinoconjunctivitis and atopic eczema: ISAAC. *Lancet* 1998; **351**: 1225–32.
65. Wilder RL. Hormones, pregnancy and autoimmune disease. *Am NY Acad Sci* 1998; **840**: 45–50.
66. Russell AS, Johnston C, Chew C, Maksymowych WP. Evidence for reduced Th-1 function in normal pregnancy: a hypothesis for the remission of rheumatoid arthritis. *J Rheumatol* 1997; **24**: 1045–50.
67. Nelson JL, Hughes KA, Smith AG et al. Maternal fetal disparity in HLA Class II alloantigens and the pregnancy induced amelioration of rheumatoid arthritis. *New Engl J Med* 1993; **329**: 466–71.
68. Strachan DP. Hay fever, hygiene, and household size. *Br Med J* 1989; **299**: 1259–60.
69. Folkerts G, Walzl G, Openshaw PJM. Do childhood infections teach the immune system not to be allergic? *Immunol Today* 2000; **21**: 118–20.
70. Shirakawa T, Enomota T, Shimazu S et al. The inverse association between tuberculin responses and atopic disorder. *Science* 1997; **775**: 77–9.
71. Herz U, Gerhold K, Gruber C, Braun A, Wahn U, Renz H et al. BCG infection suppresses allergic sensitization and development of increased airway reactivity in an animal model. *J Allergy Clin Immunol* 1998; **102**: 867–74.
72. Matricardi PM, Rosmini F, Ferrigno L, Nisini R, Rapicetta M, Chionne P et al. Cross-sectional retrospective study of prevalence of atopy among Italian military students with antibodies against hepatitis A virus. *BMJ* 1997; **314**: 999–1003.
73. Shaheen SO, Aaby P, Hall AJ, Barker DJ, Heyes CB, Shiell AW et al. Measles and atopy in Guinea-Bissau. *Lancet* 1996; **347**: 1792–6.
74. Wills-Karp M. Potential use of Th-1 promoting immunoadjuvants in the treatment of allergic disorders. Postgraduate Syllabus. Amer. Acad. Allergy, Asthma Immunol. 1999: 107–25.
75. Sigurs N, Bjarnason R, Sigurbergsson F et al. Asthma and immunoglobulin E antibodies after respiratory syncytial virus bronchiolitis: a prospective cohort study with matched controls. *Pediatrics.* 1995; **95**: 500–5.
76. Alm JS, Lilja G, Pershagen G, Scheynius A. Early BCG vaccination and development of atopy. *Lancet* 1997; **350**: 400–3.
77. Golding J. Immunisations. In: Butler N, Golding J, eds. *From Birth to Five. A Study of the Health and Behaviour of Britain's Five Year Olds.* Oxford: Pergamon, 1986, 295–319.
78. Von Hertzen LC. The hygiene hypothesis in the development of atopy and asthma—still a matter of controversy? *QJ Med* 1998; **91**: 767–71.
79. Holt PG, Sly PD, Bjorksten B. Atopy versus infectious diseases in childhood; a question of balance. *Pediatr Allergy Immunol* 1997; **8**: 53–8.
80. Bjorksten B, Naaber P, Sepp E, Mikelsaar M. The intestinal microflora in allergic Estonian and Swedish 2-year-old children. *Clin Exp Allergy* 1999; **29**: 342–6.
81. Von Ehrenstein OS, Von Mutius E, Illi S, Baumann L, Bohm O, Von Kries R. Reduced risk of hay fever and asthma among children of farmers. *Clin Exp Allergy* 2000; **30**: 187–93.
82. Riedler J, Eder W, Oberfeld G, Schreuer M. Austrian children living on a farm have less hay fever, asthma and allergic sensitization. *Clin Exp Allergy* 2000; **30**: 194–200.
83. Kilpelainen M, Terho EO, Helenius H, Koskenvuo M. Farm environment in childhood prevents the development of allergies. *Clin Exp Allergy* 2000; **30**: 201–8.
84. Baldini M, Lohman IC, Halonen M, Erickson RP, Holt PG, Martinez FD. A polymorphism in the 5' flanking region of the CD14 gene is associated with circulating soluble CD14 levels and with total serum immunoglobulin E. *Am J Respir Cell Mol Biol* 1999; **20**: 976–83.
85. Beutler B. Tlr4: central component of the sole mammalian LPS sensor. *Current Opinion in Immunol* 2000; **12**: 20–6.
86. Prescott SL, Macaubas C, Smallacombe T et al. Reciprocal age related patterns of allergen specific T cell immunity in normal VS atopic infants. *Clin Exp Allergy* 1998; **28**(suppl 5): 146–51.
87. Holt PG. Immuno-prophylaxis of atopy: light at the end of the tunnel? *Immunol Today* 1994; **15**: 484–9.
88. Iikura Y, Naspitz CK, Mikawa H, Talaricoficho S, Baba M, Sole D et al. Prevention of asthma by

88. ketotifen in infants with atopic dermatitis. *Ann Allergy* 1992; **68:** 233–6.
89. ETAC Study Group. Allergic factors associated with the development of asthma and the influence of cetirizine in a double blind, randomised, placebo controlled trial: first results of ETAC. *Pediatr Allergy Immunol* 1998; **9:** 116–24.
90. Bustos GJ, Bustos D, Bustos GJ, Romero O. Prevention of asthma with ketotifen in preasthmatic children; a 3-year follow-up study. *Clin Exp Allergy* 1995; **25:** 568–73.
91. Ciprandi G, Passalacqua G, Canonica GW. Effect of H1 antihistamines on adhesion molecules: a possible rationale for long term treatment. *Clin Exp Allergy* 1999; **29**(suppl 3): 49–53.
92. Gotzsche PC, Hammarquist C, Burr M. House dust mite control measures in the management of asthma: meta-analysis. *BMJ* 1998; **317:** 1105–10.
93. Paggiaro PL, Vagaggini B, Bacci E et al. Prognosis of occupational asthma. *Europ Respir J* 1994; **7:** 761–77.
94. Falth-Magnusson K, Kjellman N-IM. Allergy prevention by maternal elimination diet during late pregnancy—a 5-year follow-up of a randomised study. *J Allergy Clin Immunol* 1992; **89:** 709–11.
95. Saarinen UM, Kajosaari M. Breastfeeding as prophylaxis against atopic disease: prospective follow-up study until 17 years. *Lancet* 1995; **346:** 1065–9.
96. Zeiger RS, Heller S, Mellon MH, Halsey JF, Hamburger RN, Sampson HA. Genetic and environmental factors affecting the development of atopy through age 4 in children of atopic parents: a prospective randomized study of food allergen avoidance. *Pediatr Allergy Immunol* 1992; **3:** 110–27.
97. Hide DW, Matthews S, Tariq S, Arshad SH. Allergen avoidance in infancy and allergy at 4 years of age. *Allergy* 1996; **51:** 89–93.
98. Warner JO, Naspitz CK, Cropp GJA. Third international pediatric consensus statement on the management of asthma. *Pediatr Pulmonol* 1998; **25:** 1–17.
99. Abramson MJ, Puy RM, Weiner JM. Is allergen immunotherapy effective in asthma? A meta-analysis of randomised controlled trials. *Am J Respir Crit Care Med* 1995; **151:** 969–74.
100. Adkinson NF Jr, Eggleston PA, Eney D et al. A controlled trial of immunotherapy for asthma in allergic children. *New Engl J Med* 1997; **336:** 327–31.
101. Gruber W, Eber E, Mileder P et al. Effect of specific immunotherapy with house dust mite extract on the bronchial responsiveness of paediatric asthma patients. *Clin Exp Allergy* 1999; **29:** 176–81.
102. Varney VA, Hamid QA, Gaga M et al. Influence of grass pollen immunotherapy on cellular infiltration and cytokine mRNA expression during allergen induced late phase cutaneous responses. *J Clin Invest* 1993; **92:** 644–51.
103. Durham SR, Walker SM, Varga E-M et al. Long term clinical efficacy of grass pollen immunotherapy. *New Engl J Med* 1999; **341:** 468–75.
104. Bousquet J, Lockey RF, Malling HJ. WHO position paper. Allergen immunotherapy: therapeutic vaccines for allergic disease. *Europ J Allergy Clin Immunol* 1998; **53**(suppl 44): 1–42.
105. Des-Roches A, Paradis L, Menardo J-L et al. Immunotherapy with a standardised *Dermatophagoides pteronyssinus* extract VI specific immunotherapy prevents the onset of new sensitizations in children. *J Allergy Clin Immunol* 1997; **99:** 450–3.
106. Jacobsen L, Dreborg S, Moller C et al. Immunotherapy as a preventive treatment. *J Allergy Clin Immunol* 1996; **97:** 232.
107. Bergmann RL, Bergmann KE. Can we predict atopic disease using perinatal risk factors? *Clin Exp Allergy* 1998; **28:** 905–7.

20

Childhood asthma in developing countries

Pakit Vichyanond, Eugene G Weinberg, Dirceu Solé

Introduction • Prevalence • Risk factors for childhood asthma in low-income countries • Clinical presentation • Diagnosis • Treatment • Prevention of asthma

INTRODUCTION

In recent years, childhood asthma has become the major childhood chronic disease not only in developed countries but also in developing nations. This is evident from results of the recent collaborative Phase I of the International Study on Asthma and Allergic Diseases in Childhood (ISAAC), which demonstrated that prevalences of childhood asthma from most developing countries are similar to those observed in developed nations.[1] Moreover, children under 15 years of age generally accounted for 40–50% of the total population in developing countries, compared with 20% in developed countries. It is estimated that there are approximately 15 billion children under 15 years in developing countries, compared with 300 million in the developed countries.[2] These numbers accentuate the magnitude of the problem of childhood asthma in developing countries. This chapter represents a combined effort of contributors from three continents (Africa—South Africa, Asia—Thailand, and South America—Brazil) to present the current status of pediatric asthma in the developing world. Each section in this chapter will begin with an overview for developing countries, followed by discussion concerning each continent to highlight similarities and differences between continents.

PREVALENCE

The results of Phase I of ISAAC indicated that the prevalence of childhood asthma varies widely throughout the world.[1,3] Although prevalences in developing countries (10–20%) are generally lower than those in North America, Europe, and Oceania (20–30%), the results indicate that prevalences in developing nations are not as low as was once thought. There are, however, large intracontinental and intercontinental variations among developing countries, perhaps representing differences in ethnicities, cultural practices, urbanization, and the effects of industrialization influencing asthma pathogenesis.

The health problems of children in the developing world remain overwhelmingly those of poor education, poor housing, and poor nutrition. Malnutrition and the common infectious diseases still pose a huge problem. Increasingly studies in these children show that, as for children growing up in poor urban environments in countries such as the USA, poverty is associated with increased prevalence of chronic illness and increased childhood mortality.[4] Definitive evidence is lacking to link poverty and asthma prevalence but poverty has been associated with underdiagnosis and inadequate use of preventive care for asthma.

Africa

Early reports from rural Africa showed a low prevalence of asthma in young children. Various reasons have been suggested for this low prevalence. Among factors mentioned are the role of parasitic infestation, a lack of wind-borne pollination, a high death rate in young children, and the protective effect of breastfeeding. A feature of studies in Africa has been the reversal of the normal male to female ratio of childhood asthma, with the condition being as common or even more frequent in females.[5] This may result from exposure to allergens within the home or from chores such as grinding wheat or maize. The effect of urbanization appears to be very important. Comparison of asthma using the exercise challenge test in Xhosa children living in rural Transkei in South Africa revealed only one asthmatic among 671 children aged 6–9 years in the Tsolo district. Their urbanized counterparts in Guguletu in Cape Town had an asthma prevalence of 3.1%.[5] A similar study in Zimbabwe showed a prevalence of asthma of 5.9% in black children in Harare. In Wedza, a rural community 150 km away, the prevalence was 0.1%.[6] Although the exercise challenge test has its limitations, its application in matched populations as in this epidemiological study can be considered reasonably accurate. More recent questionnaire-based studies of asthma prevalence in Cape Town estimate childhood asthma prevalence at 12–15%.[7,8] Similar results for rural and urban differences (3% versus 9.5%) were reported from Kenya recently.[9]

Asia

As in other parts of the world, childhood asthma has become a very common pediatric illness in Asia. Only a decade ago childhood asthma was believed to occur at much lower frequencies among Asian children than among their Western counterparts. This perhaps owes to results of previous investigations such as ones in Thailand[10] and Taiwan[11] which indicated that the prevalence rate of childhood asthma in these countries was in the range 1–4%. Nevertheless, results of Phase I of ISAAC, utilizing a standardized epidemiological tool,[1,3,12] have indicated that childhood asthma in Asia is as common as in the rest of the world (i.e. 10–15%). An interesting distribution of prevalence rates in Asia became apparent from the ISAAC Phase I study, i.e. that prevalences in more developed nations (such as Japan, Hong Kong, Singapore, etc.) were higher than prevalence rates in China and India. Nevertheless, prevalences in Taiwan and South Korea were lower than those from Southeast Asian nations.

In Thailand, the prevalence of childhood asthma has increased three-fold in less than a decade, rising from 4.3% in 1987 to 13% in 1994.[10,13] Although there were some variations between questionnaires utilized in the two surveys, these differences are not sufficient to explain such large discrepancies. Similar increases have been observed in Taiwan and Singapore.[11,14,15] The results of the ongoing ISAAC Phase II will shed light on variations in risk factors and will help us to understand more about the pathogenesis of childhood asthma in this part of the world.

Latin America

For a long time the prevalence of asthma-related respiratory symptoms in Latin American children was unknown. The International Study of Asthma and Allergies in Childhood has for the first time facilitated the production of reliable data. The ISAAC study has been conducted in 17 centers in nine different Latin American countries, resulting in 36 264 and 52 549 written questionnaires filled out by parents of 6–7-year-old children and by adolescents aged 13–14 years, respectively.[1,16] Among adolescents, the prevalences of diagnosed asthma and of wheezing during the previous 12 months were 5.5–28% and 6.6–27%, respectively.[1,16] Among younger children, the prevalences of diagnosed asthma and of wheezing during the previous 12 months were 4.1–26.9% and 8.6–32.1%, respectively. The prevalence of asthma and asthma-related symptoms in Latin America is as high and variable as previously reported for industrialized regions, according to the ISAAC protocol.[1,16]

On the other hand, a low prevalence of asthma has been found in areas with high levels of environmental pollution, suggesting that there might be a different relationship between asthma and inhalation of polluted air in these children.[16] In addition, a high frequency of asthma detected in one region with elevated levels of parasitic intestinal infections and acute virus respiratory infections occurring early in life suggests that factors that have been considered as protective against asthma in other populations may not have the same role among Latin American children.[16]

RISK FACTORS FOR CHILDHOOD ASTHMA IN LOW-INCOME COUNTRIES

Risk factors for developing asthma in low-income countries have not been well studied. Ongoing risk factor studies from Hong Kong and Thailand indicated that sensitization to inhaled allergens, particularly from house dust mites and cockroaches, is the major risk factor for development of asthma. Low socioeconomic status itself is also a risk for asthma, as has been shown in inner-city populations in the USA. Other reported risk factors for asthma for children from developing regions are overcrowding, tobacco smoking at home, use of kerosene or wood stoves, use of fans for sleeping, living in coastal and humid areas, helminthic infections, sudden weather and temperature changes, viral infections, pneumonia, air pollution, and family history of asthma and other allergic conditions.[17,18] Most of these risk factors are clearly related to low socioeconomic status and are very similar to those mentioned in the literature as risk factors for more severe acute respiratory infections in children.

CLINICAL PRESENTATION

In a prospective follow-up of 2000 asthmatic children in Thailand, 50% manifested their initial symptoms within the first 2 years of life.[19] Since respiratory infections were the major precipitant of asthmatic attacks among these children (84.5%), it was possible that a large number of these subjects were children who wheezed during respiratory tract infection (i.e. wheezing-associated respiratory infections) or were 'early wheezers' as classified by Martinez et al.[20] It was, therefore, possible that asthma in younger children could have been overdiagnosed in Thailand. Nevertheless, a recent review of medical records from a large children's hospital in Bangkok has indicated otherwise.[21] In this review, it was apparent that asthmatic bronchitis was overdiagnosed by pediatric house officers and a thorough reclassification of diagnoses increased the clinical diagnosis of asthma among 2312 children from 52% to 80%.[21] With such contradictory results, a prospective study is urgently needed to gain further insight into the pathophysiology of early childhood wheezing in Southeast Asia. Recently, a study from Taiwan looking at Chinese children less than 2 years of age with wheezing and lower respiratory tract infections indicated that a lower value of respiratory compliance is the major risk factor, as had been observed in American children.[20,22] The issue is quite important, since the World Health Organization recommends that children with lower respiratory infections with wheeze and rapid respiratory rates be given antibiotics—and antibiotics do not have any role in therapy for genuine asthmatic attacks.

Congenital heart disease

Wheezing is a common finding in children with congenital heart disease with increased pulmonary blood flow (such as ventricular septal defects, large atrial septal defects, transposition of the great vessels, etc.). These children are prone to develop lower respiratory infections, such as by respiratory syncytial virus, which usually leads to severe narrowing of airways and resultant wheezes similar to severe asthmatic attacks. Some of these children actually developed bronchial hyperresponsiveness and responded well to corticosteroid administration. Secondary bacterial infection of the lung is common and often requires prolonged administration of antimicrobial agents along with bronchodilator and possibly corticosteroids. Such clinical scenarios are quite common in developing countries, possibly owing to a delay in the correction of congenital cardiac lesions. Such delay perhaps owes to a lack of personnel and instruments available for cardiothoracic surgery in developing countries.

Bronchopulmonary dysplasia

As in several developed nations, rapid progression in the field of neonatology in developing countries has received considerable attention not only from academic pediatricians but also from private practitioners. This has led to improved survival outcomes for premature infants with birth weight less than 1500 g. For instance, survival rates in Thailand improved from 78.6% in 1983 to 93.8% in 1990.[23] Up to 30% of these infants developed bronchopulmonary dysplasia (BPD),[24] many of whom wheezed recurrently with respiratory infections during infancy. Response to bronchodilators and anti-inflammatory agents varied considerably among these infants.[24] Most infants with BPD became asymptomatic with time.

Sinusitis

It is well established that nasal symptoms among Thai children are extremely common (almost 50% of children aged 13–14 years in Thailand reported nasal symptoms during the past 12 months in ISAAC Phase I). Reasons for the increasing prevalence rate for allergic rhinitis in Southeast Asian countries are unknown. Perhaps the overall increase in nasal symptoms among pediatric populations has led to a resultant increase in cases of sinusitis observed in this region. The true prevalence rate of sinusitis among the general pediatric population in the developing world is unknown. Nevertheless, our investigation indicated that up to 50% of children with asthma had concomitant sinusitis.[25] It is possible that sinusitis could precipitate attacks in patients with established asthma, and children with sinusitis could wheeze even without prior episodes of asthma.

Gastroesophageal reflux

The recognition of gastroesophageal reflux as a condition associated with asthma has recently been highlighted.[26] The prevalence of gastroesophageal reflux among Thai children with recurrent respiratory symptoms and recurrent pneumonia has been shown to range from 34% to 40%.[27,28]

Cough

Twenty-six percent of children in the ISAAC survey in Thailand indicated that they suffered from nocturnal cough.[13] Such a phenomenon was also observed in most countries in Southeast Asia,[1] indicating that common factors existed among these countries. Cough-variant asthma is also frequently observed in pediatric allergy clinics in Thailand. These two wheezing-associated conditions, however, have not been systemically examined in Thailand or in other countries in the region.

Parasitic infection

Despite the notion that parasitic infections are common in developing countries, parasites were infrequently found in the initial examination of 2000 asthmatic Thai children.[19] Since most of the wheezing children only exhibited signs of respiratory infections on their exacerbations, routine stool examinations are usually not carried out in asthmatics who are admitted to hospitals. Visceral larva migrans are rarely encountered despite the popularity of keeping pets such as dogs and cats in Thai homes.

DIAGNOSIS

Africa

Diagnosis of asthma in children from poorer sections of the community in South Africa is not always a simple process. In the vast majority of cases these children are black and come from disadvantaged circumstances. This is particularly so among recently urbanized children, who often live in squatter settlements. Social, financial, language, and cultural barriers create many problems. It is important to maintain a high degree of suspicion that a child presenting with wheezing may not have asthma but rather some other condition, such as tuberculosis or *Ascaris* infestation, that mimics asthma. The usual approach to the diagnosis of childhood asthma includes a careful history, physical examination, pulmonary function tests and skin tests for common allergens, and perhaps total IgE estimation and eosinophil counts. Each of these useful diagnostic aids may have its own unique difficulties in South Africa.

The history
This normally valuable approach to asthma diagnosis may have its problems. In some local dialects, no words exist for 'asthma' or 'wheezing.' A disproportionate number of families among the urban poor are headed by young, single, and poorly educated women. Children are often reared by their grandmothers while their mothers have to go out to work. Very often the child is brought to the doctor or clinic by the grandmother. Although these grandmothers are usually very caring and interested in the child's welfare, they may be unable to give a clear and concise clinical history of the child's illness. Thus one valuable pointer to asthma diagnosis, a positive family history of the illness, is often absent. Unfortunately, therefore, in many cases the history may be an unrewarding and often frustrating exercise.

Physical examination
In most cases when children suspected of having asthma are examined, no wheezing is detected on auscultation of the chest. The child is usually well enough to record a normal peak expiratory flow (PEF) when requested to blow on a mini-Wright peak flow meter. Valuable clues to the fact that the child has an atopic background, such as the presence of associated allergic rhinitis or atopic eczema, are not present in many black children with asthma. Poor growth and degree of chest deformity may bear no relation to asthma or to treatment the child may have had, but may result from poor nutrition and infections. It is essential to exclude other causes of wheezing and in this regard tuberculosis must be specifically excluded. Chest radiographs are an essential component of the examination in this context. It is also useful to examine stool specimens for the presence of *Ascaris* and other parasite infestation.

Pulmonary function tests
Common equipment available to diagnose and monitor a child with asthma are the mini-Wright peak flow meter and similar devices. It is often quite difficult to teach recently urbanized or rural children from as young as 5 or 6 years to use a peak flow meter correctly. Some problems may arise with interpretation of results. Reports have suggested that there is a difference in the normal values accepted for black and white children.[7] Our practice at Red Cross Children's Hospital has been to use standard predicted values and we have experienced no problems in the interpretation of normal and abnormal pulmonary function tests.

Skin tests
Although it is simple to perform skin prick test on African children, interpretation of results could pose a great deal of difficulty, since flare

reactions may be difficult to discern in some children with dark skins. Wheals are usually easier to see and measure; the skin is wiped with a damp cloth to allow wheals to show up more sharply.

IgE estimates and eosinophil counts

In Cape Town townships, some children are infested with *Ascaris lumbricoides* and other intestinal parasites, which leads to elevated total IgE levels and raised direct and peripheral eosinophil counts. An additional problem is that accurate normal IgE values are unavailable for black children. The normal values usually given are derived from European sources and are often of little value in African circumstances. Ethiopian children are known to have IgE levels many times higher than Scandinavian children.[8] Orren et al.,[29] using blood donor samples, found normal IgE concentrations to be three times higher in black compared with white adults. The recent introduction of the Phadiatop test has been a step forward in the screening of children for atopic disease. Studies conducted at Red Cross Children's Hospital and elsewhere in South Africa have shown a high level of sensitivity for this test. It is not influenced by parasite infestation but uses a multi-RAST system and screens each serum sample against a range of the most common allergens affecting atopic children. The chances of a truly atopic child being negative to one or other of these common allergens are very remote. The detection rate of this Phadiatop or RAST-equivalent test is therefore quite high, although the cost may be too expensive by local standards.

Tests of bronchial hyperreactivity

Sophisticated and time-consuming tests for airway hyperreactivity, such as the methacholine or histamine challenge tests, are usually not appropriate for use in busy outpatient clinics or community health centers in South Africa. Far more useful for our circumstances, although admittedly less sensitive, is the exercise challenge test. The child is encouraged to run as fast as possible on level ground for 6 minutes. A pre-exercise PEFR reading and a second reading taken at 5 minutes after the cessation of running are recorded. A positive diagnosis is made if PEFR falls by 15% or more when compared with the pre-exercise value. This test is usually performed to confirm asthma in cases in which diagnosis is uncertain. It is simple, costs nothing, and is ideal for use in developing countries.

Asia

Most pediatric asthma specialists in Thailand are familiar with Global Initiatives for Asthma (GINA), the National Asthma Education and Prevention Program (NAEEP), and the National Guidelines for Diagnosis and Treatment for Childhood Asthma. Nevertheless, general practitioners mostly concentrate on pharmacological therapies for asthma rather than on diagnosis, objectives of treatment, and prevention of asthma. This reflects an attitude among Thai physicians that asthma is readily recognized during attacks; hence possible underdiagnosis of asthma is expected in children with less obvious presentations. Only 23% of Thai pediatricians in a recent survey indicated they had used a peak flow meter in an evaluation for chronic asthma. This perhaps owes in part to the high price of peak flow meters by local standards and the relative unavailability of the device to physicians. Similarly, use of peak flow meters and spirometry is uncommon in the overall management of asthma (less than 17% of respondents used a peak flow meter in managing acute asthma and less than 25% used objective lung functions).[30] Asthma is therefore diagnosed mostly by history and physical examination, mainly during an acute attack. Complicated cases of asthma are rarely referred to specialists for further evaluation. This owes to a relative lack of knowledge among medical personnel that asthma is an inflammatory disease and could progress to a more severe condition without timely intervention with appropriate treatment.

Despite established information that up to 60–70% of asthmatic individuals in Thailand (both adults and children) are sensitized to house dust mites,[31] most physicians would consider skin testing to aeroallergens an unnecessary investigation for childhood asthma. Consequently, appropriate environmental control measures for house dust mites (such as hot washing and mattress encasing) and other allergens have received little attention from general practitioners and pulmonary specialists alike. Recently, the Phadiatop test has been evaluated in Thailand and has shown a promising sensitivity and specificity in establishing atopic status among Thai children. Nevertheless, its high cost prevents most physicians using it in the diagnosis of asthma.

In contrast to what has been reported from Africa, in an investigation of exercise-induced asthma in Thailand we found that the exercise challenge was of low sensitivity for the diagnosis of asthma in Thai children (less than 25% of asthmatics had a positive graded treadmill exercise test result).[32] We therefore do not routinely use exercise challenge in doubtful cases but prefer to proceed to methacholine testing, which we find quite simple and reproducible to carry out. Recently, we have embarked on the ISAAC Phase II investigation and have found the hypertonic saline challenge to be an even simpler test to perform than the methacholine challenge.

Latin America

Among various etiologies for asthma in Brazil, allergy has been found to be the most prominent cause. Approximately 80% of Brazilian children with asthma are sensitized to inhaled allergens, such as from house dust mites—i.e. *D. pteronyssinus* and *B. tropicalis*, cockroaches, and from cat and dog epithelia to a lesser extent.[33,34] However, considering costs, immediate hypersensitivity skin tests are thought to be more useful in identifying allergic children older than 3 years of age, owing to reduced positive rates of allergy skin tests in younger children.[35] In general, investigation of other associated diseases in Brazil included checks for sinusitis, gastroesophageal reflux, and immunodeficiencies. These should be oriented by patient's clinical history. Inquiring about passive exposure to tobacco smoke and to wood burning for the purposes of heating or cooking is important, since these are common practices particularly among low socioeconomic classes in Brazil.[36]

TREATMENT

Although international guidelines for diagnosis and management of asthma have been available for some time, these guidelines require adaptation to individual countries' practices and resources. Such adaptation has been carried out in several countries. Most of these adaptations are based on experts' opinion and have not been fully evaluated in field situations. Although emphasis has been placed on asthma education, successful attempts in this regard have been accomplished in only a few countries (such as China, the Philippines, Chile, and Indonesia). Educational materials, on the other hand, are readily available in most countries but are not distributed widely enough to reach needy patients. Environmental controls, particularly against house dust mites, are not commonly practiced, mostly because of poverty, inability to change the existing environment owing to limited resources, and lack of available materials for implementing environmental control at a reasonable cost.

Although the importance of early institution of anti-inflammatory agents is understood by most specialists in developing countries, most primary care practitioners in developing countries do not usually prescribe such forms of therapy. Compounding such a problem has been the unavailability of inhaled steroids and other anti-inflammatory agents, mostly owing to their high cost, in developing countries. Although several of these agents are on essential drug lists available to indigenous patients in some countries, a large majority of children with asthma belong to middle-class families who are not eligible for drug subsidy from the government. For such reasons, a large number of asthmatic children depend on periodic bronchodilators usage alone to control their asthma. Several utilize the emergency departments of local hospitals as their source of acute and long-term asthma care, which is hardly adequate to control their disease.

The lack of registry data on childhood asthma, including prevalence, attack rates, drug-prescribing styles among physicians, drug utilization among patients, morbidity classification, mortality, etc. in developing countries, makes it difficult to assess the economic burden of childhood asthma on these societies. Without computation of such costs, it will be difficult to persuade all stakeholders in these societies, such as the health authorities and government agencies, to understand the magnitude of the problem and to develop strategies to address it.

South Africa

Patient and parent education
One of the main problems with asthma management among the urban and rural poor, and especially the township and squatter camp dwellers, in South Africa is a lack of ready access to health care. The emergency department at the nearest hospital often serves as the location of a primary care doctor or clinic, although recently community health centers have been built close to the homes of many previously disadvantaged people. Even when services are available, some mothers have difficulty in using them. In order to reach a hospital or clinic, many mothers may take all their children (not just the one with asthma) on public transport or by township taxi. They may wait for hours for treatment in an overcrowded and overworked facility. If she works, the mother may find the clinic is not open during the hours when she is available. If there is a language problem, health care providers may not be able to translate instructions at the clinic. Most problems with inadequate access to health care result from a lack of funds on the part of both the patients and the state. Improved parent and child education, aggressive yet simple treatment protocols, and improved patient compliance will make the best use of limited funds.

Special nurse educators teaching the mother and child the correct way to use medicines and environmental control are available from several drug manufacturers. The nurses follow the children regularly and assist a great deal in improving the child's medication compliance and environmental control, especially the need to prevent exposure of the child to cigarette smoking. Simple pamphlets and illustrated booklets on asthma and its treatment have been translated into local languages and are readily available. Educational videotapes, most of which are available through asthma drug manufacturers and the Allergy Society of South Africa (ALLSA), are additional sources of information for use at clinics.

Environmental control
Children living in slum shacks have special requirements when it comes to recommending an environmental control program. Homes are often overcrowded and there may be two or three children to a bed. Furnishings may be rudimentary. Mattresses may be a piece of foam rubber and pillows are homemade and stuffed with anything from dried flowers to foam chips or feathers. Cooking activities may be carried out over open wood or coal fires or kerosene stoves and this may occur in the same room in which the children sleep. Roofs may leak; bedding is often wet and carpets are often moldy, especially in the wet Cape Town winters. Rudimentary shacks are very cold in winter and very hot in summer. These homes may be either very draughty or poorly ventilated. Cats and dogs roam freely around the dwelling. Very often the shacks do not have the benefit of electricity. Smoking among adults is extremely common. Mothers of children from such environments find instructions on environmental control, especially those relating to reduction of house dust mites, of very little use in their poor homes. Expensive measures aimed at mite reduction cannot even be considered and vacuum cleaning is not possible. The best advice that can be given is for the mother to air mattresses and bedding in the sun for prolonged periods. Pillows and duvets may be stuffed with cheap foam chips instead of feathers. Changes in cooking practices, such as con-

structing a simple outside shelter for this purpose, are useful. Parents are advised not to smoke in the child's presence and to stop the habit if possible. Cockroaches may be an important indoor allergen in poor communities in coastal cities. Suggesting to families that they should get rid of cats or dogs is not always advisable. These animals perform important functions in poor township homes. Cats control rats, mice, and other vermin. Dogs protect the family, and parents may be reluctant to act on advice to get rid of them.

Medication

Poor children are much more likely to rely on local clinics or on overburdened hospital outpatient and emergency departments than on individual medical practitioners. It is in these situations that the child requires essential asthma medications. Due regard must be paid to cultural, socioeconomic, and educational factors when prescribing these medicines. Simply following the advice of experts in asthma from overseas may not always be advisable in local circumstances. To this end the South African Childhood Asthma Working Group (SACAWG)[37] has produced simple guidelines applicable to South African circumstances for both the maintenance treatment of asthma and the treatment of acute asthma attacks.[38] These guidelines are simpler than those emanating from developed countries but still offer the child the best of currently available treatments for asthma. The limited budget of most developing countries should be reserved for the asthma drugs included in the WHO essential drugs list. Several studies in poor urban communities have shown that the principal factor related to adequate usage and adherence of medication is the simplicity of the treatment regimen.[39] Medication adherence may also be related to family function, education, and make-up and the child's personality and understanding of asthma. One study showed that children with ≥8 years of formal education are more compliant with asthma treatment than are those with less education.[40] Family characteristics that influence compliance include the number of parents present, the number of children in the family, the occurrence of illness in siblings, the educational level of the parents, communication problems, ethnic background, and socioeconomic status. Findings have sometimes been contradictory but compliance seems to be reduced when multiple caregivers are responsible for giving medication. Poor educational levels, lack of supervision, illiteracy, and the absence of electricity in many homes make it impossible for parents to administer some forms of treatment. In many cases the use of simple illustrations to explain medicine use is of great value. Graphically illustrated labeling of medicines is often of great benefit as well. Simple devices to aid the administration of medicines by inhalation are very useful. Simple spacer devices can be constructed using a 500 ml cola bottle with a hole made in it for the mouthpiece of the MDI could be used to administer β-agonists in lieu of a nebulizer. Commercial spacers with a soft facemask should accommodate all bronchodilator or anti-inflammatory MDIs by incorporating a universal fitting. A very helpful development in Cape Town has been the establishment of community health centers close to the homes of the children. Several of these clinics are now open on a 24 hour basis. Access to oxygen and nebulized bronchodilators as well as medical expertise is now available around the clock to children from poorer communities.

Asia

Prescribing styles in Thailand have concentrated more on the use of bronchodilators rather than anti-inflammatory agents despite intensive efforts over the past decade to inform medical communities in Thailand that asthma is an inflammatory disease of airways and lungs. Reasons for such practice are the myths among physicians that prophylactic agents are expensive, not cost-beneficial, and not affordable to most patients and their families. In our survey of pediatricians throughout Thailand, corticosteroids and cromolyn were chosen as elements of pharmacotherapy by only 9.6% and 2.4%, respectively.[30] The other reason for not prescribing

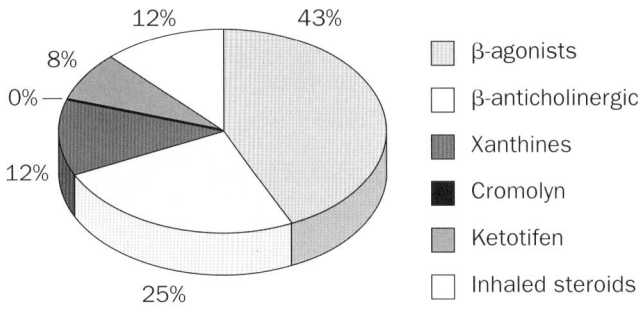

Figure 20.1 Relative market sizes of antiasthmatic drugs in Thailand, in 1997. (*Source*: Thailand Index of Medical Information 1997)

these two agents was the perceived difficulty of administering aerosol agents to children (and the lack of spacer devices). This is reflected by the fact that a large number of pediatricians chose ketotifen (up to 90.4%) as their preferred prophylactic agent for chronic asthma. In fact, the Thailand Medical Index survey in 1997 indicated that ketotifen accounted for a significant share (8%) of anti-asthmatic drugs prescribed in Thailand (Figure 20.1).

As for bronchodilator of choice for acute asthma, 81% of pediatricians chose nebulized salbutamol whereas only 13% chose subcutaneous adrenaline.[30] This has been the result of an intensive campaign on aerosol therapy over the last decade in Thailand. Similar results were seen in a review of in-hospital therapy in the largest teaching hospital in Thailand.[41] Nevertheless, over 80% still indicated their preference for aminophylline as an element of acute asthma therapy[30] despite ample information in the literature reporting theophylline's lack of efficacy in acute asthma.[42] In our survey, corticosteroids were reserved for severe attacks only, despite the need for admission.[30,41] Surprisingly, antibiotics were chosen as concomitant therapy for acute asthma by over 80% of pediatricians both in the survey[30] and the in-hospital audit[41] implying a general belief among pediatricians that bacterial pneumonia commonly coexists with asthma.

As for forms of bronchodilators prescribed for chronic asthma, oral β-agonists are the most favored group of drugs chosen (88%). Metered-dose inhalers and dry powders accounted only for small percentages of responders (7.7% and 6%, respectively). The reasons for such a prescribing style could include lack of adequate time in busy offices to teach inhaler techniques, ease of use of pills, increasing compliance with oral agents, a social myth that inhaler use is associated with a severe degree of disease condition. Pre-exercise treatment was instructed in only 19% of cases.[30] It has been well established that exercise-induced asthma is relatively uncommon among asthmatic children in Thailand, perhaps owing to the relatively high humidity in this part of the world.[32] As previously indicated, ketotifen was the most popular prophylactic agent among Thai pediatricians (preferred by 88%) whereas less than 10% preferred inhaled corticosteroids and cromolyn. Small volume spacers for infants are not popular in Thailand, being selected by only 1.2% of Thai pediatricians.

In contrast to the situation in South Africa, most essential asthmatic drugs (β-agonists and inhaled corticosteroids) are readily available for children under a subsidized program (these drugs are subsidized by government as part of Thailand's essential drug lists). Nevertheless, as in China, some families are not entitled to such assistance and would have to pay for such medications themselves. Several families opted for less expensive bronchodilators rather than anti-inflammatory agents. The relative lack of use of inflammatory agents as previously stated was due in part to the prescribing physicians not to the lack of drugs. Despite their relative lack of education, most children and families of low socioeconomic classes can be taught how to use inhalers properly.

Latin America

As in other countries, asthma guidelines did not significantly change the prevailing treatment with only bronchodilators in Brazil. Educational programs could help to reduce emergency visits and hospital admissions.[43] However, a recent cost calculation in Brazil indicated the initial costs for children 5 years and older with moderate asthma would be US$34/month and for children with severe asthma would be US$45/month. The situation in Brazil mirrors that in other Latin American countries. Given that family income averages approximately US$200, maintenance of adequate treatment for asthma is impossible. This observation can be partly confirmed by examining the data shown in Table 20.1. The percentage of sales of bronchodilators is striking, reflecting an emphasis on symptomatic treatment. On the other hand, the reduced consumption of anti-inflammatory agents suggests that:

(a) the several guidelines on the management of asthma have a low impact on Brazilian physicians' prescription habits;

(b) although physicians do follow guidelines, the very low income of most of the population does not permit acquisition of the required drugs.

The low-income population receives medical attention at National Health Units or Hospitals, where asthmatic patients can receive only oral drugs free of charge, i.e. β-agonists, aminophylline, and prednisone. Whether it would be justifiable in this situation to use long-term oral corticosteroids at the minimal dose capable of controlling the symptoms in such a population remains to be investigated.

Hospitalization for asthma is evidence of the failure of preventive treatment of this disease. In addition, hospitalization costs are high. Development of a national program for assistance to these patients, involving education as well as early institution of anti-inflammatory treatment for patients with moderate and severe asthma as priorities, will certainly modify the current status of asthma in this region, resulting in improved quality of life for these individuals.

Table 20.1 Sales (in units) of drugs used in the management of asthma in Brazil, in 1997

Drug	Total	%
β-agonists	22 436 062	61.36
Neb. solution	3 159 783	8.64
MDI	4 571 338	12.50
Xantines	9 242 180	25.28
Aminophylline	3 033 88?	8.29
Slow-release theophylline	1 367 480	3.74
Ipratropium bromide	2 517 185	6.88
Cromones	180 898	0.49
Ketotifen	1 040 655	2.84
Inhaled corticosteroids	1 144 803	3.13
Total	36 561 783	100.00

Source: Pharmaceutical Market Brazil. São Paulo: IMS Health AG, 1997.

PREVENTION OF ASTHMA

Primary prevention (preventing high-risk infants becoming sensitized) and secondary prevention (preventing sensitized children developing asthma) are not considered to be of prime priority in developing countries. This owes to physicians' lack of basic awareness and knowledge (rather than parents' awareness) about allergy prevention possibilities and strategies (food elimination, environmental control of house dust mites and cockroaches, etc.). In addition, there is a lack of basic epidemiological data regarding risk factors for asthma in children, a lack of well-laid-out preventive strategies, and a relative lack of reliable products for environmental control. In spite of limited resources for allergy prevention, certain actions could be implemented. Examples of these actions are identification of high-risk infants (e.g. those born to atopic parents), curbing exposure to parental cigarette smoking, research into methods for manipulating indoor environments, amelioration of outdoor pollution, improvement of nutrition, and control of childhood viral respiratory infections.

It should be noted that despite a relative lack of allergy preventive action by health care personnel, the public are bombarded with products advertised in simple terms as effective in preventing allergy development (tonics, health food, folk remedies, specialized vacuum cleaners, air purifiers, ozone generators, etc.). The public is quite receptive to these unproven methods and has purchased significant numbers of these products without appropriate medical advice.

Given that prophylactic agents are available to groups of children whose medical care is covered by governmental subsidy and to children of upper socioeconomic class, tertiary prevention is therefore possible in the developing world. As elsewhere in the developing world, the science of allergy and its prevention is in Asia (excepting Japan and South Korea) in its incipient stage as compared with the situation in Europe and North America. Increasing efforts to raise standards of asthma care and to produce medical personnel capable of providing care for allergic children are among the top priorities for pediatric allergy and immunology worldwide. Work on public education—in schools and communities—on asthma and allergic disorders remains a daunting challenge for developing countries in the new millennium.

REFERENCES

1. Worldwide variations in the prevalence of asthma symptoms: the International Study of Asthma and Allergies in Childhood (ISAAC). *Eur Respir J* 1998; **12**: 315–35.
2. Morley D, Lovel H. *My Name is To-day.* London: Macmillan, 1986.
3. International Study of Asthma and Allergies in Childhood Steering Committee. Worldwide variation in prevalence of symptoms of asthma, allergic rhinoconjunctivitis, and atopic eczema: ISAAC. *Lancet* 1998; **351**: 1225–32.
4. Egbuono L, Strafield B. Child health and social status. *Pediatrics* 1982; **69**: 550–7.
5. Van Niekerk CH, Weinberg EG, Shore SC, Heese H de V, Van Schalkwyk DJ. Prevalence of asthma: a comparative study of urban and rural Xhosa children. *Clin Allergy* 1979; **9**: 319–24.
6. Keeley DJ, Neill P, Gallivan S. Comparison of the prevalence of reversible airways obstruction in rural and urban Zimbabwean children. *Thorax* 1991; **46**: 549–53.
7. Ehrlich RI, Du Toit D, Jordaan E, Weinberg E. Prevalence and reliability of asthma symptoms in primary school children in Cape Town. *Int J Epidemiol* 1995; **41**: 1138–46.
8. Johansson SGO, Mellbin T, Vahlquist B. Immunoglobulin levels in Ethiopian pre-school children with special reference to high concentrations of immunoglobulin E. *Lancet* 1968; **1**: 1118–21.
9. Odhiambo JA, Ng'ang'a LW, Mungai MW, Gicheha CM, Nyamwaya JK, Karimi F et al. Urban–rural differences in questionnaire-derived markers of asthma in Kenyan school children. *Eur Respir J* 1998; **12**: 1105–12.
10. Boonyarittipong P, Tuchinda M, Balangura K, Visitsuntorn N, Vanaprapar N. Prevalences of allergic diseases in Thai children. *J Pediatr Soc Thailand* 1990; **29**: 24–32.
11. Huang JL, Hsieh KH. Increasing prevalence of childhood allergic diseases and the risk factors for the development of allergy in Taipei, Taiwan.

Presented at 5th West-Pacific Allergy Symposium, Seoul, 1–14 June 1997.
12. Asher MI, Weiland SK. The International Study of Asthma and Allergies in Childhood (ISAAC). *Clin Exp Allergy* 1998; **28**(suppl 5): 52–66, 90–1.
13. Vichyanond P, Jirapongsananuruk O, Visitsuntorn N, Tuchinda M. Prevalence of asthma, rhinitis and eczema in children from the Bangkok area using the ISAAC (International Study for Asthma and Allergy in Children) questionnaires. *J Med Assoc Thai* 1998; **81**: 175–84.
14. Goh DYT, Chew FT, Quek SC, Lee BW. Prevalence and severity of asthma, rhinitis, and eczema in Singapore schoolchildren. *Arch Dis Child* 1996; **74**: 131–5.
15. Hsieh KH, Shen JJ. Prevalence of childhood asthma in Taipei, Taiwan, and other Asian Pacific countries. *J Asthma* 1988; **25**: 73–82.
16. Mallol J, Clayton T, Asher I, Williams H, Beasley R. ISAAC findings in children aged 13–14 years—an overview. *ACI Intern* 1999; **11**: 176–81.
17. Perdomo D, Benarroch L, Marcano W, Rodriguez E, Rosales A. Allergy and parasites: an association dissoluble. *Immunologia Clinica* 1989; **89**: 223–6.
18. Valdes J, Herrara E, Riambou J, Otero R. Bronchial asthma in children: social and environmental factors that influence it. *Rev Cuba Pediatr* 1990; **62**: 365–75.
19. Tuchinda M, Habanananda S, Vareenil J, Srimaruta N, Piromrat K. Asthma in Thai children: a study of 2000 cases. *Ann Allergy* 1987; **59**: 207–11.
20. Martinez FD, Wright AL, Taussig LM, Holberg CJ, Halonen M, Morgan WJ. Asthma and wheezing in the first six years of life. *N Engl J Med* 1995; **332**: 133–8.
21. Vangveeravong M. Asthma vs asthmatic bronchitis. *Thai J Pediatr* 1999; **38**: 105–10.
22. Yau KIT, Fang LJ, Hsieh KH. Factors predisposing infants to lower respiratory infection with wheezing in the first two years of life. *Ann Allergy Asthma Immunol* 1999; **82**: 165–70.
23. Kolatat T. Neonatal mortality. In: Tuchinda M, Suvatti V, Wongjirat A, Chavalittamrong P, Jirapinyo P, eds. *Pediatrics*. Bangkok: Ruenkaew, 1997, 203–11.
24. Kolatat T. Bronchopulmonary dysplasia: BPD. In: Tuchinda M, Suvatti V, Wongjirat A, Chavalittamrong P, Jirapinyo P, eds. *Pediatrics*. Bangkok: Ruenkaew, 1997, 354–68.
25. Visitsunthorn N, Balankura K, Keorochana S, Habanananda S, Vichyanond P, Tuchinda M. Sinusitis in Thai children. *Asian Pac J Allergy Immunol* 1992; **10**: 5–10.
26. Theodoropoulos DS, Lockey RF, Boyce HW Jr, Bukantz SC. Gastroesophageal reflux and asthma: a review of pathogenesis, diagnosis, and therapy. *Allergy* 1999; **54**: 651–61.
27. Treepongkaruna S, Phuapradit P, Assadamongkok K. Gastroesophageal reflux in children with recurrent pneumonia. *Rama Med J* 1996; **19**: 92–8.
28. Aanpreung P, Vajaradul C, Keorochana SNH, Pusuwan P. Gastroesophageal reflux in children. *Siriraj Hosp Gaz* 1995; **47**(suppl 3): 25–30.
29. Orren A, Walls RS, Dowdle EB. Serum immunoglobulin E concentrations of allergic patients and blood donors: influence of allergy, sex and race on IgE values. *S Afr Med J* 1975; **49**: 1387–90.
30. Vichyanond P, Hatchaleelaha S, Jintavorn V, Kerdsomnuig S. How pediatricians manage asthma in Thailand. Manuscript in preparation.
31. Kongpanichkul A, Vichyanond P, Tuchinda M. Allergy skin reactivities among asthmatic Thai children. *J Med Assoc Thai* 1997; **80**: 89–75.
32. Vichyanond P, Anuruklekha P. Exercise-induced asthma in Thai children. Manuscript submitted.
33. Fernandez-Caldas E, Arruda LK, Sole D, Chapman MD, Platts-Mills TAE. Environmental control of mite allergy. *Pediatr Pulmonol* 1995; **11**: 47–8.
34. Santos ABR, Chapman MD, Aalberse RC, Vailes LD, Ferriani VPL, Oliver C et al. Cockroach allergens and asthma in Brazil: identification of tropomyosin as a major allergen with potential cross-reactivity with mite and shrimp allergens. *J Allergy Clin Immunol* 1999; **104**: 329–37.
35. Halasz MR, Gonsalez SL, Sole D, Naspitz CK. Specific sensitization to *Dermatophagoides pteronyssinus* and cutaneous reactivity to histamine in Brazilian children. *J Invest Allergy Clin Immunol* 1997; **7**: 98–102.
36. Sociedade Brasileira de Alergia e Imunopatologia, Sociedade Brasileira de Pediatria, Sociedade Brasileira de Pneumologia e Tisiologia. II Consenso Brasileiro no Manejo da Asma. *J Pneumol* 1998; **24**: 171–276.
37. South African Childhood Asthma Working Group. Management of childhood and adolescent asthma—1991 consensus. *S Afr Med J* 1992; **81**: 38–41.
38. South African Childhood Asthma Working Group. Management of acute asthmatic attacks in children. *S Afr Med J* 1993; **83**: 286–9.
39. Markello JR. Factors influencing pediatric compliance. *Pediatr Infect Dis J* 1985; **4**: 579–83.

40. Radu S, Becker M, Rosenstock I. Predicting mothers' compliance with pediatric medical regimens. *J Asthma Res* 1978; **15:** 133–49.
41. Visitsunthorn N, Sittichokananon N, Tuchinda M. Childhood asthma: cases admitted to Siriraj Hospital in 1992. *Siriraj Hosp Gaz* 1995; **47:** 313–21.
42. Goodman DC, Littenberg B, O'Connor GT, Brooks JG. Theophylline in acute childhood asthma: a meta-analysis of its efficacy. *Pediatr Pulmonol* 1996; **21:** 211–18.
43. Cabral AL, Gavalho WA, Chinen M, Barbiroto RM, Boueri FM, Martins MA. Are International Asthma Guidelines effective for low-income Brazilian children with asthma? *Eur Respir J* 1998; **12:** 35–40.

Index

acaricides, 240–1
accessory muscles of respiration, 198
acetylcholine, virus-induced release, 88–9
acetyl cysteine, 175
acid/base balance, in acute asthma, 194–5
action plan, 312, 320
acupuncture, 177
acute asthma, 189–209
   allergic rhinitis therapy and, 231
   assessment, 197–8
   bacterial respiratory infections and, 86
   clinical approach, 195–204
   definition, 189
   differential diagnosis, 195–6
   house dust mite exposure and, 238
   in infants and small children, 140–3
   inhalant therapy, 200, 334
   management, 199–204
   mechanical ventilation, 201–3
   outdoor air pollution and, 56, 191
   pathology, 189–90
   pharmacotherapy, 199, 200–1
   physiological characteristics, 190–5
   precipitating factors, 196–7
   risk factors, 121
   self-management plans, 312
   treatment adherence and, 198, 295–6
   viral respiratory infections and, 83, 85, 190–1
acute severe asthma
   assessment, 198
   flow rates, 191
   systemic corticosteroids, 142
   theophylline, 142–3
adenosine receptors, 162
adenotonsillectomy, 101, 108
adherence (compliance), 295–6
   acute asthma and, 198, 295–6
   in developing countries, 385
   future directions, 301–3
   holding chamber use, 336, 337
   intensive, hospital-based interventions, 303
   measurement, 296
   pharmacotherapy, 126, 162
   psychosocial factors affecting, 293–5, 297–301
adhesion molecules, 28–9, 86
adolescents
   asthma education, 321
   gender differences in asthma risk, 73
   treatment adherence, 296
adrenaline (epinephrine), 155, 288, 386
aerosol delivery, 327–46
   anatomical factors, 328
   breathing patterns and, 330
   competence and, 329
   in crying/distress, 330
   factors affecting, 328–30
   nose vs mouth-breathing and, 329–30
   systems *see* inhalant therapy, delivery devices
aetiology of asthma
   risk factors, 50–8, 67–82
   viral respiratory infections and, 54–5, 83–5, 86–93
Africa
   diagnosis of asthma, 381–2
   management of asthma, 384–5
   prevalence of asthma, 378
agammaglobulinaemia, 102, 107
age
   airways deposition and, 328, 329
   asthma exacerbations and, 121
   costs of asthma and, 349
   of onset
      asthma severity and, 58
      diagnostic labelling and, 68
   self-management behaviours, 317–22
   see also infants; school-aged children; small children
air conditioning, 241, 245
air filtration devices, 241, 243
air pollution
   in developing countries, 379
   exercise-induced asthma and, 215, 216
   indoor, 56–8, 245–6
   outdoor, 55–6, 191
airway
   anatomical changes, 328, 329
   congenital abnormalities, 104–6
   cooling, in exercise-induced asthma, 211–12
   development, 1–2
   epithelium, 25, 90–1
   malacia, 104–5, 106
   mucosal plugging, 19
   neural control, effects of viruses, 88–9
   remodelling, 25–7, 28, 29, 151
   resistance, measurement, 12
   size, gender differences, 5, 53, 73
   structure, effects of virus infections, 89
   upper, deposition of aerosols, 328, 329, 342
airway inflammation, 19–33
   in acute asthma, 189–90
   adhesion molecules in, 28–9
   airway remodelling and, 27, 28

airway inflammation *continued*
  β$_2$-agonist therapy and, 156
  BHR, atopy and asthma and, 20–2
  effects of viruses, 89–92
  exercise-induced asthma and, 212
  inhaled corticosteroids and, 158
  leukotriene modifying agents and, 169
  non-invasive markers, 30
  ontogeny, 22, 23
  proinflammatory cells, 24–5
  relevance, 29, 151
  vs sinusitis and rhinitis, 226
airway obstruction
  mechanisms of viral-induced, 87–9
  perception, 294–5
  severity, arterial blood gases and, 193–5
airway responsiveness
  acute asthma and, 190–1
  in asthmatic children, 14
  definition, 190
  in infants, 11
  in utero tobacco smoke exposure and, 57
  measurement, 10, 13, 382
  see also bronchial hyperresponsiveness
airway smooth muscle
  development, 2–3, 4
  hyperplasia, 25, 26
albuterol, *see* salbutamol
alder pollen, 262, 270
allergens, 257–78
  airborne, 53–4, 259
  in amniotic fluid, 363
  antenatal exposure, 364
  asthma exacerbations and, 191, 197
  avoidance, for asthma prevention, 370
  bronchial responses, 21–2
  cloning and sequencing, 260
  environmental control *see* environmental control
  exercise-induced asthma and, 215
  functional properties, 259–60, 261–2
  general properties, 258–60
  IgE antibodies and, 258
  immunotherapy, *see* immunotherapy
  indoor, 53–4, 56, 265–9
    environmental control, 237–45
    role in asthma, 258, 360–1, 370
  molecular biology, 260–2
  nasal provocation testing, 227
  nomenclature, 259
  outdoor, 269–71
  quantitation in environment, 258
  recombinant, 260
    clinical applications, 262–5
    expression *in vitro*, 260–2
  sources, 265–71
  structural properties, 261–2
  see also specific allergens
allergic bronchopulmonary aspergillosis, 197, 271
allergic bronchopulmonary syndrome, 197

allergic rhinitis
  asthma and, 58, 108, 223–35
    pathophysiological mechanisms, 226–9
    population studies, 74–5, 224–5
  in developing countries, 380
  inflammation in, 226
  perennial, intranasal corticosteroids, 230
  seasonal *see* hay fever
  treatment, 229–31
    antihistamines, 230–1
    antileukotriene drugs, 231
    effect on asthma outcome, 231
    intranasal corticosteroids, 229–30
allergic sensitization
  antenatal, 361–7
  asthma risk, 73–5
  in developing countries, 379, 383
  evolution into airway inflammation, 23
  four phases, 367
  genetic/environmental diversity and, 366–7
  geographical variations, 73–4
  hygiene hypothesis, 54, 367–8
  ontogeny, 361–9
  pharmacotherapy to prevent asthma, 369–70
  primary, 22
  role in asthma, 258, 359–61
  seasonal, 364
  viral infections and, 84, 85
allergy
  food, *see* food allergy
  testing, 110–11
  see also atopy
Allergy and Asthma Network, 313
Alternaria
  allergen, 74, 75, 245, 262, 271
  immunotherapy, 249
alternative medicine, 177–8
alveolar macrophages, 22, 24–5
alveolus development, 1–2
  inhaled corticosteroids (ICS) and, 161, 162
Amb a 1, 265
ambroxol, 175
ambulatory care visits, 43–6
American Academy of Allergy, Asthma and Immunology, 313
American football players, 214–15
American Lung Association, 313
American Thoracic Society (ATS), 313
  asthma definition, 37
  respiratory symptoms questionnaire, 36
aminophylline, 201, 386
anaesthesia, general, in respiratory failure, 203–4
anaphylaxis, food-induced, 281
angiogram, 106, 111
animal allergens, 241–4, 269
  environmental control, 242–4
  see also cat(s); dog(s)
animal farms, asthma risk, 78
anti-asthma medication, *see* pharmacotherapy

antibiotics
    in asthma, 85–6, 173–4
    in developing countries, 379, 386
    inhaled, 336
    for sinusitis, 231–2
anticholinergic agents
    in acute asthma, 201
    in chronic asthma, 175
    economic evaluation, 353
    in infants and small children, 141–2
    M2 receptor-specific, 177
    trial of therapy, 114
antigen-presenting cells (APCs), 22
    fetal, 363
antihistamines
    in allergic rhinitis, 230–1
    asthma prophylaxis, 369–70
    in food allergy, 288
anti-IgE therapy, 176–7, 288–9
anti-inflammatory drugs
    in developing countries, 383, 385–6, 387
    in exercise-induced asthma, 216
    in infants and small children, 122–3, 127–32
    trial of therapy, 114
    see also controller medications; corticosteroids; cromoglycate; leukotriene-modifying agents
antileukotriene drugs, see leukotriene-modifying agents
anti-reflux medication, 107
anxiety, maternal, 115
aortic arch
    double, 105
    right-sided, 110, 111
arachidonic acid, 164
arterial blood gases, in acute asthma, 193–5, 198
Ascaris lumbricoides infestations, 382
Asia
    diagnosis of asthma, 382–3
    management of asthma, 385–6
    prevalence of asthma, 40, 41–2, 378
aspergillosis, allergic bronchopulmonary, 197, 271
Aspergillus, 245, 271
Aspergillus fumigatus allergen, 261, 271
aspirin-sensitive asthma, 169
assessment
    acute asthma, 197–8
    asthma see diagnosis
association studies, genetic, 52, 71–2
asthma
    beginning, 67–8
    definitions, see definitions of asthma
Asthma and Allergy Foundation of America, 313
'asthmatic bronchitis', 38
atelectasis, 202
athletes
    asthma management, 217–18
    doping regulations, 218
    exercise-induced asthma, 214–15
atopic dermatitis (eczema), 110, 265, 369

atopy
    asthma risk, 53, 73–5
    BHR, airway inflammation and asthma and, 20–2
    diagnosis, 110, 381, 382–3
    natural history of asthma and, 58
    pharmacotherapy to prevent asthma, 369–70
    respiratory tract infections and, 55, 85
atropine, 88
auranofin, 173
auscultation, 103
Australia, asthma prevalence, 40, 41

Babyhaler, 124, 125
bacteria, allergenicity, 269
bacterial respiratory infections, asthma and, 83, 85–6
barium swallow, 105–6, 107
barotrauma, prevention, 202
BCG, 368
beclomethasone dipropionate (BDP)
    in chronic asthma, 161, 163
    delivery devices, 332–3
    dose equivalents, 152, 159
    economic evaluation, 351
    growth effects, 160
    HPA axis suppression, 159–60
    intranasal, in allergic rhinitis, 229, 230
bedding
    covers, 239, 240, 243
    in developing countries, 384
    washing, 241
behaviour (health care)
    change
        communication strategies, 314–16
        principles, 310–14
    key, 310
    psychosocial factors affecting, 207–301
    reinforcement of appropriate, 312–14
benzyl benzoate, 240, 241
β_2-agonists, 155–7
    delivery systems, 125, 332, 333, 336
    doping regulations, 218
    in exercise-induced asthma, 217
    inhaled dose delivered, 338, 339
    intravenous, 200
    long-acting inhaled, 155, 170
        combined with ICS, 170
        in exercise-induced asthma, 217
        in infants and small children, 137–40
        role in asthma therapy, 170
    mast cell actions, 24
    responsiveness, 200
    short-acting
        in acute asthma, 200
        in chronic asthma, 155–7
        in infants and small children, 140–3
        side-effects, 156
        tolerance, 156–7
    trial of therapy, 114

beta-adrenergic agonists, 155, 175
  β_2-specific, see β_2-agonists
beta-adrenoceptors, 155
BHR see bronchial hyperresponsiveness
biopsy
  in acute asthma, 189, 190
  transbronchial (TBB), 108, 112
  transthoracic, 108
birch pollen, 262, 270–1
  allergen (Bet v 1), 262, 270–1
  sensitization, 74, 364
Blatella germanica allergens, 244, 261, 266–7
  Bla g 2, 259–60, 267
  Bla g 5, 264, 267
Blomia tropicalis, 237, 266
B lymphocytes, fetal, 361–2
bone, inhaled corticosteroids (ICS) and, 160–1
books, educational, 317
boric acid, 244
Brazil see Latin America
breastfeeding, 73, 370
breathing
  exercises, 177
  patterns, aerosol delivery and, 330
breathlessness, perception of, 294–5
British Thoracic Society guidelines, 127, 137, 142, 350
bromhexine, 175
bronchi
  development, 1
  epithelium, 25, 90–1
bronchial hyperresponsiveness (BHR)
  atopy, airway inflammation and asthma and, 20–2
  β_2-agonist therapy and, 156
  mechanisms of virus-induced, 87–9
  prevalence data, 40–2, 43
  see also airway responsiveness
bronchial isomerism, left, 110
'bronchial reactivity', 21
bronchiectasis, 106
bronchiolitis, 83–4
  in asthma aetiology, 54, 76–7, 84–5
  immunomodulatory mechanisms of asthma and, 86–7
  obliterans, 196
  see also respiratory syncytial virus
bronchitis
  'asthmatic', 38
  chronic, 38
  'wheezy', 38
bronchoalveolar lavage (BAL), 109, 112
  in acute asthma, 189, 190
bronchoconstriction, suggestion-induced, 297–8
bronchodilators, 121–2
  in developing countries, 383–4, 385, 386, 387
  indications, 133
  responsiveness, in infants, 3, 11
  trial of therapy, 114
  see also β_2-agonists
bronchogenic cyst, 105

bronchomalacia, 108–9
  acquired, 108–9
  congenital, 108, 109
bronchopulmonary dysplasia
  aerosol delivery, 334, 341
  in developing countries, 380
bronchoscopy
  fibreoptic (FOB), 105, 112–13
  rigid, 107–8
Brown Norway (BN) rat, 87
bruising, easy, 161
budesonide
  in chronic asthma, 159
    growth effects, 160
    HPA axis suppression, 159
  dose equivalents, 152, 159
  economic evaluation, 350–3
  in infants and small children, 122, 132–7
    delivery devices, 123
    efficacy and safety, 132–5, 138–9
    growth effects, 135–6
    pharmacokinetics, 136
  inhaled dose delivered, 338, 341
  intranasal, in allergic rhinitis, 230
  trial of therapy, 114
bulbar palsy, 102

caffeine, 240
calycins, 267
candidate genes, 52, 70, 71
candidiasis, oropharyngeal, 158, 161
Can f 1 see dog(s), allergens
capsules, for food challenges, 286, 287
carbohydrate intolerance, 280
carbon dioxide tension ($PaCO_2$), 194
  transcutaneous, 113, 198
  in ventilated patients, 201–2
care givers
  acute asthma management, 197
  adherence to therapy, 126
  see also parents
carpets
  acaricide treatments, 240–1
  animal allergens, 243
  shampooing, 240
case–control studies, 35
castor beans, 56
cat(s)
  allergens (Fel d 1), 241–2, 261, 269
    airborne, 259
    antenatal sensitization, 364
    environmental control, 242–4
    immunotherapy, 248, 265
    sensitization predicting asthma, 369
    sensitization rates, 74, 241–2
  in developing countries, 385
  removal from home, 242–3
  washing, 243, 244
cataract, 161

catarrhal child, 101
CD4+ T-helper lymphocytes, 22
   maturation of responses, 78
   in viral respiratory infections, 87, 92
   see also Th-1 lymphocytes; Th-2 lymphocytes
CD8+ T lymphocytes, 22
   in viral respiratory infections, 87, 92
CD14, 368, 369
   gene polymorphism, 79, 368
CD16, 362
cetirizine, 29, 230, 369
C fibres, sensory, 89
chemokines, in RSV infection, 86
chest
   auscultation, 103
   deformity, 103
   palpation, 103
chest radiograph (CXR)
   in acute asthma, 198
   in asthma diagnosis, 109–10, 381
chest wall
   compliance, 2
   development, 2
   distortion in preterm infants, 2, 3
child, direct involvement, 315–16
Childhood Asthma Management Program (CAMP), 59, 143
   inhaled corticosteroids (ICS), 160
   nedocromil sodium therapy, 158
children, *see* school-aged children; small children
China, asthma prevalence, 40–2
Chlamydia pneumoniae, 86
Chlamydia trachomatis, 86
chloral hydrate, 5–6
chloride ions (Cl⁻), in exercise-induced asthma, 212
chlorine exposure, 215, 218
chlorofluorocarbons (CFCs), 152, 159, 332–3
chlorpheniramine, 230
chlorpyrifos, 244
cholinergic nerves
   in nasal-bronchial reflex, 226–7
   virus-induced activation, 88–9
chromosome 5q31, 79
chromosome 5q, 20, 71
chromosome 6, 71
chromosomes, regions implicated in asthma, 52, 71
chronic asthma
   management, 149–88
   therapeutic algorithms, 133, 151, 152
   see also episodic asthma; persistent asthma
chronic bronchitis, asthma overlap, 38
chronic obstructive pulmonary disease, inhaled corticosteroids (ICS) and, 161, 162
Churg–Strauss syndrome, 168
Ciba symposium, asthma definition, 36, 37
ciliary dyskinesia, primary (PCD, Kartagener's syndrome), 101, 102, 106–7, 112
Cladosporium
   allergen, 271

   immunotherapy, 249
clarithromycin, 174
Clean Air Act and Amendments, 55–6
clenbuterol, 218
clinical presentation, in developing countries, 379–81
clinicians *see* physicians
clubbing, digital, 103
cockroach allergens, 244–5, 257, 266–9
   airborne, 259, 268
   in developing countries, 385
   environmental control, 244–5, 268–9
   recombinant, 264
   sensitization, role in asthma, 360, 370
   structure and function, 261
cohort studies, 35–6, 38
cold air
   challenge
      exercise testing with, 214
      in infants, 10
      montelukast therapy and, 167
   exercise-induced asthma and, 211–12, 213, 215
   nasal, lower airway effects, 226–7
   protection against exposure, 216, 218
colds, viral, 101
collagen, deposition in airway wall, 25, 26
communication strategies, 314–16
community health centres, 384, 385
competence, inhalation techniques, 328, 329, 336–7
complementary medicine, 177–8
complement receptor 3 (Mac-1), 29
compliance, *see* adherence
compression pressure, in raised volume forced expiration, 8, 9
computed tomography (CT scan), 108
computer games, 317, 321
concrete operational stage, 318
congenital abnormalities, 104–6
congenital heart disease, 108, 380
consultation programs, economic studies, 354
contracts, written, 321
control, perceived, 300
controller medications, 154–5
   economic evaluation studies, 350–3
   in infants and small children, 127–40
   see also anti-inflammatory drugs
cooking
   in developing countries, 383, 384–5
   nitrogen oxides from, 56
coping styles, 300
corticosteroids (CS)
   in developing countries, 385–6
   inhaled, *see* inhaled corticosteroids
   intranasal, in allergic rhinitis, 229–30, 231
   intravenous
      in acute asthma, 199, 201
      in infants and small children, 142
   mechanisms of action, 25, 29
   mucolytic effects, 175
   oral, 170

corticosteroids *continued*
    in acute asthma, 199, 201
    in food allergy, 288
    in infants and small children, 142
    trial of therapy, 114
  resistance, 25, 161, 170–4
  systemic
    in acute asthma, 199, 200–1
    in infants and small children, 142
cost-effectiveness analysis, 348, 349–50
  controller medication, 353
  guideline development and, 354
cost-of-illness studies, 348–9
costs
  identification studies, 348–9
  treatment non-adherence, 295–6
  see also economics
cotinine, 57
cough, chronic, 99–120
  ancillary investigations, 109–13
  clinical assessment, 100–4
  in developing countries, 380
  diagnosis of asthma, 113–14
  history taking, 101–3
  maternal assessment of severity, 115
  physical examination, 103–4
  serious underlying conditions, 104–9
  significance, 100
  specificity for asthma, 114–15
  trial of asthma therapy, 113–14
creatine phosphokinase (CPK)-MB, serum, 200
cromoglycate (cromolyn)
  in chronic asthma, 157–8
  delivery devices, 332
  in developing countries, 385–6
  economic evaluations, 350, 351, 352, 353
  in exercise-induced asthma, 216, 217
  in food allergy, 288
  in infants and small children, 127–32
    indications, 133
    safety and efficacy, 127–31, 157
  inhaled dose delivered, 340
  intranasal, 229
  mode of action, 157
  nebulized, 122, 123–4
  trial of therapy, 114
cross-sectional surveys, 35, 38
croup, in asthma aetiology, 54
crying child, aerosol delivery, 330, 339
cultural beliefs, incorporating, 314
cyclic 3′,5′ adenosine monophosphate (cAMP), 177
cycling, 213, 215
cyclosporin-A (CsA), 173
cystatins, 269
cysteinyl leukotrienes (cysLT), 25, 165–6
  receptors, 166
cystic fibrosis (CF), 102, 106–7
  lung deposition studies, 340–41
  signs, 103, 104

cytokines
  in airway inflammation, 22
  blood levels, 111–12
  feto-placental, 362
  genetic polymorphisms, 20
  leukotriene modifying agents and, 169
  mast cell-derived, 24
  neonates, 362
  in virus infections, 86–7, 90–1
cytomegalovirus infection, congenital, 103

dampness, in home, 53–4
decongestants, nasal, 231
definitions of asthma
  clinical, 99–100
  epidemiological studies, 36, 37, 67–8
  genetic studies, 69, 70
  see also diagnosis
dehumidification, 241, 245
dendritic cells, 22
dermatitis, atopic, 110, 265, 369
Dermatophagoides farinae, 237, 265
Dermatophagoides pteronyssinus, 237, 265, 266
Der p 1, 257, 259, 260
  recombinant, 262
Der p 2, 259, 265
desensitization therapy, *see* immunotherapy
developing countries, 377–90
  clinical presentation, 379–81
  diagnosis of asthma, 381–3
  management of asthma, 383–7
  pharmacotherapy, 164, 383–4, 385–6, 387
  prevalence of asthma, 377–9
  prevention of asthma, 388
  risk factors for asthma, 379
development
  lung *see* lung development
  respiratory system, 1–5
dexamethasone, 169, 173
diagnosis, 99–120
  clinical categories, 99–100
  in developing countries, 381–3
  differential, 104–9
  history taking, 101–3
  investigations, 109–13
  nomenclature, 100
  physical examination, 103–4
  trial of therapy, 113–14
  see also definitions of asthma
diaphragm, development, 2, 4
diazanon, 244
diet
  elimination, 281, 287, 288
  fetal allergic sensitization and, 364–5
  maternal, avoidance of allergens, 370
digital clubbing, 103
disodium cromoglycate (DSCG), *see* cromoglycate
distressed child, aerosol delivery to, 330, 338–9

DNA vaccines, 368
    plasmid, 265, 289
doctors, *see also* physicians
dog(s)
    allergens (Can f 1), 241–2, 261, 269
        airborne, 259
        environmental control, 242–4
        immunotherapy, 248
    in developing countries, 385
    sensitization, 74
domperidone, 107
doping regulations, athletes, 218
DPIs *see* dry powder inhalers
drug therapy, *see* pharmacotherapy
dry powder inhalers (DPIs), 328, 332, 334–5
    adequacy of use, 334
    in developing countries, 386
    dose delivered, 338
    inhaled corticosteroids, 336
dust mites, *see* house dust mites
dysanapsis, 5
dysphonia, 158, 161
dyspnoea
    differential diagnosis, 195–6
    perception, 295

Early Treatment of the Atopic Child (ETAC) trial, 111
economics, 347–57
    comparative analyses, 349–50
    concepts, 348
    in developing countries, 383–4, 387
    education and consultation programs, 354
    evaluation methods, 348–50
    guideline development and, 354
    pharmacotherapy, 350–3
ECP *see* eosinophilic cationic protein
eczema, atopic, 110, 265, 369
education, 293–4, 309–26
    age 2–5 years, 317–18
    age 6–12 years, 318–21
    age 13–17 years, 321
    basic needs, 310–16
    in developing countries, 383, 384
    economic studies, 354
    future directions, 301, 302
    group programs, 316
    individualized programs, 316–17
    inhaler use, 153, 331
    key behaviour change principles, 310–14
    key behaviours, 310
    key communication strategies, 314–16
    key information, 310
    methods, 316–17
    parents, 294, 321–2
    physicians, 303
effectiveness, measures of, 349–50
electric blankets, 241
electrocardiography, in acute asthma, 200
electrostatic charge, plastic spacers, 334, 338

e-mail, 321
emergency departments
    in developing countries, 383–4, 385
    treatment non-adherence and, 295–6
emotions, health care behaviour and, 297–8
endothelins, 26
endothelium, leukocyte rolling, 29
endotoxin, 78–9, 269
endurance sports, 214–15, 217, 218
England, asthma prevalence, 40, 41
English-speaking communities, genetic diversity, 366–7
environmental control, 237–45, 258
    animal allergens, 242–4
    cockroach allergens, 244–5, 268–9
    in developing countries, 383, 384–5
    fungal allergens, 245
    house dust mites, 239–41
environmental factors
    in acute asthma exacerbations, 197
    in asthma initiation, 20, 53–8
    in exercise-induced asthma, 215
    in fetal allergic sensitization, 366–7
    see also gene–environment interactions
environmental tobacco smoke (ETS)
    asthma exacerbation and, 191, 245–6
    asthma risk and, 56, 57–8
    in developing countries, 383
    wheezing illness in childhood and, 365–6
enzymatic properties, allergens, 259–60
eosinophilic cationic protein (ECP), 76, 88, 91
    serum, 111–12, 126
    soluble (s-ECP), in exercise-induced asthma, 212
eosinophilic gastrointestinal disease, 288
eosinophils, 24
    in airway remodelling, 27
    in airway wall, 26, 29, 30
    cromoglycate actions, 157
    in exercise-induced asthma, 212
    immunotherapy and, 247
    proteins, 24, 30
    respiratory infections and, 76, 91
eotaxin, 25
epidemics, asthma, 48, 49–50
epidemiology
    bacterial infections and asthma, 85–6
    definition, 35
    economic costs of asthma, 349
    pediatric asthma, 35–66
        asthma definitions, 36, 37
        descriptive epidemiology, 38–50
        methods, 38
        problems, 36–8
        questionnaire methods, 36–8
    techniques, 35–6
    viral infections and asthma, 83–5
epidermal growth factor, 26
epinephrine (adrenaline), 155, 288, 386
episodic asthma, 178

episodic asthma *continued*
    pharmacotherapy, 156–7
    therapeutic algorithms, 133, 151, 152
    see also chronic asthma
epithelium, airway, 25, 90–1
erythromycin, 85–6, 173–4
E-selectin, 29
essential drug lists, 383, 385, 386
ethnic differences, 299
    morbidity/hospitalization data, 43, 46–7
    mortality data, 48–9
    prevalence data, 39, 40
Euroglyphus maynei, 237, 266
evidence-based medicine, 150
exacerbations of asthma, *see* acute asthma
exercise
    anti-asthma therapy before, 216–18
    challenge testing, 13, 213–14
        in developing countries, 378, 382, 383
exercise-induced asthma (EIA), 211–22
    diagnosis, 213–14
    leukotriene-modifying agents, 166–7, 169, 216, 217–18
    management, 216–18
        drug treatment, 216–18
        general measures, 216
    participation in sports and, 218–19
    pathogenesis, 166, 211–13
    physical training, athletes and sport and, 214–15
    salmeterol, 140, 217
expectorants, 175
expiratory reserve volume (ERV), 12
expiratory time, in infants, 10
extracellular matrix, break down, 27

facemasks
    crying/distressed infants, 330
    spacers/holding chambers with, 123, 124–5, 333–4
family
    aggregation studies, 52, 69
    functioning, health care behaviour and, 298–9, 385
Family Asthma Management System, 302
family history, natural history of asthma and, 58
farms, animal, asthma risk, 78
fatty acids, polyunsaturated (PUFA), 365
fears, underlying, 315
feeding problems, 102
FEF_{25-75}, in acute asthma, 191
Fel d 1 *see* cat(s), allergens
fenoterol, 49–50, 155
feto-placental unit, Th-2 cytokines, 362–3
fetus
    allergic sensitization, 361–7
        genetic/environmental diversity and, 366–7
        maternal nutrition and, 364–5
        modification, 363–4
        route, 22, 363
    chest wall development, 2
    lung development, 1–2

$FEV_{0.5}$, 9–10
$FEV_{0.75}$, 9–10
FEV_1, 12
    in acute asthma, 191
    arterial blood gases and, 193, 194
    changes in childhood, 14, 15
    in exercise-induced asthma, 214
    measurement, 9–10, 13
fibreoptic bronchoscopy (FOB), 105, 112–13
fibroblasts, 26, 27
fibronectin, 25
Finland, asthma prevalence, 40, 41
fish oil supplementation, 365
FK506, 173
FLAP (5-lipoxygenase activating protein), 164–5, 169
flow
    at a fraction of FVC, 13
    limitation, 13
    measurements, in infants, 10
    rates, in acute asthma, 191–2
flunisolide, intranasal, 229
fluticasone propionate
    dose equivalents, 152, 159
    economic evaluation, 352, 353
    growth effects, 160
    HPA axis suppression, 159–60
    salmeterol with, 170
food(s)
    adverse reactions, 280–1
    drug interactions, 168, 172–3
    pollen allergen cross-reactivity, 270
    storage, for cockroach control, 245
food allergy, 279–92
    differential diagnosis, 280–1
    future considerations, 290
    historical information, 282–3
    laboratory testing, 283–7
        food challenges, 284–7
        in vitro, 284
        in vivo, 283–4
    management, 287–9
        avoidance and interval challenge, 287
        medication, 287–8
        vaccines, 288–9
    mechanisms, 282
    natural history and prevention, 289–90
    prevalence, 279–80
    respiratory symptoms, 281
    timing of symptoms, 281–2
food challenge, 284–7
    double-blind, placebo-controlled (DBPCFC), 283, 284, 285–7
    interval, after food avoidance, 287
    open, 284–5
    oral mucosa, 283–4
    single-blind (SBFC), 285
    vehicles, 287
Food and Drug Administration (FDA), 122, 143, 168

forced expiration
   maximal expiratory flow–volume technique, 12–13
   raised volume method, 7–10
   tidal volume method, 5–6, 8
forced expiratory flow–time, 13
forced vital capacity (FVC), 10, 12
foreign body, endobronchial, 101–2, 107–8
formaldehyde, 246
formal operations stage, 321
formoterol, 170
   doping regulations, 218
   in exercise-induced asthma, 217
France, asthma prevalence, 40, 41
FRC *see* functional residual capacity
freezing, dust mites, 241
fruits
   dietary intake, 24, 364–5
   pollen allergen cross-reactivity, 270
functional residual capacity (FRC), 12
   in acute asthma, 193
   variability in infants, 6
fungicides, 245
fungi (molds)
   allergens, 245, 257, 271
      airborne, 259
      immunotherapy, 248–9
      properties, 261, 262
   allergic bronchopulmonary syndromes, 197
   asthma risk and, 53–4, 74, 75, 245
   environmental control, 245
furosemide, in exercise-induced asthma, 212, 217
FVC (forced vital capacity), 10, 12

gallamine, 88
games, educational, 317, 321
gamma scintigraphy, planar, 340
gas dilution method, 12
gastrointestinal disease, eosinophilic, 288
gastrointestinal (GI) tract
   fetal, immune function, 363
   inhaled drug dose, 335
   microbial flora, 368–9
gastro-oesophageal reflux, 102, 107, 127
   in acute asthma exacerbations, 197
   in developing countries, 380
   vs acute asthma, 196
gender differences
   airway geometry, 5, 53
   asthma risk, 52–3, 72–3, 378
   morbidity/hospitalization data, 48
   natural history of asthma, 58
gene–environment interactions, 20, 51–2
general anaesthesia, in respiratory failure, 203–4
genes
   candidate, 52, 70, 71
   strategies to identify asthma-related, 70
genetic association studies, 52, 71–2
   linkage disequilibrium, 72
   population stratification, 72

genetic diversity, allergic sensitization and, 366–7
genetic factors
   allergic rhinitis and asthma, 224
   asthma development, 20, 52, 68–72
genetic linkage analysis, 52, 70–1
genome-wide searches, 70, 71
glaucoma, 161
Global Initiative for Asthma (GINA), 313, 350, 382
glucocorticoids, *see* corticosteroids
glutathione-S-transferases (GST), 264, 267
glyceryl guaicolate, 175
GM-CSF *see* granulocyte macrophage colony-stimulating factor
goals, treatment, 311–12
gold salts, 173
grandmothers, 381
granulocyte macrophage colony-stimulating factor (GM-CSF), 20, 26
   fetal effects, 363
   in virus infections, 90
granulocytes, effects of viruses, 91–2
grass pollen, 262, 270
group instruction, 316, 320, 322
growth
   fetal, atopy risk and, 365
   inhaled corticosteroids and, 135–6, 160
growth factors, 26
guaifenasin, 175
guidelines
   in developing countries, 385, 387
   economic basis for development, 354
gut *see* gastrointestinal (GI) tract

H1-antihistamines, in allergic rhinitis, 230–1
halothane anaesthesia, 204
Harrison's sulcus, 103
hay fever (seasonal allergic rhinitis), 257, 270
   antihistamines, 230–1
   asthma risk, 53, 74–5
   intranasal corticosteroids, 229–30
   natural history of asthma and, 58
headache, intravenous immunoglobulin therapy and, 171
head circumference, at birth, 365
health belief model, 300
heart disease, congenital, 108, 380
heart rate, in exercise testing, 213–14
heat loss, respiratory, in exercise-induced asthma, 211–12
height, inhaled corticosteroids and, 135–6, 160
heliox (helium-oxygen mixture), 203
helminth infections, 363
heparin, 24
   inhaled, 217
hepatitis A, 368
hepatitis C virus, 172
herbal medicines, 177
Hering–Breuer reflex, 10
high altitude, for dust mite avoidance, 239

histamine, plasma, 284
histamine challenge testing, 10, 13, 113
  nasal, 227
history-taking, 101–3
  in developing countries, 381, 382
  in food allergy, 282–3
HLA-DR-positive cells, fetal, 363
HLA-G, 363
hoarse voice, 158, 161
holding chambers *see* spacers/holding chambers
homeopathy, 177
hormonal factors, in asthma risk, 73
horoscope effect, 364
hospitalization
  controller medication and, 353
  in developing countries, 387
  for intensive adherence interventions, 303
  in paediatric asthma, 42–8
  treatment non-adherence and, 295–6
house dust endotoxin, 78
house dust mites, 237–41, 265–6
  allergens, 257, 259, 265–6
    airborne, 259, 265
    antenatal exposure, 363
    environmental levels, 258
    immunotherapy, 248, 265
    levels of exposure, 54, 56, 238
    recombinant, 262, 263
    structure and function, 261
  allergy testing, 110
  avoidance, 239–41
    for asthma prevention, 370
    clinical trials, 238–9
    in developing countries, 384
    methods, 239–41
  sensitization
    antenatal, 361, 364
    in asthma, 238
    asthma risk, 73–4, 360, 369
    in developing countries, 382–3
housing, in developing countries, 384
humidifiers, 245
humidity, reduction, 241, 245
hydranethylnon, 244
hydro-fluoro-alkane (HFA) propellant, 152, 159, 332, 333, 334
hydro-fluoro-carbon (HFC) propellant, 332
5-hydroperoxy-eicosatetraenoic acid (5-HPETE), 165
hygiene hypothesis, 54, 77–9, 367–8
hypercapnia, 194
  permissive, 202
hyperinflation, 12, 193
hypertonic saline solution, 175, 383
hypnosis, 298
hypokalaemia, 200, 201
hypothalamic-pituitary-adrenal (HPA) axis, 159–60, 201
hypoxaemia, in acute asthma, 193

hypoxia, reduced sensitivity to, 193–4
ICAM-1, *see* intercellular adhesion molecule 1
ICS, *see* inhaled corticosteroids
identity by descent (ibd), 71
IgE, 257
  allergens and, 258
  in amniotic fluid, 363
  CD14 gene polymorphism and, 79
  cord blood levels, 362
  intravenous immunoglobulin and, 171
  maturation of responses, 78–9
  monoclonal antibodies, 176–7, 288–9
  receptors, 24–5
  RSV-specific, 55, 76
  serum total, 53, 111, 369, 382
IgG, fetal immune response and, 363–4
immediate hypersensitivity, 21, 282
immune system
  development of mature responses, 77–9
  fetal development, 361–2
immunodeficiencies, 106, 107
immunostimulatory sequences (ISS), 265, 289
immunotherapy, 246–50
  during pregnancy, 364
  efficacy, 247–9
  for food hypersensitivity, 288–9
  indications, 249–50
  mechanisms, 246–7, 371
  recombinant allergens for, 263–5
  rush, 246, 249
  safety, 249
  for tertiary prevention of asthma, 370–1
incidence
  definition, 35
  paediatric asthma, 42, 44–5
income, asthma mortality and, 49
individualized education programs, 316–17
indoor environment
  air pollution, 56–8, 245–6
  allergens, *see* allergens, indoor
infants
  aerosol therapy, 330–2, 334, 341–2
  chronic cough and/or wheezing, 99–120
  cromoglycate therapy, 127–32, 157
  inhaled corticosteroids, *see* inhaled corticosteroids (ICS), in infants and small children
  lung function data, 10–11
  lung function measurement, 5–10
  management of asthma, 121–47
  maturation of immune system, 77–9
  respiratory system development, 2–5
  of smoking mothers, 365–6
  see also neonates; preterm infants; small children
infections
  in development and course of asthma, 83–97
  in early life (hygiene hypothesis), 54, 77–9, 367–8, 369
inflammation
  airway, *see* airway inflammation

in rhinitis and sinusitis, 226
  spread from upper to lower airways, 228–9
inflammatory cells, 24–5
  effects of viruses, 91–2
inflammatory markers, diagnostic role, 111–12
inflation pressure, in raised volume forced
    expiration, 8–9, 10
influenza virus, 87, 92
information
  key, 310
  repeating, 312
inhalant therapy, 153, 327–46
  choice of drug/device combination, 335–6, 339–40
  correct technique, 294, 312
  delivery devices, 327, 330–5
    in acute asthma, 200, 334
    CFC replacement, 332–3
    in developing countries, 385, 386
    infants and small children, 123–5
    see also dry powder inhalers; metered dose
      inhalers, pressurized; nebulizers;
      spacers/holding chambers
  dose of drug, 337–42
    assessment of dose delivered, 338–9
    interpretation of studies, 336–7
    in vitro assessment, 337–8
    limitation of deposition studies, 342
    lung deposition studies, 340–1
    pharmacodynamic studies, 339–40
  education on use, 153, 331
  see also β_2-agonists; cromoglycate; inhaled
    corticosteroids
inhaled corticosteroids (ICS)
  β_2-agonist interactions, 156
  in chronic asthma, 157, 158–61
    add-on/sparing therapy, 162–70
    efficacy and safety, 158–9
    growth effects, 160
    HPA axis and, 159–60
    insensitivity, 25, 161, 170–4
    local effects, 161, 162
    plus theophylline, 163
    skeletal effects, 160–1
    therapeutic role, 161
  delivery systems, 125, 332, 334
  dose delivered, 338, 339
  dose equivalents, 152
  economic evaluation, 350–3
  in exercise-induced asthma, 216
  importance of therapy, 151
  in infants and small children, 29, 132–7
    alveolus formation and, 161, 162
    efficacy and safety, 132–5, 138–9
    growth effects, 135–6
    indications, 133
    pharmacokinetics, 136
  montelukast combined with, 169
  in preterm intubated infants, 334
  trial of therapy, 114

inhalers *see* dry powder inhalers; metered dose
    inhalers, pressurized
inner-city areas
  cockroach allergy, 266
  health care behaviours, 299
  psychosocial interventions, 302
insecticides, 244–5, 268–9
inspiratory capacity (IC), 12
inspiratory flow rates (IFR)
  in children, 327, 328
  DPI use and, 330, 334–5
  inhaled dose delivery and, 340–1
inspiratory reserve volume (IRV), 12
intensive, hospital-based adherence interventions,
    303
intensive care unit (ICU), inhalant therapy, 334
intercellular adhesion molecule 1 (ICAM-1), 28–9
  effects of viruses, 90, 92
  soluble (sICAM-1), 28–9
intercostal muscles, development, 2, 4
interferon-gamma (IFN-γ), 22, 28–9
  Alternaria sensitization and, 75
  immune system maturation and, 77, 78, 369
  TH_1/TH_2 balance and, 87, 362–3
  therapeutic use, 176
  in virus infections, 86–7, 92
interleukin-1 (IL-1), 92
interleukin-2 (IL-2), 161, 362
interleukin-2 (IL-2) receptor, soluble, 30
interleukin-4 (IL-4), 20
  antenatal exposure, 362, 363
  monoclonal antibody, 176
  in RSV infection, 86–7
  serum, 112
  in steroid-resistant asthma, 161
interleukin-5 (IL-5), 20
  monoclonal antibody, 176
  serum, 112
  in viral infections, 87
interleukin-6 (IL-6), 90, 91
interleukin-8 (IL-8), 25
  in virus infections, 90, 91, 92
interleukin-10 (IL-10), 22, 369
  feto-placental production, 362
  individual variations in response, 79
  RSV infections and, 77
interleukin-11 (IL-11), 90
interleukin-12 (IL-12), 22, 368
  recombinant human (rhIL-12), 176
  in RSV infection, 86
interleukin-13 (IL-13), 20
intermediate phenotypes, 69–70
International Classification of Disease (ICD), 48
International Consensus Report (ICR), 350
International Pediatric Consensus Statement, 137
International Study of Asthma and Allergy in
    Children (ISAAC), 35, 36–8, 40, 377, 378–9
internet web-sites, 321
interrupter technique, 113

interstitial lung disease, 108, 196
intestinal parasites, 382
intranasal corticosteroids, in allergic rhinitis, 229–30
intravenous immunoglobulins (IVIG), 170–2
iodide, 175
ipratropium bromide
   in acute asthma, 199, 201, 202
   in chronic asthma, 175
   economic evaluation, 353
   in exercise-induced asthma, 217
   in infants and small children, 141–2
isoallergens, 259
isoeffrine, 155
isoflurane anaesthesia, 204
isoprenaline (isoproterenol), 88, 155
isovolume shifts, in acute asthma, 191

Japan, asthma prevalence, 40, 41
jet nebulizers *see* nebulizers

Kartagener's syndrome (primary ciliary dyskinesia), 101, 102, 106–7, 112
ketamine anaesthesia, 204
ketotifen, 369, 386
knowledge, self-management and, 293–5

labels, diagnostic, 38, 67–8
labial testing/challenge, 283–4
lactobacilli, 368
lamina propria, eosinophil infiltration, 26, 30
lamina reticularis, thickening of, 25, 26
β-laminin, 25
language, using appropriate, 314
laryngeal cleft, 102, 107
laryngomalacia, 104–5, 106
late phase reaction, 21–2
   exercise-induced asthma, 212–13
   in food allergy, 282, 286
Latin America
   diagnosis of asthma, 383
   management of asthma, 387
   prevalence of asthma, 378–9
learned helplessness, 300
left bronchial isomerism, 110
leukocyte rolling, 29
leukotriene A_4 (LTA_4), 165
leukotriene B_4 (LTB_4), 25, 91, 165
leukotriene C_4 (LTC_4), 91, 165
leukotriene D_4 (LTD_4), 140, 165, 166
leukotriene E_4 (LTE_4), 165, 212
leukotriene-modifying agents
   in allergic rhinitis, 231
   in chronic asthma, 164–9
      administration, 167–8
      adverse reactions, 168
      drug–drug interactions, 168
      efficacy, 166–7
      food interactions, 168
   in exercise-induced asthma, 166–7, 169, 216, 217–18
   in infants and small children, 140
   mechanisms of action, 154–5, 164–6
   role in asthma therapy, 168–9
leukotriene receptor antagonists, 25, 140, 166
leukotriene receptors, 166
leukotrienes, 24, 25
   cysteinyl (cysLT), 25, 165–6
   synthesis pathway, 165
leukotriene synthesis inhibitors, 140
linkage analysis, genetic, 52, 70–1
linkage disequilibrium, 72
linolenic acid, 365
lipocalins, 267, 269
lipopolysaccharide (LPS), 78–9, 368
5-lipoxygenase, 164–5, 166
   corticosteroid therapy and, 169
   gene (ALOX5) polymorphisms, 166
Listeria monocytogenes, heat-killed, 368
liver function, leukotriene-modifying agents and, 168
locus of control, 300
loratadine, 231
lower airways, influence of upper airways, 226–9
lower respiratory infections (LRI)
   in asthma development, 75–7, 84–5
   in developing countries, 379
L-selectin, 29
lung
   aerosol deposition studies, 340–2
   compliance, in childhood, 5
lung development
   in childhood, 3–5
   inhaled corticosteroids (ICS) and, 161, 162
   in utero, 1–2
   maternal nutrition and, 365
   maternal smoking and, 366
lung disease
   chronic, of prematurity, 108
   interstitial, 108, 196
   suppurative and infective, 106–7
lung function
   in acute asthma, 191–2
   after exercise, 213, 214
   after viral respiratory infections, 55, 76–7, 84–5
   in asthmatic children, 13–15
      changes during childhood, 14–15
      variability, 13–14
   data in infants, 10–11
   maternal smoking *in utero* and, 366
   measurement
      in children aged 2–5 years, 11
      in children aged over 5 years, 11–13
      in infants, 5–10
   monitoring response to therapy, 125
   perception of reduced, 295
   respiratory symptoms and, 10–11
   tests, 113
      in acute asthma, 198
      after food challenge, 287
      in developing countries, 381

lung volumes, 12
    in acute asthma, 193
    in forced expiration methods, 8
    increase in childhood, 3–5
    landmarks, in forced expiration methods, 6, 8
lymphocyte function associated antigen 1 (LFA-1), 29
lymphocytes, immunotherapy and, 247

M_2 muscarinic receptors, 88–9
    antagonists, 177
Mac-1, 29
macrolide antibiotics, 173–4
macrophage inflammatory protein (MIP)-1α, 90
macrophages
    alveolar, 22, 24–5
    effects of viruses, 92
magnesium sulphate, intravenous, 203
major histocompatibility complex (MHC)
    class II, 22
    materno-fetal mismatching, 367
    in pregnancy, 363
male sex, asthma risk, 52–3, 72–3, 378
management of asthma
    behaviours required at different ages, 317–22
    in children aged 5 to 18 years, 149–88
    in developing countries, 383–7
    in infants and small children, 121–47
    nonpharmacological approaches, 237–56
    see also pharmacotherapy; self-management; treatment
Mantoux test, 109
mast cells, 24, 247
matrix metalloproteinases (MMPs), 26–7
mattress covers, 239, 240, 243
maximal expiratory flow rate (MEFR), 191
maximal expiratory flow–volume (MEFV) curves, 9, 191
    in acute asthma, 191, 192
    in vocal cord dysfunction, 195, 196
maximal expiratory flow–volume technique, 12–13, 191
maximal flow at functional residual capacity see V'_{maxFRC}
MDIs see metered dose inhalers, pressurized
measles, 368, 369
mechanical ventilation, 201–3
    inhalant therapy during, 334
mechanisms of asthma, 19–33
media, educational, 317
medication, see pharmacotherapy
messages, repeating, 312
metabolic acidosis, in acute asthma, 195
metaproterenol (orciprenaline), 155, 163
metered dose inhalers, pressurized (pMDIs), 327
    in acute asthma, 200, 334
    aerosol delivery, 330–2
    CFC replacement, 332–3
    competence in use, 329
    in developing countries, 386

    dose delivered, 338, 340–1
    energy source, 328
    in infants and small children, 123, 124–5
    inhaled corticosteroids, 335–6
    spacers and holding chambers see spacers/holding chambers
    treatment adherence, 295, 296
methacholine challenge testing, 13, 113, 190
    in developing countries, 383
    in infants, 10
methotrexate (MTX), 172–3
methylprednisoline (MPn)
    in acute asthma, 199, 201
    in infants and small children, 142
    macrolide antibiotics and, 173–4
methylxanthines, 175
    see also aminophylline; theophylline
MHC see major histocompatibility complex
microbial burden in early life, 54, 77–9, 367–8
microbial flora, gut, 368–9
milk hypersensitivity, 279, 280
mites
    house dust, see house dust mites
    storage (nonpyroglyphic), 266
molds, see fungi
monocytes, 24–5, 92
montelukast
    adverse effects, 168
    in chronic asthma, 167, 168
    combined with ICS, 169
    drug interactions, 168
    efficacy, 167
    in exercise-induced asthma, 216
    indications, 169
    in infants and small children, 123, 140
    mechanism of action, 165, 166
morbidity, paediatric asthma, 42–8
mortality, 35
    paediatric asthma, 48–50
        in different countries, 49, 50, 51
        New Zealand epidemic, 49–50
        time trends, 48–9
    psychological factors, 295
    see also near-fatal asthma
mothers
    exaggeration of child's symptoms, 115
    factors affecting asthma risk, 73
    smoking, 56, 57–8, 366
    see also parents; pregnancy
Mothers of Asthmatics, Inc., 313
motivation
    adherence see adherence
    for behaviour change, 310–11
mouse urinary protein, 259, 261, 269
mouth breathing, 229, 330
mucolytics, 175
Munchausen's syndrome by proxy, 115
muscarinic receptor antagonists, 175, 177
myeloperoxidase, soluble (s-MPO), 212

myopathy, 202

nasal-bronchial reflex, 226–7
nasal decongestants, 231
nasal lavage, 112
nasal obstruction
   mouth breathing caused by, 228
   treatment to alleviate, 231
nasal polyps, 103, 104
National Ambulatory Medical Care Survey
      (NAMCS), 46, 349
National Asthma Campaign - Australia, 313
National Asthma Campaign - United Kingdom, 313
National Asthma Education and Prevention
      Program, 294, 313, 350, 382
National Center for Complementary and Alternative
      Medicine, 178
National Cooperative Inner-City Asthma Study, 302
National Health Interview Survey (NHIS), 39, 349
National Health and Nutrition Examination Surveys
      (NHANES), 39
National Heart, Lung and Blood Institute (NHLBI)
   asthma definitions, 37
   medication guidelines, 123, 127, 132, 137, 141, 142
National Hospital Ambulatory Medical Care Survey
      (NHAMCS), 46
National Hospital Discharge Survey (NHDS), 42–3,
      349
National Institute of Child Health and Human
      Development (NICHHD), 143
National Jewish Medical and Research Center Lung
      LINE, 313
National Medical Expenditure Survey (NMES), 349
natural history of asthma, determinants, 58–9
natural killer (NK) cells, 77
near-fatal asthma
   physiological aspects, 193–4
   psychosocial factors, 295
   risk factors, 197–8
Nebuhaler, 125, 338
nebulizers, 114, 327, 330–2
   competence in use, 330
   crying/distressed infant, 330
   dose delivery, 123–4, 338, 340–1
   for infants and small children, 123–4
nedocromil sodium
   in chronic asthma, 158
   in exercise-induced asthma, 216, 217
   in infants and small children, 127, 133
neonates
   aerosol therapy, 334, 340–1
   airway abnormalities, 104–5
   allergic sensitization, 361, 362
   chest wall movement, 2
   immaturity of immune response, 77
   see also infants; preterm infants
neuraminidase, 88
neurokinin A, 89
neurological problems, 102

neuropeptides, 89
neutrophils, 24, 25
   in airway remodelling, 27
   effects of viruses, 91
   in exercise-induced asthma, 212
New Zealand
   asthma epidemic, 49–50, 51
   asthma prevalence, 40, 41
NF-κB, 91
nitric oxide (NO)
   exhaled, 30, 167
   nasal, 106, 112
   in virus infections, 89
nitrogen dioxide, 56, 191, 246
nitrogen oxides, 56
nitrous oxide, 246
nocturnal asthma, PEFR variability, 192
nonadrenergic, noncholinergic neurons, 89
nonpharmacological management, 237–56
nose
   breathing, aerosol delivery and, 329
   exclusion of foreign material, 328, 330
   regulation of lower airways, 226–9
nuclear factor kappa B (NF-κB), 91
nurses
   education by, 317, 322, 384
   school, 320–1
nutrition, maternal, 364–5

obesity, asthma risk, 73
obstructive sleep apnoea (OSA), 101, 105, 108
occupational asthma, 266, 370
oesophageal disease, 107
oral allergy syndrome, 270
oral mucosa, food challenge, 283–4
orciprenaline (metaproterenol), 155, 283–4
Osler, William, 19
outcome measures, 354
outpatient care data, 43–6
ovalbumin, hen's egg, 361, 363
oximetry, 198
oxygen radicals, 24
oxygen tension
   in acute asthma, 193–4, 194
   transcutaneous, 113, 198
oxygen therapy, 199
ozone, 56, 191, 246

pamphlets, educational, 317
'panic–fear' personality, 297
parainfluenza virus (PIV), 83
   airway inflammation and, 90, 91, 92
   airway responsiveness and, 88–9
   in asthma aetiology, 54, 84
   rat model of infection, 87
paralysis, therapeutic, 202
parasitic infections, 380–1, 382
parasympathetic nerves, virus-induced activation,
      88–9

parents
    adherence to therapy, 126
    asthma education, 294, 321–2
    atopy in, 53
    psychological problems, 298–9
    reports of asthma, 38
    smoking, 56, 57–8, 365–6
    treatment adherence, 302
    see also mothers
particle size, airway deposition and, 328, 329
pathology
    acute asthma, 189–90
    asthma, 19–20
peak expiratory flow (rate) (PEF, PEFR), 381
    monitoring, 13, 192, 200, 312
    variability, 192
peak flow meters, 192, 381, 382
pectus carinatum, 103
Pedipress, Inc., 313
Penicillium, 245
Per a 1, 267
perception, symptom, 294–5
Periplaneta americana allergens, 244, 261, 266–7
persistent asthma, 178
    management algorithms, 133, 151, 152
    see also chronic asthma
personality, health care behaviour and, 297
pesticides, 240–1, 244–5, 268–9
pets
    allergens, 241–2
    control of allergens, 242–4
    removal from home, 110–11, 242–3
    see also cat(s); dog(s)
Peyer's patches, fetal, 363
pH, arterial, 194–5
Phadiatop test, 382, 383
pharmacodynamic effects, inhalant therapy, 327, 338–9
pharmacoeconomic analysis, 348
pharmacokinetic studies, inhaled drugs, 341
pharmacotherapy
    acute asthma, 199, 200–1
    chronic asthma, 149–88
        aims, 153
        algorithm (stepwise approach), 151, 152
        classes of medications, 154–5
        complementary and alternative medicine, 177–8
        future perspectives, 175–7
        guidelines, 150–1
        inhaled corticosteroids, 158–61
        mucolytics and expectorants, 175
        muscarinic receptor antagonists, 175
        nedocromil sodium, 158
        routes of administration, 153
        short-acting beta-agonists, 155–7
        sodium cromoglycate, 157–8
        in steroid-resistant patients, 170–4
        steroid-sparing/add-on therapy, 162–70
        in developing countries, 164, 383–4, 385–6, 387

economic evaluation studies, 350–3
exercise-induced asthma, 216–18
in infants and small children, 121–47
    adherence, 126
    confounding factors, 126–7
    delivery devices, 123–5
    indications and timing, 122
    issues specific to this age group, 122–7
    long-term control medications, 127–40
    monitoring response, 125–6
    quick-relief medications, 140–3
    range of medications available, 122–3
    research needs, 143
    stepwise approach, 133
inhaled see inhalant therapy
tertiary prevention of asthma, 369–70
trial of, 113–14
pharyngeal-bronchial reflexes, 227
pharyngomalacia, 104–5
phenotype
    asthma
        components, 100
        in genetic studies, 69, 70
        see also definitions of asthma
    intermediate, 69–70
phosphodiesterase (PDE) inhibitors, 162, 177
phospholipase A2, 164
physical examination, 103–4
    in developing countries, 381, 382
physical training, exercise-induced asthma and, 214–15
physicians
    communication with child, 315–16
    delivery of education, 316–17
    patient relationships, 300–1, 314–15
    reports of asthma, 38
    training, 303
pillow covers, 239, 240, 243
placenta, cytokine production, 362–3
plan
    action, 312, 320
    treatment, 311–12, 322
planar gamma scintigraphy, 340
plasmid DNA vaccines, 265, 289
platelet-activating factor, 92
play, education via, 318
plethysmography, 5–6, 12, 191
pneumonitis
    chronic, of infancy, 108
    nonspecific interstitial, 108
pneumotachograph, 10
pollen, 257, 269–71
    allergens, 262, 270–1
    immunotherapy, 246, 247–8
    sensitization, 74, 369
        antenatal, 362
    role in asthma, 258
    see also hay fever
polymerase chain reaction (PCR), 109

polyunsaturated fatty acids (PUFA), 365
positive end-expiratory pressure (PEEP), intrinsic, 202
positron emission tomography (PET), 340
postmortem studies, 19, 189–90
postnasal drip, 101, 108
    inflammatory material, 228
potassium iodide, 175
potassium, serum, 200
poverty
    asthma prevalence and, 378
    health care behaviour and, 299
pranlukast
    adverse effects, 168
    mechanism of action, 165, 166
predictive markers, asthma, 29, 30, 359, 369
prednisolone
    in acute asthma, 199, 201
    in infants and small children, 142
prednisone
    in acute asthma, 199, 201
    in infants and small children, 142
pregnancy
    allergen avoidance, 370
    as allergic phenomenon, 362–3
    maternal nutrition, 364–5
    maternal smoking, 57, 366
    primary prevention of asthma, 364
    see also fetus
pre-operational stage, 318
preschool children, *see* small children
pressure-support ventilation, 202–3
pressurized metered dose inhalers (pMDIs) *see* metered dose inhalers, pressurized
preterm infants
    chest wall movement, 2, 3
    cromolyn therapy, 130
    in developing countries, 380
    inhaled corticosteroids (ICS) for intubated, 334
prevalence, 35
    food allergy in asthma, 279–80
    paediatric asthma, 38–42, 43
        in developing countries, 377–9
        in different countries, 40, 41–2
        time trends, 39, 40, 77
preventers, 154
prevention
    asthma, 359–76
        in developing countries, 388
        targets, 371–2
    food allergy, 289–90
    primary, 68, 359
        in pregnancy, 364
        targets, 371, 372
    secondary, 68, 359, 369
        targets, 371, 372
    tertiary, 359, 369–71
        allergen avoidance, 370
        in developing countries, 388

        immunotherapy, 370–1
        pharmacotherapy, 369–70
        targets, 371–2
Preventive Allergy Treatment study (PAT), 371
primary ciliary dyskinesia (PCD, Kartagener's syndrome), 101, 102, 106–7, 1112
proinflammatory cells, 24–5
prospective cohort studies, 36
prostaglandin D_2, 24
prostaglandin E_2, 92, 166
9α, 11β prostaglandin F_2, 212
prostanoids, 25
proteolytic enzymes, 259–60
pseudo-bulbar palsy, 102
pseudoephedrine, 231
psychological problems
    interventions, 301–2, 303
    near-fatal asthma and, 295
    parents, 298–9
psychosocial factors
    acute asthma exacerbations, 198
    asthma treatment outcomes, 293–307
pulmonary artery sling, 105, 106
pulmonary aspiration, nasal secretions, 228
pulmonary function, *see* lung function
pulmonary oedema, 108
pulsus paradoxus, 198

questionnaires, in epidemiological studies, 36–8

racial differences *see* ethnic differences
radioallergosorbent testing (RAST), 110–11, 284
ragweed allergen, 262, 265, 270
raised volume forced expiration, 7–10
    compression pressure, 9
    inflation pressure, 8–9
    parameters used, 9–10
    practical considerations, 10
    recommended standard pressures, 9
RANTES, 25, 90, 92
rapid-eye-movement (REM) sleep, 2, 3
rat urinary protein, 259, 261, 269
reassurance, 315
referral to specialists, 354
reinforcement, appropriate behaviour, 312–14
relaxation training, 295, 298
relievers (quick-relief medications), 140–3, 154
residual volume (RV), 12
    in acute asthma, 192, 193
respiratory alkalosis, 194, 195
respiratory distress syndrome (RDS), 334
respiratory failure, refractory, 203–4
respiratory symptoms
    ancillary investigations, 109–13
    days free of, 354
    differential diagnosis, 104–9
    exaggeration, 115
    in food allergy, 281

history taking, 101–3
lung function data and, 10–11
perception, 294–5
physical examination, 103–4
questionnaires, 36–8
see also cough, chronic; wheeze
respiratory syncytial virus (RSV), 83–4
   airway inflammation and, 90, 91, 92
   allergic sensitization and, 84, 85
   in asthma aetiology, 54–5, 75–7, 84
   immunomodulatory mechanisms in asthma and, 86–7, 368
respiratory system, development, 1–5
respiratory tract infections, 83–97
   in asthma development, 54–5, 75–7, 83–6
   asthma exacerbations and, 85, 86
   in developing countries, 379
   passive smoking and, 57
   physical exercise during, 215, 216, 218
   recurrent suppurative, 106–7
retinoids, 364
reverse transcription polymerase chain reaction (RT-PCR), 85
rheumatoid arthritis, 366–7
rhinitis
   allergic, *see* allergic rhinitis
   from birth, 101, 108
rhinovirus (RV) infections
   airway inflammation and, 90, 91, 92
   in asthma development, 55, 85
   asthma exacerbations and, 85
   bronchial hyperresponsiveness and, 87
rib cage, paradoxical movement in infants, 2, 3
rimiterol, 155
risk factors
   acute asthma exacerbations, 121
   asthma development, 50–8, 67–82
      in developing countries, 379
      methodological issues, 35–6, 67–8
rodents, 269
role-playing scenarios, 320, 321
roxithromycin, 174
RSV, *see* respiratory syncytial virus
running, 213, 214

saccharine test, 106
salbutamol (albuterol)
   in acute asthma, 199, 200, 202
   in chronic asthma, 155
   delivery devices, 125, 333
   in developing countries, 386
   doping regulations, 218
   in exercise-induced asthma, 217
   in infants and small children, 141, 142
   inhaled dose delivery, 339–41
   nebulized, 200
salmeterol
   in chronic asthma, 170
   doping regulations, 218
   in exercise-induced asthma, 140, 217
   in infants and small children, 137–40
SAY (Support for Asthmatic Youth), 321
school-aged children (over 5 years)
   acute asthma, 189–209
   aerosol delivery, 329, 330
   asthma education, 318–21
   lung function measurement, 11–13
   management of chronic asthma, 149–88
school-based asthma education, 320–1, 322
seasonal allergic rhinitis, *see* hay fever
seasonal asthma
   allergens causing, 270
   antihistamine therapy, 230–1
   intranasal corticosteroids, 229–30
selectins, 29
self-management
   behaviours at different ages, 317–22
   education *see* education
   future directions, 301–3
   knowledge and skill and, 293–5
   psychosocial factors affecting, 297–307
   skills, 293–5, 312
   training, 302
self-monitoring, 312
self-regulation model of behaviour change, 311
Sendai virus, 88–9
sensory C fibres, 89
severe combined immunodeficiency, 107
severity of asthma, determinants, 58–9
sex differences, *see* gender differences
siblings, number of, 84
silica particles, 226
single photon emission computed tomography (SPECT), 340
sinusitis (paranasal)
   in acute asthma exacerbations, 197
   asthma and, 223–35
      historical considerations, 223–4
      pathophysiological mechanisms, 226–9
      population studies, 225
   in developing countries, 380
   inflammation in, 226
   medical treatment, 231–2
   surgical therapy, 232
skiers, cross-country, 215
skills, self-management, 293–5, 312
skin, thinning, 161
skin prick tests, 110–11
   in developing countries, 381–2, 383
   food allergy, 283
   recombinant allergens, 263
sleep apnoea, obstructive (OSA), 101, 105, 108
small children (aged 2-5 years)
   aerosol delivery, 330–2, 338
   asthma education, 317–18
   chronic cough and/or wheezing, 99–120
   cromoglycate therapy, 127–32, 157
   exercise-induced asthma, 214

inhaled corticosteroids, *see* inhaled corticosteroids (ICS), in infants and small children
lung function measurement, 11–13
management of asthma, 121–47
treatment adherence, 302
see also infants; school-aged children
smoke
   tobacco, *see* environmental tobacco smoke
   wood, 246
smoking
   during pregnancy, 57, 366
   natural history of asthma and, 58–9
   parental, 56, 57–8, 365–6
   passive *see* environmental tobacco smoke
snoring, 101
social support, 299, 312–14
socioeconomic status, asthma risk and, 379
sodium cromoglycate, *see* cromoglycate
soft furnishings, 241
South Africa *see* Africa
South African Childhood Asthma Working Group, 385
soybeans, 56
spacers/holding chambers, 114, 333
   in acute asthma, 200, 334
   aerosol delivery, 333–4
   in developing countries, 385
   dose delivery and, 338, 340–1
   electrostatic charge, 334, 338
   for infants and small children, 123, 124–5
   inhaled corticosteroid delivery, 332
   non-adherence, 337
specialists, referral to, 354
spirometry, 13, 191
sports
   exercise-induced asthma and, 214–15
   participation in, 218–19
sputum induction, 175
STAR strategy, 320
steroid-dependent asthma, food hypersensitivity, 288
steroid-resistant asthma, 25, 161, 170–4
steroids *see* corticosteroids
steroid sparing agents, 170–4
storage mites, 266
storytelling, 318
stress
   health care behaviour and, 297–8
   vocal cord dysfunction and, 195
stridor, 100, 104–5
subclavian artery, aberrant, 105, 111
substance P, 89
suggestion-induced bronchoconstriction, 297–8
summer camps, 321
sunlight, dust mite exposure, 241, 384
surfactant, maternal nutrition and, 365
swallowing, incoordinate, 102, 107
sweat test, 106
Sweden
   allergic sensitization and asthma, 74
   asthma prevalence, 40, 41
swimming, 214, 215
symptom-free days, 354
symptoms *see* respiratory symptoms

tachyphylaxis, *see* tolerance
Tahiti, asthma prevalence, 40, 41
tannic acid, 240–1, 243–4
Tc_2 T cells, in viral respiratory infections, 87
tenascin-c, 25
terbutaline
   in acute asthma, 199
   in chronic asthma, 155, 175
   doping regulations, 218
   in exercise-induced asthma, 217
Th-1 inflammatory response, 54
   development in early life, 78, 367–8, 369
   induction strategies, 265, 289
   in pregnancy, 366–7
   in viral infections, 87, 92
Th-1 lymphocytes, 22, 54
Th-2 inflammatory response, 54
   allergen immunotherapy and, 247, 371
   development in early life, 78, 362–3, 368–9
   genetic diversity and, 367
   in rhinitis and sinusitis, 226
   in viral infections, 86, 87, 92, 368
Th-2 lymphocytes, 22, 24
Thailand *see* Asia
T-helper lymphocytes
   in primary sensitization, 22
   see also Th-1 lymphocytes; Th-2 lymphocytes
theophylline
   in acute asthma, 142–3, 201
   adverse reactions, 163–4
   in chronic asthma, 162–4
   in developing countries, 164, 386
   in infants and small children, 137, 142–3
   interactions, 164
   mechanisms of action, 154, 162–3
therapeutic alliance, 301, 309
thromboxane B_2, 25, 92
tidal breathing
   aerosol delivery during, 329, 333–4
   assessments, 7
tidal volume (TV), 12, 113
   inhaled dose delivery and, 341
tidal volume forced expiration, 5–6, 8
tiotropium bromide, 177
tissue inhibitors of matrix metalloproteinases (TIMPs), 26–7
T lymphocytes
   activated, 112
   cyclosporin A actions, 173
   primary sensitization, 22
   responses to viral infections, 87, 92
tobacco smoke, environmental *see* environmental tobacco smoke
tolerance

β_2-agonists, 156–7, 170
   in exercise-induced asthma, 217
Toll-like receptor 4, 368
total lung capacity (TLC), 12
   in acute asthma, 192, 193
   measurement in infants, 8–9
toys, 241, 318
T_{ptef}/T_E, 7
tracheo-oesophageal fistula, H-type, 102, 107
transbronchial biopsy (TBB), 108, 112
transcutaneous oxygen/carbon dioxide tensions, 113, 198
transforming growth factor beta, 26
transmission disequilibrium test (TDT), 72
treadmill running, 213
treatment
   adherence see adherence
   early, 359
   natural history of asthma and, 59
   outcomes, psychosocial factors mediating, 293–307
   plans, 311–12, 322
   see also management of asthma; pharmacotherapy; self-management
tree pollen allergens, 262, 270
troleandomycin (TAO), 173–4
tropomyosins, 268
tuberculin responsiveness, 368
tuberculosis (TB), 109, 381
Tucson Children's Respiratory study, 36, 44, 45, 54–5
tumour necrosis factor-α (TNF-α), 25, 28–9
   in virus infections, 92
Turbuhaler, 338, 339, 341
twin studies, 52, 68–9

United States
   incidence data, 42, 44–5
   morbidity/hospitalization data, 42–8
   mortality data, 48–9
   prevalence data, 39, 40
upper airways, deposition of aerosols, 328, 330, 340–42
upper airways disease
   asthma and, 108, 223–35
      effects of nasal and sinus therapies, 229–32
      historical considerations, 223–4
      pathophysiological mechanisms, 226–9
      population studies, 224–5
   inflammation in, 226
   see also allergic rhinitis; rhinitis; sinusitis
upper respiratory tract infections, bronchial responses, 87
urban areas, 266, 378
   see also inner-city areas

vaccines
   DNA see DNA vaccines
   for food hypersensitivity, 288–9
vacuum cleaning, 240
vaporizers, 245

vascular cell adhesion molecule 1 (VCAM-1), 29
vascular rings, 105–6, 110
vasculitis, systemic, 168
VATER/VATERLS spectrum, 110
vegetables, 24, 364
ventilation
   domestic, 241, 245
   mechanical see mechanical ventilation
   pressure-support, 202–3
very late antigen 4, 29
videos, educational, 317, 320, 321, 384
viral respiratory infections, 83–97
   airway inflammation and, 89–92
   allergic sensitization and, 84, 85
   in asthma development, 54–5, 83–5
   asthma exacerbations and, 83, 85, 190–1
   in athletes, 216
   immunomodulatory mechanisms in asthma and, 86–7
   mechanisms of airway obstruction and asthma, 87–9
   rat model of airway dysfunction, 87
visceral larva migrans, 381
vital capacity (VC), 12
   in acute asthma, 193
vitamin A, 365
V'_{maxFRC}
   challenge testing, 10
   gender differences in infants, 5
   measurement in infants, 5–6
   predicting later respiratory function, 11
   variability in infants, 6
vocal cord dysfunction (VCD), 195–6
volatile organic compounds, 246
volume–time measurements, raised volume forced expiration method, 9–10
von Ebner's gland protein (VeGh), 269

warm-up, pre-exercise, 216
water loss, in exercise-induced asthma, 212
web-sites, internet, 321
weed pollen allergens, 262, 270
weight, inhalation therapy and, 328
wheeze
   airway responsiveness, 11
   ancillary investigations, 109–13
   bronchodilator responsiveness, 11
   clinical assessment, 100–4
   in developing countries, 379, 381
   diagnostic approaches, 99–120
   differential diagnosis, 195–6
   food-induced, 281
   history taking, 101–3
   immunopathology, 29
   indications for therapy, 122
   in infants of smoking mothers, 365–6
   labelling issues, 38, 67–8
   markers of airway inflammation, 30
   mother's assessment of severity, 115

wheeze *continued*
　　nomenclature, 100
　　physical examination, 103–4
　　predicting later asthma, 29, 30
　　prediction from V'_{maxFRC} in early life, 11
　　respiratory infections and, 75–7
　　serious underlying conditions, 104–9
　　trial of asthma therapy, 113–14
'wheezy bronchitis', 38
wood smoke exposure, 383, 384
World Health Organization, asthma definition, 37

zafirlukast, 167–8
　　drug interactions, 168
　　efficacy, 166
　　food interactions, 168
　　indications, 169
　　in infants and small children, 140
　　mechanism of action, 165, 166
zileuton, 168
　　adverse effects, 168
　　drug interactions, 168
　　in exercise-induced asthma, 216
　　mechanism of action, 165, 166